Strauss's FEDERAL DRUG LAWS *and* EXAMINATION REVIEW

Strauss's
FEDERAL DRUG LAWS and EXAMINATION REVIEW

Steven Strauss, Ph.D., R.Ph.

Professor of Pharmacy Administration, Emeritus
Arnold & Marie Schwartz College of Pharmacy and Health Sciences
Long Island University, Brooklyn, New York

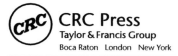

CRC Press
Taylor & Francis Group
Boca Raton   London   New York

CRC Press is an imprint of the
Taylor & Francis Group, an **informa** business

Library of Congress Cataloging-in-Publication Data

Main entry under title:
Strauss's Federal Drug Laws and Examination Review—Fifth Edition, Revised

Full Catalog record is available from the Library of Congress

Visit the CRC Press Web site at www.crcpress.com

© 2000 by Steven Strauss, Ph.D., R.Ph.
First CRC reprint 2002
Originally Published by Technomic Publishing

No claim to original U.S. Government works
International Standard Book Number 1-56676-978-7
Library of Congress Card Number 00-101295
Printed in the United States of America   6 7 8 9 0
Printed on acid-free paper

Table of Contents

Introduction to the Fifth Edition, Revised

This revised fifth edition maintains and enhances the features that made the previous five best selling and highly acclaimed editions (formerly entitled *Strauss's Pharmacy Law and Examination Review*) so popular among pharmacy law faculty, students, and candidates for pharmacist licensing examinations. In fact, the book has set the standard for excellence for pharmacy law publications since it was first published in 1988. And now, with periodic revisions it brings you the very latest in pharmacy law to help you prepare for the "boards."

The book's extensive editorial contents and multiple-choice review questions accurately mirror the subjects and format of the Multistate Pharmacy Jurisprudence Examination™ (MPJE™) and state law pharmacist licensing examinations.

The editorial matter reflects the need for new and expanded information to keep abreast of legal and regulatory developments.

This new revised edition contains:

- Expanded list of controlled substances.
- Additional legal citations, with commentary.
- Expanded glossary of acronyms.
- One revised chapter.
- Additional commentary relating to compounding and manufacturing.
- Alternative to methadone to treat heroin addicts.

In addition, a thank you to everyone who offered suggestions and recommendations on how to improve this book.

STEVEN STRAUSS
Brooklyn, NY

Multistate Pharmacy Jurisprudence Examination and MPJE are trademarks owned by the National Association of Boards of Pharmacy.

CHAPTER 1

The Legislative Process

THE FEDERAL REGISTER SYSTEM*

Steven Strauss, Ph.D., R.Ph.

In the surge of New Deal legislation enacted in the early 1930's, Congress delegated more and more responsibility to federal departments and agencies in the form of authority to issue detailed regulations dealing with complex social and economic issues. As more and more regulations were written, a serious communications problem developed. The number of regulations was expanded rapidly, but since there was no central publication system, there was no efficient way for citizens to know about regulations which affected them.

Congress recognized this communications gap and enacted the Federal Register Act, which became law on July 26, 1935 [1]. The Act established a uniform system for handling agency regulations by providing for:

• Filing of documents with the Office of the Federal Register;

• Placement of documents on public inspection;

• Publication of documents in the *Federal Register*; and

• After a 1937 amendment, a permanent codification or numerical arrangement of rules in the *Code of Federal Regulations*.

Publication in the *Federal*

Register has certain legal effects. Publication:

• Provides official notice of a document's existence and its contents;

• Establishes the accuracy of the text;

• Indicates the date of the regulation's issuance; and

• Provides *prima facie* evidence acceptable to a court of law.

Several important new dimensions were added to the Federal Register System by the Administrative Procedure Act, which became law on June 11, 1946 [2].

This Act:

• Introduced as a general requirement (but with some stated exceptions) the right of the public to participate in the rulemaking process by commenting on proposed rules;

• Required that the effective date for a regulation be not less than 30 days from the date of publication unless there was good cause for an earlier date; and

• Provided for publication of agency statements of organization and procedural rules.

From the mid-1930's until the late 1960's, the Federal Register Act and the Administrative Procedure Act defined the basic functions of the *Federal Register*.

Since the late 1960's, however, these functions have been ex-

panded because the roles of the agencies have become far more extensive than ever before. These different roles have reflected and created various social and legal changes. Both the volume of regulations issued and the number of citizens who might be directly affected by a regulation have increased dramatically.

As a result, on March 24, 1978, then-President Carter issued an order [3] directing executive agencies to improve their existing and future regulations through a variety of procedures. The aim, without creating economic pressures, was to publish regulations that are simple and clear as possible, and to achieve legislative goals effectively and efficiently.

Agencies were directed to publish, at least semi-annually, agendas of significant regulations under development or review, to give the public adequate notice to become involved in the rule-making process.

The Executive Order also:

• Sought more control by agency heads;

• Established criteria determining the significance of regulations;

• Extended the opportunity for public participation; and

• Imposed a 60 day minimum comment period for significant regulations at the proposed rule stage.

*Reprinted with permission from *U.S. Pharmacist* (October 1983).

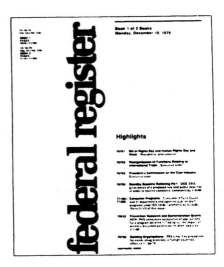

FIGURE 1.

Definition

The Federal Register System is comprised primarily of two major federal government publications, the *Federal Register* (*FR*) (Figure 1) and the *Code of Federal Regulations* (*CFR*) (Figure 2). The two publications complement one another to provide an up-to-date version of any federal government agency regulation. To understand the System, one needs to understand each separate publication as well as the relationship between the two of them.

The *FR* is a serial publication which contains, as determined by the Federal Register Act:

• Presidential documents—documents signed by the President and submitted to the Office of the Federal Register (OFR) for publication;

• Rules and Regulations—regulatory documents having general applicability and legal effect;

• Proposed Rules—notices to the public of the proposed issuance of rules and regulations;

• Notices—documents other than rules and proposed rules that are applicable to the public; and

• Sunshine Act Meetings—notices of meetings published pursuant to the government in the Sunshine Act [4].

The *FR* is published each official federal government work day, i.e., it is published daily, five days a week. The *FR* is the daily newspaper of the federal government which keeps the *CFR* up-to-date.

The *Code of Federal Regulations* is an annually revised codification of the general and permanent rules published in the *FR* by the federal government's executive departments and agencies. The *CFR* is divided into 50 titles which represent broad areas subject to federal government regulation (Table 1).

There are approximately 145 *CFR* volumes.

For example, the Food and Drug Administration (FDA) and Drug Enforcement Administration (DEA) regulations are in Title 21, Food and Drugs. Each Title is further subdivided into chapters, subchapters, parts, subparts, and sections (Figure 3).

Regulations appearing in the *Federal Register* are cited by volume and page number, as 59 FR 67151 (Figure 4). Volume 1 was published on March 14, 1936; the 48th volume corresponds to the year 1983.

In order to determine the latest version of a rule, both the *FR* and *CFR* must be used together.

The *FR* and *CFR* are usually available at libraries which are designated as depositories for federal government publications. In addition, they may be available at main branches of public libraries, law school and university libraries, and some local congressional offices. A list of depository libraries is available from the U.S. Government Printing Office.

Rulemaking

A government agency enacts rules and regulations because many of the statutes (Acts) passed

FIGURE 2.

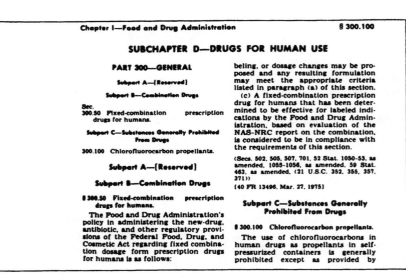

FIGURE 3.

Table 1
List of Code of Federal Regulations (CFR) Titles [5]

1. General Provisions	19. Customs Duties	36. Patriotic Societies and Observations
2. The Congress	20. Education	37. Pay and Allowances of the Uniformed Services
3. The President	21. Food and Drugs	
4. Flag and Seal, Seat of Government, and the States	22. Foreign Relations and Intercourse	38. Veterans' Benefits
5. Government Organization and Employees	23. Highways	39. Postal Service
6. Surety Bonds (repealed by the enactment of Title 31)	24. Hospitals and Asylums	40. Public Buildings, Property, and Works
7. Agriculture	25. Indians	41. Public Contracts
8. Aliens and Nationality	26. Internal Revenue Code	42. The Public Health and Welfare
9. Arbitration	27. Intoxicating Liquors	43. Public Lands
10. Armed Forces	28. Judiciary and Judicial Procedure	44. Public Printing and Documents
11. Bankruptcy	29. Labor	45. Railroads
12. Banks and Banking	30. Mineral Lands and Mining	46. Shipping
13. Census	31. Money and Finance	47. Telegraphs, Telephones, and Radiotelegraphs
14. Coast Guard	32. National Guard	
15. Commerce and Trade	33. Navigation and Navigable Waters	48. Territories and Insular Possessions
16. Conservation	34. Navy (eliminated by the enactment of Title 10)	49. Transportation
17. Copyrights	35. Patents	50. War and National Defense
18. Crimes and Criminal Procedure		

Each volume of the *CFR* is revised at least once each calendar year and issued on a quarterly basis approximately as follows:
Title 1 through Title 16   as of January 1
Title 17 through Title 27   as of April 1
Title 28 through Title 41   as of July 1
Title 42 through Title 50   as of October 1
The appropriate revision date is printed on the cover of each volume. Each year's cover is a different color for quick reference.

by the legislative branch of government are written in general terms (Figure 5). These Acts do not consider the required and necessary details to put statutes into effect. Such responsibility is delegated to the government agency that will be held responsible for the Act. The agency that puts the law into effect has to make rules to provide the details. These rules interpret the statute and have the same effect as the Act of the legislature, but cannot supersede it.

It is important for the public to understand the regulatory process of the federal agencies, and how to participate in that process. Public involvement, from the earliest point possible, is necessary in order to allow that the public viewpoint be heard in the agency decision making on regulations. Not only is this in the public interest, it is a basic right (Figure 6).

In rulemaking, every voice is important. Agencies cannot count the number of comments received as if they were votes. An agency must consider each issue and use its expertise to reach a solution that meets the letter and spirit of the law. Each comment is analyzed for new information and new issues. Although it may be useful to be the 10,000th comment to say the same thing, it is just as important to be the one comment in 10,000 to present new information or raise an issue that the agency has not considered.

Agencies must give the public an early and meaningful opportunity to participate in the development of agency regulations (Figure 7). They shall consider a variety of ways to provide this opportunity, including:

• Publishing an advance notice of proposed rulemaking;

• Holding open conferences or public hearings;

• Sending notices of proposed regulations to publications likely to be read by those affected; and

• Notifying interested parties directly.

Each agency has the option to prepare its documents for publication in the *FR* in whatever way is most suitable to its needs. The major requirement is conformity to the preamble requirements and the *CFR* codification system, while at the same time following the basic rulemaking process. Regardless of agency publication differences, the public generally has its first opportunity to comment at the "proposed rule" stage or earlier if there is what is referred to as an "intent to publish" or an "advance notice of proposed rulemaking" document published.

Proposed Rule: Document[s] in-

FIGURE 4.

Rulemaking Process

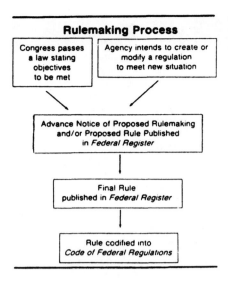

FIGURE 5.

tended by an agency to result in new rules are published in the *FR* (Figure 8). These notices, by inviting comments, offer the public the opportunity to participate in the rulemaking process, prior to adoption of the final rule, which has the effect of law. The proposed rule may be a guideline of how a section of a statute will be interpreted for compliance.

An agency would follow these steps in publishing a proposal:

• Notice of the proposed rule is published in the *FR*;

• Interested persons are given the opportunity to submit written or oral data, views, and arguments. A time limit, which may range from 60 days to possibly one year, is set for comments;

• When the comment period for a particular proposal has expired, all comments are carefully analyzed. An agency is required to balance the favorable and unfavorable comments against one another, consider all supporting facts, reasons, research, or other evidence and arrive at an equitable decision.

Final Rule: When the decision has been made, the rule is published in its final form in the *FR*, with the date it will become effective (Figure 9).

The regulations or rules, which are synonymously used in the *FR*,

Stages in Rulemaking for Maximum Participation

What the public can do	Stages in rulemaking Information published in the Federal Register	How to locate published information in the Federal Register
Monitor pending regulatory authority	Agency semiannual agendas	FR Contents, FR Index, LSA
	Regulatory Council's Calendar of Federal Regulations	FR Contents, FR Index
Make oral or written comments	Advance notices of proposed rulemaking, proposed rules, meetings, public hearings, open conferences, interim rules, final rules	FR Contents, FR Reminders, FR Index, LSA
Review comments made by others	Advance notices of proposed rulemaking, proposed rules, meetings, public hearings, open conferences, interim rules, final rules	Document preamble, especially "ADDRESSES"
Obtain more detailed information	Advance notices of proposed rulemaking, proposed rules, meetings, public hearings, open conferences, interim rules, final rules	Document preamble, especially "FOR FURTHER INFORMATION CONTACT"
Monitor significant regulations	Agency semiannual agendas	FR Contents, FR Index, LSA
	Regulatory Council's Calendar of Federal Regulations	FR Contents, FR Index

FIGURE 6.

DEPARTMENT OF AGRICULTURE

Office of the Secretary

[7 CFR Subtitle A]

Title IV, Agricultural Credit Act of 1978; Regulations To Govern Emergency Conservation Programs

AGENCY: Department of Agriculture.

ACTION: Advance Notice of Proposed Rulemaking and Request for Public Comment.

SUMMARY: The Department of Agriculture gives advance notice of forthcoming decisions leading to the implementation of Title IV of the Agricultural Credit Act of 1978, Pub. L. 95-334.

DATE: Comments and suggestions should be submitted on or before August 8, 1979.

ADDRESS: Comments and suggestions should be addressed to Mr. Arnold Miller, Office of the Secretary, Department of Agriculture, Room 117-A, Washington, D.C. 20250. (202) 447-3465.

The Secretary has directed that implementation of the programs authorized by Title IV be carried out with a view toward ensuring that they are efficiently administered, uniformly responsive in emergencies, and limited to practices and measures that are environmentally and economically supportable. In order to achieve these goals, public comment is requested on such issues as: (1) The criteria to be

Comments and suggestions made in response to this notice should be received by August 8, 1979, in order to be sure of receiving consideration in connection with development of the proposed rules.

FIGURE 7. Advance notice of proposed rulemaking.

CONSUMER PRODUCT SAFETY COMMISSION

16 CFR Part 1700

Human Prescription Drugs in Oral Dosage Forms; Exemption of Prednisone Tablets From Child-Protection Packaging Requirements

AGENCY: Consumer Product Safety Commission.

ACTION: Proposed rule.

SUMMARY: The Commission proposes for public comment an exemption from child-protection packaging requirements for prednisone in tablet form when dispensed in packages containing no more that 105 mg. of the drug. Prednisone is an anti-inflammatory steroid drug. The Commission believes that child-resistant packaging is unnecessary to protect children who ingest the drug in quantities of 105 mg. or less from serious illness or injury.

FIGURE 8. Proposed rules.

CONSUMER PRODUCT SAFETY COMMISSION

16 CFR Part 1700

Human Prescription Drugs in Oral Dosage Forms; Exemption of Prednisone Tablets From Child-Protection Packaging Requirements

AGENCY: Consumer Product Safety Commission.

ACTION: Final rule.

SUMMARY: The Commission exempts prednisone in tablet form when dispensed in packages containing no more than 105 milligrams of that drug from requirements for child-protection packaging. Information available to the Commission indicates that child-protection packaging is not required to protect children who may ingest the drug in quantities of 105 milligrams or less because of the low toxicity of prednisone and the lack of adverse human experience associated with that drug.

DATE: The exemption is effective September 14, 1982.

FIGURE 9. Date rule becomes effective in final form.

properly issued have the "force and effect of law" because they are a direct line from the Congress (slip law).

Finally, the text of the rule will be incorporated into the agency's regulations in the *CFR*, when it is next revised and republished, which normally happens once a year.

Petitions: Once a rule is in effect, any interested party can petition an agency head or similar officer (Commissioner) to establish, amend, or revoke a rule or any part thereof.

The petitioner should state the problem or circumstance which requires action, and then propose what the new rule should include. Such a proposal/petition should be based on sound and supportable facts, on the needs of the public, and on reasonable grounds for compliance. If the agency head finds the petition has reasonable merit, notice of its filing and availability is published in the *FR* with a request for public comment within a time limit. An agency may also publish simultaneously its own version of such a proposal, for public comment, in which case the response to both proposals would be weighed in preparing a final regulation.

Interim or Temporary Rule: These regulatory documents are effective as of the day of enactment but for a short or definable period of time. They have the same effect as a final rule in that they amend the *CFR* and give an effective date. However, in issuing an interim or temporary rule, the agency often asks for public comments and acts upon any received before issuing the final rule. If no changes occur due to the comments received, or if the publication date for the *CFR* volume in which the regulation belongs is reached, the rule will automatically appear in the *CFR* as originally published unless the regulation expires prior to the *CFR* publication.

Notices: These are documents printed in the *FR* that inform the public about hearings, investigations, committee meetings, agency

---

Table 2

Agencies of the Federal Government Generating Subject Matter in the Federal Register of High Interest to the Profession of Pharmacy

Centers for Disease Control (CDC)
Availability/status of biological products for disease control related to distribution by pharmacists and information to pharmacists;
Consumer Product Safety Commission (CPSC)
Safety of drugs, packaging, poison control
Drug Enforcement Administration (DEA)
Controlled substances; changes in scheduling drugs
Environmental Protection Agency (EPA)
Chemical problems of concern to pharmacy practice and industry
Federal Trade Commission (FTC)
Advertising, labeling, unfair practices
Food & Drug Administration (FDA)
New drug evaluation, Drug Efficacy Study Implementation (DESI), bioequivalence, good manufacturing practices, biologicals, patient package inserts (PPIs)
Health Care Financing Administration (HCFA)
Medicaid/Medicare
National Center of Health Services Research
Grants, manpower
National Center for Health Statistics (NCHS)
Data on health manpower
National Institutes of Health (NIH)
Studies related to clinical trials, carcinogens
Presidential Proclamations
Of interest to health field or to pharmacists in general
Public Health Service (PHS)
Protection of human subjects, health planning; health education

---

decisions and rulings, delegation of authority, filing of petitions, applications, and agency statements of organization and function. Types of notices vary. Some examples include:

Notice of Intent: These invite public comment at the earliest opportunity. Such notices state an agency's intention to develop a proposal to change or issue a new regulation. They also identify the issues for public comment. This type of notice may be issued as a press release, or as an announcement at public meetings or offered as a study draft. The purpose of the study draft is to foster comments and ideas, before a formal proposal is made, from those who may be affected (Figure 10).

Notice of Public Meeting or Briefing: Used by an agency to explain significant issues to the public. An agency may schedule public meetings before developing a proposal or after a program change is proposed. Such meetings or briefings provide for an open discussion of the anticipated effects and purpose of the proposed action. A press release by the agency serves to notify interested parties of the date, time, and place for meetings.

Notice of Public Hearing: The public hearing is a legal process used in administering an agency's regulatory program. A hearing may also be scheduled to obtain public viewpoints concerning an agency's

---

DEPARTMENT OF AGRICULTURE

Soil Conservation Service

Batavia Kill Watershed, New York; Intent To Prepare Environmental Impact Statement

AGENCY: Soil Conservation Service, U.S. Department of Agriculture.

ACTION: Notice of Intent to Prepare and Environmental Impact Statement.

FOR FURTHER INFORMATION CONTACT: Mr. Robert L. Hilliard, State Conservationist, Soil Conservation Service, U.S. Courthouse and Federal Building, 100 S. Clinton Street, Room 771, Syracuse, New York 13260, telephone number (315) 423-5493.

NOTICE: Pursuant to Section 102 (2)(C) of the National Environmental Policy Act of 1969; the Council on Environmental Quality Guidelines (40 CFR Part 1500); and the Soil Conservation Service Guidelines (7 CFR Part 650); the Soil Conservation Service, U.S. Department of Agriculture, gives notice that an environmental impact statement is being prepared for the remaining works of improvement in the Batavia Kill Watershed, Greene County, New York.

The environmental assessment of this federally-assisted action indicates that

FIGURE 10. Notice of intent.

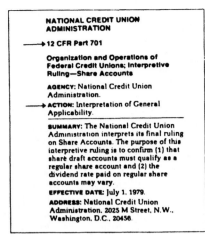

FIGURE 11.

programs and issues. An official record of evidence composed of either oral or written testimony on specified program proposals is maintained.

There are times, however, when legal constraints prohibit the presiding officer from considering comments from the general public. For example, during a formal evidentiary hearing or a hearing before a public board of inquiry only evidence on the record, i.e., witnesses called by either party and subject to cross examination or exhibits presented by either party and admitted into evidence, may be weighed in reaching a decision. From the time that a notice of opportunity is published in the *FR* for such a hearing, the presiding officer is prohibited from receiving ex *parte* (off the record) communications on any issue presented at the hearing. However, interested parties may at any time submit comments to the hearing clerk or to the parties included in the hearing.

Notices are not codified in the *CFR*.

Finally, the rules and regulations category also includes documents that have no regulatory text and do not amend the *CFR* but either affect an agency's handling of its regulations or are of continuing interest to the public in dealing with an agency. In this category are general policy statements, interpretations of agency regulations, and statements of organization and function (Figure 11).

References

1. 44 U.S.C. Chapt. 15.
2. 5 U.S.C. 551 et seq.
3. Executive Order (EO), 43 FR 12661, March 24, 1978.
4. 5 U.S.C. 551b (c)(3).
5. American Pharmacy NS 22(2):6, 1982.

HOW A BILL BECOMES A LAW*

Hon. Robert H. Michel of Illinois, Minority Whip, House of Representatives

Mr. Michel. Mr. Speaker, those of us in Congress are so close to the legislative process that we sometimes forget that the way in which a bill becomes law is not clearly understood by many of our fellow Americans. I receive inquiries from time to time about the process in the hope it may be useful to anyone who is interested in the machinery of Government.

How a Bill Becomes Law

Our[s] is a government "of the

*Reprinted with permission from *NARD Journal* (October 1979).

people, by the people, for the people." It is not a pure democracy. It is a republic in a democracy. It is a representative democracy.

Our laws are the embodiment of the wishes and wants, the ideas of the American people as expressed through their Representatives in the Congress: 435 in the House of Representatives and 100 in the Senate. Any Member of the House or Senate may introduce a bill embodying a proposed law or revision of existing laws at any time when his respective house is in session. When introduced the bill will be entered in the *Journal of the House*, and the title and sponsor of

it printed in the *Congressional Record* of that day.

The Deliberative Stage

The committee's deliberations are the most important stage of the legislative process. It is here that detailed study of the proposed legislation is made and where people are given the right to present their views in public hearings. When the chairman has set a date for public hearings it is generally announced by publication in the *Congressional Record*.

Copies of the bill under consideration by the committee are customarily sent to the executive departments or agencies concerned with the subject matter for their official views to be presented in writing or by oral testimony before the committee. The number of witnesses—pro and con—heard by the committee is largely dictated by the importance of the proposed legislation and degree of public interest in it.

Testimony Heard

The transcript of the testimony taken is available for inspection in the individual committee offices. Quite frequently, dependent on the importance of the subject matter, the committee hearings on a bill are printed and copies made available to the public.

After conclusion of the hearings, the committee proceeds to meet in executive session (sometimes referred to as "markup" sessions) to discuss the bill in detail and to consider such amendments as any member of the committee may wish to offer. Each committee has its own rules of procedure but they generally conform to the rules of the House itself.

The Committee Vote

By a formal vote of the committee, it decides whether to report favorably to the House the bill with or without committee amendments. A committee report must accompany the bill, setting forth the nature of the bill and reasons for the committee's recommended approval. The report sets forth specifically the committee amendments and, in compliance with the rules of each House, indicates all changes the bill would make in existing law. Any committee member, individually or jointly, may file additional supplemental or minority views to accompany the majority committee report. The committee report, accompanying the bill, is viewed by the courts and the ad-

ministrative agencies as the most important document as to the intent of the Congress in proposed legislation.

After Reporting

When a bill is reported by the committee it is placed on the appropriate calendar. The majority leadership decides how and when the bill will be considered on the floor. In general the bill is allowed to remain on the calendar for several days to enable members to become acquainted with its provisions.

In both the House and the Senate innumerable measures of relatively minor importance are disposed of by unanimous consent. In the Senate, where debate is unlimited, major bills are brought up on motion of the majority leader and in the House are called up under a privileged resolution reported from the Rules Committee which fixes the limits of debate and whether amendments may be offered from the floor. The Rules Committee resolution is called a "rule" for consideration of a bill: a "closed rule" if no amendments are allowed, as is generally the case in tax bills, and an "open rule" if amendments can be offered.

Reaching Consensus

While there are distant differences between the House and Senate procedures, in general a bill is debated at length with the proponents and opponents presenting their views to acquaint the membership, as well as the general public, with the issues involved, and all with a view to arriving at the consensus. Amendments are frequently offered to make the measure more in conformity with the judgment of the majority. In the course of consideration of the bill there are various parliamentary motions, in both the House and the Senate, which may be offered to determine the sentiment of the

members with respect to the pending legislation. The measure may be postponed to some future date or referred back to the committee which reported it.

With the conclusion of general debate and the reading of the bill for amendments, the question becomes whether the House or Senate, as the case may be, will pass the bill in its final form. The *Congressional Record* of the day the bill was under consideration will set forth the verbatim debate on the bill and the disposition made of such amendments as were offered.

After Passage

With the passage of a bill by either body, it is messaged to the other with the request that they concur. If no action has been taken on the like measure by the body receiving the message, the bill is usually referred to the appropriate committee of that body for consideration. Hearings are again held and the bill reported for floor action. On relatively minor or noncontroversial matters, the Senate or the House accepts the measure as messaged to it by the other body.

If there are substantial differences between the House and Senate versions of a given bill, the measure is sent to a conference committee which is appointed by the Speaker and the President of the Senate from the ranking committee members of each body having original jurisdiction over the bill. The object of the conference committee is to adjust the differences between the two bodies, and to report back to each its agreement. The report of the conference committee must be in writing and signed by those agreeing thereto and must have the signature of the majority of the conference of each House.

Conference Report

The report of the conference

committee cannot be amended and must be accepted or rejected by each House as it stands. If either House finds itself unable to accept the conference committee report, a further conference is usually requested.

When the bill has been agreed to in identical form by both bodies a copy of the bill is enrolled, signed by the Speaker and by the President of the Senate, for presentation to the President. The bill becomes law with the President's signature of approval, or it may become law without his signature if he does not return it, with his objections, to the Congress within 10 days of its presentation to him.

If the President should return the bill, with his objections, to the originating body of the Congress, his veto may be overridden by two-thirds of both the House and Senate, respectively, voting to have the measure become law, the President's objections to the contrary notwithstanding. Both the President's veto message and a record of the vote of the individual Members in the motion to override are required by the Constitution and set forth in the *Congressional Record*.

ENACTMENT OF A FEDERAL LAW*

David Forbes, Ph.D., R.Ph. and Steven Strauss, Ph.D., R.Ph.

Few subjects fascinate, and infuriate, the public at large more than their government and how it operates. The President, Congress, the Supreme Court and the federal bureaucracy are targets of criticism from nearly everyone. And yet, few really know or understand how the federal government functions. Compounding the public's uncertainty of government is the fact that it is dynamic.

"All legislative powers herein granted shall be vested in a Congress of the United States, which shall consist of a Senate and a House of Representatives" [1]. The Senate and House enact federal criminal law and laws governing operations of federal departments and agencies [2]. Basic to this authority is the "power of the purse." The Congress alone has the constitutional authority to levy taxes [3]. Consequently, revenues can be spent only if authorized and appropriated by the Congress. As part of the legislative role, its major function, the Congress also holds investigative powers. It can hold hearings, subpoena witnesses, and compel them to testify. In addition to its legislative and investigative functions, Congress exercises other authority granted it by the Constitution, such as "to fix the standard of weights and measures" [4] and "to regulate commerce with foreign nations and among the several States" [5]. In fact, the Federal Food, Drug, and Cosmetic Act was enacted on the basis of the federal government's constitutional authority to control interstate commerce.

Although all the powers of Congress are of vital concern, this article will limit itself to the basic federal legislative process. The term "house" and "chamber" are used interchangeably to designate either the Senate or the House of Representatives.

Sources of Legislation

A legislative proposal or bill may originate in a number of ways (Figures 1 and 2). A member of Congress may develop the idea for a piece of legislation. Lobbying groups for business, civil rights, farm, labor organizations and the like, are another source of legislation. Citizens, either as individuals or groups, also may propose legislation. The idea for a possible law, or even a draft of a suggested law also can originate with a professional association (APhA, NARD, PMA), the officials at any government level or agency (FDA, DEA, OSHA), a governor of a state or even the President of the United States. The U.S. Constitution provides that the President "shall from time to time give to the Congress information of the State of the Union, and recommend to their consideration such measures as he shall judge necessary and expedient" [6]. In fact, each year the President outlines his legislative program in the State of the Union, Budget and special messages. The President fulfills this duty either by personally addressing a joint session of the two Houses or by sending messages in writing to the Congress or to either body, which are

*Reprinted with permission from *U.S. Pharmacist* (January 1982).

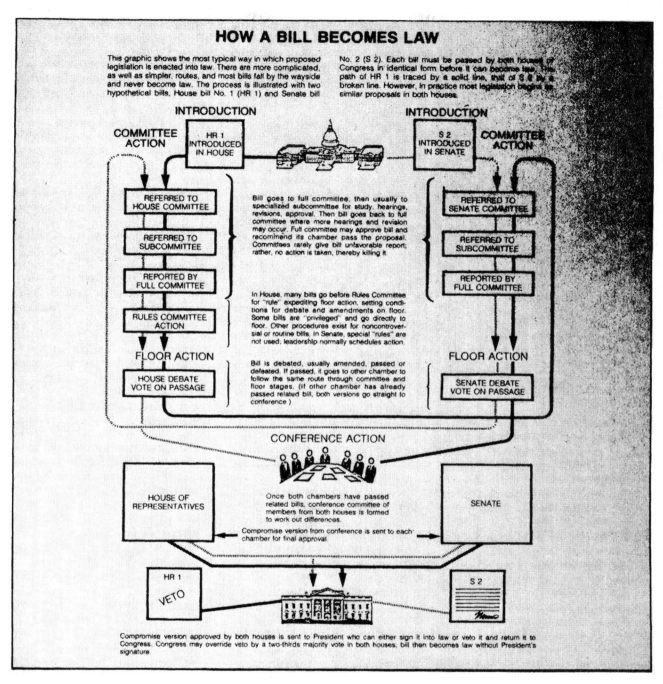

HOW A BILL BECOMES LAW

This graphic shows the most typical way in which proposed legislation is enacted into law. There are more complicated, as well as simpler, routes, and most bills fall by the wayside and never become law. The process is illustrated with two hypothetical bills, House bill No. 1 (HR 1) and Senate bill No. 2 (S 2). Each bill must be passed by both houses of Congress in identical form before it can become law. The path of HR 1 is traced by a solid line, that of S 2 by a broken line. However, in practice most legislation begins as similar proposals in both houses.

INTRODUCTION

COMMITTEE ACTION

HR 1 INTRODUCED IN HOUSE

INTRODUCTION

S 2 INTRODUCED IN SENATE

COMMITTEE ACTION

REFERRED TO HOUSE COMMITTEE

REFERRED TO SUBCOMMITTEE

REPORTED BY FULL COMMITTEE

RULES COMMITTEE ACTION

Bill goes to full committee, then usually to specialized subcommittee for study, hearings, revisions, approval. Then bill goes back to full committee where more hearings and revision may occur. Full committee may approve bill and recommend its chamber pass the proposal. Committees rarely give bill unfavorable report; rather, no action is taken, thereby killing it.

REFERRED TO SENATE COMMITTEE

REFERRED TO SUBCOMMITTEE

REPORTED BY FULL COMMITTEE

In House, many bills go before Rules Committee for "rule" expediting floor action, setting conditions for debate and amendments on floor. Some bills are "privileged" and go directly to floor. Other procedures exist for noncontroversial or routine bills. In Senate, special "rules" are not used; leadership normally schedules action.

FLOOR ACTION

HOUSE DEBATE VOTE ON PASSAGE

FLOOR ACTION

SENATE DEBATE VOTE ON PASSAGE

Bill is debated, usually amended, passed or defeated. If passed, it goes to other chamber to follow the same route through committee and floor stages. (If other chamber has already passed related bill, both versions go straight to conference.)

CONFERENCE ACTION

HOUSE OF REPRESENTATIVES

Once both chambers have passed related bills, conference committee of members from both houses is formed to work out differences.

Compromise version from conference is sent to each chamber for final approval.

SENATE

HR 1 VETO

S 2

Compromise version approved by both houses is sent to President who can either sign it into law or veto it and return it to Congress. Congress may override veto by a two-thirds majority vote in both houses; bill then becomes law without President's signature.

FIGURE 1.

then referred to the appropriate committees. Executive departments and agencies also transmit to the Congress drafts of proposed legislation to carry out the President's program. (Perhaps with some minor deviations, this basic procedure is followed by legisla-tures at other levels of government.)

Introduction of Bills

After they are drafted, legislative bills may be introduced in either or both chambers of the legislature (Congress), e.g., the Senate or the House of Representatives. One notable exception is that all bills for raising revenues shall originate only in the House, but the Senate may propose or concur with amendments, as on other bills. These bills are introduced by the

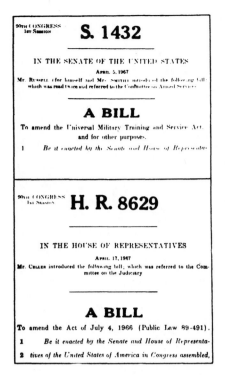

FIGURE 2.

chairman of the committee or subcommittee having jurisdiction over the subject. For example, the Senate committees dealing with health matters include the Finance Committee-Subcommittee on Health and the Human Resources Committee-Subcommittee on Health and Scientific Resources. In the House it is the Ways and Means Committee-Subcommittee on Health and the Interstate and Foreign Commerce Committee-Subcommittee on Health and Environment. Sometimes, committees consider proposals that have not been formally introduced in bill form. In such cases the committee formulates its own bill. (This is usually done with revenue bills.)

Joint resolution is a term that is sometimes used synonymously for bill. A joint resolution requires the approval of both Houses and the signature of the President, just as a bill does, and has the effect of law if approved. They are identified as "H.J. Res." or "S.J. Res."

In addition, a distinction must be made between public and private bills. A private bill, unlike a public bill, instead of pertaining to matters of public interest and affecting generally all persons, e.g., the public at large, affects only a particular person. Such bills confer privileges, benefits or an exemption upon some person.

No matter how a legislative proposal originates, it can be introduced only by a Senator or Congressman. Bills may be jointly sponsored or co-sponsored, and carry several names, although such sponsorships are not necessary to the legislative process. Examples of co-sponsored bills which became federal law are the Durham-Humphrey Amendments and the Kefauver Harris Amendments to the Federal Food, Drug, and Cosmetic Act. On the other hand, the Delaney Amendment to this Act was sponsored by Congressman Delaney who was the chairman of a select committee to investigate the use of chemicals in foods.

Co-sponsorship has advantages. The Senator and Congressman co-sponsoring the proposed legislation become partners, each giving active support for the bill in their respective chambers. Standing committees of both chambers can conduct simultaneous studies and hearings, thus preparing both for possible concurrent action, which speeds the legislative process.

The U.S. Senate consists of 100 elected Senators, two from each of the 50 states [7]. The House of Representatives consists of 435 elected representatives (Congressmen), whose seats are apportioned among the states based upon the population of a given state [8]. Therefore, the legislative branch of the United States government is comprised of 535 elected public officials.

A Senator introduces a bill by seeking recognition from the presiding officer of the Senate (the Vice President of the United States) [9], or the president *pro tempore*, in the absence of the Vice President. If there is an objection by any Senator the introduction of the bill is postponed until the next working day. If there is no objection, the bill is read twice by name (title) and referred to the appropriate committee.

In the House of Representatives a Congressman introduces a bill by handing it to the Clerk of the House or by placing it in a container, called the "hopper", at the side of the Clerk's desk in the House Chamber. At this point the bill has, in legislative parlance, been "dropped in the hopper." When introduced, the bill's title and sponsor(s) will be entered in the *Journal of the House* [10] and printed in the *Congressional Record* of that day. (*The Congressional Record* is a compilation of the daily proceedings of the U.S. Congress. Likewise, state legislatures publish similar journals.) A House bill is considered "read" for the first time when it is referred to the appropriate committee. At this point the bill is ready for discussion, study, possible amendment, and finally a vote.

In order to identify bills besides title and sponsor(s), they are numbered consecutively in the order in which they are introduced in a given session of Congress. A bill originating in the House of Representatives is designated by the letters "H.R." followed by a number that it retains throughout its parliamentary stages, e.g., H.R. 8629. A senate bill is identified by the letter "S." followed by a number, e.g., S. 1432 (Figures 1 and 2).

Copies of the bill under consideration by the committee are customarily forwarded to the executive department or agencies concerned with the subject for their official views to be presented in writing or oral testimony before the committee.

Committee Action

The committee's deliberations are the most important stage of the legislative process because it provides for detailed study of the proposed legislation. Standing committees conduct in-depth public hearings (hearings also may be closed), sample public opinion, and consult with regulatory agency officials and experts in the private sector.

After the public hearings are concluded, committee members meet in closed (executive) session to "mark-up" a bill, e.g., review it section by section, in detail, voting on proposed changes. It is during this state that lobbyists exert their greatest efforts to influence committee members' votes.

When the deliberative process is completed, the full committee makes its recommendation on whether or not to report a bill to its respective chamber for final action. A bill which does not receive a majority of the committee's votes is "killed" or deferred for further study. It should be noted that a great number of bills are "killed" or defeated in committee because they duplicate other bills which are "reported out of committee". Other bills are not reported because they treat only a portion of a problem which requires a more comprehensive solution.

If voted out of committee, the committee issues a report which must accompany the bill, setting forth the nature of the bill and reasons for the committee's approval. The report sets forth specifically the committee's amendments and, in compliance with the rules of the Congress, indicated changes the bill would make in existing law. Any committee member, individually or jointly, may file additional supplemental or minority views to accompany the majority committee report. The committee report accompanying the bill is viewed by the courts and the administrative agencies as the most important document as to the intent of the Congress in proposed legislation [11].

Committees are comprised of members of both major political parties. Meetings are presided over by the Chairman, who is a member of the majority party. Detailed records are kept of committee actions by the committee counsels and clerks who report such actions

to the *Congressional Record*, which in turn, records all legislative actions of the Congress.

Floor Action

This step in the legislative process is the most interesting and the most complex [12].

When a bill is "reported out of committee" it is placed on the calendar for debate on the floor. A calendar is printed for each day of the week and is the daily guide to the legislative action. When the presiding officer of either chamber calls it into session, the clerk reads the calendar, bill by bill. The first bills read by the Clerk are those newly reported by committees and are listed "on the order of second reading." These bills are then advanced to the "third order of reading," which means they will be ready for action on the following working day. The "active" Calendar of Bills, which was previously advanced to "the order of third reading" is then considered.

Bills must be available to a legislator for at least several days to enable him/her to deliberate, in effect to become acquainted with its contents. If a legislator desires to debate a bill, he/she requests that it be "laid aside" for consideration after action has concluded on non-controversial items which are disposed of by unanimous consent. Every legislator is permitted an opportunity to express an opinion during debate. In the Senate debate is unlimited. However, it can be terminated by "cloture", which requires a three-fifths majority of the entire Senate. In the House, debate is limited by the Rules Committee. An "open rule" permits amendments, a "closed rule" does not. The presiding officer of the Senate and the Speaker of the House, preside over floor debates, recognize members for arguments on a bill, and make all rulings. Debate is generally concluded first by the Minority Leader and then by the Majority Leader in the respective Houses.

When a bill is finally ready for

action, with or without debate, it may be voted upon different ways. The Senate has three different methods of voting: an untabulated voice vote, a standing vote, and a recorded roll-call ("long roll call") whereby each Senator must announce his vote as a "yes" or "no".

The House has four different methods of voting, one or more which may be used in deciding a single issue. The four methods are: voice vote, standing vote, teller vote, and roll-call vote.

The voice vote is the usual method of voting when a proposition is first considered. The presiding officer calls for "yes" or "no" votes which decide the result. If the result of the voice vote is in doubt or if a further test is required, then a standing vote is demanded. In this case the members stand and are counted by the presiding officer. A standing vote is sometimes referred to as a "division vote" because only vote totals are announced; there is no record of how individual members voted.

The teller vote may be utilized upon demand of one-fifth of a quorum. The chair appoints two tellers from opposite sides of the aisle and directs the Representatives to pass between them up the center aisle of the House to be counted. The "ayes" pass through first, then the "nays". The votes of individual members are not announced.

Under the roll call vote, the Clerk of the House calls each member's name, and each answers "yea" or "nay". If a representative does not want to vote, an answer of "present" is sufficient. In the House, roll-call votes are recorded electronically. Each member is assigned a personal wallet-size voting card which is inserted into one of 44 voting terminals. A computer provides a summary of votes on a lighted scoreboard, and projects the vote of each member.

Once a bill has passed one chamber, it is sent to the other. Frequently, the House and Senate pass different versions of a bill. When this happens, a "conference committee" of Senators and Representatives must resolve the difference (Figure 3). The compromise version must then be re-passed by both chambers before it is sent to the President for his signature [13].

Enrollment

When the two legislative bodies reach agreement on an identical bill, it is delivered to the Enrolling Clerk of the House or the Secretary of the Senate when that bill has originated in that body. A final copy of the bill is prepared for forwarding to the Government Printing Office (GPO) for "enrollment", which means historically "written on parchment", e.g., printed on parchment paper. Upon receipt of the enrolled bill from the GPO, it is presented to the Speaker of the House for his signature. All bills, regardless of the body in which they originated, are signed first by the Speaker and then by the President of the Senate. After both signatures are affixed, the bill is presented to the President.

Presidential Action

The President has ten days (Sunday excepted) after the enrolled bill has been presented to him in which to act upon it [14]. Copies of enrolled bills are usually transmitted by the White House to the various agencies which have an interest in the subject, so that they may advise the President [15].

If the President approves the bill, he signs it, giving the date, and returns it to the chamber in which it originated [Figure 3(a)]. The enrolled bill is then delivered to the Administrator of the General Services Administration, who designates it as a public or private law and assigns it a number. An official copy is sent to the GPO to be used in making the "slip law", which is the first official publication of the statute [Figure 3(b)].

In the event the President does not favor a bill and vetoes it, he

---

90TH CONGRESS } HOUSE OF REPRESENTATIVES { REPORT
1st Session   No. 346

AMENDING AND EXTENDING THE DRAFT ACT AND RELATED LAWS

JUNE 8, 1967.—Ordered to be printed

Mr. RIVERS, from the committee of conference, submitted the following

CONFERENCE REPORT

[To accompany S. 1432]

The committee of conference on the disagreeing votes of the two Houses on the amendment of the House to the bill (S. 1432) to amend the Universal Mili-

---

Ninetieth Congress of the United States of America   *(a)*

AT THE FIRST SESSION

Begun and held at the City of Washington on Tuesday, the tenth day of January, one thousand nine hundred and sixty-seven

An Act

To amend the Act of July 4, 1966 (Public Law 89-491).

Be it enacted by the Senate and House of Representatives of the United States of America in Congress assembled, That the Act of July 4, 1966 (80 Stat. 259), is hereby amended as follows:

Public Law 90-187   *(b)*
90th Congress, H. R. 8629
December 12, 1967

An Act
_____ 81 STAT. 567

To amend the Act of July 4, 1966 (Public Law 89-491).

Be it enacted by the Senate and House of Representatives of the United States of America in Congress assembled, That the Act of July 4, 1966 (80 Stat. 259), is hereby amended as follows: American Revolution Bicenten-

---

Public Law 93-190   *(c)*
93rd Congress, S. 2641
December 18, 1973

An Act

To confer jurisdiction upon the district court of the United States of certain civil actions brought by the Senate Select Committee on Presidential Campaign Activities, and for other purposes.

Be it enacted by the Senate and House of Representatives of the United States of America in Congress assembled, That (a) the District U.S. District

---

Public Law 93-148   *(d)*
November 7, 1973
93rd Congress, H. J. Res. 542

CARL ALBERT
Speaker of the House of Representatives.

JAMES O. EASTLAND
President of the Senate pro tempore.

IN THE HOUSE OF REPRESENTATIVES, U.S.,
November 7, 1973.

The House of Representatives having proceeded to reconsider the resolution (H. J. Res. 542) entitled "Joint resolution concerning the war powers of

---

FIGURE 3.

must return it, with his objections ("veto message"), "to that house in which it shall have originated, who shall enter the objections at large on their journal, and proceed to reconsider it" [Figure 3(c)]. If after such reconsideration two-thirds of that house shall agree to pass the bill, it shall be sent, together with the objections, to the other house, by which it shall likewise be reconsidered, and if approved by two-thirds of that house, it shall become law, without again being presented to the President of the United States. If, upon reconsideration by either house, the bill does not receive the two-thirds affirmative vote to pass over the objections of the President, the President's veto is sustained and the bill does not become law.

If any bill is not returned by the President within ten days (Sundays excepted) after it has been presented to him, the same shall be a law, in like manner as if he had signed it [Figure 3(d)]. If the Congress is adjourned which prevents the return of a bill with objections by the President, the bill cannot become law, and is referred to as a "pocket veto".

Publications

One of the important steps in the enactment of a valid law is the requirement that it shall be made known to the people who are bound by it, by publishing it immediately upon enactment.

The Administrator of General Services Administration (GSA), who is responsible for publishing the statute, assigns it either a public or a private law number, starting at the number "1", for each two year term of Congress. For example, the first public law of the 97th Congress is designated Public Law 1, 97th Congress or PL 97-1.

For the purpose of providing a permanent collection of the laws of each session of the Congress the bound volumes, which are referred to as the *United States Statutes at Large*, are prepared by

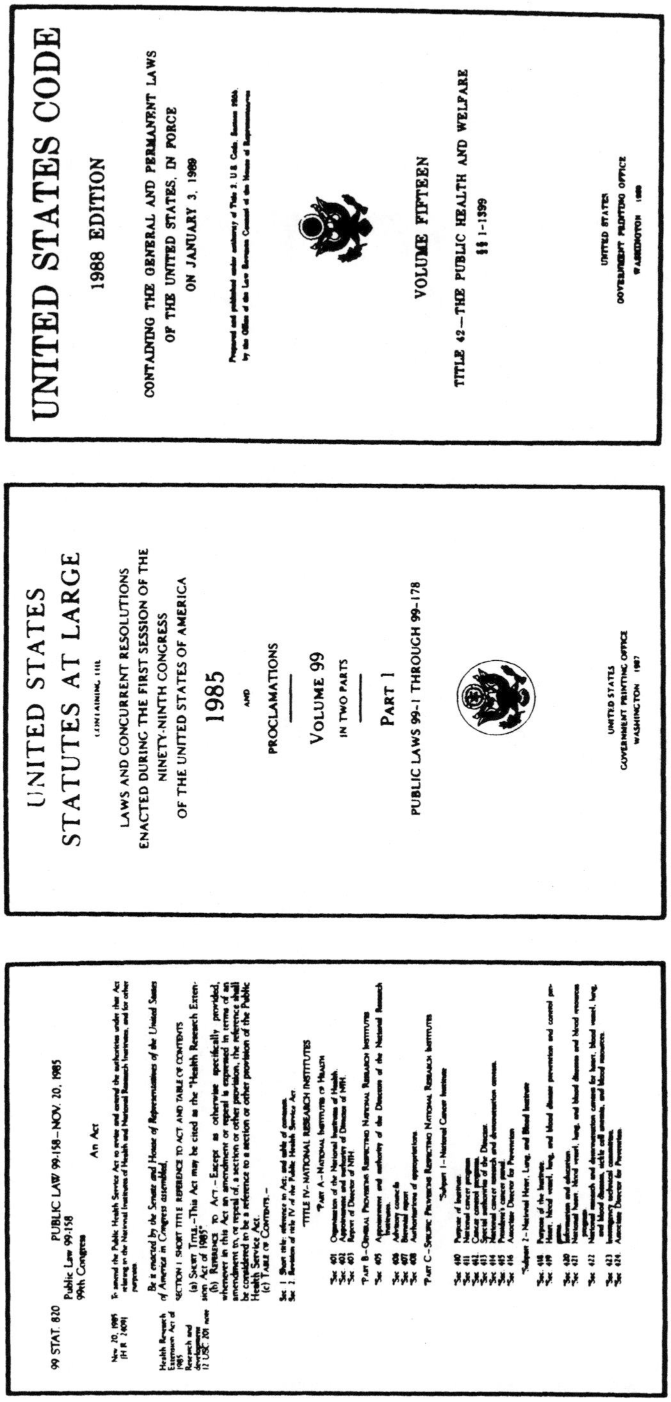

Legislation is published first as a slip law. This is a printing, in pamphlet form, of a law as enacted by Congress and signed by the President. Marginal notes and citations are added, and it is published by the Office of the Federal Register.

These slip laws are compiled annually by the Office of the Federal Register as a volume of the *United States Statutes at Large*, a chronological compilation of all private and public laws of one session of Congress.

Finally, the law is codified in the *United States Code*. This publication, arranged by subject matter, is fully revised every six years. Between revisions, annual cumulative supplements are issued. The *United States Code* is not an Office of the Federal Register publication; it is prepared by the Office of the Law Revision Counsel of the House of Representatives.

Legislation is implemented by Federal agencies' regulations.

FIGURE 4. Parallel codification of legislation and regulations.

Legislation is implemented by Federal agencies' regulations.

Public Health

code of federal regulations

42

PARTS 61 TO 299
Revised as of October 1, 1991

After publication in the *Federal Register* as a final rule, regulations are then codified in the annual *Code of Federal Regulations* (*CFR*). The *CFR* is cited by title and part number such as 42 CFR Part 64.

federal register

Wednesday
June 26, 1991

SECOND CLASS NEWSPAPER

Regulations appearing in the *Federal Register* are cited by volume and page number such as 56 FR 29187, beginning with volume 1 in 1936 and changing with each calendar year.

[Billing Code 4160-01]

DEPARTMENT OF HEALTH AND HUMAN SERVICES

Public Health Service

42 CFR Parts 4, 60a, and 64

RIN 0905-AA59

National Library of Medicine Programs

AGENCY: Public Health Service, HHS.

ACTION: Final rule.

SUMMARY: These regulations govern the programs of the National Library of Medicine (NLM). The regulations (1) permit the Regional Medical Libraries to recover part or all of the costs of providing photocopies of biomedical materials; (2) improve readability of the regulations; and (3) update reference to statutory authorities and uniform administrative requirements.

EFFECTIVE DATE: These regulations are effective [Federal Register please insert the date of publication].

FOR FURTHER INFORMATION CONTACT: Mr. John J. Migliore on (301) 496-6076.

SUPPLEMENTARY INFORMATION: These regulations, which pertain to the National Library of Medicine in whole or in part, were proposed for revision as part of the Department's effort to simplify and update its regulations. The notice of proposed

Proposed rules and final rules are drafted as agency documents, submitted to the Office of the Federal Register, edited to conform to a common style, and published in the *Federal Register.*

FIGURE 4 (continued).

---

the GSA. The *Statutes* are only a chronological arrangement of the laws exactly as they were enacted.

The *United States Code* is a consolidation and codification of statutes arranged according to subject matter. For example, Title 21 contains legislation pertaining to drugs and Controlled Substances, while Medicaid legislation is contained in Title 42 of the *U.S. Code.* New statutes are continually integrated into the existing *U.S. Code.*

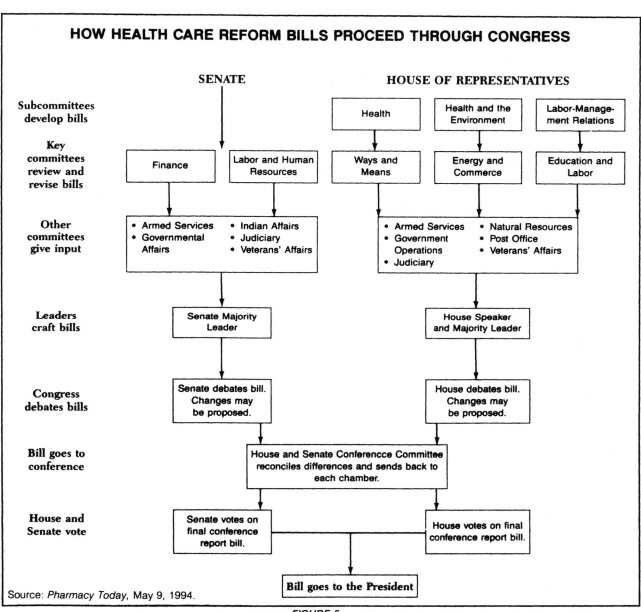

HOW HEALTH CARE REFORM BILLS PROCEED THROUGH CONGRESS

	SENATE	HOUSE OF REPRESENTATIVES

Subcommittees develop bills

Health • Health and the Environment • Labor-Management Relations

Key committees review and revise bills

Finance • Labor and Human Resources • Ways and Means • Energy and Commerce • Education and Labor

Other committees give input

- Armed Services
- Governmental Affairs
- Indian Affairs
- Judiciary
- Veterans' Affairs

- Armed Services
- Government Operations
- Judiciary
- Natural Resources
- Post Office
- Veterans' Affairs

Leaders craft bills

Senate Majority Leader • House Speaker and Majority Leader

Congress debates bills

Senate debates bill. Changes may be proposed. • House debates bill. Changes may be proposed.

Bill goes to conference

House and Senate Conferencce Committee reconciles differences and sends back to each chamber.

House and Senate vote

Senate votes on final conference report bill. • House votes on final conference report bill.

Bill goes to the President

Source: *Pharmacy Today*, May 9, 1994.

FIGURE 5.

15

References

1. United States Constitution, Art. I, Sect. 1.
2. Ibid, Art. I, Sect. 8 (18).
3. Ibid, Art. I, Sect. 8 (1); 16th Amend.
4. Ibid, Art. I, Sect. 8 (5).
5. Ibid, Art. I, Sect. 8 (3).
6. Ibid, Art. II, Sect. 3.
7. Ibid, Art. I, Sect. 3 (1); 17th Amend.
8. Ibid, Art. I, Sect. 2 (3); 14th Amend., Sect. 2.
9. Ibid, Art. I, Sect. 3 (4).
10. Ibid, Art. I, Sect. 5 (3).
11. Michel, RH: "How a bill becomes a law," NARD J 101(10):57, 1979.
12. United States Constitution, Art. I, Sect. 5 (2).
13. Ibid, Art. I, Sect. 7 (2).
14. Ibid, Art. I, Sect. 7 (2).
15. Ibid, Art. II, Sect. 2 (1).

THE STATUTE OF LIMITATIONS*

David Brushwood, J.D., R.Ph. and Maven J. Myers, J.D., Ph.D.

One of the legal technicalities which may deprive a litigant of the right to assert a legitimate claim is the *statute of limitations*. A potential trap to the unwary patient who intends to file a malpractice claim against a pharmacist, the statute of limitations is a legislative enactment peculiar to each jurisdiction which declares that no lawsuit may be successfully prosecuted unless initiated within a specific time after the plaintiff's right to sue has accrued. Thus, the patient's case may be forever barred if he waits too long to file the lawsuit, even if the pharmacist's negligence is beyond question.

Virtually every legal action, whether criminal, administrative, or civil, must be initiated within a specified time following the occurrence of the act giving rise to the legal action. Although this article will be limited to a discussion of the tort statute of limitations as it applies to pharmacist malpractice lawsuits, the reader is cautioned that other legal proceedings in which pharmacists may become involved also are subject to statutes of limitations.

*Reprinted with permission from *U.S. Pharmacist* (June 1983).

The General Statutory Framework

Statutes of limitations in tort law vary in length depending on the basis of liability, the type of claim, and the nature of the interest invaded. A typical statute of limitations reads:

> Civil actions . . . can only be commenced within the period prescribed . . . after the cause of action shall have accrued [1].

One of the first points a lawyer determines when he undertakes to represent a client is the applicable statute of limitations for the client's claim. If a lawyer fails to do this, it may expose the lawyer to liability for malpractice.

The express language of the preceding quoted statute indicates that the statute of limitations commences when a cause of action "accrues," i.e., comes into existence as a legally enforceable claim. Since damages are an essential part of a cause of action based on negligence, most courts have held that the statute commences when there has been an actual injury to the plaintiff's person or property. But this may not be the case in a pharmacist malpractice lawsuit. Actions against pharmacists are usually governed by a special statute of limitations which applies to health care providers.

A typical statute of this type reads:

> A cause of action arising out of the rendering or the failure to render professional services by a health care provider shall be deemed to have accrued at the time of the occurrence of the act giving rise to the cause of action, unless the fact of injury is not reasonably ascertainable until some time after the initial act, then the period of limitation shall not commence until the fact of injury becomes reasonably ascertainable to the injured party [2].

In the case of pharmacist malpractice, the general rule would indicate that if it can be determined that the injury occurred on the date the medication was dispensed, that would be the date on which the statute of limitations would begin. When the statutorily specified period of time has passed, following the accrual of the cause of action, the right to maintain a lawsuit expires. Then, no matter how meritorious a claim may be, that particular claim is forever barred.

Certain events may interrupt the statute of limitations. The statute of limitations is in most instances interrupted due to the inability of the plaintiff to bring suit through no fault of his own. Two examples which illustrate when the statute of limitations is interrupted are (1) absence of the defendant from the jurisdiction, and (2) fraudulent concealment from the plaintiff of the existence of plaintiff's cause of action. Any period during which the statute of limitations is interrupted extends the time within which a lawsuit may be filed after the cause of action accrues.

The Discovery Rule

In most jurisdictions, the statute of limitations in health professional malpractice cases is relatively short. In 39 states it is three years or less [3]. Yet damage resulting from an act of malpractice involving the sale of drugs does not always manifest itself within a short period of time. Some drugs, such as diethylstilbestrol, allegedly cause harm which does not become obvious until many years or decades after the occurrence of the negligent act which is said to have caused the harm. Without some type of exception to the general rule, many victims of drug induced personal injuries would lose their right to sue before they even discovered that any injury existed.

The Court of Appeals of Georgia ruled on this aspect of a pharmacist malpractice case in 1977 [4]. The facts of the case showed that the patient, who suffered from steroid-induced glaucoma, had last had a steroid prescription filled at the defendant's pharmacy in February, 1971. A suit was filed against the defendant pharmacist in July, 1975. The applicable Georgia statute of limitations provided that "actions for injuries to the person shall be brought within two years after the right of action accrues" [5].

Without some type of health care provider exception to the general rule, the right of action would have accrued when the pharmacist sold (dispensed) the medication to the patient in February, 1971. By that analysis, it would have been

too late, after February 1973 to bring a lawsuit against the pharmacist. But the patient was able to show that she was unable to discover the source of her problems until October, 1973. At that time, an ophthalmologist diagnosed her steroid-induced glaucoma. Less than two years after this diagnosis, the pharmacist was named as a defendant in the lawsuit.

The court ruled that this case fell within the doctrine of "continuing tort" [4]. The statute of limitations was interrupted until the discovery of the injury. Upon discovery, the cause of action was complete, and two years later the action would be barred if it was not on file. Since the pharmacist had in fact been sued within two years after the discovery of the damage, the patient was allowed to proceed with the lawsuit. The court thus recognized the "discovery rule" as an exception to the general rule that a legal action accrues when a negligent act occurs and causes damage.

Courts in other jurisdictions have dealt with the statute of limitations in drug and latent injury cases in a variety of different ways. The most restrictive view taken by a court is that the discovery rule simply does not apply. In jurisdictions which adopt this view, the statute of limitations begins at the time the injury occurs, *not* when the plaintiff discovers the cause of the injury [6]. Even if the drug has a slowly evolving toxicity, the statute of limitations under the restrictive view begins either at the time of sale or at the time of ingestion of the drug, not when the injury becomes evident.

An alternative approach adopted by some courts is that the statute of limitations begins when the injury is discovered by the plaintiff, rather than when the injury occurs [7]. A patient may suffer tissue damage as the result of ingesting a drug, but be asymptomatic for a period of time. The statute of limitations begins only when the patient discovers there is an injury. The patient does not have to know the cause of the injury or that there is a

right to file a lawsuit against a particular defendant. All that is required is that the injury be apparent, and that the injured party should know that somebody, somewhere may be legally liable for the injury. As soon as the fact of injury becomes known to the plaintiff, the statute of limitations begins.

Still another view which some courts favor is that a cause of action accrues only when the victim discovers or should discover the nature or cause of the disability or impairment [8]. This is a variation of the discovery rule. Simply discovering that an injury exists is not enough to start the statute of limitations. Some courts hold that the statute of limitations does not begin until the plaintiff discovers that the injury was caused by the drug which the defendant manufactured, prescribed, or dispensed. There must be discovery of both the injury itself and the cause of the injury for the statute of limitations to begin. This is probably the most liberal approach. Rarely would a statute of limitations defense be successful in a jurisdiction where the courts have adopted this view.

Since there are so many different concepts governing the statute of limitations, it is crucial for a pharmacist's defense attorney to understand the position which courts in the jurisdiction have adopted with regard to latent injury cases. The statute of limitations is a collection of concepts which can close the door to litigation or keep it open, depending on the facts of the case and the relevant judicial interpretations. The discovery rule exception is a "foot-in-the-door" which keeps the door to litigation open for plaintiffs who have suffered a latent toxicity to a drug.

Statutes of Repose

Some states have enacted legislation which provides for another limitation period which limits the length of time the discovery rule can extend the accrual date of a cause of action. For example, a general malpractice statute of limitations provides a two year period, with a discovery exception postponing the statute until a plaintiff discovers, or through the exercise of reasonable diligence should discover, an injury [9]. An additional statute of repose would provide that in no event could a cause of action be brought more than four years after the act causing the injury occurred.

As is the case with a statute of limitations, the additional statute of repose may bar a cause of action before a latent injury becomes apparent to the patient. The statute of repose operates to restrict access to the courts afforded by the discovery rule [10]. On constitutional grounds, certain statutes of repose in drug product liability cases against manufacturers have been invalidated, because they violate the constitutional guarantee of free access to the courts [11].

Medical Malpractice Statutes of Limitations and Statutes of Repose

Apparently in response to the "medical malpractice crisis" of the 1960's, 48 states developed statutes of limitation and statutes of repose which are specifically applicable to medical malpractice cases [12]. Special medical malpractice statutes usually afford the physician preferred status among personal injury defendants. Of the 48 special malpractice statutes, five have a longer limit than the otherwise applicable statute of limitations, 16 have a shorter limit, and 23 are the same [3]. Thirty-six have some type of discovery rule, and most of those with a discovery rule have a repose period. Many of the special statutes of repose are shorter than the general statutes of repose, in effect making latent injury lawsuits against physicians more difficult to sustain.

Medical malpractice is sometimes defined within the statute to include pharmacist malpractice, but in most statutes there is no specific definitional guidance. Al-

though there is no crisis in pharmacy malpractice, as in medicine, pharmacists would do well to argue for inclusion with the special status granted to the medical profession. The benefits legislatively bestowed upon physicians could prove to be the turning point in a pharmacist's effort to avoid liability.

In a 1961 Ohio case, a pharmacist made precisely that argument in an effort to defend himself on the basis of a one-year limitation period applicable to malpractice actions [13]. The patient sued the pharmacist more than one year after an allegedly negligent act occurred. The trial court dismissed the lawsuit based on the malpractice statute of limitations. The dismissal of the lawsuit against the pharmacist was affirmed by the Ohio Court of Appeals. The appellate court reasoned that the patient had come to the pharmacist clothed in the doctor–patient relationship. If the allegations contained in the patient's petition had been proven to be true, the pharmacist would have been liable for malpractice, so the one year statute of limitations was held to apply just the same as it would have applied to a physician.

In a more recent case, the United States Court of Appeals for the Eleventh Circuit reached the same conclusion [14]. The facts in the recent case showed that, over two years after the plaintiff's last purchase from a pharmacy, a lawsuit was filed claiming that the pharmacy lacked the necessary physician's authorization to issue the plaintiff's last six prescription refills. Even if proven at trial, this assertion alone would not necessarily have been sufficient to warrant a verdict for the patient. But the pharmacy opted to assert a procedural technicality, in an attempt to avoid going to trial at all. The pharmacy sought to dismiss the action, relying on a statute which said, "An action for medical malpractice shall be brought within two years after the date on which the negligent or wrongful act or omission occurred."

The patient's attorney argued that the statute of limitations for medical malpractice was inapplicable, because a pharmacist is not engaged in "the practice of medicine" as defined by statute. The court reasoned, however, that a narrow definition of "the practice of medicine" is not inconsistent with a broad definition of "medical malpractice." The court pointed to the definition of "medical malpractice," which did not expressly include pharmacists, but nonetheless stated that "any claim for damages arising out of prescriptions, rendered by a person authorized by law to perform such service" was to be considered a medical malpractice claim. The court noted that the applicable law historically had allowed medical malpractice suits against dentists and hospitals. Therefore, the court upheld the dismissal of the lawsuit against the pharmacist.

The statute of limitations is a procedure upon which a lawsuit may be resolved other than on the actual merits of the case. The statute of limitations serves a useful and well-recognized purpose: It prevents plaintiffs from delaying claims until the facts grow stale and memories fade, thereby delaying the defense from utilizing available material in trial preparation.

The discovery rule has contributed to the rapid rise in the cost of medical malpractice insurance. Many pharmacist malpractice policies are issued on what is called an "occurrence" basis. This means that the policy covers the pharmacist's conduct during a given year even though a claim based on that conduct may not arise for many years. Because of this fact, actuarial projections call for very high premiums. Many insurance companies have begun to issue malpractice insurance policies on a "claims made" basis. These policies would cover only claims filed against the pharmacist that year regardless of when the act of malpractice occurred.

For plaintiffs whose rights are

jeopardized by the statute of limitations the discovery rule is a powerful ally. Defendants have available an opposite, yet equal, doctrine in the statute of repose. Just as the law can create a right of action, the law can limit or overtly deny that right. The statute of limitations and other technical requirements may operate to bar a plaintiff's claim. Consequently, all personal injury claims should be referred to an insurer or a private attorney prior to any payment or other settlement.

References

1. Kan. Stat. Ann. § 60–510.
2. Kan. Stat. Ann. § 60–513(c).
3. McGovern, Francis E., The Status of Statutes of Limitations and Statutes of Repose in Product Liability and Toxic Substances Litigation, Toxic Substances Litigation, Practicing Law Institute, 1982.
4. Piedmont Pharmacy, Inc. v. Patmore, 240 SE 2d. 888 (Ga. App. 1977).
5. Ga. Code Ann. § 3–1004.
6. See: Berry v. G. D. Searle, 309 N.E. 2d 550 (Ill., 1974).
7. See: Steiner v. Ciba-Geigy Corp., 364 So. 2nd 47 (Fla. App. 1978).
8. See: Sindell v. Abbott Labs., 149 Cal. Rptr. 138 (1978).
9. Kan. Stat. Ann. § 60–513(a).
10. Kan. Stat. Ann. § 60–513(c).
11. Diamond v. Squibb & Sons, Inc. 397 So. 2d 671 (Fla. 1981); Bolick v. American Barmag Corp., 284 S.E. 2d 188 (N.C. App. 1981).
12. Fagan, Thomas H., The Medical Malpractice Statute of Limitations: The Severance of the Long Tail of Liability, Illinois Bar Journal, 70: 114 (Oct. 1981).
13. Boudot v. Schwallie, 178 N.E. 2d 599 (Ohio App. 1961).
14. Faser v. Sears, Roebuck & Co., 674 F. 2d 856 (11th Cir. 1982).

QUESTIONS: CHAPTER 1

1. What is the term used to designate the draft of proposed legislation?
   a. Common law
   b. Article
   c. Bill
   d. William
   e. Short title

2. Rules and regulations are promulgated by the:
   a. U.S. Congress
   b. State legislature
   c. Mayor of a municipality
   d. Food and Drug Administration (FDA)
   e. Executive order

3. A statute law that is enacted by a municipality is referred to as a(n):
   a. Ordnance
   b. Case law
   c. Municipal law
   d. Ordinance
   e. Ordinary law

4. The final step in the federal government's rulemaking process involves:

    a. The FDA issuing an interim rule

    b. Publication of the final rule in the *FR*

    c. Congress having its law published in the *CR*

    d. Codification in the *CFR*

    e. Publication in the *NYS Register*

5. A legislature that consists of two legislative chambers or "houses" is said to be:

    a. Bicameral

    b. Bicentennial

    c. Bilingual

    d. Bicamelar

    e. Bicarbonate

6. Which of the following is considered the "daily newspaper" of the federal legislature?

    a. *Congressional Record*

    b. *Code of Federal Regulations*

    c. *Government Manual*

    d. *Federal Register*

    e. *The Daily Federal Government Record*

7. The final act in the legislative process by which a bill becomes a statute requires:

    a. Passage of the bill by both houses of the legislature

    b. The government's chief executive officer's signature

    c. Cosponsorship of a senator

    d. Floor debate

    e. Approval of the appropriate legislative committee

8. Documents intended by a federal government agency to result in new regulations are published in the *Federal Register* and are referred to as:

    a. Notice of rulemaking

    b. Proposed regulations

    c. New federal regulations

    d. Notices

    e. Petitions

9. An annually revised publication which contains federal government agency regulations is the:

    a. *Record of Federal Regulations, as Amended*

    b. *Congressional Record*

    c. *Federal Register*

    d. *Code of Federal Register*

    e. *Code of Federal Regulations*

10. A request or application to a federal government agency by a person requesting the establishment, amendment, or revocation of a regulation is known as a:

    a. Notice of intent

    b. Petition

    c. Proposal

    d. Probate

    e. Peremptory challenge

11. The laws that pertain to the administrative aspects of its enforcement are referred to as:
   a. Substantive law
   b. Adjective law
   c. Statute law
   d. Civil law
   e. Regulatory law

12. The publication that provides all the official notices and proposed and final regulations issued by federal agencies of government is referred to as:
   a. *CFR*
   b. *FR*
   c. *CL*
   d. *CR*

13. A preliminary section of a statute which declares its enactment and serves to identify it is known as:
   a. Grandfather clause
   b. Enacting clause
   c. Santa clause
   d. Severability clause
   e. Identification clause

14. The state in which you practice pharmacy regulates the profession of pharmacy by the authority granted it by the:
   a. Interstate commerce clause
   b. Governor
   c. Board of pharmacy
   d. U.S. Constitution
   e. Intrastate commerce clause

15. Which of the following is considered the "daily newspaper" of the U.S. government agencies?
   a. *Congressional Record*
   b. *Code of Federal Regulations*
   c. *Government Manual*
   d. *Federal Register*
   e. *The Daily Federal Government Record*

16. Which of the following is the component of a statute which prevents it from being declared unconstitutional in its entirety simply because some segment of it may be under challenge?
   a. Severability clause
   b. Repealing clause
   c. Clause of taking effect
   d. Santa clause
   e. Enacting clause

17. The "daily newspaper" of the U.S. Congress is the:
   a. *Congressional Record*
   b. *Code of Federal Regulations*
   c. *Congressional Report*
   d. *Federal Register*
   e. *The Daily Federal Government Record*

18. The words which refer to actions of a government agency that extend beyond its legal authority as defined by statute is/are:

   a. Nondelegation doctrine
   b. Unconstitutional
   c. Ultra vires
   d. Duces tecum
   e. Misfeasance

19. The first official publication of a statute is in the form generally known as the:

   a. Slip law
   b. Session law
   c. Enrolled bill
   d. Statute-at-large
   e. Statutory law

20. The chronological arrangement of federal statutes is referred to as:

   a. *Code of Federal Laws*
   b. *United States Code*
   c. *Congressional Directory*
   d. *United States Statutes-at-Large*

21. A compilation of United States statutes by subject is called the:

   a. *United States Statutes-at-Large*
   b. *United States Code*
   c. *Federal Registry of Statutes*
   d. *Code of Federal Statutes*

22. Which one of the following may be considered the daily supplement to the *Code of Federal Regulations?*

   a. *United States Code*
   b. *Federal Register*
   c. *Congressional Daily Record*
   d. *Code of Federal Register*

23. Which one of the following contains a consolidation and codification of the general and permanent statutes of the United States arranged according to subject matter?

   a. *Code of Federal Regulations*
   b. *United States Code*
   c. *United States Statutes-at-Large*
   d. *Congressional Record*

CHAPTER 2

The Judicial System

WHAT TO EXPECT WHEN A LAWSUIT IS STARTED*

J. L. Fink III, B.S. Pharm., J.D., R.Ph.

The courts are being called upon more frequently to decide cases involving pharmacy and pharmacists and the pharmacist should understand some of the basic procedures involved. The procedures which lead to trial can be quite complex and often are as important if not more important than what occurs at trial. Many decisions which are made in framing the complaint or answer, considering pretrial motions, and conducting discovery and depositions are critical to the outcome of the case. This article reviews the procedure followed by the courts of most states hearing civil lawsuits, i.e., malpractice, breach of contract, etc.

Consulting an Attorney

The first step in initiating or defending a lawsuit is hiring and consulting with an attorney. Pharmacists should retain an attorney upon whom to call for legal advice on a regular basis. The services of an attorney were probably retained for purchasing a home or a pharmacy and thus pharmacists have already had some contact with a lawyer. The need for legal advice is underscored by increasing govern-

*Reprinted with permission from U.S. Pharmacist (Jan., Nov./Dec. 1979).

mental intervention in the practice of pharmacy. The time may come when a pharmacist will need legal advice on matters pertaining to legality of an inspection, etc., and an attorney with whom the pharmacist has dealt with in the past will be more likely to provide aid on a sometimes urgent basis.

It is important to select an attorney who is conversant with the type of problem with which an individual is confronted. The attorney who handles delinquent accounts receivable may not be suitable to litigate a malpractice violation. Assistance in locating an attorney with specific qualifications may be obtained by contacting the local bar association.

The attorney can counsel the plaintiff whether or not a claim has merit and is worth the cost. He can also advise a defendant of any defenses and whether the plaintiff's suit has merit. The attorney can estimate the amount of time the case will involve and can advise what to expect in court with a particular case.

It is best to reach an agreement with an attorney about the amount of compensation and method of payment, and the expenses that are anticipated and expected at the outset of the lawsuit or defense. This will prevent misunderstandings later which could be unpleas-

ant for the client and the attorney. Some attorneys handle certain types of litigation on a contingent fee basis, i.e., their compensation is based on a percentage of the amount awarded in the lawsuit. Other types of legal matters may be charged on an hourly fee or on a flat fee basis, e.g., $250 for a simple will.

Initiating the Lawsuit

To initiate a lawsuit the plaintiff (complainant, petitioner) and his attorney draft a complaint and file it with the clerk of court. The complaint outlines the plaintiff's case and sets forth certain facts which the plaintiff believes to be true. The clerk then issues a summons with a copy of the complaint. Receipt of the summons and complaint, either by mail or from a process server, is often the first time the defendant knows that he is being sued. The defendant has a stated period of time, usually 30 days or less, to respond to the allegations in the complaint. If the defendant does not respond in time, he loses by default. If he responds, he may admit to or deny the statements in the plaintiff's complaint or assert new facts in the answer as a defense. If the defendant denies the allegations in the response, the burden of proof is placed on the plaintiff at trial to prove the allegations to be true.

Pre-Trial Motions

An alternative to answering the complaint is for the defendant to address certain motions to the court. Usually, motions of objection will be filed before the answer. For example, the defendant may assert that the action was brought in the wrong court or that he was improperly served with notice of the suit. If the objection is sustained, the suit may end there, or the plaintiff may be permitted to correct the mistake. Another objection is the motion to dismiss, known as *demurrer*. This means that the defendant is saying that even if all the facts alleged by the plaintiff are true, the latter is still not entitled to any legal relief.

If new facts are presented in the answer filed by the defendant, the plaintiff must file a reply and either admit or deny the new facts that the defendant has presented. The complaint, the defendant's response, and the plaintiff's reply constitute the *pleadings* which compose the boundaries for the trial.

The defendant may also file a *counterclaim* or *cross complaint* alleging that the plaintiff owes him money or damages, and that such liability should be offset against any claim which the plaintiff has.

Once the pleadings are completed, either party may make a *motion for judgment on the pleadings*. This is a request that the judge review the papers filed and decide the case on the basis of the claims made. If the judge does so, that may end the case.

Another pre-trial motion which may be encountered is the *motion for summary judgment*. In most courts the lawsuit may be shortened by presenting to the court sworn statements or affidavits which show that a claim or defense is false or a sham. However, this approach cannot be used when there is substantial dispute concerning the facts to be proved by use of the affidavits. Granting of a motion for summary judgment made by either party may end the suit at that stage.

Often, a *pre-trial conference* will be held by the judge and attorneys representing the parties. The purpose of this meeting is to narrow the focus of the trial by eliminating matters that are not in dispute and agreeing to what issues remain for trial. While the pre-trial conference is not intended to settle the case out of court, frequently the attorneys for the parties to the suit recognize that the differences between their clients are not insurmountable or that the arguments on one side are not as meritorious as was thought. This should lead to a settlement, helping to eliminate the backlog of cases in the courts.

Pre-Trial Procedures

Rules of legal procedure in the federal courts and most state courts now permit the parties to engage in a pretrial process known as *discovery*. This is the opportunity for one party to inquire of the other and his witnesses about anything related to the lawsuit. The attorney may ask the adverse party the names of witnesses, ask the adverse party and the witnesses what they know about the case, examine records or papers, and even have an examination of the physical or mental condition of a party when this has a bearing on the lawsuit. Due to the rules permitting discovery, surprise, which used to be a prime tool of the trial attorney, has virtually disappeared from the litigation process. Each side will know what evidence the opposition tends to introduce and what their witness will say on the witness stand.

One last pre-trial procedure is known as *deposition*. Usually witnesses testify in court at the time of trial. However, sometimes it may be necessary to obtain testimony out of court prior to trial. This is usually done when the witness is aged, infirm or about to leave the state or country and will not be present when the trial occurs.

Beginning the Trial

On the date set for trial, both parties appear in court with their attorneys. The judge calls the court to order and begins selection of the jury if it is to be a trial by jury. Use of a jury is not mandatory in a civil case. If plaintiff and defendant agree, the trial can proceed without a jury.

The role of the jury in a trial is to determine the facts in dispute; the judge decides questions of law. For example, assume that a contract case arises in which a letter admittedly was written by the defendant in response to an offer made by the plaintiff, and the plaintiff is suing the defendant, alleging that the letter constituted acceptance of the offer and a contract resulted. Whether the wording of the letter constitutes an acceptance of the plaintiff's offer is a question of law to be answered by the judge. On the other hand, it may be admitted by the defendant that such a letter would constitute an acceptance of the offer had it been written, but he alleges that no such letter was ever written. This is a question of fact for the jury to determine.

Jury Selection

If it is to be a trial by jury, the selection of the jury begins with the clerk of courts preparing a list of eligible jurors, usually from a list of local property owners or from the roll of registered voters. A large number of potential jurors is called to the courthouse and when a case has been assigned by the presiding judge to a courtroom for trial, a smaller group of potential jurors is sent to that location. The names of the prospective jurors are placed on slips of paper and placed in a shuffling device. The clerk of the court then selects a sufficient number of slips to complete the jury. The traditional jury was composed of 12 persons. However, the U.S. Supreme Court has ruled that number to be wholly without significance and many states now authorize use of juries of less than 12 people in all or some civil trials. The jury at trial is known as a *petit jury* because it has fewer members than a *grand jury* used in a criminal case to determine whether sufficient evidence exists to refer a case for trial. Following their selection, potential jurors must swear to give true answers to all questions the attorneys ask of them for the attorneys and the judge to determine whether they qualify to serve as jurors.

Addressing questions to the prospective jurors to determine whether they qualify is known as *voir dire examination*. After questioning the jury candidate, if the attorney feels that the person should not serve, he can challenge the nominee juror. If such a person is prejudiced or related to one of the attorneys or parties to the case, the attorney can *challenge for cause*. Another potential juror will then be called for *voir dire*.

In addition to the challenges for cause, which are unlimited in number, the attorney may have a certain juror dismissed without stating a reason. This is known as a *preemptory challenge* and the number allowed each side is usually set by court rule, ranging from two to six per party to the suit. The process of *voir dire* continues until a jury panel is chosen.

Opening Statements

After the jury has been selected, the attorneys make their *opening statements*, the plaintiff's attorney going first. This is presentation to the jury of an outline of what the issues are and how the attorney will attempt to prove his case so that they may follow the case. The attorney for the defendant has the option of making his opening statement immediately after the plaintiff's counsel, or he may reserve it until he begins to present his defense arguments.

Presentation of Each Side's Case

The plaintiff has the burden of proving his case in most situations.

Accordingly, his case is presented first, and the plaintiff's attorney has the opportunity to make the last statement to the jury at close of trial.

The plaintiff's attorney calls the first witness and asks questions related to the case. This is known as *direct examination* since the attorney is questioning his own witness. Once he has finished, the attorney for the defendant has an opportunity to ask questions of the same witness. This is known as *cross-examination* since the attorney is questioning a witness for the opposite side. Following the cross-examination, the attorney for the plaintiff may ask the same witness further questions to preempt some of the points made by the defense attorney in his examination. This is known as *redirect examination*. The defense attorney has the same option following redirect, known as *recross examination* of a witness. Usually, however, the attorneys will attempt to limit redirect and recross because this may confuse the jurors (and irritate them).

Once the first witness for the plaintiff has completed his testimony, subsequent witnesses are called until the plaintiff has completed presenting its witnesses. The defense then begins to call its witnesses, having first opportunity to question each, with the attorney for the plaintiff conducting the cross-examination. The opportunity for redirect and recross is the same.

A witness who refuses to appear in court may be directed to do so by a *subpoena*. He may also be ordered to bring relevant documents to court by a *subpoena duces tecum*. If the subpoena is disobeyed, the witness may be found in contempt of court just as may be a witness who refuses to testify, unless the Fifth Amendment is pleaded concerning self-incrimination. Again, there may be little surprise since the witness will probably have reviewed with the attorney who is calling him as a witness all points on which he'll

be expected to testify on both direct and cross-examination.

Pharmacists may be called upon to provide expert testimony at trial, i.e., some testimony related to their professional knowledge. The testimony of an *expert witness* is admissible as evidence once the judge rules that the individual is qualified to testify as an expert. If the judge is of the opinion that the witness is more knowledgeable about a topic than the judge or jury, questioning of the witness about his professional credentials, expertise, etc., will then take place.

The expert witness may be asked to explain the day to day procedures in order to establish the standard of practice within his profession and/or specialty. Moreover, the expert witness, because of his qualification may be permitted professional opinions and may be asked for an opinion(s) concerning the procedures in the factual situation undergoing trial.

Once the witnesses for both sides have been presented, each attorney presents a *summation*, attempting to once again outline for the jury what he feels he has established. The attorney for the plaintiff follows the attorney for the defense at this point, having last opportunity for a presentation to the jury.

Motions during Trial

If the plaintiff is dissatisfied with the way his case is developing, he may wish to stop the trial to begin again at a later date. This is known as a *voluntary nonsuit*. The judge also has this option, known as an *involuntary nonsuit*. If the defendant feels that the evidence and testimony of the plaintiff does not entitle the defendant to recover, he may make a motion for *compulsory nonsuit*. If granted by the judge, the case will end. Sometimes, despite the best efforts of the judge to prevent introduction of inflammatory or prejudicial testimony or evidence, such matters will be presented during trial by one of the attorneys or a witness.

One example of this may be the use of an enlarged, full-color photograph of a badly mutilated body. If the judge feels that the matters are so overwhelming that the jury will be unable to ignore them in reaching their decision, he may declare a *mistrial*. The latter may also occur when a juror is guilty of misconduct, e.g., reading a newspaper account of the trial after the jury has been sequestered.

It is customary for attorneys to make *motions for directed verdicts* following completion of evidence at the trial. This is a request to the judge to rule in their favor due to the fact that the case as shown by the opposing side does not support recovery on his part.

During presentation of evidence and testimony, the attorneys may object to certain testimony or evidence which the opposing side is attempting to have introduced for the jury's consideration. The *objections* are based on rules of evidence which have evolved over centuries of Anglo-American legal history. If the judge feels the objection is valid, he rules it *sustained*. If it is invalid, he *overrules* the objection. It is important that objections be raised at the proper moment for if the objection was not made in a timely fashion by the attorney, he forever loses the right to object to the testimony or evidence. This may be crucial if the case is appealed because the appellate court can only consider whether evidence or testimony was proper if an objection was raised at trial.

Instructions to the Jury

Summation by the attorneys is followed by *instruction of the jury* or *charge to the jury* by the judge. The latter presents an overview of the evidence presented at trial as well as an explanation of the applicable law, such as definitions of legal terms, applicable legal rules and principles, etc.

Verdict

After the judge's charge the jury retires to the jury room to deliberate how the evidence relates to the law as explained by the judge. The *verdict* represents the jury's opinion following detailed discussion and analysis of the information presented to them. In a civil case, the jury's decision is based on a *preponderance of the evidence* that is just sufficient to favor one party over the other. This is in contrast to the requirement of proof beyond a reasonable doubt in criminal cases. If the jury cannot reach agreement on a verdict after a stated period of time established by court rules, e.g., several days, a mistrial will be declared and a new trial ordered. However, not all states require unanimous decisions from juries. Some state statutes authorize verdicts by five-sixths of the jury, i.e., ten out of twelve, or majority verdicts.

Motions after the Verdict

Following the jury's report of its verdict, a party may move for a new trial if dissatisfied with the verdict or if the amount of damages appears extravagant. If it is clear that the jury made a mistake, such as awarding an amount of damages that is clearly excessive, or that new evidence is available which could not have been available sooner, the judge will grant the *motion for a new trial*, and another trial will be held before a new jury, and perhaps a new judge. If the jury's verdict is clearly wrong as a matter of law, the judge may enter a judgment contrary to the verdict. This is known as a *judgment non obstante verdicto* (not withstanding the verdict) or *judgment n.o.v.*

Judgment

The judge enters a judgment conforming to the verdict, unless a new trial has been granted, a mistrial declared or motion for *judgment n.o.v.* entered. Generally, the winning party will be awarded "costs" as well as the amount requested for damages. "Costs" include fees for filing papers with the court, witness fees, jury fees, etc. "Costs" do not include attorney's fees nor compensation lost due to participation in the trial or in preparation for trial. The pharmacist should be certain that these expenses are covered by his insurance policies because they can be substantial and the amount awarded as "costs" will represent only a small portion of the actual expense of going to court.

Collecting the Judgment

After a judgment has been entered, the losing party should (and will generally) comply with the order of the court. If there is noncompliance, the winning party may initiate action to recover the amount due. It will require going to court again to obtain a *writ* to direct the sheriff or similar officer to take some official action.

A *writ of execution* is a written order from the judge to the sheriff authorizing him to seize property belonging to the person in debt, sell it, and use the money to pay the judgment. In most states the defendant is permitted an exemption of several hundred dollars and certain articles, such as personal clothing and tools used in his trade.

A *writ of replevin* authorizes the sheriff to seize and return to a person something that is rightfully his. A *writ of garnishment* is an order that funds owed the debtor, e.g., salary, be seized to satisfy the judgment. Most states have a limit on the amount which can be seized pursuant to a writ of garnishment.

Small Claims Court

One forum which pharmacists may use if available in their area is the *small claims court*. This generally features the most informal proceedings and an attorney is often not required. A judge or justice of the peace, rather than a jury, hears the case and usually renders an immediate decision. One limiting factor is the amount of claim which can be brought into this court—in most states $1,000 is the limit. However, this alternative might be useful for the pharmacist attempting to collect past due accounts receivable.

A case in small claims court is initiated by filing papers with the clerk's office. Due to the nature of the court, i.e., people presenting their own claims, the personnel in the clerk's office of this court are accustomed to assisting those filing papers. Such assistance may not be so readily attained in a "standard" court.

Conclusion

Serious contemplation should be given to alternative approaches before a suit is filed for it can involve a great commitment of time and money. An understanding of the working of the courts may assist the pharmacist to evaluate the alternatives.

The American legal system is based on the adversary approach to resolution of problems. Each party presents its case in a manner most favorable to its position to an impartial trier of fact and law upon which a decision is reached. While far from perfect, this system appears to be advantageous for resolving disputes and certainly is superior to trial by ordeal or other methods used in some societies.

WHAT TO EXPECT WHEN A LAWSUIT IS STARTED. II: THE APPEALS PROCESS*

Steven Strauss, Ph.D., R.Ph.

Once a trial is complete and the verdict rendered, a party to the suit may choose an appeal. In civil cases, either side may do so. In criminal cases, usually only the defendant can appeal [1]. The lawyer for the aggrieved (e.g., appellant, loser) party in the trial court may take several important measures to carry out his client's appeal [3]. He must file the motion for new trial if it is a prerequisite to appeal (as it is, for example, where jury misconduct is alleged); he must give notice of appeal within a limited time, usually 30 days, and he must file an appeal on behalf of the client, guaranteeing payment of certain administrative costs of appeal. The amount of the bond varies, e.g., in the federal courts this bond is usually $250, unless the court fixes a different amount [4]. An appeal does not prevent the enforcement of the trial court's judgment pending the appeal. The reason is obvious. An aggrieved party could appeal merely to delay enforcement of the judgment although he has no hope of obtaining a reversal. However, an appellant can prevent enforcement during the appeal by filing a *supersedeas bond*, which is a bond of sufficient dollar amount to guarantee compliance with the judgment if it is affirmed on appeal [2]. In many cases the cost of this bond is an adequate deterrent to frivolous appeals.

There are two primary methods of appellate court review. One is by appeal wherein the aggrieved party in the lower court, assuming his lawyer properly perfects the appeal, has a right to have the higher court consider the claimed errors on their merits. The other is *certiorari*, which is an order to the lower court to transfer the case to the higher court for its consideration of alleged errors made below. Review by *certiorari* is not a *right* of the aggrieved party, but is *discretionary* with the higher court [2]. Whether its discretion is exercised in favor of granting *certiorari* usually turns on the general importance of the issues in the case as well as on the apparent correctness or incorrectness of the decision of the lower court. Whatever the method of review, the attorney for the aggrieved party must do more than just show that error was committed during the trial. The appellate court must be convinced that the error denied the appellant substantial justice in the case, or to put it another way, the attorney must demonstrate that any error which did occur was not harmless. This is a heavy burden to carry, and in most cases the appellate court's judgment affirms the judgment of the lower court, either because there was no error, or because the errors committee were harmless.

*Reprinted with permission from *U.S. Pharmacist* (November/December 1979).

One of the advantages of appellate court review is that instead of having just one judge consider the alleged errors as is normally the case in the trial court, an appellate court consists of three or more judges.

Except for a few instances in which an appeal is taken from a trial court to the next higher trial court and retried totally, the appellate court decides the case on the basis of the record of the trial proceedings. The appeals process is not a new trial. The appellate court does not hear witnesses, nor does it consider new evidence; in short, it does not hold another trial. The record, the recorded history of this trial, may include the testimony at trial taken down by the court reporter and reduced to written form, the documents and things introduced into evidence, transcriptions of other proceedings that occurred during trial, plus the complaint and answer, the jury verdict, the judgment, and the other papers filed with the clerk of the trial court. From all of this comes the record on appeal [5]. The lawyer for the appellant has the responsibility for designating the parts of the record that he wants the court reporter and the clerk to prepare for appeal, and the lawyer for the successful party, e.g., appellee, can request such additional portions of the record as he believes are necessary [6]. (In the Federal system the record on appeal must be filed in the U.S. Court of Appeals within 40 days after notice of appeal is filed unless additional time is granted to the appellant [7].) Many appellate courts require that the records be printed.

The appellant's lawyer must now prepare his appellate court brief, which is a written document that sets forth the reason for the appeal. First, he specifies the errors upon which he relies for a reversal or modification of the lower court's judgment. Then he considers each point or error and cites legal references he depends on to support his contentions. He develops the legal principles that he asserts are established by the cases and other cited authorities, and applies these principles to the issues he has raised as bases for reversal or modification. The attorney's arguments, if accepted by the court, should result in a reversal or modification of the judgment of the trial court. Most courts permit the appellant 30 days after the record is filed, to file his brief. The court rules may also require that the brief be printed (typed), and of course a copy of the brief must be sent to the appellee's lawyer. The appellee's lawyer is entitled to file a reply brief prior to oral argument. His brief presents the countervailing authorities and arguments. In most appellate courts oral argument is granted only if requested by one of the attorneys. In most appellate courts the judges have studied the case prior to the time of oral argument. (An *argument* is intended to establish a position and to induce belief [2].) The time granted for oral argument is rarely more than 30 minutes to each side. Probably the greatest value of oral argument lies in the opportunity for the lawyer to answer questions posed by the various judges. Complete preparation in terms of knowing the record and the applicable law is essential if the lawyer expects to do a creditable job of answering the questions of the judges [8].

The judgment and opinion of the appellate court normally is not rendered for weeks, sometimes months, pursuant to oral argument. The process of decision varies from court to court, but the following items are usually present. After oral argument the appellate judges deliberate in private. The judges may vote on the judgment to be rendered and choose one of their number to write the court's opinion. In some courts a straw vote may be taken at this point, with a final vote only after an opinion has been written and circulated among the judges. If there is disagreement in conference, one of the judges may be selected to write and circulate a dissenting opinion. Often there must be compromise among the judges in order to reach an acceptable solution. Finally, a majority reach agreement on the correct judgment in the case, and usually a majority also agrees as to the opinion explaining the court's decision on each of the issues before it. In a difficult and protracted case this may require a great deal of time, and all the while the judges are also hearing oral arguments in other cases, reading other briefs, studying proposed opinions by other members of the court in this or other cases, and working on other opinions.

When the appellate court decision is announced, a copy of the opinion is sent to each lawyer in the case. The aggrieved party is given a limited time in which to file a motion for rehearing, and the successful party may file a reply if desired. In the overwhelming number of cases the motion for rehearing is overruled, and the appellate court's judgment is now final. In the few cases where the motion is successful the court will write a new opinion, and the same rehearing process is again available to the appellant.

If the first appeal is not to the highest appellate court in the system, and in many states and in the federal system there are intermediate appellate courts, review may not be available by appeal or *certiorari* to the highest appellate court. The Supreme Court of the United States stands at the very pinnacle of review in the federal system and in each state court system on federal question issues. The procedures for review by a second appellate court are less burdensome on the lawyer for the appellant since the record is already in existence. However, the lawyer must make sure that he complies with all of the court's rules pertaining to the filing of appeals, the record, bond or deposit for costs, and briefs. Here again the lawyer for the other party has the burden of making the proper objection if the rules are not being followed.

Eventually, the lawyer for the losing party exhausts all possible avenues for further review of his client's case, and the judgment of an appellate court becomes final. The clerk of that court on request of the lawyer for the successful party issues a mandate, which is an order to the trial court stating that the case has now been finally decided and instructing the trial court as to its future action. Judgment of the trial court may be affirmed, modified, or reversed; or a new trial may be ordered. The opinion of the appellate court gives reasons for the decision made by that court, but the mandate is official order that controlls

the subsequent actions of the trial court. If the mandate orders the entry of a final judgment for one of the parties, the judgment will be entered by the trial court and will then be enforced like any other trial court judgment that has become final.

Settlement of the lawsuit at any time prior to the opinion of the highest court is always a possibility. There is no legal impediment to settlement after the highest court has rendered an opinion, but as a practical matter settlement is usually impossible because one of the parties has now lost all bargaining power. A substantial number of lawsuits are settled while on appeal (out-of-court settlement), and upon notification of this fact the

appellate court dismisses the appeal because there is no longer a case or controversy to be decided; the particular case is *moot* [2].

References

1. U.S. News & World Report. The ABC's of How Your Government Works. May 9, 1977.
2. Gifis SH: *Law Dictionary*. Woodbury, NY, Barron's Educational Series, Inc. 1975.
3. Rules of Appellate Procedure for the Federal Courts #3.
4. Ibid. #7.
5. Ibid. #10.
6. Ibid. #10b.
7. Ibid. #11.
8. Ibid. #28.

GIVING LEGAL REFERENCES A FAIR TRIAL*

Joseph L. Fink III, B.S. Pharm., J.D., R.Ph.

The system of symbols and references used by lawyers to indicate where the law can be found in reference books may appear complex, but it really is not. Pharmacists should not be intimidated by the unique reference format for legal materials. A brief review of this shorthand way of indicating references will make pharmacy law more readable and may make it easier for you to understand some of the references used in this publication.

Statutes enacted by legislatures usually are compiled into reference books and are divided into

---

*Reprinted with permission from *Legal Aspects of Pharmacy Practice* (Feb./March 1983).

"titles" and "sections." For example, the Federal Food, Drug, and Cosmetic Act begins at 21 USC §321. If you wanted to locate this statute, you would look for the United States Code (USC), Title 21, Section 321. In federal statutes, the title number precedes the USC designation and the section number follows ("§" means section and "§§," sections).

Regulations adopted by administrative agencies clarify the meaning of statutes and give the administrative details that help to make the statute work. Proposed federal regulations are published daily in the *Federal Register*. These references are cited by volume number, page, and year, e.g., 48 Fed Reg 28704 (1980).

The *Federal Register* lists regulations both when proposed and when finally adopted. A period for public comment occurs between these two publication dates. The initial notice includes an address to which remarks about the proposed regulation can be sent. Once finalized, regulations appear in the appropriate section of the *Code of Federal Regulations* (*CFR*)—the "official" source of administrative regulations that is revised and issued annually. Citations include title number and section, e.g., 21 CFR §120.201. Of the numerous books comprising the complete *Code of Federal Regulations*, the volume that is particularly relevant to daily pharmacy practice is 21 CFR §§1300 to end, which contains the federal regulations pertaining to controlled substances.

Decisions in court cases usually are referred to by names of the parties involved, separated by a small "v," meaning versus, e.g., *Miller v White*. In a trial court decision, the first name in the case title is the person bringing suit; so here Miller (the plaintiff) is suing White (the defendant). If one of the parties appeals the decision of the trial court, the appellate court decision will carry the name of the person filing the appeal first. Therefore, on appeal, the case could be either *Miller v White* or *White v Miller*.

Sometimes a case designation will change. For example, if a government official is sued in his official capacity, not personally, and he subsequently leaves office, the name of his successor may be

THE FEDERAL AND STATE JUDICIAL SYSTEM.

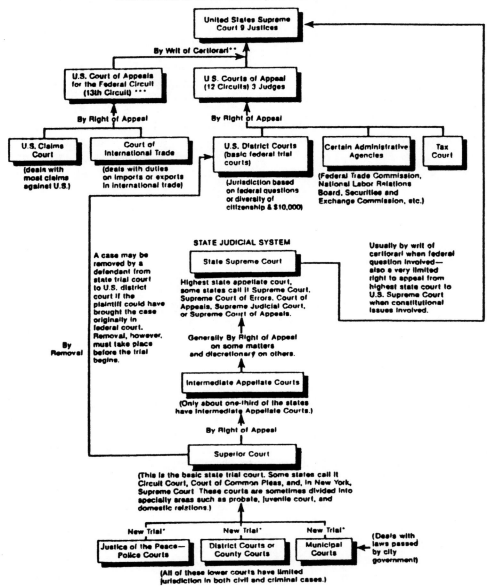

*A number of states do not provide for a new trial with these lower courts, but instead allow appeal by right directly to the appellate courts.

**An appeal to the United States Supreme Court may be taken as a matter of right if any federal court has held a federal statute invalid in a civil action to which the United States is a party or if a federal court of appeals has held a state statute unconstitutional or repugnant to a federal statute or treaty.

***Exclusive nationwide jurisdiction of patent appeals, federal contract appeals, and court of International Trade and Claims Court Appeals.

Reprinted with permission from W. T. Schantz and J. E. Jackson, *The American Legal Environment—Individuals, Business Law and Government*, Second edition. St. Paul, MN: West Publishing Co. (1984).

substituted. Hence, the case could be listed with one name at the trial court level and with a different one when referring to the appeal. For example, a case involving the HEW secretary could be *Smith v Califano* at first and later become *Smith v Schweiker*.

Courts have two types of authority to decide cases: *in personam* jurisdiction over persons, and *in rem* jurisdiction over things. Therefore, case titles do not always include persons' names. For example, if an automobile is used to transport narcotics, the court will have jurisdiction over the car, and a suit might be filed to seize it. This can result in some strange case names: one was known as *1962 Ford Thunderbird v Division of Narcotic Control*.

In a citation to a case decision, the name of the case is followed by an indication of where the decision is located in legal reference books. For example, *US v Sullivan*, 332 US 689 (1948), means that this case can be found in volume 332 of *United States Reports* on page 689. The date of the decision provides immediate identification of its age.

Many sets of reference works contain reports of case decisions. Some report cases from a number of different courts, so additional information is needed to indicate which court decided the case. An example of this is the *Federal Reporter* system, which includes decisions of all twelve US Courts of Appeals. A typical citation in these volumes is 215 F2d 881 (8th Cir 1974). The country is divided into twelve circuits, and the Circuit Court that decided the case is indicated in parentheses, here, the eighth circuit. There also are regional reporters, which publish decisions from state courts. Here, the state is indicated in parentheses, e.g., 212 SE2d 458 (NC 1959). This tells the reader that the case was decided in North Carolina and indexed in "SE2d," the *Southeastern Reporter*, second series. (A second set of volume numbers was begun when the first set was exhausted.)

Legal reference citations are consistent and relatively simple. Understanding them should make your reading about pharmacy law that much easier.

QUESTIONS: CHAPTER 2

1. The litigants involved in a lawsuit are the:
   a. Plaintiff and complainant
   b. Villain and plaintiff
   c. Plaintiff and petitioner
   d. Plaintiff and defendant
   e. Defendant and pleader

2. Which of the following is an appeals court?
   a. Surrogate court
   b. Village court
   c. U.S. District Court
   d. Court of original jurisdiction
   e. U.S. Circuit Court

3. Which of the following does *not* belong?
   a. *United States Reports*
   b. *Supreme Court Reporter*
   c. *United States Law Week*
   d. *Supreme Court Bulletin*
   e. *Federal Reporter 2nd Series*

4. Generally, federal district courts have exclusive jurisdiction over such matters as:
1) Bankruptcy proceedings
2) Cases arising under copyright law
3) Cases arising under patent law
4) Cases involving a fine, penalty, or forfeiture under federal law
5) Violations involving the Federal Food, Drug and Cosmetic Act

   a. 1), 2) and 4) are correct.
   b. 1), 3) and 4) are correct.
   c. 1), 2), 4) and 5) are correct.
   d. 2), 3) and 5) are correct.
   e. 1), 2), 3), 4) and 5) are correct.

5. A detailed statement of the claim that appears in the legal complaint is known as the:

   a. Answer
   b. Demurrer
   c. Laundry list
   d. Bill of particulars
   e. In rem

6. The venue of a legal case is the place where the:

   a. Defendant in the case resides
   b. Appeal in the case is heard
   c. Court may hear the case
   d. Complainant in the case resides
   e. Defendant and the petitioner reside

7. Any law which fixes the time within which parties must take judicial action to enforce their rights is referred to as:

   a. Show cause order
   b. Injunction
   c. Law of time
   d. Statute of limitations
   e. Obiter dictum

8. The initial formal written statement in legal form of the allegations against a pharmacy intern or a pharmacist is known as the:

   a. Answer
   b. Tort
   c. Complaint
   d. Bill of particulars
   e. Demurrer

9. The term that best describes a person who provides testimony (testifies) is:

   a. Fiduciary
   b. Plaintiff
   c. Deponent
   d. Tort-feasor
   e. Ex officio

10. A pharmacist who decides to initiate a civil lawsuit in a court of law must:
   a. Hire and consult an attorney
   b. Draft a complaint and file it with the clerk of the court
   c. File for probate
   d. Request a show cause order
   e. Attempt an out-of-court settlement

11. A registered pharmacist who appears for a hearing before the state board of pharmacy for alleged violations of the state pharmacy act may be referred to as the:
   a. Respondent
   b. Petitioner
   c. Complainant
   d. Fiduciary
   e. Appellee

12. A judicial remedy which requires that a party refrain from conduct that is contrary to law is known as:
   a. Subpoena
   b. Injunction
   c. Prosecution
   d. Incarceration
   e. Arraignment

13. Court procedures are intended to:
   1) Determine facts with the presentation of evidence
   2) Decide which facts apply to the case
   3) Utilize the appropriate law
   4) Formally decide the outcome of a case

   a. 1) and 2) are correct.
   b. 1), 2) and 3) are correct.
   c. 2), 3) and 4) are correct.
   d. 1), 2) and 4) are correct.
   e. 1), 2), 3) and 4) are correct.

14. Which of the following is the court of last resort?
   a. U.S. District Court
   b. U.S. Court of Claims
   c. U.S. Circuit Court
   d. U.S. Court of Appeals
   e. U.S. Supreme Court

15. Which one of the following U.S. courts is not common to the others?
   a. Tax Court
   b. Court of Claims
   c. Customs Court
   d. District Court
   e. Court of Customs & Patent Appeals

16. The right to fair and equal treatment under the law is referred to as:
   a. Procedural law
   b. Adjective law
   c. Civil rights
   d. Equal rights
   e. Due process of law

17. An example of a nominal award granted by a court is:
   a. $5.00
   b. $5,000.00
   c. One week imprisonment
   d. One year imprisonment
   e. a. and c.

18. A written court order which demands that a pharmacist produce certain designated documents or evidence in court, such as prescription records, is referred to as:
   a. Subpoena ad testificandum
   b. Complaint
   c. Summons
   d. Subpoena duces tecum
   e. Injunction

19. The inherent power of a court to hear and decide a case is referred to as:
   a. Venue
   b. Jurisdiction
   c. Due process
   d. Stare decisis
   e. Fair hearing

20. The term that best describes the law dealing with the relationship between private parties is:
   a. Civil law
   b. Public law
   c. Common law
   d. Due process of law
   e. Criminal law

21. Which court has jurisdiction to review, affirm, reverse, or modify the judgment of a lower court?
   a. Contempt of Court
   b. District Court
   c. Surrogate's Court
   d. Appellate Court
   e. Court of original jurisdiction

22. The process of examining witnesses and the revelation of documents pertinent to a law case prior to trial is referred to as:
   a. Demurrer
   b. Discovery
   c. Pretrial conference
   d. Pretrial motions
   e. Adjudication

23. In which one of the following federal courts can an individual citizen or a corporation sue the federal government?

    a. District Court
    b. Supreme Court
    c. Tax Court
    d. Court of Claims
    e. Customs Court

24. The removal of a lawsuit from one particular geographical location to another is known as a *change of*
_____:

    a. Address
    b. Location
    c. Jurisdiction
    d. Venue
    e. Court

25. The person who files a lawsuit is referred to as the:

    a. Villain
    b. Respondent
    c. Deponent
    d. Plaintiff
    e. Persona non grata

26. Which one of the following federal courts is a trial court?

    a. District Court
    b. Circuit Court
    c. Supreme Court
    d. Court of Appeals

27. Which one of the following federal courts is the "lowest" in the federal judicial system?

    a. District Court
    b. Circuit Court
    c. Supreme Court
    d. Court of Appeals

28. How many judges are there in the U.S. Supreme Court?

    a. Three
    b. Five
    c. Seven
    d. Nine

29. The name of the person(s) which appears first in the caption related to a lawsuit is referred to as the:

    a. Defendant
    b. Respondent
    c. Complainant
    d. Fiduciary

30. The person(s) who initiates a lawsuit may be referred to as:

    a. Defendant

    b. Plaintiff

    c. Respondent

    d. Expert witness

31. The person(s) who is party to and responds to a lawsuit may be referred to as:

    a. Plaintiff

    b. Complainant

    c. Petitioner

    d. Respondent

32. The identifying mark assigned by the court clerk to an individual case is known as the:

    a. "Next" number

    b. Assignment code

    c. Docket number

    d. Summons

33. Who nominates and appoints U.S. federal judges?

    a. President of the United States

    b. Vice president of the United States

    c. Justices of the U.S. Supreme Court

    d. The political party in power

34. In a trial by jury, who determines the facts relevant to the case?

    a. Judge

    b. Jury

    c. Prosecution

    d. Defense attorney

CHAPTER 3

The Compendia and the *USP DI*

PRACTICAL USES FOR THE *USP:* A LEGAL PERSPECTIVE*

Joseph Valentino, J.D., R.Ph.

I think it is important for students to understand how the *USP* fits in with the various regulatory schemes and for them to have a perception of the underlying scientific basis for the rules under which they are practicing, perhaps by rote. *USP* has a program in which students, interns, or externs are invited to visit *USP* headquarters, and we provide them with a series of presentations regarding the history and activities of the Convention. Some of you may have participated in one of these visits. It always impresses *USP* staff as to how many misconceptions there are about *USP* and that in many cases the students indicate they haven't been taught how the *USP* relates to the law at all. Or, put another way, how the law relates to the *USP*, since the law came later. Before I get into the regulatory scheme of things, I would just like to point out two different areas in which *USP* is involved which might be helpful to you.

The first of these is drug nomenclature. The *Federal Food, Drug and Cosmetic Act* mandates that a drug label bear an established name. Under Section 502(e), an established name is defined as (*i*) the official name

given by the FDA, or, if none, (*ii*) the name in an official compendium, or if none, (*iii*) the common or usual name. Aside from its compendial role in establishing drug nomenclature, USPC also plays a vital role in the USAN Council (along with the AMA, APhA, and FDA) and publishes *USAN and the USP Dictionary of Drug Names.* FDA has indicated via 21 CFR 299.4 that all who are concerned with the prescription, dispensing, use, sale or manufacture of drugs may, in the absence of designation of an official name by the FDA, rely on the names in this volume as being the established name, under the Federal Act. As an aside, from a legal perspective, I find the USAN Council procedure interesting since it has its own hearing and appeals procedures.

A second activity which *USP* is involved in is the area of Material Safety Data Sheets. In November 1983, the Occupational Safety and Health Administration (OSHA) published a regulation (29 CFR Part 1910) requiring that Material Safety Data Sheets (MSDS) accompany hazardous chemicals used by employees in certain industries. There is a question as to what extent drugs are covered under the regulation. I don't think they are exempt from the MSDS requirements, but my purpose here is not

to talk to you about the OSHA requirement, only to inform you that as part of its chemical reference standard program, *USP* has developed approximately 900 of these material safety sheets. As state and even municipal right-to-know laws are passed, and the pharmacist is sought out as a reliable source of information, this may be a source of unbiased information your students should be aware of.

The *USP/NF* itself incorporates information unrelated to its standards setting role per se which I believe can be helpful in teaching a course of pharmacy law.

1. *USP* has abstracted and "corrected" those parts of the Controlled Substances Act Regulations believed to be of most concern to practitioners and students of pharmacy. We also keep them up-to-date on an annual basis. We have done the same for the Poison Prevention Packaging Act and regulations.

2. We've also abstracted those portions of the Federal Food, Drug and Cosmetic Act relating to human drugs. In this regard, I believe we incorporated the Drug Price Competition Act, even before the government publication did.

3. Along these lines we have also placed in *USP* the Good

*Reprinted with permission from the *American Journal of Pharmaceutical Education* (Spring 1987).

Manufacturing Practice Act regulations of the FDA on the theory that the principles embodied therein would be helpful to practitioners.

If you notice, I have mentioned the *USP/NF*. The two compendia remain separate for legal reasons but were combined in 1980 under the cover in response to the professions' expressed desire for only one book. With the combining, the scope of the two texts was changed. The *USP* contains monographs for active substances and dosage forms. The *National Formulary* contains inactive ingredient monographs. In this regard, *USP's* scope has been expanded to provide standards for "all drugs," not just those of greatest medical merit.

An important point to remember, and which is often confused by students and pharmacists, is that the *USP/NF* are not published in response to any statute. Rather the statutes govern the enforcement agencies and indicate to those bodies what aspects of the *USP/NF* to enforce.

In 1820, when *USP* was founded, the United States was basically a country of immigrants. Physicians, depending upon their background, would prepare drugs under the same name utilizing different ingredients or methods. Preparations of differing compositions with potentially different effects were being dispensed or sold under the same name. To solve the problem, the professions of pharmacy and medicine met in convention to elect scientific experts and authorized them to publish a Pharmacopeia which contained formulations and methods of preparation to which they would adhere in their respective practices. Thus, USPC was designated the professional fact-finding body; it gave definition to the terms used in medical and pharmaceutical practice; it defined the drugs used in their practice. This helps explain why the system is constitutional and changes in *USP* or *NF* can be enforced without changes in the enforcement statute.

The law operates on the facts. The law remains constant. The facts, like a speed limit for automobiles, can change.

A common misconception that I've come across is the belief that a drug has to be labeled *USP* or *NF* to be subject to the standards. Just the opposite is true. Drugs do not have to be labeled with the initials "USP" or "NF" to be subject to their standards. Section 502(e) requires a drug to bear its established name. If a drug bears a *USP* title, or purports to be or represents itself to be the official article it must in fact be the *USP* article, and Section 501(b) of the *FD&C Act* provides that it meet the *USP* standards of strength, quality, purity or state on its label that it's not *USP;* because otherwise, everyone will think it is the *USP* article.

In order to determine if an article complies with the *USP* standard, the *USP* method of analysis must be utilized. The government (federal or state governments under most state food and drug acts) can tell *USP* if the method of analysis is insufficient. If the Committee or Revision fails to improve it within a reasonable time, the FDA or the respective state agency can publish a regulation prescribing an adequate method. Thus, the reason the scheme is constitutional is because the adulteration provision is based on a misbranding concept. A company need not produce the *USP* product, it need only produce a truthfully labeled product which will not mislead anyone. The government agency is not irrevocably bound to the *USP* method; they can be overridden. It's never happened, but it's theoretically possible.

Under the federal law dispensing is at the established name level not the brand name level. To gain the exemption provided by Section 503(b) of the federal law from the full disclosure requirements and other labeling provisions, the pharmacist must dispense the "same" drug called for in the prescription.

Now I realize the "buzz words" of today are therapeutic equiva-

lents and bioequivalents and pharmaceutical equivalents under state pharmacy selection acts. But if the products aren't the same ones called for in the prescription as defined by *USP*, if they aren't "compendial equivalents," this level of "sophistication" isn't reached. The article is misbranded. What do I mean—Digitoxin is not Digoxin; Quinine is not Quinidine; Conjugated Estrogens aren't Esterified Estrogens; Prompt Phenytoin Capsules are different from Extended Phenytoin Capsules; Delayed Release Aspirin Tablets (formerly Enteric Coated Aspirin Tablets) are not Aspirin Tablets. *USP* can differentiate or not depending upon the need. The committee can look at an item with a 10 power or 100 power lens to determine whether or not it should be considered "the same."

USP standards are directed to giving reasonable certainty to transactions involving the drug. A transaction includes not only commercial transactions, but the taking of the drug by patients—the therapeutic transaction. If the different manufactured products of the drug are not equivalent for the purposes of the transactions, *USP* will change the standards to make them equivalent or require different names or differentiation in the labeling. This is directly opposite to the approach fostered by the FDA's "orange book," i.e., everything is inequivalent, unless the government says it's equivalent.

As I mentioned, standards give "reasonable certainty to the transaction"—most pharmacists take this for granted and don't understand the importance *USP* plays in commercial transactions, both nationally from the wholesale-retail level to the bulk production level and even to the international level. For the most part pharmacists don't compound and just aren't concerned anymore with the actual chemical standards applied to their products in their daily practice. All they want is for someone to say the products are "OK" to use, whatever that means.

Three items pharmacists are somewhat more concerned with are packaging, labeling and preservation or storage of drugs. The *USP* packaging requirements are enforceable down to the dispensing levels. What are some of the practical things *USP* has accomplished and is working on relative to packaging, which pharmacists or students should at least know about?

In the early seventies, *USP* became concerned about the efects on drug quality from the container-closures systems brought into being by tamper resistant packaging requirements and provided moisture permeation requirements for multiple unit containers for oral solid dosage forms. This precipitated a change in the entire plastic containers industry and the containers utilized by pharmacists from polystyrene to polypropylene.

Following this, *USP* became concerned with characterizing the moisture permeation of a single-unit and unit-dose containers. *USP* did not establish requirements for these containers because of the state of the industry. Only a nomenclature scheme was established, so that pharmacists could communicate with their suppliers and uniformly judge the characteristics of films they were using and containers they were utilizing for repackaging. Along these lines, here are two recent items which you should be aware of.

1. Scheduled to be published in the Fourth Supplement to *USP* is a chapter on "Patient Med Paks." The chapter provides requirements and guidelines for pharmacists for placing multiple drug dosage forms in customized patient packages. I suggest you review it relative to your state law.
2. *USP* is currently exploring establishment of standards or test procedures for plastic containers for the dispensing of liquids by pharmacists. This is an example where many pharmacists have just accepted without question what has been presented to them by industry.

Labeling

USP labeling requirements are usually directed to the drug's characteristics or to the safety of the user. Unlike packaging requirements, *USP* labeling requirements do not apply to the dispensed drug under Federal law. Enforcement of prescription labeling requirements is dependent upon the particular state statute.

What are some interests from a practical legal perspective here? Since 1976 *USP* has required that dosage forms bear an expiration date. *USP* defined what is meant when an expiration date is expressed only in terms of the month and year. *USP* prohibited pharmacists' dispensing from containers without expiration dates.

What is the pharmacist's responsibility when a drug is repackaged for dispensing? *USP XXI* indicates pharmacists should consider placing a suitable beyond-use date on the label. *USP* indicates that the maximum beyond-use date shall be one year or the expiration date on the manufacturer's container, whichever is less. Is this effected under your state pharmacy statutes?

Aside from its direct enforcement, *USP/NF* help give definition as to what constitutes good pharmacy practices and establish prescribing-dispensing conventions. What is a cool place? Does an elixir contain alcohol or doesn't it? Why can the pharmacist dispense a 60 mg tablet when the prescription calls for 1 grain which is equivalent to 65 mg.?

Riff v. Morgan Pharmacy, Superior Court of Pennsylvania

I'm sure you will be hearing about and discussing this case. I'd like to bring to your attention a major point mentioned in a minor footnote. For those of you not familiar with the facts, this is a case regarding a prescription for Cafergot Suppositories (a Brand of Ergotamine and Caffeine). The physician prescribed the insertion of one suppository every *four hours* for headache. The pharmacist did not warn the patient not to exceed two suppositories per attack nor more than five suppositories in one *week*. The pharmacy also refilled the Rx. The patient received an overdose and suffered damage to a foot due to diminished blood supply. The patient sued the pharmacy, and the physician experts testified that the toxic properties of Cafergot suppositories were well known and that instructions as to proper dosage and warning were listed in the standard reference books which all pharmacists were required by law to maintain.

The footnote to the case indicated the texts the pharmacists were required to have were the *U.S. Pharmacopeia*, the *National Formulary*, and a reference publication such as the *Physician's Desk Reference (PDR)*.

The filling of the prescription in this case occurred in 1979, before the compendia were combined, and thus both *USP* and *NF* were relevant to establishment of the standard of care issue. The *NF* indicated the maximum dosage was 6 mg of Ergotamine. The Dispensing Information in the *USP Supplement* reminded the pharmacist to explain the dosage schedule to the patient. Subsequently, this type of information was removed from *USP/NF* and placed in *USP DI*. The Court also mentioned *PDR*. But *PDR* contains full disclosure information usually much more information than a non-prescribing pharmacist would act upon. The court simply noted that all 3 texts agreed on the dosage. In this instance, failure to provide the information was evidence of negligence. What about the opposite situation where *USP DI* does not contain the side effect or adverse reaction as clinically significant? Could this be a defense for the pharmacist? Approximately 10 states now mandate that pharmacies have on hand the *USP DI*.

There is dictum by the court in the decision that it is for the medical community to determine what degree of vigilance is required, and that they (the professions) are in the best position to balance the interests and prescribe a standard of conduct which is consistent with the best interests of the patient. The Committee of Revision intends that *USP DI* serve that purpose.

You should be aware that the *USP* Board of Trustees has directed staff to put in the *USP DI* all those *USP/NF* standards that specifically apply to the pharmacy at the dispensing level. Because *USP DI* has been designed to serve as the new "convention" between medicine and pharmacy to meet the new, modern need for a biprofessional counseling medium, the Board of Trustees has directed staff to work with Boards of Pharmacy to recognize and/or require *USP DI* and its patient information materials, wherever appropriate. It is hoped that reprinting in *USP DI* all of the drug standards and pharmacy practice requirements in *USP/NF* that are specific to the dispensing situation this will lessen the financial burden on pharmacists.

Any thoughts or suggestions you have along these lines would be welcome.

THE COMPENDIA AND THEIR ROLE IN DRUG REGULATION*

Joseph G. Valentino

The challenge of the eighties for the United States Pharmacopeia may be the challenge of returning to the twenties—the 1820s, that is. Although *USP* is now more sophisticated in its specification terminology than it was 161 years ago and although industry and government have become directly involved in the drug production picture, today's practitioners face the same problems that their 1820 counterparts did. Preparations of differing compositions with potentially different therapeutic effects being sold or dispensed under the same name. The problem then, as now, was a lack of adequate identification. That is, when a pharmacist dispenses a particular brand or dosage form that a physician has prescribed, will it always be therapeutically equivalent to the product originally specified? Different batches of product from the same manufacturer may not be identical, and different brands of the same generic drug may lack uniformity.

PRINCIPLES OF THE PHARMACOPEIA

The preface of that first pharmacopeia in 1820 outlined three functions necessary for solving the main problems of the day: (1) to select those drug substances with the most fully established utility, (2) to form from those substances preparations and compositions that would use their therapeutic powers to best advantage, and (3) to distinguish those substances by convenient and definite names in order to minimize confusion between physicians and apothecaries.

The first function, selection of drug substances, translates today into FDA's safety and efficacy determinations, based on clinical evidence supplied mainly by the pharmaceutical manufacturers.

The second function, the forming of preparations, has evolved into standardization of the dosage forms to ensure predictable therapeutic action. Lacking the scientific expertise to provide chemical tests that would precisely identify a final drug product, the founders of *USP* standardized a drug by specifying its formulation and by outlining procedures for its manufacture. This method of standardization assumed that as long as knowledgeable and competent persons followed directions, they would produce the desired preparation, and the preparation would produce the desired therapeutic effect. On this basis, the products were considered equivalent. We might call this method "standardization by fiat."

This manner of standardization was customary until about 1880, when another method of standardization—end-product testing by measurement of a substance's interaction with a particular environ-

---
*Reprinted with permission from *Pharmaceutical Technology* (April 1981).

ment—gained ascendancy. Such end-product testing could be "absolute," measuring a definite property, or "comparative," evaluating a substance against a reference standard. The environment could be chemical, physical, or biological. The method assumed that identical substances under identical conditions would react in an identical manner. The main problem was to define adequately the substance's environment test in order to distinguish consistently between the article desired and a noncomplying or undesired article, and at the same time, to allow for therapeutically insignificant differences so that every manufacturer would not be required to use the same formulation and the same manufacturing procedure.

The third function, identification of substances by individual names, professed a basic and important principle—distinguishing articles by name to prevent confusion between physicians and pharmacists.

Because no governmental enforcement existed in 1820, physicians and pharmacists obligated themselves as professionals to utilize and to be bound by *USP* determinations. Uniformity was encouraged by the representation theory of the USPC, the implicit officiality of *USP,* and the understanding that utilization of *USP* terminology without further specification meant that the *USP* product was intended. Thus, *USP* developed into a fact-finding body that gave meaning to the identity of drug products, and its pharmacopeia became a dictionary governing the terminology in interprofessional transactions. The current *FD&C Act,* which incorporated the *USP* and *NF,* is based on this concept. For example, Section 501(b) of the *FD&C Act* states that a drug identified in *USP* shall comply with *USP's* standards of strength, quality, and purity. This also explains why a manufacturer can produce a noncompendial item utilizing a compendial name, provided the article is labeled "not *USP*" and provided the extent of difference is in-

dicated on the label. FDA, as a regulatory agency empowered to enforce drug standards, can inform *USP* when its methods of analysis are inadequate, but there is no express provision for overruling *USP* if FDA considers its standards inappropriate.

USES OF THE COMPENDIA

Government Drug Standards

The U.S. government's utilization of drug standards established by a nongovernmental body dates back 133 years, when Congress enacted the *Drugs and Medicines Act of 1848.* This act was directed at imported drugs and was based on the standards of strength and purity established by the *USP* or by the Edinburgh, London, French, or German pharmacopeias and dispensatories.

The definition of adulteration based on *USP* monograph standards was also used in several state statutes in the late 1800s and early 1900s. Thus, when the *Pure Food and Drugs Act* was adopted by Congress in 1906, the expertise of the official-compendia compilers was already generally recognized and accepted. The standards of strength, quality, and purity contained in both the *USP* and the *NF* are made enforceable by the 1906 act, the first overall national drug legislation. The *FD&C Act of 1938* also made compendial labeling and packaging specifications enforceable.

Biologicals

Biologicals, however, were subject to the *Virus, Serum, and Toxin Act of 1902,* a special statute enacted to ensure the safety, purity, and potency of serums and vaccines injected through the skin directly into the circulatory system. These were regarded as needing more rigid standards than drugs administered topically or orally.

Early compendia did not discuss injections, however. In fact, the U.S. Pharmacopeial Convention

(USPC) at that time voted against instructing the Committee of Revision to include serums, even though their use had become extensive during the previous decade. Although the eighth revision of the *USP* recognized serum antidiphthericum, its standard of strength was defined by the U.S. Public Health and Marine Hospital Service's criteria. According to the scheme of biological regulation that is in effect today, both the product and its manufacturer are individually licensed.

Insulin

The insulin amendments to the *FD&C Act* were passed in response to the expiration of the patent on insulin in 1941. The patent had been held by the University of Toronto. Licensing arrangements required that U.S. manufacturers first assay and standardize each batch and then submit a sample to the University of Toronto Insulin Committee. This arrangement was due to end in December 1941, when the patent was to expire.

Fearing a possible flood of imports of substandard insulin and concerned with maintaining the existing quality of insulin, *USP* called a conference of U.S. and Canadian experts on insulin control and standardization. At first, it was proposed that *USP* establish an insulin board, a certification agency to which manufacturers would submit protocols for the potency. Since *USP* had no laboratory facilities of its own, the plan envisioned that *USP* would contract a laboratory to test for the insulin board, which would in turn bill the manufacturer. Only the laboratory in Toronto was in a position to proceed with the necessary testing, however, and the idea of authorizing a Canadian laboratory to approve *USP* products was questioned.

After Dr. H. O. Calvery, chief of FDA's Division of Pharmacology, appeared before the USPC Board of Trustees, the trustees recommended that *USP's* Committee of

Revision be asked to move quickly toward the establishment of insulin standards. In addition, they suggested that protocols be submitted to FDA, which would then test materials and approve their release. Thus, nearly 40 years ago, USPC's Board of Trustees attempted to use *USP's* authority to confer certification authority upon FDA. This method of control was deemed necessary because it was believed that postmarketing methods based on compendial standards, while effective for most medicinal substances, would not give the needed protection to diabetics. That was because the release of an insulin either too weak or too strong might result in many deaths before it could be discovered and banned from the market.

Needless to say, the government did take over certification of insulin, although Section 506(b) of the *FD&C Act* required that government regulations prescribe no standard of identity, strength, quality, or purity different from that in an official compendium. It is clear that FDA's authority resulted from cooperation between the two bodies and probably because *USP* was in the forefront. *USP* has not yet established standards for the newer purified insulins, however, and FDA is seeking to control them not through the public certification procedures that Congress established but through the New Drug Application (NDA) procedures. Thus, one challenge of the eighties is to develop public standards (suitable for certification purposes) for the newer purified insulins.

Antibiotics

To ensure the continued quality of penicillin after termination of special wartime control, certification of antibiotic drugs began in 1945. Because penicillin was administered to extremely ill patients, and the physician had to wait 12 to 18 hours before the effect on the patient became clear, it was important for the drug to be potent and safe. FDA, anticipating increases in

the production of and demand for penicillin, also maintained that it would lack adequate resources to collect and examine representative postmarketing samples to guarantee public safety. Therefore, the safety and potency of penicillin had to be ensured before marketing.

The reasons given for not referring to compendial standards were that (1) the whole standardization program was subject to such wide changes that freezing it in a *USP* monograph was not desirable at that time (the *USP* was published at ten-year intervals then), and (2) *USP* had no facilities for maintaining and distributing the reference-standard material essential for conducting the tests. At the time, FDA assured *USP* that this was a unique instance and that the agency had no intention of substituting government standards for those prescribed by the compendia.

Despite these early assurances, the Kefauver-Harris Amendments of 1962 changed the *FD&C Act* to require that all antibiotics for human use be certified. The amendments further provided that the standards of strength, quality, and purity for certifying antibiotics were to be those prescribed by government regulation rather than those of the official compendia.

Naturally, USPC's Board of Trustees opposed this move, claiming that there was no evidence of any failure in the present system. *USP* pointed out that of the twelve basic antibiotics in the compendia only four were subject to certification and that the record for the other eight antibiotics indicated that the certification procedure was unnecessary and its cost unjustified. *USP* also maintained that the conditions that originally existed to justify penicillin certification no longer existed. Nevertheless, *USP's* views did not prevail. The law was specifically amended to provide that antibiotics would be subject to standards promulgated by the secretary of HEW and not those promulgated by the official compendia.

Section 507 of the act requires the certification of batches of antibiotics, measured against a governmentally established monograph providing tests for strength, quality, and purity. The initial request for certification is functionally equivalent to an NDA. Once a monograph has been established, however, subsequent requests for certification of the drug (either later batches by the same manufacturer or batches made by another manufacturer) are measured against the monograph and need not contain independent data establishing safety or efficacy. The monograph supplies the entire test. Despite being published by FDA in the *Federal Register*, the standards have been criticized as being outdated and inaccessible for continuous scientific criticism and comment. In particular, some say that the standards fail to incorporate newer chemical methods and depend too heavily on microbiological methods.

In response to this criticism, a joint *USP*-FDA committee was formed to revise the standards, expose them to continuous scientific review, and publish them in the *USP*. The idea was that the end-product standards could in time be deleted from the *Code of Federal Regulations (CFR)*, which then would simply make reference to the *USP*. Despite the desirability of this plan for both FDA and *USP* (and probably the industry as well), it was rejected by FDA's general counsel on the grounds that any proposed change would have to be subjected to the *Federal Register* process that allows public comment, even though such opportunity would be afforded through the *USP* process as for all other drugs. Nevertheless, the joint committee intends to seek publication of improved specifications and methods of analysis in both *Pharmacopeial Forum* and *Federal Register*, and eventually in the *USP* and the *CFR*. As part of the program, *USP* assumed sole distribution of antibiotic reference standards substances in 1978.

A second issue has now arisen—the applicability of compendial specifications to decertified antibiotics (those not subject to Section 507 standards). This novel question has not been officially answered by FDA. Although the continuing need for certification as a means of ensuring the quality of many antibiotics has been criticized, the decertification process has been held up; therefore, answering this question has been given low priority by the FDA general counsel. It is my understanding that the reason for the delay is neither scientific nor legal, but bureaucratic. The jobs of more than 100 people within the agency are dependent upon the certification process and the fees obtained therefrom. Even if these people could be given other jobs, new money would have to be found to pay them. Existing budgetary restraints therefore prohibit any large-scale decertification at this time, and the U.S. public must continue to pay for this unnecessary governmental "service."

Another challenge of the eighties for *USP*, then, is to provide improved standards and methods so that FDA may eventually be able to regulate antibiotics in the same way as it does all other drugs.

New Drugs

Substitution, insofar as the *FD&C Act* is concerned, is determined at the established-name level. To gain the exemption from full disclosure on the prescription label, provided by Section 503(b)(2), a pharmacist must dispense the same drug called for in the prescription.

The goal of *USP* is the same today as it was in 1820: to ensure that drug products with the same name are identical and that different products have different names. Supposing that identical articles produced under GMPs will react the same under identical conditions, then it must be assumed that pharmaceutical equivalents are bioequivalents and are, therefore, therapeutic equivalents. If supposed pharmaceutical equivalents are found not to be bioequivalent or therapeutically equivalent, then *USP* would conclude that the articles were insufficiently characterized or distinguished. Thus, there is a standards problem to be solved. For example, two separate monographs covering prompt and extended phenytoin sodium capsules have been introduced into the *USP* in place of the single monograph for phenytoin sodium capsules that previously encompassed all such preparations. This was because tests showed that two types of capsules existed that were not pharmaceutical equivalents.

Aside from adequate labeling, FDA's definition of therapeutic equivalence encompasses three basic elements: pharmaceutical equivalence, bioequivalence, and GMPs. FDA has sought to allow new brands of drug products to be marketed without therapeutic trials if certain bioequivalency requirements are met. Further, FDA has sought to gain control over such new brands through the NDA process, even though the substance in appropriate dosage forms is recognized as safe and effective. FDA maintains that there may be bioequivalency differences that relate to the therapeutic safety and efficacy of the drug.

The NDA procedure, introduced in 1938, was not intended as a horizontal standardization procedure covering different manufacturer's brands of the same drug but was designed to ensure uniformity of a single manufacturer's product. This was accomplished by requiring manufacturers to submit evidence demonstrating that the drug was adequately tested and was safe for the purposes intended. It then required a freezing of the manufacturing procedures to ensure that the marketed product corresponds to the one that had been investigated and approved. This is a form of vertical standardization.

For evidence of this intent to effect only vertical standardization, one need only look at the wording of the statute outlining NDA requirements. First, there is no corresponding adulteration provision for a product that fails to meet the standards contained in its NDA procedure. Second, there is no exemption from compendial requirements (unlike antibiotics).

In 1962, efficacy (in addition to safety) was made a requirement of new drug products, retroactive to 1938. FDA then contracted with the National Research Council of the National Academy of Sciences to review the efficacy of those drugs that were introduced on the market only as "safe" under the new drug procedures from 1938 to 1962. FDA declared that the efficacy conclusions would be applicable to all "identical, related, or similar" drug products and revoked all advisory letters for "me too" products that had been issued over the years. FDA took the position that all reviewed drugs would henceforth remain new drugs, and introduced the Abbreviated New Drug Application (ANDA) concept to allow the marketing of additional brands without subjecting them to full safety and efficacy study.

Consistent with FDA concepts of pharmaceutical equivalency, Section (314)(1)(f) of the *CFR* now requires an ANDA to contain satisfactory information to ensure that the drug dosage form and components will comply with the specifications and tests in *USP*. That is further evidence that the NDA process has been transformed from vertical to horizontal standardization, designed to control different manufacturers' brands of the same drug product.

In order to expand its regulatory control, FDA attempted to distinguish a middle ground between compendial tests (mostly chemical) and full-scale clinical tests designed to demonstrate safety and efficacy. But the distinction was not clear. At first FDA sought to persuade *USP* that its standards were applicable only to in vitro testing. There was, however, adequate evidence that the compendia had in the past provided in vivo testing utilizing animals and, in one instance involving liver preparations, utilizing human subjects. In any event, such a dichotomy would later prove unworkable if FDA itself were to establish in vitro requirements and procedures in lieu of in vivo methods. More recently, FDA's staff has attempted to justify this philosophy by distinguishing *USP* dissolution standards ("only" quality standards) from FDA dissolution standards (intended to ensure "bioequivalency").

In 1973, FDA published a proposed regulation to require bioavailability testing for certain drug products. The agency stated that until recently it was believed that in vitro testing of drug products for potency, content uniformity, disintegration time, and dissolution rate was sufficient to ensure a uniform quality for all formulations of the same drug, and FDA then would require bioavailability testing to be done instead of full clinical trials.

In 1977, FDA published final regulations, modifying them to include bioavailability and bioequivalency requirements. The agency's declared purpose was to ensure that all drugs intended to be used interchangeably and that had known or potential bioequivalence problems would be identified and tested to determine that they were bioequivalent. FDA also maintained that by approving a drug product, it ensures that the product is safe and effective, meeting all applicable standards of identity, strength, quality, and purity. The purpose of the regulations, according to FDA, was to ensure that these *standards* include a bioequivalence requirement.

FDA indicated that, because of recent advances in biopharmaceutics and pharmacokinetics, the standards for certain drug products should be amended to include bioequivalence requirements. This would ensure that drug products intended to be used interchangeably meet the same standards.

Thus, the issue became one of standards. From *USP's* perspective, a logical resolution of the bio-equivalency issue was clear—upgrade the standards in the official compendia. But the issue evidently is no longer one of mere standards setting.

In the *Lannett* case, the issue of whether certain drugs were new drugs, and therefore subject to FDA premarketing clearance, was raised. Lannett argued that considerations of bioavailability and bioequivalence were irrelevant to determining whether its articles were new drugs, while FDA's position was that bioavailability and bioequivalency were applicable to the determination as to general recognition of safety and efficacy.

Now comes a problem for *USP*. To give substance to its position, FDA has attacked *USP's* processes and standards as insufficient to provide continuing assurance of once-proven safety and efficacy. To demonstrate to the courts that new brands of previously marketed drugs should be subjected to the NDA process and FDA's bioequivalency standards, the agency has to claim that *USP* standards defining articles bearing the same official name do not ensure uniformity of transaction. FDA must also maintain that drugs that meet its specifications published in the *Federal Register* will be equivalent despite the fact that those requirements may be the same as would appear in the compendia.

The controversies surrounding the *Lannett, Premo,* and *Pharmadyne* cases seem based not on the scientific potential of *USP* standards to ensure the equivalency of marketed products but on FDA's desire to gain control of as many drugs as possible through NDA procedures.

What are the advantages of subjecting a new brand of drug to the NDA procedure when the basic substance in a comparable dosage form has been found safe and effective? What can FDA do under the NDA procedure that it couldn't accomplish otherwise?

1. FDA can require the submission of adverse-reaction reports. However, in this instance we are concerned with drugs in which at least one brand has been on the market for a number of years. It is unlikely, then, that new information will be obtained from this procedure.

2. FDA can require manufacturers to submit paper work in a uniform manner, thus avoiding the need to ferret out certain information through inspections.

3. FDA can increase its power over pharmaceutical manufacturers. A firm for which drug approval can be withheld is more likely to comply with FDA requests promptly, regardless of the firm's reservations about their scientific necessity or validity. The manufacturer usually finds it cheaper to comply with such requests rather than delay marketing a drug for further discussions.

4. Requiring a test under NDA procedures allows FDA to avoid the need to justify it to *USP's* Committee of Revision.

Over the years, FDA seems to have experienced an internal ambivalence. One faction within the agency attempts to degrade the compendial standards in order to provide their own dissolution specifications (in the name of bioequivalency) in order to gain regulatory control. A second faction recognizes that dissolution specifications are basically akin to the quality standards traditionally established by *USP.*

Undoubtedly, there are those who privately believe that the compendia should not establish dissolution specifications for the articles contained in them. If "pharmaceutical equivalence" were adequate to ensure bioequivalency and therefore therapeutic equivalence, wouldn't this weaken FDA's reason for establishing new drug bioequivalency requirements? Furthermore, on a practical basis, would a court of law uphold an FDA requirement involving dissolution specifications if *USP* provided a different standard?

Clearly, dissolution testing remains a problem area between FDA and *USP,* while much of the industry acts as an interested bystander, although less than eager to provide data to either body for establishing dissolution standards. Consequently, an additional challenge of the eighties is to divorce the desires of the government for greater regulatory control from the standards-setting role of *USP/NF*.

CMED PROGRAM

In 1974, the Congress' Office of Technology Assessment issued its report on drug bioequivalence, which seems to reflect a basic misunderstanding of the role of compendial tests in ensuring the quality of products. The report criticized *USP* for matters that were properly within the province of FDA's control of GMPs. For example, *USP* was criticized for having a disintegration test that took 30 minutes to run—a period long enough, it claimed, for the manufacture of hundreds of thousands of tablets! In addition, *USP* was criticized for failing to have adequate statistical sampling procedures, when in fact the compendia had never professed to publish a sampling procedure for batch release purposes.

FDA, it appears, recognized the important role of the compendia and the tremendous resources it would take to replace them, as well as the unfairness of the report. Responding to the political pressures of the time, the agency decided that the better course of action would be to work with the newly combined compendia to "improve" their standards and methods. This eventually led to the formation of the Compendial Liaison Staff by the Bureau of Drugs.

At the same time, there were many other pressures on FDA to ensure the quality and interchangeability of multisource drug products. Among them were the repeal of the antisubstitution statutes, the increasing amount of dollars paid for drugs under Medicare and Medicaid, the Maximum Allowable Cost (MAC) program, and the government-wide purchasing programs.

For many drugs on the market there were no NDAs or bioequivalency requirements readily forthcoming. With older NDA's, the specifications and methods may have become outdated because they were never subjected to continuous open, scientific review. Finally, different NDAs for the same drug contained varying specifications and methods since different NDA reviewers looked at specific manufacturer's formulations and in some instances probably ignored compendial requirements. Justifying these actions at the time by silently deciding *USP* standards and methods were minimal or inadequate, these reviewers gave precedence to NDA methods. And who was there to object? After it was decided to continue using the compendia, however, it was necessary to rely on compendial standards. To declare that, overall such standards were inadequate would jeopardize these programs. Furthermore, FDA might have been criticized for having allowed this situation to develop, especially since the agency had been charged by law with responsibility for cooperating with the official compendia, and, to our knowledge, there was no repeal of Section 501(b) with respect to the new drug process.

In January 1979, FDA publicly declared that significant improvements had been made in the compendia since 1974, and except for identified problems of bioequivalence, the agency stated that it was unaware of any therapeutically significant differences existing among compendial drugs. The year before, FDA had launched its Compendial Monographs Evaluation and Development (CMED) program to develop proposed monographs for *USP* where none existed, to evaluate existing compendial monographs, and, where necessary, to develop or improve analytical testing methods to ensure they were suitable "for regulatory use." Still another challenge of the eighties, then, is to undo the damage caused by the Office of Technology Assessment report and by a period of FDA aloofness, while restoring compendial standards to their proper perspective within and without FDA.

INDEPENDENCE OF THE COMPENDIA

If the purpose of standardization is to give reasonable certainty to a transaction involving the product, then FDA's activities may be having exactly the opposite effect. By indicating that it can ensure therapeutic equivalence only for those drugs over which it has NDA-approval authority, FDA may have created unnecessary suspicion and confusion among health professionals concerning those items not subject to the NDA process. If not, how can one explain the cry from professionals for the requirement that labels bear an approved NDA number as if this would be a panacea, even though little public information is available about the specifications contained in an NDA?

The challenge of the 1980s, then, is the challenge of the 1820s, if drug products are to be deemed equivalent while public and professional confidence is restored.

The lessons of history seem to demonstrate that if we are to maintain the nongovernmental compendial system, which has worked so effectively, then it must remain strong and independent and be in the forefront of new developments. The government seems always ready to fill an apparent vacuum. If the compendia are to be free of the bureaucratic, political, or commercial winds blowing at a given time, they must continue to be capable of devising standards and specifications independently.

USP-NF

The major tools at the disposal of practicing pharmacists and physicians are nationally established and recognized standards embodied in a set of books developed and produced by a nongovernmental organization, the United States Pharmacopeial Convention, Inc. (USPC). The USPC is voluntarily supported by the professions of pharmacy and medicine.

Since the Food and Drugs Act of 1906, the federal government has been empowered to enforce the standards of the *United States Pharmacopeia (USP)* and the *National Formulary (NF)*. Pursuant to the terms of the Federal Food, Drug, and Cosmetic Act of 1938 (the Act), the Food and Drug Administration (FDA) enforces the standards established in the *USP* and the *NF* by the *USP* Committee of Revision. Neither the American Pharmaceutical Association (APhA), the former owner of the *NF*, nor the USPC, which now owns both books, is mentioned in the Act, only the books themselves.

Not everything in the *USP-NF* is enforceable under the Act, only the standards of strength, quality, purity, packaging, labeling, and where applicable, bioavailability. In addition to drugs, the *USP-NF* also provides standards for devices, diagnostics, and nutritional supplements.

The main volume of the *USP-NF* is published every five years. The current revision (edition), *USP 24/NF 19* is official from January 1, 2000 for the next five years, until December 31, 2004.

Proposals for revisions are published bimonthly in *Pharmaceutical Forum (PF)*.

In setting standards, the elected members of the *USP* Committee of Revision make the decisions to revise or not revise, to add to or to delete from the *USP-NF*. Decisions by the Committee do not have to be pre-approved by the FDA before they are enforceable. The Committee makes its decisions in revising the *USP/NF* standards and the law authorizes FDA to enforce the law based on those standards.

USP-NF Supplements are published twice a year, and contain all the approved changes to the *USP-NF*.

An article is recognized as "official" when a monograph for the article is published in the *USP-NF*, including its supplements, addenda, or interim revisions, and an official date is generally or specifically assigned to it.

USP-NF provides:

- Legally recognized standards for drugs and excipients
- Specifications for packaging, labeling, and storage
- Tests and assays for strength, quality, purity, and identity, as well as specifications for reagents, indicators, and solutions
- Standards for medical devices, diagnostics, botanicals used as dietary supplements, and vitamins and minerals
- An article may appear in the *USP* if it has an FDA-approved or *USP DI*–accepted use. A product with no FDA-approved or *USP DI*–accepted use may be included in the *NF* if the product has been used extensively without a significant safety risk.

USP DI

The first edition of the *USP DI* was published as one book in 1980; it has been published every year since then. The current *USP DI* consists of three volumes.

USP DI is continuously reviewed and revised and is intended for use by prescribers, dispensers, and consumers of medications. The information is developed by the consensus of the USP Committee of Revision and its Advisory Panels and anyone, including users of medicines, may contribute through review and comment on drafts of the monographs when they are published for comment in the *USP DI Review*.

for the Health Care Professional, contains:

- Medically accepted uses covering both labeled (FDA approved) and unlabeled indications. (Unlabeled uses are included when consensus indicates such use to be current practice.)
- A general index including established names, categories of use, cross-references by brand names, and older nonproprietary names.
- An indication index for quick access to drugs used in treatment, prevention, or diagnosis of specific disease.
- Primary and secondary Veterans Administration drug classification designations.
- Information for both United States and Canadian medicines by categories:
  - Indications
  - Pharmacology
  - Precautions, contraindications, drug interactions
  - Side/adverse effects
  - Patient consultation
  - Dosing information
  - Dosage forms

Volume II, titled *Advice for the Patient—Drug Information in Lay Language,* contains:

- General information about using medicines properly.
- Discussions of commonly and not-so-commonly used medicines.
- Information relating to categories listed in Volume I in lay language.

Volume III, titled *Approved Drug Products and Legal Requirements,* contains:

- The contents of *Approved Drug Products with Therapeutic Equivalence Evaluations* (the "Orange Book")
- *USP/NF* dispensing requirements for labeling, packaging, storage, and quality
- Federal Food, Drug, and Cosmetic Act provisions relating to drugs for human use
- Portions of:
  - Federal Controlled Substances Act and regulations
  - Poison Prevention Packaging Act and regulations
  - Current Good Manufacturing Practice (GMP) regulations

USP DESIGNATION

Questions have been received through the *USP* Drug Product Problem Reporting Program (DPPR) asking the difference between a product that bears the "USP" designation on its label and a product that does not. Pharmacists wonder whether the presence or absence of the "USP" designation is any indication of differing product quality.

The *United States Pharmacopeia (USP)* sets the public standards for the strength, quality, purity, packaging, and labeling, and where applicable, bioavailability of drug products available in the United States. If a *USP* monograph exists for a drug product, the drug product is subject to the *USP* standards set for it. This is required by the Federal Food Drug and Cosmetic (FD&C) Act and by various state laws as well. This is true whether or not the article bears the initials "USP" on the label.

When a product label bears the "USP" designation, it simply is an express representation that a product meets *USP* standards. In addition to *USP* standards, the specifications contained in the NDA/ANDA for a drug product (private standards) also apply. If a drug product differs from existing *USP* standards of strength, quality, or purity, the product label must state "Not *USP*" and plainly state its difference from the official product.

For drug products where no monograph exists the *USP* or its *Supplements,* the product must only meet the criteria set forth in its NDA/ANDA. "Old drugs" that are not in the *USP,* and do not have an NDA/ANDA, need only meet their labeled criteria. For example, if a product is labeled as "Sterile Nose Drops" the product *must* be sterile.

It is also worth noting that some official dosage forms are not regulated as drug products, e.g., certain official vitamin/mineral products are regulated as foods. Therefore, *USP* standards may be enforced differently by the Food and Drug Administration (FDA). However, any product that bears "USP" on its label, whether regulated by the FDA as a food, drug, or even a medical device or cosmetic, must meet *USP* standards.

The standards set forth in the *USP* are applicable not only at the time of manufacture, but throughout the product's shelf-life. Patients have the right to expect that the medication dispensed to them complies with applicable legal requirements. In selecting drug products, pharmacists are urged to check the *USP* and its *Supplements* or the *USP DI* to see if a monograph exists. If so, all products in the marketplace bearing the same generic name as the monograph should meet the requirements set forth therein. If there is ever any question about whether a particular drug product meets pharmacopeial standards, USP recommends that pharmacists obtain assurance from the manufacturer that its product does, in fact, meet compendial standards.

QUESTIONS: CHAPTER 3

1. The task of selecting appropriate nonproprietary names for newly discovered chemical agents (drugs) rests primarily with:

    a. FDA-USP/NF

    b. *USP-NF*

    c. USP-NF Revision Committee

    d. USAN Council

    e. U.S. Pharmacopoeial Convention, Inc.

2. The standards set forth in the *USP-NF* are enforced by the:

    a. *USP-NF*

    b. USP Committee of Revision

    c. FDA and *USP-NF*

    d. FDA

    e. United States Pharmacopeial Convention, Inc.

3. The *USP-NF* are designated as official compendia under federal and state statutes and contain enforceable drug standards and specifications for:

    a. Strength, quality, purity, storage

    b. Strength, quality, purity, packaging, labeling, bioavailability

    c. Strength, quality, purity, packaging, labeling, storage, bioavailability

    d. Strength, quality, packaging, labeling

    e. Strength, quality, purity, packaging, labeling, patient information

4. The latest edition of *USP-NF* is:

    a. 23/18

    b. 24/19

    c. 22/26

    d. 22/17

    e. 25/26

5. Standards in the *USP* and *NF* are established by the:

    a. Commissioner of FDA

    b. Secretary of HHS

    c. American Pharmaceutical Association

    d. Employees of the USPC

    e. USP Committee of Revision

6. The federal government has been empowered to enforce the standards in the *USP* and *NF* since:

    a. 1820

    b. 1906

    c. 1938

    d. 1951

    e. 1962

7. Before they are enforceable, revisions in *USP-NF* standards must be approved by:

    a. The U.S. government

    b. The commissioner of FDA

    c. The USP Committee of Revision

    d. A congressional USP watchdog committee

    e. The Secretary of DHSS

8. The United States Pharmacopeial Convention's printed vehicle for generating public review of and comments on text being proposed for inclusion in the *USP DI* is:

    a. *USP DI Supplements*

    b. *USP DI Review*

    c. *USP DI Update*

    d. *USP DI Public Commentary Notice*

    e. *USP DI Pharmaceutical Forum*

9. Which of the following is false regarding the *USP* and *NF*?

    a. They affect pharmacists by way of state and federal laws covering adulteration and misbranding.

    b. They primarily safeguard and benefit the profession of pharmacy.

    c. They affect pharmacists by way of state laws governing pharmacy practice.

    d. They are produced by an organization that cannot make manufacturers obey its standards.

    e. They must be purchased by pharmacies, not pharmacists.

10. According to the USP, when a drug is repackaged for dispensing by the pharmacist, the maximum beyond-use date placed on the label shall be:

    a. The first date of the month following the dispensing

    b. The last day of the month following the dispensing

    c. One year from the date of dispensing

    d. The expiration date on the manufacturer's label

    e. One year from the date of dispensing *or* the expiration date on the manufacturer's label, whichever occurs first

11. The *USP* and *NF* received legal recognition by the U.S. government with the enactment of the:

    a. Pure Food and Drugs Act of 1906

    b. Food, Drug, and Cosmetic Act of 1938

    c. Drugs and Medicines Act of 1848

    d. Durham-Humphrey Amendments to the FDCA in 1951

    e. Kefauver-Harris Amendments to the FDCA in 1962

12. Proposals to revise or add to or to delete items from *USP-NF* are published in the bimonthly:

    a. *USP-NF Supplements*

    b. *USP Public Commentary Notice*

    c. *Pharmacopoeial Forum*

    d. *USP-NF Proposed Revisions and Comments*

    e. *USP-NF Review*

13. The main volume of the *USP-NF* is published every:

    a. Year
    b. Two years
    c. Three years
    d. Four years
    e. Five years

14. The *USP-NF* are published and marketed by the:

    a. U.S. Food and Drug Administration
    b. U.S. Government Printing Office
    c. U.S. Pharmacopeial Convention, Inc.
    d. Drug Compendia Association, Inc.
    e. USP-NF Publications Company, Ltd.

15. *USP-NF Supplements* are issued:

    a. Every year
    b. Biennially
    c. Semi-annually
    d. Every month
    e. Bimonthly

16. Which of the following is the printed vehicle through which the *USP DI* is revised and kept current?

    a. *USP DI Supplements*
    b. *USP DI Review*
    c. *USP DI Update*
    d. *UDP DI Pharmacy Forum*
    e. *USP DI Leaflets*

17. The first edition of the *USP DI* was published in:

    a. 1960
    b. 1962
    c. 1970
    d. 1975
    e. 1980

18. How many volumes comprise the *USP DI*?

    a. 2
    b. 3
    c. 4
    d. 5
    e. 6

19. What is the latest edition of the *USP DI*?

    a. Eighteenth
    b. Nineteenth
    c. Twentieth
    d. Twenty-first
    e. Twenty-third

20. The *USP DI* is published:

    a. Once a year

    b. Biennially

    c. Every two years

    d. Whenever necessary

    e. Every five years

21. What is the title of Volume I of the *USP DI*?

    a. *Approved Drug Products and Legal Requirements*

    b. *Advice for the Patient—Drug Information in Lay Language*

    c. *Drug Information for the Health Care Professional*

    d. *Encyclopedia of Medical Terms for the Pharmacist*

    e. *Drug Information for the Health Care Practitioner*

22. What is the title of Volume II of the *USP DI*?

    a. *The Pharmacist's Answer Book*

    b. *Approved Drug Products and Legal Requirements*

    c. *Drug Information for the Health Care Professional*

    d. *Advice for the Patient—Drug Information in Lay Language*

    e. *Drug Information for the Health Practitioner*

23. What is the title of Volume III of the *USP DI*?

    a. *Drug Information for the Health Care Practitioner*

    b. *The Pharmacist's Answer Book*

    c. *Legal Requirements for Dispensing Prescription Drugs*

    d. *Drug Information for the Patient*

    e. *Approved Drug Products and Legal Requirements*

24. Which of the following are legally recognized by the Federal Food, Drug, and Cosmetic Act?

    1) *United States Pharmacopeia*

    2) *National Formulary*

    3) *Homeopathic Pharmacopeia of the United States*

    4) *United States Pharmacopeia Drug Information*

    5) *USP DI*

    a. 1), 2), 3) and 5)

    b. 1) and 2)

    c. 1), 2) and 3)

    d. 1), 2) and 4)

    e. 1), 3) and 5)

25. *The National Formulary* contains monographs for:

    a. Active substances

    b. Excipients

    c. Patient information

    d. FDA approved drug products

CHAPTER 4

The Controlled Substances Act

HOW TO VERIFY A DEA REGISTRATION NUMBER*

Have you ever been suspicious of a Drug Enforcement Administration registration number and wish you had a way of checking it? There is a way to do just that according to information supplied by DEA.

The DEA registration numbers are unique, nine-character numbers consisting of two alphabet characters followed by 7 digits. The number is a great deal more than a randomly assigned serial number, however.

The first position is either a "B" or an "R" the former designating a dispenser of controlled substances, the latter referring to a registrant engaged in distribution. The second position is derived from the first letter of the registrant's last name, or if a registrant business name starts with numbers (as in 38th Street Pharmacy), the digit "3" appears.

---

*Reprinted from Drug Enforcement Administration literature.

The third to eighth positions are a six-digit, computer-generated number for each "B" or "R" group, unique to a particular registrant.

The ninth position—and a key in verification—is a computer-calculated check digit.

This right-most digit is automatically generated as the result of the summing of odd-numbered digits (1st, 3rd and 5th), and then adding to that sum the sum of the even-numbered digits (2nd, 4th and 6th) multiplied by 2. When the two numbers are added together, the right-most digit in the result should correspond with the check digit. For example, in the case of a fictitious DEA registration number, BC235614n:

1. Add 1st, 3rd, 5th digits $(1 + 3 + 5 = 9)$.

2. Add 2nd, 4th, 6th digits $(2 + 4 + 6 = 12)$, and multiply by 2 $(12 \times 2 = 24)$.

3. Add the two results $(9 + 24 = 33)$; the right-most digit, 3, becomes the check digit.

Therefore, in this case the complete DEA registration number would be BC 1234563.

While the check digit verification is not 100% foolproof, DEA points out, it does assure greater accuracy and helps to detect transpositions of invalid numbers. Numbers failing the test should be further verified by the pharmacist.

For example:

Take DEA NUMBER
1234563
$1 + 3 + 5 \ = \ 9$
$2 + 4 + 6 \times 2 \ = \ 24$
TOTAL $=$ 33

FIGURE 1. The last digit in the total is "3," which corresponds to the last digit in the DEA number 1234563.

MID-LEVEL PRACTITIONER CATEGORY*

The Drug Enforcement Administration (DEA) has released its final rule amending Title 21, *Code of Federal Regulations (CFR)*, Parts 1301 and 1304, regarding the definition and the registration of a new category of DEA registrants, entitled "mid-level practitioners (MLPs)," who are permitted to dispense controlled substances by the state in which they practice.

The final rule, which was published in the June 1, 1993 *Federal Register*, defines a "mid-level practitioner" as

an individual practitioner [as defined in §[1304.02(d)], other than a physician, veterinarian, or podiatrist, who is licensed, registered, or otherwise permitted by the United States or the jurisdiction in which he/she practices, to dispense [federal definition] a controlled substance in the course of professional practice.

The registration requirement applies to

. . . any person who administers, prescribes, or dispenses directly, i.e., affects the physical delivery of a controlled substance to the ultimate user or its agent . . . unless exempted by law or pursuant to Title 21, Code of Federal Regulations (CFR), § 1301.24#1301.29 . . .

Some examples of mid-level practitioners cited by the DEA are nurse practitioners, nurse midwives, nurse anesthetists, clinical nurse specialists, and physician assistants. Because there are wide variations between states regarding the prescribing authority of various MLPs, the newly established category serves to eliminate any questions regarding the practitioner's medical practice or activities, and whether or not the individual is allowed to handle controlled substances by the state in which he or she practices.

According to the DEA, this category was created because the Agency felt it was important to alert the appropriate individuals who have the responsibility for verifying authorization to dispense controlled substances that there may be a restriction on the authority of the individual whose application they are reviewing.

In order to separate the registrations of mid-level and traditional practitioners, the DEA added a new type of DEA number. Registration numbers issued to MLPs will now begin with the letter "M," while DEA numbers issued to traditional registrants will continue to begin with the letters "A" or "B." The "M" alerts pharmacists and wholesalers of the need to verify that the state authorizes these registrants to engage in specific controlled substance transactions.

A provision has also been included that requires MLPs to maintain documents required by the state in which the individual is practicing and that describe the conditions and extent of that individual's authority to dispense controlled substances. The documents should be kept readily available for inspection and copying by DEA authorities. Examples of such documentation are practice agreements, practice guidelines, and protocols.

An explanation of the conditions under which MLPs may conduct research as a coincident activity to their registration is included in 21 CFR, Part 1301. This rule states that,

A person registered to dispense controlled substances in Schedules II through V shall be authorized to conduct research and to conduct instructional activities with those substances, except that a mid-level practitioner, as defined in § 1304.02(f), may conduct research

coincident to his/her practitioner registration only to the extent expressly authorized by state statute.

The section also clarifies the exemption of MLPs in institutions and agents or employees of registered practitioners from the registration requirements. Generally, a mid-level practitioner may dispense, administer, and prescribe controlled substances under the registration of the hospital or institution where the MLP is employed without an individual registration to do so. This provision also applies to interns, residents, foreign-trained physicians, physicians on staff at a Veteran Administration facility, and physicians who are agents or employees of the Health Bureau of the Canal Zone government.

A related section of the rule addresses individual practitioners who are agents or employees of another practitioner registered to dispense controlled substances. When acting in the usual course of the individual practitioner's employment, such mid-level practitioners may administer and dispense controlled substances under the registration of the employer or principal practitioner if the individual MLP is authorized or permitted to do so by the jurisdiction in which he or she practices.

A major area of concern was the definition of the term "dispense." The DEA clarified that the federal definition of the term "dispense," as specified in the Controlled Substances Act, applies in this ruling. The question of whether an individual who administers but does not prescribe controlled substances is considered to be "dispensing" was also addressed. According to the DEA, dispensing includes the acts of administering and prescribing controlled substances, either as individual or combined acts.

Another area addressed was the

*Reprinted with permission from *National Pharmacy Compliance News* (November 1993).

granting of controlled substance privileges to mid-level practitioners by providing them with a DEA registration number. The commentors held that MLPs do not have the education and experience to properly dispense controlled substances, that registering MLPs will overburden state regulatory forces, and that by issuing registration numbers to MLPs, the DEA is condoning the expanding privileges of MLPs in prescribing controlled substances.

In response, the DEA reiterated that the requirement for a registration issued to an individual whom the state has approved to handle controlled substances has already been established under federal legislation. Registration of MLPs by the DEA occurs after the state has made its determination regarding prescribing authority. The state is also given the authority to set standards for medical practice, such as educational standards.

TRANSMISSION OF PRESCRIPTIONS FOR CONTROLLED SUBSTANCES BY FACSIMILE

The Drug Enforcement Administration (DEA) has issued a rule that allows controlled substance prescription orders to be transmitted from a prescriber to a dispensing pharmacy by facsimile. This rule will facilitate delivery of prescription orders in situations where medication needs change quickly and prescribers' orders must be communicated rapidly.

The rule, published in the May 19, 1994 *Federal Register*, specifies that *faxed prescription orders must contain all information required on written prescription orders except the prescriber's signature*. It "requires that the *original written prescription be presented and verified against the facsimile when the prescription is dispensed*, and that the original document be properly annotated and retained for filling."

The rule places additional responsibilities on the pharmacist to ensure the authenticity of a facsimile and prevent forgeries. The pharmacist must check that each faxed prescription order has been issued for a legitimate medical purpose by a practitioner acting in the usual course of professional practice. To prevent diversion of controlled substances through forgeries, DEA suggests that pharmacies maintain a file of practitioners' FAX numbers, verify the originating FAX number when a prescription order is received, and phone the practitioner's office to double-check that the prescription order was both written and transmitted from there.

The DEA specified *two exceptions* to the revised rule:

Currently a pharmacist may dispense Schedule II drugs only pursuant to a written prescription that has been signed by the prescriber. Orally transmitted prescriptions for Schedule II drugs are allowed only in emergency situations subject to certain specific limitations. The transmission of a Schedule II prescription from the prescriber to the pharmacy is now allowed, but DEA requires that the original written prescription be presented and verified against the facsimile at the time the substances are actually dispensed and that the original document be properly annotated and retained for filing.

21 CFR 1306.11(a)

The regulations allow two exceptions to the requirements for Schedule II prescriptions. The *first* of these applies to pharmacies providing home infusion/intravenous pain therapy, where it is not necessary for the original prescription to be delivered to the pharmacy either prior to or subsequent to the delivery of the medication to the patient's home. The facsimile of the prescription is treated as the original document by the home infusion pharmacy and must contain all information required by 21 CFR 1306.05(a), including the date issued; full name and address of the patient; and the name, address, and DEA registration number and signature of the prescribing practitioner, as well as any state labeling requirements. *This exception is not extended to oral dosage forms.*

21 CFR 1306.11(e)

Fax Prescription to Pharmacy

Schedule II
- OK to transmit.
- Original Rx must be presented to the pharmacist prior to dispensing

Schedule III–IV–V
- OK to transmit.
- Original Rx does not have to be presented to the pharmacist prior to dispensing; fax copy can serve as the original.

Note: States may have regulations more stringent than those of the DEA, and the above may not apply.

Fax—Schedule II

When is a facsimile (fax) prescription acceptable as an original written prescription?

(1)   When compounded for the direct administration to a patient by parenteral, intravenous, intramuscular, subcutaneous or intraspinal infusion.   21 CFR 1306.11(e)

(2)   When written for a resident of a Long Term Care Facility (LTCF).   21 CFR 1306.11(f)

(3)   When written for a patient residing in a hospice certified by Medicare under Title XVIII or licensed by the state. The prescription must indicate that the patient is a hospice patient. (Note: A hospice patient may reside in his/her residence or a long-term care facility; *reside* is not intended to be "venue specific".)   21 CFR 1306.11(g)

The *second* exemption applies to Schedule II prescriptions written for patients in long-term care facilities, which are filled and delivered to the facility by a consulting pharmacy. As in the case of the home infusion pharmacists' exemption, these facsimiles would be treated as original documents (original written prescriptions).

21 CFR 1306.11(f)

The facsimile of a prescription for a Schedule II narcotic substance written for a patient residing in a hospice certified by Medicare under Title XVIII or licensed by the state may serve as the original prescription. The practitioner or the practitioner's agent will note on the prescription that the patient is a hospice patient.   21 CFR 1306.11(g)

In allowing these exemptions, DEA's intent is to facilitate the prescription communication process in both the home infusion and long-term care environments where patients' medication needs can change rapidly. Implementation of these proposed exemptions would eliminate the need to treat such long-term care and home infusion prescriptions as "emergency prescriptions," which, as defined by 21 CFR 1306.11(d), are limited as to the quantity that may be dispensed. Under current regulations, pharmacists are responsible for ensuring that controlled substance prescriptions "have been issued for a legitimate medical purpose by an individual practitioner acting in the usual course of his professional practice."

Some measures to be considered in authenticating prescriptions received by facsimile equipment would include maintenance of a physician's facsimile number reference file, verification of the telephone number of the originating facsimile equipment; and/or telephone verification with the physician's office that the prescription was both written and transmitted by the prescribing practitioner. Although such measures parallel efforts currently employed in verifying the authenticity of prescriptions transmitted by traditional means, the requirement of this proposal places an additional responsibility on the pharmacist to take efforts to ensure that the facsimile has been initiated by the prescriber.

Practitioners should be aware, however, that where an individual state's law or regulations are more stringent than the federal requirements, the state requirements would apply.

Facilitating the transmission of prescription orders will substantially eliminate the need for "emergency prescriptions," which limit prescribed quantities of Schedule II medications to amounts required for an emergency's duration for patients in long-term-care facilities and for patients receiving home-infusion and intravenous pain therapy.

FEDERAL COMPREHENSIVE DRUG ABUSE PREVENTION AND CONTROL ACT OF 1970 (P.L. 91-513)

SCHEDULES OF CONTROLLED SUBSTANCES

The controlled substances that come under jurisdiction of the Federal Comprehensive Drug Abuse Prevention and Control Act of 1970 (P.L. 91-513) are divided into five schedules. Examples of controlled substances and their Schedules are listed in Table 1.

RETAIL DISTRIBUTION RESTRICTIONS FOR SCHEDULE V SUBSTANCES

Schedule V controlled substances of any controlled substance listed in Schedule II, III, or IV which is not a prescription item under the Federal Food, Drug, and Cosmetic Act may be dispensed without a prescription order at retail, provided that:

1. Such dispensing is made only by a pharmacist and not by a nonpharmacist employee even if under the direct supervision of a pharmacist. However, after the pharmacist has fulfilled professional and legal responsibilities, the actual cash, credit transaction, or delivery may be completed by a nonpharmacist.

2. Not more than 240 mL (8 fluid ounces) or not more than 48 solid dosage units of any substance containing opium, nor more than 120 mL (4 fluid ounces) or not more than 24 solid dosage units of any other controlled substance, may be distributed at retail to the same purchaser in any given 48-hour period without a valid prescription order.

3. The purchaser at retail is at least 18 years of age.

4. The pharmacist requires every purchaser of a controlled substance under this section not known to him to furnish suitable identification (including proof of age where appropriate).

5. The pharmacist requires every purchaser at retail of a Schedule V controlled substance not known to the pharmacist to furnish suitable identification (including proof of age where appropriate).

6. A Schedule V bound record book is maintained which contains the name and address of the purchaser, name and quantity of controlled substance purchased, date of each sale, and initials of the dispensing pharmacist. This record book shall be maintained for a period of two years from the date of the last transaction entered in such record book, and it shall be made available for inspection and copying by officers of the United States, authorized by the Attorney General.

7. Other Federal, state, or local law does not require a prescription order. 21 CFR 1306.32

SYMBOLS AND LABELING

Each commercial container of a controlled substance is required to have on its label a symbol designating to which Schedule it belongs. the symbol for Schedule I through V controlled substances is as follows:

Ⓒ or C-I
Ⓒ or C-II
Ⓒ or C-III
Ⓒ or C-IV
Ⓒ or C-V

These symbols are not required on prescription containers dispensed by a pharmacist to a patient in the course of sound professional practice. 21 CFR 1302.03

WHAT THE PRESCRIPTION MEDICATION LABEL MUST CONTAIN

The pharmacist dispensing a prescription order for a controlled substance must affix to the container a label showing the pharmacy name and address, the serial number and date of initial dispensing, the name of the patient, the name of the practitioner issuing the prescription order, and direction for use and cautionary statements, if any, contained in the prescription order as required by law.

The label of any drug listed as a "Controlled Substance" in Schedules II, III, or IV of the Controlled Substances Act shall, when dispensed to or for a patient, contain the following warning:

CAUTION: Federal law prohibits the transfer of this drug to any person other than the patient for whom it was prescribed.

21 CFR 1308 et seq.

REGISTRATION

Every pharmacy engaged in distributing or dispensing any controlled substance must register with the Drug Enforcement Administration. The registration must be renewed every three years and the certificate of registration must be maintained at the registered location and kept available for official inspections. If a person owns and operates more than one pharmacy, each place of business must be registered.

Every pharmacy will receive a reregistration application once every three years approximately 60 days before the expiration date of the registration. If such reregistration forms are not received within 45 days before the expiration date of the registration, the pharmacy must request the

---

AS A RULE . . .	
Anabolic steroids are Schedule III	Amphetamines are Schedule II
Barbiturates are Schedule IV	Narcotics are Schedule II
Benzodiazepines are Schedule IV	Opiates are Schedule II

NOTE . . .

The following barbiturates are Schedule II
  Amobarbital   Secobarbital
  Pentobarbital   Any combination of the above, e.g., Tuinal

Controlled substances having the same names but in different dosage forms may be in different Schedules (their potencies and formulations may also be different)

  Ex: Tylenol w/Codeine tablet   C-III
       Tylenol w/Codeine Elixir   C-V
       Pentobarbital capsule   C-II
       Pentobarbital rectal suppository   C-III

Table 1
The Schedules for Controlled Drugs.

The basic structure of *Federal* law consists of five classifications or "schedules" of controlled substances. The degree of control, the conditions of record-keeping, the particular order forms and prescriptions required, and other regulatory requirements all hinge on these classifications. Following are the five schedules, their criteria and some specific drugs that are included in each of the schedules.

Schedule I
Drugs included in this schedule are considered to have:
- A high potential for abuse.
- No currently accepted medical use in the United States.
- A lack of accepted safety for use under medical supervision.
  Examples: Hallucinogenic substances, methaqualone, heroin, and certain narcotics (various opiates and their derivatives). Among those drugs categorized as hallucinogenic are: LSD, marijuana, mescaline, peyote.

Schedule II
Drugs are included in this schedule upon finding that:
- The substance has a high potential for abuse.
- The substance has a currently accepted medical use in the United States or a currently accepted medical use with severe restrictions.
- The abuse of the drug may lead to severe psychological or physical dependence.
  Examples:

Amobarbital and salts (Amytal)	MS Contin
Amphetamines	Opium Tincture
Cocaine	ORLAAM
Codeine Sulfate, Phosphate	Oxycodone (Roxicodone)
Dihydromorphinone	Oxymorphone (Numorphan)
Fentanyl (Sublimaze)	Pentobarbital and salts (Nembutal)
Hydromorphone (Dilaudid)	Percocet
Mepergan	Percodan
Mepergan Fortis	Percodan-Demi
Meperidine (Demerol)	Secobarbital and salts (Seconal)
Methadone (Dolophine)	Sufentanil (Sufenta)
Methamphetamine (Desoxyn)	Tuinal Pulvules
Methylphenidate (Ritalin)	Tylox
Morphine (Pantopon)	

Schedule III
Drugs are included in this schedule upon a finding that:
- The substance has a potential for abuse but less than those drugs listed in Schedules I and II.
- The substance has a currently accepted medical use in the United States.
- Abuse of this drug may lead to moderate or low physical dependence or high psychologic dependence.
  Examples are:

Anabolic steroids (Halotestin, Winstrol)	Percogesic w/Codeine
Aprobarbital (Alurate)	Phenaphen 650 w/Codeine
Benzphetamine (Didrex)	Phendimetrazine (Plegine)
Brontex Tablet	Testoderm, Androderm
Butabarbital (Butisol)	Thiopental (Pentothal)
Deconamine CX	Triaminic Expectorant DH
Dronabinol (Marinol)	Tylenol w/Codeine Tablet
Empirin w/Codeine Tablet	Tussend Expectorant
Fiorinal	Tussend Syrup
Fiorinal w/Codeine	Tussionex Suspension
Hycodan Syrup, Tablet	Synalgos-DC
Hycomine Syrup	Vicodin, Vicodin ES
Ketamine (Ketalar)	Vicodin Tuss Expectorant
Nembutal Rectal Suppository	Vicoprofen
Paregoric	

Table 1 (continued)
The Schedules for Controlled Drugs.

Schedule IV

Drugs are included in this schedule upon finding that:
- The substance has a low potential for abuse relative to those in Schedule III.
- The substance has a currently accepted medical use in the United States.
- Abuse of the drug may lead to limited physical or psychological dependence relative to controlled substances in Schedule III.

Examples:

Alprazolam (Xanax)	Lorazepam (Ativan)
Butorphanol (Stadol)	Mazindol (Mazanor, Sanorex)
Chloral hydrate (Noctec)	Meprobamate (Miltown, Equanil)
Chlordiazepoxide (Librium)	Modafinil (Provigil)
Clonazepam (Clonopin)	Oxazepam (Serax)
Clorazepate (Tranxene)	Paraldehyde
Darvocet-N	Pentazocine (Talwin NX)
Diazepam (Valium)	Phenobarbital (Luminal)
Diethylpropion (Tenuate, Tepanil)	Phentermine HCl (Fastin)
Ethchlorvynol (Placidyl)	Phentermine Resin (Ionamin)
Ethinamate (Valmid)	Prazepam (Centrax)
Fenfluramine (Pondimin)	Propoxyphene (Darvon, Compound)
Flurazepam (Dalmane)	Temazepam (Restoril)
Halazepam (Paxipam)	Triazolam (Halcion)

Schedule V

Drugs are included in this schedule upon finding that:
- The substance has a low potential for abuse relative to Schedule IV.
- The substance has a currently accepted medical use in the United States.
- The substance has limited physical or psychologic dependence relative to controlled substances listed in Schedule IV.

Drugs included in this Schedule contain limited quantities of such narcotics as codeine, dihydrocodone, ethylmorphine, or diphenoxylate. Generally, these products are antitussives and antidiarrheals. Some drug products in Schedule V must be sold pursuant to prescription only; some may be sold OTC, depending on state law.

Examples are:

*Actifed w/Codeine Cough Syrup	*Phenergan w/Codeine Syrup
Ambenyl Cough Syrup	*Phenergan VC w/Codeine Syrup
Brontex Liquid	Robitussin A-C Syrup
Calcidrine Syrup	Robitussin-DAC Syrup
Cheracol Cough Syrup	Triaminic Expectorant w/Codeine
*Dimetane-DC Cough Syrup	Triaminic Expectorant DH Liquid
*Lomotil	Tussar-2 Cough Liquid
Novahistine Expectorant Liquid	Tussar SF Syrup
Novahistine DH Liquid	Tussi-Organidin NR
Pediacof Syrup	*Tylenol w/Codeine Elixir

*Requires Rx.
Source: 21 CFR 1308.11 through 1308.15 (5/91).

---

reregistration forms by writing to the Registration Unit, Drug Enforcement Administration, P.O. Box 28083, Central Station, Washington, D.C. 20005, or from any DEA field office.

Public Interest Provision

The 1984 Diversion Control Amendments give the Attorney General authority to deny an application for registration if it is determined that the issuance of such registration would be inconsistent with the public interest. In determining the the public interest, the following factors shall be considered:

1. The recommendation of the appropriate State licensing board or professional disciplinary authority.

2. The applicant's experience in dispensing, or conducting research with respect to controlled substances.

3. The applicant's conviction record under Federal or State laws relating to the manufacturer, distribution, or dispensing of controlled substances.

4. Compliance with applicable State, Federal, or local laws relating to controlled substances.

5. Such other conduct which may threaten the public health and safety.

New Registrations

Pharmacies that seek to become

**Table 2
Controlled Substances—Criteria for Inclusion.**

The major criteria for inclusion of a drug under the federal Controlled Substances Act are:

— the actual or relative potential for the abuse of the drug
— its known pharmacological effects
— its scientific background
— the history and current pattern of abuse of the drug
— the scope, duration and significance of abuse of the drug
— the risk to public health involved
— the potential of the drug producing psychic or physiological dependence liability
— whether the drug is an immediate precursor of a substance already controlled.

The principal criterion, however, is its *actual or relative potential for abuse.*

This criterion is derived from the following:

— Evidence that individuals are taking the drug in amounts sufficient to create a hazard to their health or to the safety of other individuals or of the community; *or*

— Significant diversion of the drug from legitimate channels; *or*

— A finding that individuals are using a drug on their own initiative, without the advice and/or prescription of a physician; *or*

— A finding that the drug is so related to existing restricted drugs that it will have the same potential for abuse.

There are two points relating to the foregoing criteria that should be defined.

— *Potential* rather than *actual* abuse. In considering a drug for control, it would not be necessary to prove that abuse exists but only that there are indications of a *potential* for abuse.

— *Substantial evidence of potential for abuse.* This means more than a few isolated incidences of abuse. The documentation of several hundred thousand dosage units of drug having been diverted would be *substantial* evidence of abuse, despite the use of many millions of dosage units of the same drug, used legitimately in the same time period.

**Table 3
The Prescription Label.**

The prescription label must be affixed to the immediate container, i.e., vial, bottle, jar, tube, in which the drug is dispensed.

Pursuant to federal law, the information required on the prescription label for a controlled substance dispensed by the pharmacist in an out-patient setting shall contain the following information:

1. Name of the pharmacy
2. Address of the pharmacy
3. Serial number of the prescription
4. Date the prescription is filled
5. Directions for use as may be stated in the prescription, and cautionary statements, if any
6. Name of the prescriber
7. Name of the patient
8. The statement "Caution: Federal law prohibits the transfer of this drug to any person other than the patient for whom it was prescribed"   (21 CFR 1306.14 and 1306.24)

Information *Not* Required:

1. Age of patient
2. Quantity of drug dispensed
3. Number of authorized refills remaining
4. Dispenser's (pharmacist's) name or initials
5. Pharmacy's DEA registration number
6. Prescriber's DEA registration number

Note: a. State laws may require additional information on the prescription label.
        b. Statement #8 above not required on Schedule V drug prescription labels.

Table 4
Special Warning Statement.

The following statement must be included as part of the prescription label when dispensing certain controlled substances.

"CAUTION: FEDERAL LAW PROHIBITS THE TRANSFER
OF THIS DRUG TO ANY PERSON OTHER THAN
THE PATIENT FOR WHOM IT WAS PRESCRIBED"

- Required for Schedule II, III, IV substances.
- Not required for Schedule V substances.
- Not required for controlled substances dispensed for use in clinical investigations which are "blind."

Note: The caution statement is commonly a part of a pharmacy's printed prescription label, which is used for all prescriptions dispensed. This type of prescription label should not be used when dispensing non-controlled drug products. The inclusion of the caution statement on the prescription label when dispensing a non-controlled drug product may constitute misbranding under federal law.

---

registered for the first time must request a registration application for new registrants from the Drug Enforcement Administration, Registration Unit.

Any pharmacy engaged in co-op buying of controlled substances must register as a distributor with the Drug Enforcement Administration.

In order to be registered as a distributor, a pharmacy must meet the security requirements as set forth for a distributor (wholesaler) and keep records required of a distributor.

An affidavit system for expediting pharmacy applications may be used to expedite obtaining a DEA registration number for either a new pharmacy or for the transfer of ownership of an existing pharmacy. Additional information may be obtained from any DEA office or 21 CFR 1301.38 of the DEA regulations.

Change of Business or Professional Address

The 1984 Diversion Control Amendments require that every registrant including pharmacies notify DEA of any change of business or professional address. Notification must be made, and the application approved prior to the anticipated move. 21 CFR 1304 et seq.

RECORDS

Every pharmacy engaged in handling controlled substances must keep complete and accurate records of all receiving and dispensing transactions. All such records shall be maintained for a period of two years.

All inventories and records of controlled substances in Schedule II must be maintained separately from all other records of the registrant. All inventories and records of controlled substances in Schedules III, IV, and V must be maintained separately or must be in such form that they are readily retrievable from the ordinary professional and business records of the pharmacy.

All records pertaining to controlled substances must be made available for inspection and copying by duly authorized officials of the Drug Enforcement Administration.

When a registrant first engages in business and every two years thereafter, a complete and accurate inventory of all stocks of controlled substances on hand must be made. This inventory record shall be kept by the registrant for a period of two years. Pharmacies are not required to submit a copy of the inventory to the Drug Enforcement Administration.

Central Record Keeping

Central record keeping permits are not issued by the DEA. A registrant desiring to maintain required records at a location other than the registered location must notify the nearest DEA field office. Unless the registrant is informed by DEA that the permission to keep central records is denied, the registrant may maintain central records 14 days after notifying DEA. 21 CFR 1304.04

If records are kept at a central location, the registrant must provide the records to the registered location within two (2) days at DEA's request, or allow DEA to inspect the records at the central location without notification (warrant).

Executed DEA 222 order forms, prescriptions, and inventory records must be kept at the pharmacy.

Transfer of Prescription Information

DEA allows the transfer of prescription renewal information for Schedules III, IV, and V controlled substances between pharmacies if permissible under state law. However, pharmacies sharing a real-time, on-line electronic database may transfer up to the maximum refills permitted by law and the prescriber's authorization. Transfers are subject to the following requirements:

(1) The transfer is communicated directly between two licensed pharmacists and the transferring pharmacist records the following information:

(i) Write the word "VOID" on the face of the invalidated prescription.

(ii) Record on the reverse of the invalidated prescription the name, address and DEA registration number of the pharmacy to which it was transferred and the name of the pharmacist receiving the prescription information.

(iii) Record the date of the transfer and the name of the pharmacist transferring the information.

(b) The pharmacist receiving the transferred prescription information shall reduce to writing the following:

(1) Write the word "transfer" on the face of the transferred prescription.

(2) Provide all information required to be on a prescription pursuant to 21 CFR 1306.05 and include:

(i) Date of issuance of original prescription;

(ii) Original number of refills authorized on original prescription;

(iii) Date of original dispensing;

(iv) Last refill date, and date(s) and locations of previous refill(s);

(v) Pharmacy's name, address, DEA registration number and prescription number from which the prescription information was transferred;

(vi) Name of pharmacist who transferred the prescription.

(vii) Pharmacy's name, address, DEA registration number and prescription number from which the prescription was originally filled;

(3) The original and transferred prescription(s) must be maintained for a period of two years from the date of last refill.   21 CFR 1306.25

Continuing Records to Be Kept by a Pharmacy

Every pharmacy must maintain a current, complete and accurate record of each controlled substance received.

Copy 3 of executed order forms retained by the pharmacy which have been completed as described under section entitled "Order Forms" will constitute a pharmacy's receiving records for Schedule II controlled substances. Invoices for Schedules III, IV, and V controlled substances will be considered as complete receiving records if the actual date of receipt is clearly recorded on the invoices by the pharmacist or other responsible individual.   21 CFR 1305 et seq.

ORDER FORMS

A triplicate order form is necessary for the transfer of controlled substances in Schedules I and II. Pursuant to the Controlled Substances Act, the use of the order forms are for Schedules I and II drugs only. A registrant desiring DEA order forms can obtain them by requesting them on the initial application form or from the Drug Enforcement Administration, Registration Unit, P.O. Box 28083, Central Station, Washington, D.C. 20005.

Once a registrant has obtained DEA order forms a separate requisition form, DEA-222A, will be mailed to the registrant in order to request additional books. No charge is made for order forms.

DEA order form books consist of seven sets of order forms. Each pharmacy is allowed a maximum of six books at one time unless it can show that its needs exceed this limit. In such case, the pharmacy should contact the field office of DEA serving its area.

DEA 222 is an accountable form and the number in the lower right corner, which is printed in red, is an internal control number used by the DEA's Computer Operations Office. This control number ensures that all of these forms, whether printed and issued, or destroyed in the production process, are accounted for.

The number on the lower left side of the form is the specific number of the order form, the second copy of which must be forwarded by the supplier to the DEA office in the area in which the supplier is lo-

cated. This number is used to associate a specific purchase or sale of a controlled substance between a DEA registrant and a pharmaceutical supplier.

In summary, both numbers are used for control purposes. The first number, in red, tracks the blank form and the second number tracks the actual controlled substances transaction.

Proper Completion of DEA Form 222

When a registrant issues an order form for Schedule I and II controlled substances and after the items are received, the number of packages and the date such packages were received must be recorded on the retained copy. A space is provided for this on the DEA order form. The order form must be completed properly and bear no material alteration or erasure. A distributor is obligated to refuse the form if it is not properly completed, or if it bears material alteration or erasure. It may also be refused when it is not completed correctly.

Title 21 of the *Code of Federal Regulations (CFR)*, Section 1305.06(b) states that only one item shall be entered on each numbered line. It further states that the total number of items ordered shall be noted on the order form in the space provided. On the current version of DEA Form 222, the aforementioned "space provided" is termed "number of lines completed." When the above requirements are followed to the letter, there is no discrepancy between

---

DEA 222 order forms for carfentanil, etorphine hydrochloride, and diprenorphine hydrochloride shall contain only these substances in reasonable quantities. These substances can be purchased from a supplier by a veterinarian engaged in zoo and exotic animal practice, wildlife management programs and/or research.   21 CFR 1305.16(b)

Carfentanil citrate is a narcotic analgesic.

Etorphine hydrochloride is a highly potent narcotic analgesic. It is used with acepromazine maleate as a sedative to assist in the control of large animals, and with methotrimeprazine for small animals.

Diprenorphine hydrochloride is a narcotic antagonist used in veterinary medicine to reverse the effects of etorphine hydrochloride.

See Reverse of PURCHASER'S Copy for Instructions	No order form may be issued for Schedule I and II substances unless a completed application form has been received. (21 CFR 1305.04)	OMB APPROVAL No. 1117-0010
TO: (Name of Supplier) Towne Wholesale Drugs, Inc.	STREET ADDRESS 695 Commercial Way	
CITY and STATE Anytown, U.S.A.	DATE March 5, 1986	TO BE FILLED IN BY SUPPLIER SUPPLIERS DEA REGISTRATION No PT0008976

No of Packages	Size of Package	Name of Item	National Drug Code	Packages Shipped	Date Shipped
3	100	Sod. Pentobarbital cap. 100 mg		3	3/25/86
2	100	Secobarbital cap. 100 mg.		2	3/25/86
		VOID FOR OFFICIAL USE ONLY			

2 ◄ NO. OF LINES COMPLETED	SIGNATURE OF PURCHASER OR HIS ATTORNEY OR AGENT	*Bob Richard*
Date Issued 2/25/86	DEA Registration No BR1234567	Name and Address of Registrant Richard's Drugs, Inc. 672 Broadway Anytown, USA
Schedules 2, 2N, 3, 3N, 4 and 5		
Registered as Retail Pharmacy	No of this Order Form P05612345	

U.S. OFFICIAL ORDER FORMS - SCHEDULES I & II
DRUG ENFORCEMENT ADMINISTRATION
SUPPLIER'S COPY 1

29353018

Sample Form DEA 222 "Order Form"

the number of items ordered and the number of lines completed.

Problems in interpretation have been encountered when the purchaser either uses more than one line to describe an item or voids an item. In the first instance, the correct interpretation would be to list the number of items ordered on the form in the space labeled "number of lines completed." DEA Form 222 will be revised in its next printing to rename the heading "number of items ordered."

The issue of voided lines on the order form is a bit less clear-cut in its interpretation. In strictly interpreting the regulations, the only conclusion that can be reached which is not open for interpretation is that a supplier may not fill an order form which "shows any alteration, erasure, or change of any description" (21 *CFR* 1305.11(2)). In fact, instructions provided on the reverse side of the DEA Form 222 advise the purchaser not to make erasures or alterations. They state that if an error should be made, all copies of the form should be voided and kept on file.

In addition, the regulations imply that only a supplier, not a purchaser, may void an item on a DEA Form 222, Section 1305.15(a) of the regulations states:

A purchaser may cancel part or all of an order on an order form by notifying the supplier in writing of such cancellation. The supplier shall indicate the cancellation on Copies 1 and 2 of the order form by drawing a line through the canceled items and printing "canceled" in the space provided for number of items shipped.

Consequently, only the supplier has the authority to indicate the cancellation on the order form.

A separate but related issue has also been raised regarding generic substitution on order forms. DEA policy does not preclude generic substitution of identical products provided that the name and National Drug Code number of the actual product shipped is reflected on the form. Therefore, it would be acceptable to make a substitution provided that the customer agrees to accept a generic rather than a brand name product, the generic product of a manufacturer other than the one specified, or a brand name product rather than a generic one. Therefore, the purchaser will not be required to submit a new DEA Form 222 to accommodate such a change.

Power of Attorney

Any registrant (pharmacy) may authorize one or more individuals

whether or not located at the registered location, to obtain and execute order forms by granting a power of attorney to each such individual. *The power of attorney must be signed by the same person who signed the most recent application for registration or reregistration.* It must contain the signature of the individual being authorized to obtain and execute order forms. Any power of attorney may be revoked at any time by the person who signed the power of attorney. It will be necessary to grant a new power of attorney upon the reregistration of a purchaser only if the application for reregistration was signed by a different person. The power of attorney should be filed with executed order forms. The power of attorney is not submitted to DEA. DEA does not provide power of attorney forms (see Figure 1).

21 CFR 1305.07

Lost or Stolen Order Forms

If a purchaser ascertains that an unfilled order form has been lost, he shall execute another in triplicate and a statement containing the serial number and date of the lost form, and stating that the goods covered by the first order form were not received through loss of that order form. Copy 3 of the second form and a copy of the statement shall be retained with Copy 3 of the order form first executed. A copy of the statement shall be attached to Copies 1 and 2 of the second order form sent to the supplier. If the first order form is subsequently received by the supplier to whom it was directed, the supplier shall mark upon the face thereof "Not accepted" and return Copies 1 and 2 to the purchaser, who shall attach it to Copy 3 and the statement.

Whenever any used or unused order forms are stolen or lost (other than in the course of transmission) by any purchaser or supplier, he/she shall immediately upon discovery of such theft or loss, report the same to the Special Agent in Charge of the Drug Enforcement

Administration in the Divisional Office responsible for the area in which the registrant is located, stating the serial number of each form stolen or lost. If the theft or loss includes any original order forms received from purchasers and the supplier is unable to state the serial numbers of such order forms, he/she shall report the date or approximate date of receipt thereof and the names and addresses of the purchasers. If an entire book of order forms is lost or stolen, and the purchaser is unable to state the serial numbers of the order forms contained therein, he/she shall report, in lieu of the numbers of the forms contained in such book, the date or approximate date of issuance thereof. If any unused order form reported stolen or lost is subsequently recovered or found, the Special Agent in Charge of the Drug Enforcement Administration in the Divisional Office responsible for the area in which the registrant is located shall immediately be notified.

If any unused order form reported stolen or lost is later recovered or found, the pharmacy shall immediately notify the DEA Divisional Office.   21 CFR 1305.12

PRESCRIPTION ORDERS

21 CFR 1306 et seq.

Who May Issue

A prescription order for a controlled substance may be issued only by a physician, dentist, podiatrist, veterinarian or other registered practitioner who is:

1. Authorized to prescribe controlled substances by the jurisdiction in which licensed to practice;

2. Either registered under the Controlled Substances Act or exempted from registration (military and Public Health Service physicians).   21 CFR 1306.03

Purpose of Issue

A prescription order for a controlled substance to be effective must be issued for a legitimate medical purpose by a physician acting in the usual course of sound professional practice. The responsibility for the proper prescribing and dispensing of controlled substances is upon the prescribing physician, but a corresponding liability rests with the pharmacist who dispenses the prescription order. A request purporting to be a prescription order issued not in the usual course of professional treatment or in legitimate and authorized research is not a prescription order within the meaning and intent of Section 309 of the Controlled Substances Act. The person knowingly dispensing such a purported prescription order, as well as the person issuing it, will be subject to the penalties provided for violations of the provisions of law relating to controlled substances.

21 CFR 1306.04

Execution of Prescription Orders by Practitioners

All prescription orders for controlled substances shall be dated as of, and signed on, the day when issued and shall bear the full name and address of the patient, and the name, address, and DEA registration number of the practitioner. A practitioner may sign a prescription order in the same manner as a legal document would be signed;

Filing of Prescriptions for Controlled Substances

Pursuant to federal law, prescriptions for controlled substances may be filed in one of the following three ways:

1. A pharmacy can maintain *three* separate files:
   A file for Schedule II drugs
   A file for Schedule III-IV-V drugs
   A file for non-Schedule drugs

2. A pharmacy can maintain *two* separate files:
   A file for all Schedule II drugs
   A file for Schedule III-IV-V drugs and non-Schedule drugs

   If this method is used, the Schedule III-IV-V prescriptions must be stamped with the letter C in red ink, not less than one inch high, in the lower right corner. This distinctive marking makes the records "readily retrievable" for inspection.

3. A pharmacy can maintain *two* separate files:
   A file for Schedule II-III-IV-V drugs
   A file for non-Schedule drugs

   If this method is used, the Schedule III-IV-V prescriptions must be stamped with the letter C in red ink, not less than one inch high, in the lower right corner.

   If a pharmacy employs an ADP [automated data processing] system or other electronic recordkeeping system for prescriptions which permits identification by prescription number and retrieval of original documents by prescriber's name, patient's name, drug dispensed, and date filled, then the requirement to mark the hard copy prescription with a red "C" is waived.

   The stamped C may still be required, however, in states that have more stringent regulations than those of the federal government.

Source: 21 CFR 1304.04.

——————— (Name of registrant)
——————— (Address of registrant)
——————— (DEA registration
number)
I, ——————— (name of person
granting power), the undersigned, who is
authorized to sign the current application
for registration of the above-named registrant under the Controlled Substances Act
or Controlled Substances Import and
Export Act, have made, constituted, and appointed, and by these presents, do make,
constitute,   and   appoint
——————— (name of attorney-in-
fact), my true and lawful attorney for me in
my name, place, and stead, to execute applications for books of official order forms and
to sign such order forms in requisition for
Schedule I and II controlled substances, in
accordance with section 308 of the Controlled Substances Act (21 U.S.C. 828) and
part 305 of Title 21 of the Code of Federal
Regulations. I hereby ratify and confirm all
that said attorney shall lawfully do or cause
to be done by virtue hereof.

———————————————————
(Signature of person granting power)
I, ——————— (name of attorney-
in-fact), hereby affirm that I am the person
named herein as attorney-in-fact and that
the signature affixed hereto is my signature.

———————————————————
(Signature of attorney-in-fact)
Witnesses:
1. ———————————————.
2. ———————————————.
Signed and dated on the ——— day of
———————. (year) at ———————.

NOTICE OF REVOCATION

The foregoing power of attorney is hereby
revoked by the undersigned, who is authorized to sign the current application for registration of the above-named registrant
under the Controlled Substances Act of the
Controlled Substances Import and Export
Act. Written notice of this revocation has
been   given   to   the   attorney-in-fact
——————— this same day.

———————————————————
(Signature of person revoking power)
Witnesses:
1. ———————————————.
2. ———————————————.
Signed and dated on the ——— day of
———————. (year) at ———————.

FIGURE 1. Examples of power of attorney
for DEA order forms.

for instance, J. H. Smith or John H. Smith. Where an oral order is not permitted (Schedule II), a prescription order must be written with ink or indelible pencil or typewritten and must be manually signed by the practitioner issuing such prescription order. The prescription order may be prepared by a secretary or agent for the signature of the practitioner, but the practitioner is responsible in case the prescription order does not conform in all essential respects to the law and regulations.

No prescription order for a controlled substance in Schedule II

may be refilled. Such prescription orders must be kept in a separate file, or as outlined in the "Filing of Prescription Orders for Controlled Substances" section below. Prescription orders for controlled substances in Schedule III or IV may be issued either orally or in writing by a practitioner and may be refilled if so authorized. Such prescription orders may not be dispensed more than six months after the issue date or be refilled more than five times after the issue date. If a practitioner wishes a patient to continue on the medication, a new prescription order is required. Oral prescription orders must be promptly committed to writing and filed by the pharmacist.

A prescription order for a controlled substance listed in Schedule V may be refilled only as authorized by the practitioner on the prescription order. If no such authorization is given, the prescription order may not be refilled. For items which may be sold over-the-counter, however, the burden of determining the propriety of the dispensing is upon the pharmacist.

A prescription order written for office stock of "medical bag" use is not valid. Orders for Schedule II substances must be placed pursuant to an official order form.

Oral Authorization for a New Prescription

The authority for prescribing controlled substances is vested only in the practitioner and cannot be delegated to anyone else. However, nurses or staff members receiving calls from pharmacists regarding a new prescription may act as the practitioner's agent and transmit the practitioner's order.

Recording Refills

When a prescription order for any controlled substance in Schedule III or IV is refilled, the following must be entered on the back of that prescription oder: the dispensing pharmacist's initials, the date the prescription order was refilled,

and the amount of drug dispensed on such refill. If the pharmacist merely initials and dates the back of the prescription order, the pharmacist shall be deemed to have dispensed a refill for the full face amount of the prescription order.

21 CFR 1306.21

Partial Dispensing of Schedule II Controlled Substances Prescription Orders

The partial filling of a prescription for a controlled substance listed in Schedule II is permissible, if the pharmacist is unable to supply the full quantity called for in a written or emergency oral prescription and a notation is made of the quantity supplied on the face of the written prescription (or written record of the emergency oral prescription). The remaining portion of the prescription may be filled within 72 hours of the first partial filling; however, if the remaining portion is not or cannot be filled within the 72-hour period, the pharmacist shall so notify the prescriber. No further quantity may be supplied beyond 72 hours without a new prescription.

A prescription for a Schedule II controlled substance written for a patient in a Long Term Care Facility (LTCF) may be filled in partial quantities to include individual dosage units. Both the pharmacist and the prescribing practitioner have a corresponding responsibility to assure that the controlled substance is for a terminally ill patient or for patients in hospice or patients in home-care who have a medical diagnosis documenting a terminal illness. This authority *does not apply to other classes of patients,* such as patients with severe intractable pain who are not diagnosed as terminal. A prescription that is partially filled and does not contain the notation "terminally ill" or "LTCF patient" shall be deemed to have been filled in violation of the Act. For each partial filling, the dispensing pharmacist shall record on the back of the prescription (or on another appropriate record, uniformly maintained, and readily retrievable) the date of the partial filling, quantity dispensed, remaining quantity authorized to be dispensed, and the identification of the dispensing pharmacist. The total quantity of Schedule II controlled substances dispensed in all partial fillings must not exceed the total quantity prescribed. Schedule II prescriptions for patients in a LTCF or patients with a medical diagnosis documenting a terminal illness shall be valid for a period not to exceed 60 days from the issue data unless sooner terminated by the discontinuance of medication.

Information pertaining to current Schedule II prescriptions for patients in a LTCF or for patients with a medical diagnosis documenting a terminal illness may be maintained in a computerized system if this system has the capability to permit:

(1) Output (display or printout) of the original prescription number, date of issue, identification of prescribing individual practitioner, identification of patient, address of the LTCF or address of the hospital or residence of the patient, identification of medication authorized (to include dosage, form, strength and quantity), listing of the partial fillings that have been dispensed under each prescription and the information required in §1306.13(b).

(2) Immediate (real time) updating of the prescription record each time a partial filling of the prescription is conducted.

(3) Retrieval of partially filled Schedule II prescription information is the same as required by §1306.22(b) (4) and (5) for Schedule III and IV prescription refill information. 21 CFR 1306.13

Partial Dispensing of Schedules III and IV Controlled Substance Prescription Orders

Partial dispensing of a Schedule III or IV controlled substance is permitted if the pharmacist dispensing or refilling the prescription order sets forth the quantity dispensed and initials the back of the prescription order. The partial dispensing may not exceed the total amount authorized in the prescription order. The dispensing of all refills must be within the six-month limit. 21 CFR 1306.23

Emergency Dispensing of Schedule II Controlled Substances

In the case of a bona fide emergency situation, as defined by the Secretary of Health and Human Services, a pharmacist may dispense a Schedule II controlled substance upon receiving oral authorization of a prescribing physician provided that:

1) The quantity prescribed and dispensed is limited to the amount adequate to treat the patient during the emergency period. Prescribing or dispensing beyond the emergency period must be pursuant to a written prescription order.

2) The prescription order shall be immediately reduced to writing by the pharmacist and shall contain all information, except for the prescribing physician's signature.

3) If the prescribing physician is not known to the pharmacist, the pharmacist must make a reasonable effort to determine that the oral authorization came from a physician, by verifying the physician's telephone number with that listed in the directory and by making other good faith efforts to insure proper identity.

4) Within seven (7) days after authorizing an emergency oral prescription, the prescribing individual practitioner shall cause a written prescription order for the emergency quantity prescribed to be delivered to the dispensing pharmacist. The prescription order shall have written on its face "Authorization for Emergency Dispensing." The written prescription order may be delivered in person or by mail, but **if delivered by mail it must be postmarked within the 7 day period**. Upon receipt, the dispensing pharmacist shall attach this prescription order to the oral emergency prescription order which had earlier been reduced to writing. *The pharmacist shall notify the nearest office of DEA if the prescriber fails to deliver a written prescription order. Failure of the pharmacist to do so shall void the authority conferred to dispense without a written prescription order of a prescriber.*

For the purpose of authorizing an oral prescription order of a controlled substance listed in Schedule II of the Controlled Substances Act, the term *emergency situation* means those situations in which the prescribing physician determines that:

1) Immediate administration of the controlled substance is necessary for the proper treatment of the intended ultimate user; and

2) No appropriate alternative treatment is available, including administration of a drug which is not a controlled substance under Schedule II of the Act; and

3) It is not reasonably possible for the prescribing physician to provide a written prescription order to be presented to the person dispensing the substance, prior to the dispensing.

An emergency means a situation where a quantity of a controlled substance may be dispensed by a pharmacist to a patient who does not have an alternative source for such substance reasonably available, and the pharmacist cannot obtain such substances through normal distribution channels within the time required to meet the immediate needs of the patient for such substance. 21 CFR 1306.11(d)

Computerization of Prescription Information

A pharmacy is permitted to use a data processing system as an alternative method for the storage and retrieval of prescription order refill information for controlled substances in Schedules III and IV.

The computerized system must

provide immediate retrieval (via CRT display or hard-copy printout) of original prescription order information for those prescription orders which are currently authorized for refilling. The information which must be readily retrievable from this type of system must include, but is not limited to, data such as: the original prescription number; date of issuance of the prescription order by the physician; full name and address of the patient; the physician's name and DEA registration number; the name, strength, dosage form and quantity of the controlled substance prescribed; and the total number of refills authorized by the prescribing physician.

In addition, the system must provide immediate retrieval of the current refill history for Schedule III or IV controlled substance prescription orders that have been authorized for refill during the past six months and backup documentation to show that the refill information is correct. The backup documentation must be stored in a separate file at the pharmacy and be maintained for a two-year period from the dispensing date.

21 CFR 1306.22

Return of Controlled Substances to Supplier

Any pharmacy lawfully in possession of a controlled substance listed in any schedule may return that substance (without being registered as a distributor) to the person from whom it was obtained or to the manufacturer of the substance. The controlled substance may be returned provided that a written record is maintained which indicates the date of the transaction; the name, form, and quantity of the substance; the name, address, and registration number, if any, of the person making the return; and the name, address, and registration number, if known, of the supplier or manufacturer. In case of returning a controlled substance listed in Schedule II, a triplicate order form shall be issued by

the supplier to the pharmacy in the transfer of such substance. This also applies to any other registrant who returns controlled substances to a supplier.

Distribution by a Pharmacy

A phsarmacy (as well as all physician registrants) registered to dispense a controlled substance may distribute (without being registered to distribute) a quantity of such substances to a physician for the purpose of dispensing by that physician provided that the following conditions are met:

1) The pharmacy or physician to which the controlled substance is being distributed is registered under the Act to dispense that controlled substance.

2) The distribution is recorded as being distributed by the pharmacy and the receiving pharmacy or physician records the substance being received. The pharmacy distributing a controlled substance must record the name of the substance, the dosage form, the quantity and the name, address, and DEA registration number of the pharmacy or physician to whom it is distributed on an official triplicate order form.

3) If the substance is listed in Schedule I or II, the transfer must be made on an official triplicate order form.

4) The total number of dosage units of controlled substances distributed by a pharmacy may not exceed 5 percent of all controlled substances dispensed by the pharmacy during the 12-month period in which the pharmacy is registered. If at any time it does exceed 5 percent, the pharmacy is required to register as both a distributor and pharmacy.

Controlled Substance Security

The Drug Enforcement Administration requires pharmacies to keep Schedules II, III, IV, and V controlled substances in a locked

cabinet or dispersed through the non-controlled stock to deter theft. An electronic alarm system is recommended.

Disposal of Controlled Substances

A pharmacy to dispose of any excess or undesired stocks of controlled substances is required to contact their state agency or nearest DEA office for disposal instructions and to request the necessary form (DEA-41).

The DEA office will advise the registrant of the procedures to be followed which will consist of one of the four courses of action listed below.

1. The pharmacy will be advised that the drugs may be destroyed by two responsible parties employed or acting on behalf of the registrant. This course of action will be used when there are factors that preclude an on-site destruction witnessed by DEA personnel, such as the firm's history of compliance and the abuse potential of the drugs involved.

2. The pharmacy will be advised to forward the excess of undesired stocks of controlled substances to the appropriate state agency for destruction. In lieu of actual surrender to the state agency, destructions witnessed by state personnel are acceptable.

3. The pharmacy will be advised to hold the substances until DEA personnel can witness the destruction of the substances. DEA personnel will date and sign the reports or forms after witnessing the destruction.

4. The pharmacy will be advised to forward the substances to the DEA Field Office which serves the area in which the registrant is located. Upon receipt of the substances, the DEA Field Office will verify the actual substances submitted. If errors are found, a corrected from must be prepared and the registrant duly notified. The original form will be returned to the registrant.

Regardless of the destruction procedures used, three copies of DEA Form-41 are required. The procedures established for destruction shall not be construed as affecting or altering in any way the disposal of controlled substances through procedures in laws and regulations adopted by any state.

21 CFR 1307.21, 1307.22

Controlled Substance Theft

A pharmacy involved in theft or significant loss of controlled substances must upon discovery notify the nearest DEA office in addition to reporting such theft or loss by completing DEA Form-106. The Code of Federal Regulations implements CSA requirements that notification be made.

Such reports shall contain the following information:
1. Name and address of firm.
2. DEA registration number.
3. Date of theft.
4. Local police department notified.
5. Type of theft (night break-in, armed robbery, etc.).
6. Listing of symbols or cost code used by pharmacy in marking containers (if any).
7. Listing of controlled substances missing through theft or significant loss.

The pharmacy is required to prepare the report in triplicate and retain the third copy for its records and forward the original and duplicate copy to the nearest DEA office.

Distribution upon Discontinuance or Transfer of Business

The 1984 Diversion Control Amendments require that registrants must notify DEA of any change of professional or business address. Notification to DEA must be made prior to the anticipated move.

A registrant discontinuing controlled substances business, and who does not transfer such business activities to another person shall return the certificate of registration and any unexecuted triplicate order forms to the Registration Branch, Drug Enforcement Administration, Department of Justice, Post Office Box 28083, Washington, D.C. 20005. If a registrant discontinues controlled substances business and transfers such business activity to another person, the certificate of registration and any unexecuted triplicate order forms are also required to be returned. It is recommended that unused order forms be marked "VOID" by the registrant prior to being sent to DEA. The new owner requires a new registration.

A registrant discontinuing controlled substances business altogether, or transferring it to another person, shall submit in person or by registered mail the following information to the nearest DEA office at least 14 days before the date of the proposed transfer:
1. The name, address, registration number of the pharmacy discontinuing business;
2. The name, address, registration number of the person acquiring the pharmacy;
3. Whether the business activities will be continued at the location registered by the person discontinuing business or moved to another location. If the latter, the address of the new location shall be stated:
4. The date on which the transfer of controlled substances will occur.

On the day of transfer of the controlled substances, a complete inventory of all controlled substances being transferred shall be taken. This inventory shall serve as the final inventory of the registrant who is transferring the controlled substances and the initial inventory for the registrant receiving such controlled substances, and a copy of the inventory shall be included in the records of each. It is not necessary to file a copy of the inventory with the DEA. Transfers of any substances listed in Schedule II require the use of triplicate order forms. The order forms of the registrant receiving the controlled substances are to be used for the transfer.

On the date of the transfer of the controlled substances, all records required to be kept by the registrant transferor with reference to the controlled substances being transferred shall be transferred to the registrant transferee. Responsibility for the accuracy of records prior to the date of transfer remains with the transferor, but responsibility for custody and maintenance shall be upon the transferee.

INTERNS, RESIDENTS, AND FOREIGN PHYSICIANS

Any physician who is an intern, resident, foreign physician, or physician on the staff of a Veterans Administration facility (exempted from registration), may dispense, administer, and prescribe controlled substances under the registration of the hospital or other institution in which the physician is employed provided that:
1. The dispensing, administering, or prescribing is in the usual course of sound professional practice;
2. The physician is authorized or permitted to do so by the state where practicing;
3. The hospital or institution has verified that the physician is permitted to dispense, administer, or prescribe controlled substances within the state;
4. The physician acts only within the scope of employment in the hospital or institution;
5. The hospital or other institution authorizes the physician to dispense or prescribe under its registration and assigns a specific internal code number for each physician so authorized. An example of a specific internal code number is as follows:

Hospital DEA Registration Number	AB1234567—012	Physician's Hospital Code Number

6. A current list of internal codes and the corresponding individual practitioners is kept by the hospital or other institution and is made available at all times to other regis-

trants and law enforcement agencies upon request for the purpose of verifying the authority of the prescribing individual practitioner.

Pharmacists should contact the hospital or other institution for verification if they have any doubts in dispensing such prescription orders.   21 CFR 1301.24

Military and Other Personnel

Any official of the U.S. Army, Navy, Marine Corps, Air Force, Coast Guard, Public Health Service, or Bureau of Prisons who is authorized to prescribe, dispense, or administer, but not to procure or puchase, controlled substances in the course of official duties is not required to be registered with DEA.
                                          21 CFR 1301.25

INVENTORY REQUIREMENTS

Initial Inventory

A registrant is required to take an initial inventory on the date when controlled substances activities are first engaged. In the event that no controlled substances are on hand at the initial inventory a zero inventory is to be recorded.

The inventory record must:

1. List the name, address, and DEA registration number of the registrant.

2. Indicate the date and the time the inventory is taken, i.e., opening or close of business.

3. Be signed by the person or persons responsible for taking the inventory.

4. Be maintained at the location appearing on the registration certificate for at least two years.

5. Keep records of Schedule II drugs separate from all other controlled substances.   21 CFR 1304.12

Biennial Inventory

Every two years following the date of the registrant's initial inventory, a new inventory must be taken. The information required on the biennial inventory is the same as that for the initial inventory. Biennial inventories of controlled substances may be taken on any date which is within two years of the previous biennial inventory date.   21 CFR 1304.11

When taking the inventory of Schedule II controlled substances, an exact count or measure must be made. When taking the inventory of Schedules III, IV, and V controlled substances, an estimated count may be made. If the container holds more than 1,000 dosage units, an exact count must be made if the container has been opened.   21 CFR 1304.17

Newly Controlled Substances

Occasionally a drug that has not been previously controlled will be placed in one of the drug schedules or a controlled substance will be moved into a higher or lower schedule. In either of these cases, the drug must be inventoried as of the effective date of transfer, and this inventory added to the biennial inventory record.   21 CFR 1304.14

THE PHARMACIST'S CORRESPONDING RESPONSIBILITY FOR CONTROLLED SUBSTANCE PRESCRIPTION ORDERS

Title 21, Code of Federal Regulations, Sections 1306.04 provides, in part, that:

"A prescription for a controlled substance to be effective must be issued for a legitimate purpose by an individual practitioner acting in the usual course of his professional practice. The responsibility for the proper prescribing and dispensing of the controlled substances is upon the prescribing practitioner, *but a corresponding responsibility rests with the pharmacist who fills the prescription.* An order purporting to be a presentation issued not in the usual course of professional treatment or in legitimate and authorized research is not a prescription within the meaning and intent of Section 309 of the Act (21 USC 829) and the person knowingly filling such a purported prescription, as well as the person issuing it, shall be subject to the penalties provided for violations of the provisions of law relating to controlled substances."

A pharmacist is required to exercise sound professional judgment with respect to the legitimacy of prescription orders dispensed. The law does not require a pharmacist to dispense a prescription order of doubtful origin. To the contrary, the pharmacist who deliberately turns the other way when there is every reason to believe that the purported prescription order had not been issued for a legitimate medical purpose may be prosecuted, along with the issuing physician, for knowingly and intentionally distributing controlled substances, a felony offense which may result in the loss of one's business or profession.

CONTROLLED SUBSTANCE REGISTRANT PROTECTION ACT OF 1984

On May 31, 1984, Congress approved the Controlled Substance Registration Protection Act of 1984. Robberies, burglaries and assaults perpetrated on pharmacists and other registrants are a serious problem in the United States. These crimes result in property loss and sometimes serious injury to professionals and innocent bystanders. The proceeds from thefts and robberies serve to fuel the drug abuse problem.

The Controlled Substance Registrant Protection Act of 1984 mandates federal investigation if any of the following conditions are met:

1. Replacement cost of the controlled substance taken is $500 or more.

2. A registrant or other person is killed or suffers "significant" bodily injury during the commission of the controlled substance robbery or theft.

3. Interstate or foreign commerce is involved in planning or executing the crime.

The penalties for violating the Act's provisions are as follows:

1. Conviction for commission of burglary or robbery can result in a maximum $25,000 fine and/or 20 years imprisonment.

2. Conviction for use of a dangerous weapon in the commission of the crime can result in a maximum $35,000 fine and/or 25 years imprisonment.

3. If death results from the crime, the convicted person can receive a maximum $50,000 fine and/or life imprisonment.

Emergency Oral Prescription—Schedule II

- The pharmacist must make a reasonable, good faith effort to identify the prescriber, if not known;
- The pharmacist must immediately write the prescription in proper form;
- The quantity is limited to treating the patient during the emergency period;

- The prescriber is required to deliver a written "follow-up" prescription *within seven (7) days* after authorizing the emergency oral prescription;
- If the pharmacist does not receive the "follow-up" prescription, the nearest DEA office must be notified.

Written Prescriptions Controlled Substances

Pursuant to *federal regulations,* all prescriptions for controlled substances must contain the following:

- date when issued (signed) by prescriber
- full name of patient
- address of patient
- name of drug
- strength of drug (if applicable)
- dosage form
- quantity prescribed
- directions for use
- name of prescriber
- address of prescriber
- DEA registration of prescriber
- prescriber's signature

Prescriptions shall be *written* with:

- ink
- typewriter
- indelible pencil
- non-erasable ball point pen

Prescriptions shall be *signed* with:

- ink
- indelible pencil
- non-erasable ball point pen

Prescriptions may be prepared by an employee or agent for the signature of the prescriber, but the prescribing practitioner is responsible in case the written prescription does not conform in all essential respects to the law.

A corresponding liability results upon the pharmacist who dispenses a prescription not prepared as mandated by law.

Source: 21 CFR 1306.05.

QUESTIONS: CHAPTER 4

MISCELLANEOUS

1. Generally speaking, which of the following persons can prescribe controlled substances?

    a. Pharmacist
    b. Nurse
    c. Optometrist
    d. Medical doctor
    e. Psychologist

21 CFR 1306.03(a)

2. A written prescription for a controlled substance shall contain:
1) The date of its issue
2) The prescriber's signature
3) The patient's full name and address
4) The prescriber's DEA registration number
5) The prescriber's name and office address

    a. 1), 2), and 5) are correct.
    b. 1), 2), and 3) are correct.
    c. 1), 2), 3), and 4) are correct.
    d. 1), 2), 3), and 5) are correct.
    e. 1), 2), 3), 4), and 5) are correct.   21 CFR 1306.05(a)

3. A prescription for a controlled substance shall be written with:

    a. Ink
    b. Ink, indelible pencil
    c. Ink, pencil, typewriter
    d. Ink, pencil, indelible pencil, typewriter
    e. Ink, indelible pencil, typewriter, non-erasable ball-point pen   21 CFR 1306.05(a)

4. Which federal government agency is responsible for the enforcement of the Controlled Substances Act?

    a. DEA
    b. FDA
    c. BNDD
    d. FBI
    e. FTC   21 CFR 291.501

5. The total number of dosage units of all controlled substances distributed to DEA registrants by a practitioner during the twelve-month period in which the practitioner is registered to *dispense* cannot exceed _____ percent of the total number of dosage units of all controlled substances distributed *and* dispensed during this time period:

    a. 5
    b. 10
    c. 12
    d. 15
    e. 20   21 CFR 1307.11(a)(4)

6. The DEA is a component of the:

    a. Department of Customs and Immigration
    b. Department of Health and Human Services
    c. Department of Justice
    d. Department of Health, Education and Welfare
    e. Federal Bureau of Investigation   21 CFR 291.501

7. The Drug Enforcement Administration is the federal government agency responsible for enforcement of the:

    a. Food, Drug and Cosmetic Act, as Amended
    b. Poison Prevention Packaging Act
    c. Consumer Product Safety Act
    d. Controlled Substances Act
    e. Federal Hazardous Substances Act   21 CFR 291.501

8. "Caution: Federal law prohibits the transfer of this drug to any person other than the patient for whom it was prescribed." This statement is required as part of the prescription label for:
   1) Schedule II narcotics
   2) Schedule II non-narcotics
   3) Schedule III drugs
   4) Schedule IV drugs
   5) Schedule V prescription drugs

      a. 1) and 2) are correct.
      b. 1), 2), and 3) are correct.
      c. 1), 2), 3), and 4) are correct.
      d. 3), 4), and 5) are correct.
      e. 1), 2), 3), 4), and 5) are correct.   21 CFR 290.5

9. Generally speaking, which of the following can prescribe controlled substances?

      a. DVM
      b. DMD
      c. DDS
      d. MD
      e. All of the above   21 CFR 1306.03(a)

10. A prescription for a controlled substance:
   1) Must be issued only for a legitimate medical purpose
   2) Must be issued only by a DEA registered physician acting in the usual course of his/her profession
   3) May be communicated by the office nurse to the pharmacist if so authorized by the prescriber
   4) May be issued to an addict for detoxification purposes
   5) May be issued by the prescriber to obtain such drugs for dispensing to patients in the office

      a. 1), 2), and 3) are correct.
      b. 1), 2), 3), and 4) are correct.
      c. 2), 3), and 4) are correct.
      d. 3), 4), and 5) are correct.
      e. 1), 2), 3), 4), and 5) are correct.

11. An M.D. prescribed 360 Phenobarbital tablets 30 mg for her pet cat, two tablets to be given three times a day with milk:

      a. The dose is too high and should be lowered.
      b. The prescription is illegal.
      c. The prescription should be limited to a 30-day supply.
      d. Phenobarbital may be given without milk.   21 CFR 1301.22(a)(3)

SCHEDULES OF CONTROLLED SUBSTANCES

1. Controlled substances are divided into five schedules based on:

      a. Relative potential for abuse
      b. Currently accepted usual adult dose
      c. Currently accepted average adult dose
      d. USAN classification
      e. Chemical classification   21 U.S.C. 812

2. Drugs which have a currently accepted medical use in the United States and have a high abuse potential with severe psychic or physical dependence liability are included in:

    a. Schedule I
    b. Schedule II
    c. Schedule III
    d. Schedule IV
    e. Schedule V   21 U.S.C. 812

3. Drugs which have a currently accepted medical use in the United States and an abuse potential which may lead to a limited physical or psychological dependence are included in:

    a. Schedule I
    b. Schedule II
    c. Schedule III
    d. Schedule IV
    e. Schedule V   21 U.S.C. 812

4. An example of a Schedule I drug is:

    a. Heroin
    b. Codeine
    c. Cocaine
    d. Oxycodone
    e. Morphine   21 CFR 1308.11

5. An example of a Schedule II drug is:

    a. Marijuana
    b. Meperidine
    c. Mescaline
    d. Methaqualone
    e. Methyprylon   21 CFR 1308.12

6. Drugs which have a currently accepted medical use in the United States and have a low abuse potential and limited physical or psychological dependence are included in:

    a. Schedule I
    b. Schedule II
    c. Schedule III
    d. Schedule IV
    e. Schedule V   21 U.S.C. 812

7. Drugs which have accepted medical use in the United States and a potential for abuse which may lead to moderate or low physical dependence or high psychological dependence are included in:

    a. Schedule I
    b. Schedule II
    c. Schedule III
    d. Schedule IV
    e. Schedule V   12 U.S.C. 812

8. The person having authority to reschedule a controlled substance is the:

    a. Commissioner of FDA
    b. Secretary of the Department of Health and Human Services
    c. Attorney General of the United States
    d. Director of the FBI
    e. Administrator of the Bureau of Narcotics and Dangerous Drugs   21 U.S.C. 811(a)

9. Drugs which do not have a currently accepted medical use in the United States, have a high potential for abuse, and lack safety for use under medical supervision are included in:

   a. Schedule I
   b. Schedule II
   c. Schedule III
   d. Schedule IV
   e. Schedule V   21 U.S.C. 812

10. An example of a Schedule IV drug is:

   a. Amytal Pulvule 65 mg
   b. Tylenol with Codeine No. 4 tablet
   c. Lomotil tablet
   d. Darvon-N tablet
   e. Terpin Hydrate with Codeine Elixir   21 CFR 1308.14

11. The person having authority to remove controls over a controlled substance is the:

   a. Commissioner of FDA
   b. Secretary of the Department of Health and Human Services
   c. Attorney General of the United States
   d. Director of the FBI
   e. Administrator of the Bureau of Narcotics and Dangerous Drugs   21 U.S.C. 811(a)

12. An example of a Schedule V drug is:

   a. Robitussin A-C Syrup
   b. Valium 2 mg tablet
   c. Fiorinal capsule
   d. Seconal Pulvule 100 mg
   e. Meprobamate 400 mg tablet   21 CFR 1308.15

13. An example of a Schedule III drug is:

   a. Amobarbital sodium capsule 200 mg
   b. Amphetamine tablet 5 mg
   c. Tylenol with Codeine No. 3 tablet
   d. Nembutal capsule 100 mg
   e. Phenobarbital tablet 15 mg   21 CFR 1308.13

14. The person having authority to classify a drug as a controlled substance is the:

   a. Commissioner of FDA
   b. Secretary of the Department of Health and Human Services
   c. Attorney General of the United States
   d. Director of the FBI
   e. Administrator of the Bureau of Narcotics and Dangerous Drugs   21 U.S.C. 811(a)

15. According to federal law, in which schedule would the following prescription be included?

Rx Codeine Sulfate   grains (X)
         Actifed Syrup   qs 240 mL
              Sig: Two teasp. q 4 hrs.

   a. Schedule I
   b. Schedule II
   c. Schedule III
   d. Schedule IV
   e. Schedule V   21 CFR 1308.15

16. An example of a Schedule II drug is:

    a. Tylox capsule

    b. Fioricet w/Codeine capsule

    c. Triaminic Expectorant liquid

    d. Propoxyphene HCl compound
21 CFR 1308

17. An example of a Schedule V drug is:

    a. Tylenol w/Codeine Elixir

    b. Tylenol w/Codeine No. 2 tablet

    c. Tylenol w/Codeine No. 3 tablet

    d. Tylenol PM, Extra Strength Tablet
21 CFR 1308

SCHEDULE II

1. If the pharmacist cannot supply the balance of a partially filled prescription for a C-II drug within the 72-hour period of the first partial filling, the pharmacist shall:

    a. Notify the prescriber.

    b. Notify the nearest office of the DEA.

    c. Notify the prescriber *and* the nearest office of the DEA.

    d. Tell the patient to obtain a new written prescription.

    e. There is no need to do anything.
21 CFR 1306.13(a)

2. In an emergency, the pharmacist is legally permitted to dispense a C-II drug upon receiving oral authorization from a prescriber:

    a. A 24-hour supply of the drug if used in accordance with directions

    b. A 72-hour supply of the drug if used in accordance with directions

    c. A 5-day supply of the drug if used in accordance with directions

    d. An amount adequate to treat the patient during the emergency period
21 CFR 1306.11(d)(1)

3. The prescriber of an emergency oral prescription for a C-II controlled substance is required to provide a written prescription to the pharmacist within _____ after having authorized such prescription:

    a. 24 hours

    b. 48 hours

    c. 72 hours

    d. 7 days

    e. 30 days
21 CFR 1306.11(d)(4)

4. What is the pharmacist required to do upon receiving an emergency oral authorization to dispense a Schedule II controlled substance?

1) Immediately reduce the prescription to writing.

2) Make a reasonable effort to determine that the oral authorization came from a DEA registered practitioner.

3) Make a good faith effort to insure proper identity of the prescriber.

4) Verify the prescriber's telephone number with that listed in the telephone directory.

    a. 1), 2), and 3) are correct.

    b. 2), 3), and 4) are correct.

    c. 1), 3), and 4) are correct.

    d. 1), 2), and 4) are correct.

    e. 1), 2), 3), and 4) are correct.
21 CFR 1306.11(d)(3)

5. If a pharmacist does not receive a written prescription as a follow-up to an emergency oral prescription for a Schedule II substance, the pharmacist must notify the nearest DEA office within:

    a. 72 hours

    b. 5 days

    c. 14 days

    d. 30 days

    e. A time is not specified in the regulations.   21 CFR 1306.11(d)(4)

6. The dispensing of a Schedule II substance is permissible if the pharmacist is unable to supply the full quantity prescribed to an outpatient. The remaining portion of the prescription may be dispensed within _____ of the first partial filling:

    a. 24 hours

    b. 72 hours

    c. 5 days

    d. 7 days

    e. 60 days   21 CFR 1306.13(a)

7. What is the pharmacist required to do upon receiving the written follow-up prescription to an emergency oral prescription for a C-II drug?

    a. Throw away the emergency oral prescription which had been reduced to writing.

    b. Keep the written follow-up prescription and send the *written* emergency oral prescription to DEA.

    c. Place the written follow-up prescription in the controlled substances prescription file.

    d. Attach the follow-up prescription to the *written* emergency oral prescription and place both in the C-II prescription file.   21 CFR 1306.11(d)(4)

8. Federal regulations permit the partial filling of a Schedule II controlled substance. The balance of the prescription may be supplied to a patient in a nursing home within:

    a. 5 days

    b. 7 days

    c. 30 days

    d. One month

    e. 60 days   21 CFR 1306.13(a)

9. Partial filling of a prescription for a Schedule II controlled substance to a patient in an LTCF is permitted. Such prescription shall be valid from the issue date for a period of:

    a. 24 hours

    b. 7 days

    c. 30 days

    d. 60 days

    e. 90 days   21 CFR 1306.13(b)

10. For each partial filling of a C-II drug for a patient in an LTCF, which of the following is the pharmacist required to record on the reverse side of the written prescription (or on another appropriate record):

    1) The date of the partial filling

    2) Quantity dispensed

    3) Remaining quantity authorized to be dispensed

    4) Identification of the dispenser

    a. 1) and 2) are correct.

    b. 1), 2), and 3) are correct.

    c. 1), 2), and 4 are correct.

    d. 2), 3), and 4) are correct.

    e. 1), 2), 3), and 4) are correct.   21 CFR 1306.13(b)

11. An emergency oral prescription for a Schedule II drug product is limited to:

    a. A 72 hours supply.

    b. A 5 days supply.

    c. A 7 days supply.

    d. An adequate amount to treat the patient during the emergency period.   21 CFR 1306.11

12. Which one of the following prescriptions cannot be refilled?

    a. Schedule V

    b. Schedule IV

    c. Schedule III

    d. Schedule II

    e. Schedule I   21 CFR 1306.12

13. For which of the following may a pharmacist dispense a prescription pursuant to an oral order from a duly authorized prescriber?

    1) Schedule II

    2) Schedule III

    3) Schedule IV

    4) Schedule V

    a. 1) is correct.

    b. 1) and 2) are correct.

    c. 2), 3), and 4) are correct.

    d. 1), 2), 3), and 4) are correct.   21 CFR 1306.21

14. A duly authorized practitioner may obtain C-II drug products "for office use" by:

    a. Utilizing a "KOW"

    b. Writing a prescription with a patient's name on it

    c. Using a DEA Form 222

    d. Calling the pharmacy with an emergency oral order

    e. Writing a prescription with the notation "for office use"   21 CFR 1306.04(b)

15. What must the pharmacist do if the prescriber of an emergency oral prescription for a C-II drug product is not known to him/her?

    1) Nothing

    2) Make a resonable effort to determine that the oral authorization came from a DEA registered practitioner

    3) Make good faith efforts to insure prescriber's identity

    4) Verify prescriber's address and telephone number in the telephone directory

    5) Call the regional DEA's "hot line" to request information

    a. 1) is correct.

    b. 1) or 5) is correct.

    c. 2), 3), and 4) are correct.

    d. 1) or 4) or 5) are correct.

    e. 2), 3), and 5) are correct   21 CFR 1306.11(a)(3)

SCHEDULES III AND IV

1. You, the pharmacist, receive a written prescription for a C-IV drug with authorization from the prescriber to refill it once. What information is required to be entered on the reverse side of the prescription at the time of the refill?
1) Date of dispensing the refill
2) Initials of the dispensing pharmacist
3) The distributor's name, if a generic drug
4) Amount dispensed
5) Price charged the patient for the prescription, if a partial refill

    a. 1), 2), 3), and 4) are correct.
    b. 1), 2), and 4) are correct.
    c. 1), 3), and 4) are correct.
    d. 1), 2), 4), and 5) are correct.
    e. 1), 2), 3), 4) and 5) are correct.   21 CFR 1306.22(a)

2. The transfer of original prescription information for a controlled substance listed in Schedule III, IV, or V for the purpose of refill dispensing is permissible between pharmacies provided:
1) It is on a one-time basis.
2) Both the original and transferred prescription are maintained for a period of two years from the date of the last refill.
3) The transfer is communicated directly between two licensed pharmacists.
4) The procedure allowing the transfer prescription information is permitted pursuant to state or other applicable law.

    a. 1) and 2) are correct.
    b. 1), 2), and 3) are correct.
    c. 1), 3), and 4) are correct.
    d. 2), 3), and 4) are correct.
    e. 1), 2), 3), and 4) are correct.   21 CFR 1306.26

3. What is the maximum number of times and for how long may a written prescription for either a C-III or C-IV drug be refilled from the date of issue?
    a. Up to 6x within 5 months
    b. As often as indicated by the prescriber up to 6x within 5 months
    c. Up to 5x within 6 months.
    d. As often as indicated by the prescriber up to 5x within 6 months.
    e. As often as indicated by the prescriber up to 6 months.   21 CFR 1306.22(a)

4. For how long a period of time is a written or oral prescription for a C-III or C-IV drug valid after it is issued by the prescriber?
    a. 72 hours
    b. 5 days
    c. 30 days
    d. One month
    e. six months   21 CFR 1306.22(a)

5. You receive a valid prescription for Fiorinal w/Codeine No. 1 Capsule, DTD No. 20. You have only ten capsules in stock. Pursuant to federal law, how much time do you have to supply the balance of ten capsules to the patient?
    a. 72 hours
    b. 5 days
    c. 30 days
    d. 60 days
    e. 6 months   21 CFR 1306.22(a)

SCHEDULE V

1. An OTC Schedule V product may be sold by a pharmacist to an individual who is at least _____ years of age:

    a. 16
    b. 18
    c. 21
    d. 30
    e. 60

21 CFR 1306.32 (a) and (c)

2. A person purchasing a Schedule V drug product which is not a prescription, must be at least _____ years of age:

    a. 16
    b. 18
    c. 19
    d. 21

21 CFR 1306.32

3. C-V controlled substances which do not require a prescription consist mainly of preparations containing narcotic ingredients and are generally used as:

    a. Antitussives
    b. Analgesics
    c. Antidiarrheals
    d. a. and c.
    e. All of the above

21 CFR 1306.32(b)

4. Which one does not belong?

    a. Novahistine DH
    b. Lomotil
    c. Dilaudid
    d. Opium Tincture
    e. Paregoric

21 CFR 3106.32(b)

5. An OTC Schedule V product is sometimes referred to as an:

    a. Excepted prescription drug
    b. Exempt narcotic
    c. Excluded non-narcotic over-the-counter substance
    d. Class A drug
    e. Class B drug

6. Which of the following is *not* required to be entered in the bound record book for the sale of OTC Schedule V controlled substances?

    a. Name and address of purchaser
    b. Intended use
    c. Date of purchase
    d. Signature or written initials of the dispensing pharmacist
    e. Name and quantity of controlled substance purchased

21 CFR 1306.32(e)

7. A Schedule V drug may be sold without prescription at retail provided that:
1) The sale is made by a pharmacist.
2) The purchaser is at least eighteen years of age.
3) Not more than 240 mL of any substance containing opium is sold to the purchaser in any 48-hour period.
4) Suitable identification is provided by the purchaser if not known to the pharmacist.
5) Not more than 24 dosage units of any other controlled substance (other than opium) is sold to the purchaser in any 48-hour period.

    a. 1), 2), 3), and 5) are correct.
    b. 1), 2), 4), and 5) are correct.
    c. 1), 3), and 5) are correct.
    d. 1), 2), and 4) are correct.
    e. 1), 2), 3), 4), and 5) are correct.   21 CFR 1306.32

8. Which of the following may be sold as OTC Schedule V drugs?
1) Brontex liquid
2) Brontex tablet
3) Robitussin AC
4) Lomotil tablet
5) Paregoric

    a. 1) and 3) are correct.
    b. 1), 2), and 3) are correct.
    c. 2), 3), and 5) are correct.
    d. 1), 2), 3), and 4) are correct.
    e. 1), 2), 3), 4), and 5) are correct.   21 CFR 1306.32(b)

9. Which of the following is required to be entered in the Schedule V bound record book when an OTC Schedule V product is sold at retail?
1) Name and address of purchaser
2) Name and quantity of the product purchased
3) Date of sale
4) Age of purchaser
5) Initials or name of dispensing pharmacist

    a. 1), 2), and 3) are correct.
    b. 1), 2), 3), and 5) are correct.
    c. 2), 3), 4), and 5) are correct.
    d. 1), 2), 3), 4), and 5) are correct.
    e. 1), 2), 3), and 4) are correct.   21 CFR 1306.32(e)

10. A prescription for a controlled substance listed in Schedule V may be refilled:
    a. Indefinitely
    b. Indefinitely, but only the number of times authorized by the prescriber
    c. Indefinitely, but only as authorized by the prescriber up to 5 times
    d. Five times within six months from the date of issue of the prescription, as authorized by the prescriber
    e. Only as expressly authorized by the prescriber on the prescription   21 CFR 1306.31(a)

11. Who is permitted to sell Schedule V non-prescription drugs?
    a. Pharmacist
    b. Pharmacy intern
    c. Pharmacy technician
    d. All of the above
    e. Pharmacist and pharmacy intern   21 CFR 1306.32(a)

12. What is the maximum quantity of an OTC Schedule V drug product containing opium that is permitted to be sold in any 48-hour period?

    a. 60 cc

    b. 120 cc

    c. 240 cc

    d. 480 cc   21 CFR 1306.32(b)

13. What is the maximum number of dosage units of a Schedule V drug product containing a controlled substance other than opium that may be sold at retail within any given 48-hour period?

    a. 12

    b. 24

    c. 36

    d. 48   21 CFR 1306.32(b)

14. A 21-year-old customer with suitable identification wants to purchase Robitussin AC Syrup. What is the most that the pharmacist may sell this person without a prescription?

    a. Cannot sell, because product requires either a written or oral prescription

    b. 60 cc

    c. 120 cc

    d. 240 cc   21 CFR 1306.32(b)

REGISTRATION

1. How often must a pharmacist register his/her pharmacist's license with the Drug Enforcement Administration?

    a. Annually

    b. Biennially

    c. Every five years

    d. Every three years   21 U.S.C. 827(a)

    e. A pharmacist need not register the license with DEA   21 CFR 1301.24(b)

2. The ABC Hospital Medical Center operates a central pharmacy within the hospital, a satellite pharmacy on the fourth floor of the hospital, and an outpatient pharmacy in a building which houses the hospital's clinic three miles from the central location. How many DEA pharmacy registrations must the ABC Hospital Medical Center apply for?

    a. One

    b. Two

    c. Three   21 U.S.C. 823(f)

    d. None, because hospitals are exempt   21 CFR 1301.23(a)

3. The DEA registration alpha-numeric *number* consists of:

    a. Seven alpha-numeric characters

    b. Two alphabet characters + 9 digits

    c. Two digits + 7 alphabet characters

    d. Two digits + 9 alphabet characters

    e. Two alphabet characters + 7 digits

4. The second position of the DEA alpha-numeric registration number refers to the:

    a. Type of registrant, i.e., dispenser or distributor

    b. First initial of the registrant's first name

    c. Last initial of the registrant's last name

    d. First initial of the registrant's last name

    e. Last initial of the registrant's first name

5. The first position *B* of the DEA alpha-numeric registration number identifies a:

    a. Registrant engaged in the distribution of controlled substances
    b. Pusher of controlled substances
    c. Dispenser of controlled substances
    d. Consumer of controlled substances
    e. Pharmacist who fills prescriptions of controlled substances

6. The DEA registration is terminated when the registrant:

    a. Dies, e.g., a physician
    b. Goes out of business, e.g., a pharmacy
    c. Ceases legal existence, e.g., a partnership
    d. Discontinues professional practice, e.g., a physician
    e. All of the above   21 CFR 1301.62

7. Any person who is registered with DEA may apply to be re-registered not more than _____ before the expiration date of the registration:

    a. 14 days
    b. 30 days
    c. 45 days
    d. 60 days
    e. 3 months   21 CFR 1301.31(b)

8. Every pharmacy in the United States registered with DEA must re-register:

    a. Annually
    b. Biennially
    c. Triennially
    d. There is no need to re-register.

9. Any member of the U.S. military who is authorized to prescribe, dispense, or administer a controlled substance in the course of official duties is required to register with DEA:

    a. Annually
    b. Biennially
    c. Triennially
    d. Such persons are exempt from registration.   21 CFR 1301.25(a)

10. How soon before the proposed transfer of business activities must a pharmacy-registrant submit required information to the regional DEA administrator either in person, or by registered or certified mail, return receipt requested?

    a. 7 days
    b. 10 days
    c. 14 days
    d. 30 days
    e. 72 hours   21 CFR 1307.14

11. Any physician who is not registered with DEA and who is a resident in a hospital may administer and prescribe controlled substances, provided that:

    a. The physician is authorized to do so by state authority where he is practicing.
    b. The physician acts only within the scope of employment in the hospital.
    c. The hospital authorizes the physician to administer and prescribe under its registration.
    d. The hospital assigns a special internal code for each physician.
    e. All of the above   21 CFR 1301.24

12. How soon before discontinuing business activities is a pharmacy-registrant required to report such intent to the regional DEA administrator either in person, or by registered or certified mail, return receipt requested?

    a. 7 days

    b. 10 days

    c. 14 days

    d. 30 days

    e. 60 months

21 CFR 1307.14

13. Which of the following is a valid DEA registration?

    a. John Mortrin, MD   AM 1854911

    b. Winthrop A. Stearns, DDS   BW 1977036

    c. Vi Syneral, DVM   VS 1874321

    d. Alpha Beta Drug Wholesaler   RB 8346000

14. Which of the following is a valid DEA registration?

    a. B.A. Demerol, MD   BD 1854911

    b. I.V. Morphine, OD   AI 1977036

    c. U.R. Numorphan, DO   UR 1874331

    d. James H. Geritol, DMD   BG 18174456

15. Manufacturers and distributors of controlled substances are required to register with DEA:

    a. Annually

    b. Biennially

    c. Triennially

    d. There is no need to register with DEA.

21 U.S.C. 827

ORDER FORMS

1. Which of the following, among other things, must be recorded on the retained copy of the federal order form when a Schedule II substance is received by the purchaser (pharmacist)?

    a. Size of package(s) and date received

    b. Signature of person checking order

    c. Name of product received

    d. Number of packages received and date on which received

    e. Size of package and quantity received

21 CFR 1305.09(e)

2. Which of the following does *not* require a federal triplicate order form?

    a. Amytal sodium

    b. Codeine sulfate powder

    c. Lomotil tablet

    d. Tuinal Pulvule

    e. Percodan tablet

21 CFR 1308.15(c)(4)

3. Which of the following does *not* require a federal triplicate order form?

    a. Phenobarbital tablet

    b. Codeine sulfate powder

    c. Seconal Pulvule

    d. Demerol tablet

    e. Nembutal capsule

21 CFR 1308.15(c)(2)

4. Pursuant to federal law, what is the supplier of a Schedule II drug required to do with the order form?
   a. Retain copy 1, and send copy 2 to DEA.
   b. Retain copy 2, and send copy 1 to DEA.
   c. Retain copy 1 and copy 2.
   d. Retain copy 1, and return copy 2 to purchaser.
   e. Return copy 2 to purchaser, and send copy 1 to DEA.   21 CFR 1305.09(d)

5. The copy of an endorsed federal order form for a Schedule II controlled substance shall be retained by the purchaser (from the last date of entry) for:
   a. 30 days
   b. One month
   c. 6 months
   d. 2 years
   e. 5 years   21 CFR 1305.13(c)

6. The pharmacist places an order for a Schedule II controlled substance with a source of supply. Pursuant to federal law, what is the pharmacist required to do?
   a. Retain copy 1, send copy 2 to DEA, and send copy 3 to supplier.
   b. Retain copy 2, send copy 3 to DEA, and send copy 1 to supplier.
   c. Retain copy 3, and send copy 1 and copy 2 to supplier.
   d. Retain copy 2, and send copy 1 and copy 3 to supplier.
   e. Retain copy 3, send copy 1 to DEA, and send copy 2 to supplier.   21 CFR 1305.09(a)

7. According to federal regulations, if a vendor cannot supply the entire order for a Schedule II drug product, within what period of time may the balance of said order be shipped to the purchaser?
   a. 72 hours from date order was issued by purchaser
   b. 30 days from date order was issued by purchaser
   c. 60 days from date order was issued by purchaser
   d. 60 days from date order was shipped by vendor
   e. 60 days from date order was received by vendor   21 CFR 1305.09(b)

8. Which of the following may sign an order form for a Schedule II drug?
   a. Staff pharmacist
   b. Pharmacy intern
   c. Community pharmacy owner
   d. Hospital administrator
   e. Person who signed the most recent DEA application for re-registration of the pharmacy
          21 CFR 1305.07

9. The controlled substance order form is intended only for ordering _____ drugs:
   a. Schedule I only
   b. Schedule II only
   c. Schedule I and II
   d. Schedule II, III, and IV
   e. Schedule V   21 CFR 1305.03

10. You make a mistake on a DEA triplicate order form by indicating the right quantity but the wrong medication on one line. Everything else on the form has been filled out correctly. How does DEA law advise you to handle this?

    a. Erase the error and write in the correct quantity on each copy of the form.

    b. Draw a line through the line with the error and rewrite the correct quantity and medication on the next blank line.

    c. Void the entire order form and send copies 1 and 2 to the DEA.

    d. Void the entire form, send copies 1 and 2 to the DEA, and retain copy 3 on file available for inspection for two years.

    e. Void the entire form, and retain copy 1, copy 2, and copy 3.　21 CFR 1305.11(a)

11. The controlled substance order form must be prepared by use of:

    a. Typewriter

    b. Pen

    c. Indelible pencil

    d. Non-erasable ball-point pen

    e. All of the above　21 CFR 1305.06(a)

12. Which of the following DEA authorized registrants is permitted to purchase reasonable quantities of either etorphine hydrochloride or diprenorphine using the triplicate federal order form?

    a. Community pharmacist

    b. Hospital pharmacist

    c. Veterinarian engaged in exotic animal practice

    d. Osteopathic physician

    e. Veterinarian engaged in farm animal practice　21 CFR 1305.16(b)

13. If an order for a Schedule II substance cannot be filled for any reason, the supplier shall:

    a. Return copy 1 to purchaser, and retain copy 2.

    b. Return copy 2 to purchaser, and retain copy 1.

    c. Retain copy 1, and send copy 2 to DEA indicating why the order was not filled.

    d. Return copy 1 and copy 2 to purchaser, and indicate why the order was not filled.

    e. Request copy 3 from purchaser, retain copy 1, send copy 2 to DEA, and indicate why the order was not filled.　21 CFR 1305.11(b)

14. If the DEA registration of any purchaser terminates for any reason, all unused triplicate order forms shall be:

    a. Destroyed by the registrant

    b. Returned to the nearest DEA office

    c. Surrendered to a DEA agent at the registrant's location

    d. Passed on to the new owner of the registered location (pharmacy)

    e. None of the above　21 CFR 1305.14

15. Copy 2 of the triplicate order form for a Schedule I drug shall be forwarded by the supplier to DEA:

    a. Within 72 hours after order was shipped to purchaser

    b. Within 60 days after order was shipped to purchaser

    c. By the 15th day of the month following the month in which shipment was made to purchaser

    d. At the close of the month in which shipment was made to purchaser

    e. Within six months from the date the order form was issued by the purchaser　21 CFR 1305.09(d)

16. If an unfilled order form for a Schedule II drug has been lost, the purchaser shall:

    a. Execute another order form and send copy 1 and copy 2 to the supplier:

    b. Issue a written statement containing the serial number and date of the lost form, and indicate that the drugs from the first order were not received.

    c. Attach copy 3 of the second order form to copy 3 of the lost order form.

    d. Attach the copy of the written statement in b. above to copy 1 and copy 2 sent to supplier.

    e. All of the above   21 CFR 1305.12(a)

17. Which of the following must be included on the order form for a Schedule II drug at the time the order is issued by the purchaser:

    1) Total number of item(s) ordered
    2) Date of the order
    3) Name of the drug
    4) The name and address of the supplier
    5) Signature of the person authorized to place the order

    a. 2), 3), and 4) are correct.

    b. 1), 3), and 5) are correct.

    c. 1), 2), 3), and 4) are correct.

    d. 1), 2), 3), 4), and 5) are correct.   21 CFR 1305.06

18. If an order for a Schedule II drug cannot be filled for any reason, and copy 1 and copy 2 of the order form are returned to the purchaser by the supplier, what should the purchaser do?

    a. Attach copy 1 and copy 2 to copy 3.

    b. Attach copy 1 to copy 3, and send copy 2 to DEA.

    c. Attach copy 2 to copy 3, and send copy 1 to DEA.

    d. Send copy 1, copy 2, and copy 3 to DEA with supplier's statement why the order was not filled.

    e. The purchaser shouldn't do anything.   21 CFR 1305.11(c)

19. The controlled substance order form is not valid beyond _____ after its execution by the purchaser:

    a. 72 hours

    b. 10 days

    c. 30 days

    d. 60 days

    e. 6 months   21 CFR 1305.09(b)

20. A purchaser may cancel part or all of an order for a Schedule II drug by:

    a. Notifying the nearest DEA office in writing

    b. Notifying the supplier by telephone

    c. Notifying the supplier in writing and including copy 3 of the triplicate order form

    d. Notifying the supplier in writing

    e. Notifying the supplier in writing and requesting that copy 1 and copy 2 of the triplicate order form be returned   21 CFR 1305.15(a)

21. How many lines are there on a DEA Form 222 order form?

    a. Three

    b. Five

    c. Nine

    d. Ten

    e. Twelve   21 CFR 1305.06(b)

22. How many drugs may be ordered on a DEA Form 222?

    a. Three
    b. Five
    c. Nine
    d. Ten
    e. Twelve

21 CFR 1305.06(b)

23. What is the minimum number of Form 222 that may be obtained from DEA?

    a. Three
    b. Five
    c. Seven
    d. Ten
    e. Twelve

21 CFR 1305.05(a)

24. How many copies does the triplicate DEA Form 222 contain?

    a. One
    b. Two
    c. Three
    d. Five

21 CFR 1305.05(a)

25. What information is imprinted on Form 222 when sent by the DEA to the registrant?
  1) Serial number of form
  2) Name and address of registrant
  3) Authorized activity and schedule of the registrant
  4) Date forms are issued by DEA to registrant
  5) DEA registration number

    a. 1) and 2) are correct.
    b. 1), 2), and 3) are correct.
    c. 2) and 3) are correct.
    d. 2), 3), and 4) are correct.
    e. 1), 2), 3), 4), and 5) are correct.

21 CFR 1305.05(d)

26. For how long a period of time must Copy 3 of DEA Form 222 be available for inspection?

    a. Six months
    b. One year
    c. Two years
    d. Five years

21 CFR 1305.13(c)

27. Where must Copy 3 of DEA Form 222 be kept?

    a. Registered location
    b. Corporate headquarters of the chain drugstore
    c. Either corporate headquarters or registered location of chain drugstore
    d. Office at home of pharmacy owner
    e. Nowhere, form may be discarded after order is received

21 CFR 1305.13(c)

28. Which of the following controlled substances must be ordered by themselves when a DEA Form 222 is used?
1) Opium
2) Carfentanil
3) Diprenorphine HCl
4) Etorphine HCl
5) Diacetylmorphine

    a. 1) and 2) are correct.

    b. 2) and 3) are correct.

    c. 2), 3) and 4) are correct.

    d. 1), 4), and 5) are correct.

    e. 4) and 5) are correct.
21 CFR 1305.16

29. Which of the following controlled substances cannot be ordered with any other controlled substance, using a DEA Form 222?
1) Opium
2) Carfentanil
3) Diprenorphine HCl
4) Marijuana
5) Heroin

    a. 1), 4), and 5) are correct.

    b. 1) and 2) are correct.

    c. 2), 3), and 5) are correct.

    d. 2) and 3) are correct.

    e. 4) and 5) are correct.
21 CFR 1305.16

30. Schedule II substances may be ordered from a vendor by utilizing:
1) Telephone
2) FAX
3) U.S. Mail
4) Semaphore
5) E-mail

    a. 1) and 3) are correct.

    b. 1), 2), 3), and 5) are correct.

    c. 3) is correct.

    d. 5) is correct.

    e. 1) is correct.
21 CFR 1305.09(a)

31. What must the registrant do if a DEA Form 222 is imprinted incorrectly?

    a. Correct the error using a typewriter or ink pen

    b. Telephone DEA and correct error with DEA's authorization

    c. No need to do anything

    d. Return the form to DEA
21 CFR 1305.05(d)

32. What is the supplier required to do if part or all of a C-II drug order is cancelled by the purchaser?

    a. Return original and copy 2 of order form to purchaser

    b. Indicate the cancellation of the order on the original and copy 2

    c. Notify DEA of the cancellation

    d. a. and b. are correct.

    e. b. and c. are correct.
21 CFR 1305.15(a)

33. When is the "DEA Copy" of the triplicate order form required to be sent to the agency?
1) Immediately after the order is filled
2) At the end of each day
3) By the 15th day of the month following the month in which the order was filled
4) At the close of the month during which the order was filled
5) At the close of the month during which the 60 day validity period expires

    a. 1) is correct.
    b. 2) is correct.
    c. 3) is correct.
    d. 4) is correct.
    e. 4) and 5) are correct.

21 CFR 1305.09(d)

INVENTORY

1. Every inventory of controlled substances shall be kept by the DEA registrant at the registered location and be available for inspection for at least _____ from the date of such inventory:

    a. Six months
    b. Two years
    c. Three years
    d. Five years
    e. Indefinitely

21 CFR 1304.04(a)

2. Unless the registrant is informed by DEA that the permission to keep central records is denied, the registrant may begin to maintain such central records of controlled substances _____ after notifying DEA:

    a. 2 days
    b. 5 days
    c. 7 days
    d. 14 days
    e. One month

21 CFR 1304.04(a)

3. Central record keeping requirements for controlled substances do not include:
1) Executed triplicate order forms
2) Prescriptions
3) Inventories

    a. 1) and 2) are correct.
    b. 1) and 3) are correct.
    c. 2) and 3) are correct.
    d. 1), 2), and 3) are correct.

21 CFR 1304.04(b)(1)

4. To which federal government agency is the biennial controlled substance inventory sent?

    a. FDA
    b. FBI
    c. BNDD
    d. DEA
    e. To no agency

5. A DEA registrant who elects to maintain central records of controlled substances is required to deliver all or any part of such records to the registered location within _____ business days after a written request from DEA:

    a. 2
    b. 5
    c. 7
    d. 14
    e. 30   21 CFR 1304.04(b)(3)

6. When a controlled substance is reclassified to a Schedule II from a Schedule IV it must be inventoried:

    a. Biennially on May 1st
    b. Annually on May 1st
    c. Within 6 months of May 1st
    d. As of the effective date of transfer
    e. Within 6 months from the date it is so classified   21 CFR 1304.14

7. A prescription for a controlled substance may be filed in one of the following three ways. Which is correct?
  1) A pharmacy can maintain three separate files—a file for Schedule II drugs dispensed, a file for Schedules III, IV, and V drugs dispensed, and a file for prescription orders for all noncontrolled drugs dispensed.
  2) A pharmacy can maintain two files—a file for all Schedule II drugs dispensed and another file for all other drugs dispensed including those in Schedules III, IV, and V. If this method is used, the prescription orders in the file for Schedules III, IV and V must be stamped with letter *C* in red ink, not less than one inch high, in the lower right corner. This distinctive marking makes the records *readily retrievable* for inspection.
  3) A pharmacy can maintain two files—one file for all controlled drugs in all schedules and a second file for all prescription orders for noncontrolled drugs dispensed. If this method is used, the prescription orders for drugs in Schedules III, IV, and V in the controlled drug prescription file must be stamped with the red letter *C* not less than one inch high in the lower right corner, as previously mentioned.

    a. 1) is correct.
    b. 2) is correct.
    c. 3) is correct.
    d. 2) and 3) are correct.
    e. 1) and 2) and 3) are correct.   21 CFR 1304.04(h)(2)

8. The initial inventory record of controlled substances must:
  1) List the name, address, and DEA registration number of the registrant.
  2) Indicate the date and the time the inventory is taken, i.e., opening or close of business.
  3) Be signed by the person or persons responsible for taking the inventory.
  4) Be maintained at the location appearing on the registration certificate for at least two years.
  5) Keep records of Schedule II drugs separate from all other controlled substances.

    a. 1), 2), and 3) are correct.
    b. 1), 3), and 4) are correct.
    c. 2) and 4) are correct.
    d. 2), 4), and 5) are correct.
    e. 1), 2), 3), 4), and 5) are correct.   21 CFR 1304.11–13

9. When taking the inventory of a Schedule III controlled substance:

   a. An exact count or measure must be made.

   b. An exact count must be made of solid dosage forms only.

   c. An estimated count or measure is permitted unless the container holds more than 1,000 dosage units.

   d. An estimated count or measure is permitted unless the container holds less than 1,000 dosage units.

   e. An estimated count or measure is permitted unless the container holds more than 1,000 dosage units of a tablet or capsule, in which case an exact count must be made if the container has been opened.

10. In regard to the inventory of controlled substances, which is correct?

   1) Every two years following the date of the registrant's initial inventory, a new inventory must be taken.

   2) The information required on the biennial inventory is the same as that for the initial inventory.

   3) The biennial inventory date may be changed by the registrant to fit the regular general physical inventory date, if any, so long as the date is not more than six (6) months from the biennial date that would otherwise apply.

   4) The actual taking of the inventory should not vary more than four (4) days from the biennial inventory date.

   5) A registrant desiring to change the biennial inventory date must notify in advance the nearest DEA office of the date on which the inventory is to be taken.

   a. 1) and 2) are correct.

   b. 1), 2), and 4) are correct.

   c. 1), 2), 3), and 4) are correct.

   d. 1), 3), 4), and 5) are correct.

   e. 1), 2), 3), 4), and 5) are correct.

21 CFR 1304.11–13

CHAPTER 5

Poison Prevention Packaging Act

Introduction

The U.S. Consumer Product Safety Commission (CPSC) has the responsibility for enforcing the provisions of the Poison Prevention Packaging Act (PPPA) and its regulations at 16 *CFR* 1700. As part of its responsibilities, the CPSC investigates suspected violations of the special packaging (Child-Resistant Packaging, abbreviated as "CRP") requirements for prescription drugs being dispensed by the nation's retail pharmacists to consumers. The Commission also conducts inspections of pharmacies to check on complaints with the special packaging requirements at 16 *CFR* 1700.14(a)(10).

Recent compliance activity with a chain store pharmacy corporation and review of reports of investigations and inspections during 1990 and 1991 revealed that there is an apparent misconception on the part of pharmacists in many areas of the country regarding their responsibility to comply with the special packaging requirements for the PPPA.

The mandatory safety standard at 16 *CFR* 1700.14(a)(10) requires that "Any drug for human use that is in a dosage form intended for oral administration and that is required by Federal law to be dispensed only by or upon an oral or written pre-

scription of a practitioner licensed by law to administer such drug shall be packaged in accordance with the provisions of Part 1700.15(a), (b), and (c). . . ." There is an exception to this requirement for 17 specific drugs listed in Part 1700.14(a)(10).

Section 4(b) of the PPA (15 U.S.C. 1473) provides an exemption for drugs which are subject to the special packaging standards and which are dispensed pursuant to an order of a physician, dentist, or other licensed medical practitioner authorized to prescribe. Such prescription drugs may be dispensed in noncomplying packages "only when directed in such order or when requested by the purchaser."

Many pharmacists interviewed by CPSC investigators in recent years have indicated that they do not use child-resistant packaging with many of the prescriptions they dispense because the customers are "senior citizens" or have at some time in the past requested regular closures on their prescription drug containers. Some pharmacies, at some point, enter names of patients requesting non CRP in the pharmacy's computer or in a log book where the request may reside unchanged for an indefinite period (possibly as long as the individual remains a patron at the pharmacy.)

The purpose of the PPPA and the mandatory standard at 16 *CFR* 1700.14 is to *prevent* or minimize the risk of serious personal injury or serious illness to children under five (5) years of age by requiring hazardous household substances, including prescription drugs to be packaged in special child protection packaging. The exemption (Section 4(b) of the PPPA) to the standard for prescription drug packaging is meant to be the exception *not* the rule.

A patient who previously requested non child-resistant packaging may change his or her mind about use of CRP, but the patient has no obligation to spontaneously inform the pharmacist of the change in CRP preference. It is the responsibility of the dispensing pharmacist who packages the prescription drug to ensure that it is placed in CRP unless a specific request for non CRP has been initiated by the purchaser or the prescriber.

The dispensing pharmacist should keep in mind that it is not up to the pharmacist to decide whether to use CRP or non CRP on prescription drugs, although the pharmacist may specifically ask the consumer in those cases where a past prescription has been requested in non child-resistant packaging.

Finally, for their own protection and to help insure that the law is complied with, pharmacists should institute some form of record keeping procedure to document each request they receive for non child-resistant packaging for prescription drugs. The CPSC suggests that pharmacists include a waiver signed either by the patient or the caregiver.

Note: The U.S. Consumer Product Safety Commission (CPSC) has reversed its recent policy on pharmacists' duties regarding child-resistant caps; while pharmacists had been required to ask patients whether or not they want child-resistant caps each time they have a prescription dispensed, CPSC now states that patients can give pharmacists a "blanket" waiver requesting that all future medications be placed in non child-resistant packages.

(Many pharmacists have used blanket waivers since child-resistant packaging was required, but CPSC recently said they were not valid.)

CPSC points out that a single request from a patient to dispense a specific prescription in a non child-resistant bottle is enough for the pharmacist to assume that the patient always wants his or her medication placed in a non child-resistant container.

POISON PREVENTION PACKAGING ACT, PART I*

Steven Strauss, Ph.D., R.Ph.

The purpose of the Poison Prevention Act of 1970 (PPA) [1] is to prevent accidental poisoning of young children. Ingestion of a potentially hazardous substance is the most common medical emergency facing young children. The Act, and regulations issued under the Act, adopt special packaging as the means to reduce injury or illness of young children arising from the use, handling or ingestion of toxic or harmful household substances. Specific substances or categories of substances that must comply with these standards are named in both the Act and the regulations. The Act became effective on December 30, 1970 and was enforced and administered by the Food and Drug Administration (FDA). Responsibility for the Act was transferred from the FDA to the Consumer Product Safety Commission (CPSC) on May 14, 1973 [2].

The Commission is composed of five members appointed by the President of the U.S., by and with the advice and consent of the Senate, for terms of seven years.

The purpose of the Consumer Product Safety Commission is:

• To protect the public against unreasonable risks of injury associated with consumer products;

• To assist consumers in evaluating the comparative safety of consumer products;

• To develop uniform safety standards for consumer products and to minimize conflicting State and local regulations; and

• To promote research and investigation into the causes and prevention of product-related deaths, illnesses, and injuries [3].

The Act regulates, among other things, certain OTC and Rx substances, and requires that such substances be packaged for consumer use in special packages that will make them significantly difficult for children under the age of five years to open, but not difficult for adults. The child-resistant container for these substances must be sufficiently difficult so that they cannot be opened by 80 percent of children under five years of age but they must allow access to at least 90 percent of adults, who will then be able to open and properly close the package conveniently. The law does *not* require that the packaging be so difficult to open that *no* children can gain access to the contents [4]. The special packaging referred to is sometimes called "safety closures" or "child-resistant containers," not "child-safety" nor "child-proof".

Pursuant to the PPPA, the Commission (CPSC) has authority to grant exemptions from special packaging standards.

An exemption is made in the PPPA for OTC products for elderly or handicapped persons; the exemption allows the manufacturer of such products to market one size of container with non-complying packaging. Such a package must have the printed statement: THIS PACKAGE FOR HOUSEHOLDS WITHOUT YOUNG CHILDREN or if the package is small: PACKAGE NOT CHILD-RESISTANT [5].

The law places the liability on the person who supplies the pack-

*Reprinted with permission from *U.S. Pharmacist* (May 1980).

age in the form it is likely to be used by the consumer. All prescription drugs subject to a child-resistant packaging standard that are distributed to pharmacies shall be in child-resistant packaging if the immediate packages in which the drugs are distributed by the manufacturers are intended to be the packages in which the drugs are dispensed to the consumer [6]. This means safety closures are not required on manufacturer's packages of 100's, 500's, 1000's, etc., designed to be used by the pharmacist for dispensing smaller quantities in individual prescription containers. For drug products packaged in containers which are intended by the manufacturer to be dispensed to the consumer in the original package, the obligation to provide special packaging rests with the manufacturer. Prescription drugs packaged and dispensed in violation of any applicable regulations pursuant to the PPA are deemed to be misbranded under the Federal Food Drug & Cosmetic Act. The misbranding of any drug is prohibited by the latter Act and is subject to penalties of imprisonment for not more than one year or a fine of not more than $1,000, or both.

Remember, it is necessary to package all oral prescription products, with certain exemptions in safety closure containers, and OTC drugs if they are dispensed as a prescription.

The use of an "exemption statement" in the patient medication profile or any facsimile will not suffice. The exemption must be handled on a prescription-by-prescription basis in the community pharmacy. The practice of obtaining blanket orders and requests for non-complying packaging is meant to be the exception rather than the rule, and because changing circumstances in a household may present young children with the opportunity to gain access to prescription drugs.

The PPPA also states that the prescription "may be dispensed in noncomplying packages only when directed on such order (by the prescribing physician) or when requested by the purchaser" [7]. The pharmacist may post a sign or inform a patient of the options under the law. A pharmacist should not solicit patient requests for non-complying containers to evade the intent of the law, but may inform the patient of a choice of container. A patient may only exercise this right if aware of it. However, there is nothing in the law which indicates that pharmacists may encourage or "invite" the use of non-complying packaging. The U.S. Consumer Product Safety Commission indicates the purchaser may make such a request on an oral basis, but this leaves the pharmacist open to possible legal entanglements. Therefore, it is suggested that one of the forms in Figure 1 be utilized.

The statements could be implemented by using a rubber stamp on the reverse side of the prescription blank or actually imprinted on the pharmacy's blanks. In the event of a delivered prescription with no personal patient–pharmacist contact, the dispensing pharmacist could print the patient's name and initial it, using his initials.

Where prescription packaging is used only in institutional practices, such as a nursing home or hospital, it is not deemed necessary to dispense the medication in safety closure containers. In these instances the medications are kept under lock and remain under the direct supervision of professional personnel and are not in the hands of the consumer. Should the patient be discharged from the institution it would then be necessary for the medication to be properly packaged, unless the patient or physician requests otherwise.

Pursuant to the *Code of Federal Regulations* "Special packaging for substances subject to the provisions of this paragraph shall not be used" [8]. Because safety closures

---

Suggested Authorization for Exemption Forms

Form A
I request that this medication not be placed in a safety container.

_____ _____
Signature   Date

Form B

Pursuant to Section 4(b) of the Poison Prevention Packaging Act of 1970 and the regulations thereunder, I hereby request that the medication dispensed to me for use by me and/or my family be packaged and dispensed in non-safety packages.

_____ _____
Signature   Date

In the case of a telephoned prescription, the pharmacist may want to document the fact that the prescriber requested a noncomplying container. The pharmacist could complete this form and place it on file with the prescription:

Form C

Pursuant to Section 4(b) of the Poison Prevention Packaging Act of 1970 and the regulations thereunder, I certify that dispensing in non-complying packaging was requested by the prescriber.

_____ _____
Signature   Date

FIGURE 1.

can lose their effectiveness through repeated use, especially when made of plastic, *new* packaging (cap and container) must be used when prescriptions are refilled. However, when glass containers are used, using new caps for refills fulfills the poison prevention packaging requirements.

Child resistant containers or container caps may be recognized by their brand names, such as: CR-1® (Kerr Glass), Screw-Lok®, Safti-Collars® and Clin-Loc® (all Owens-Illinois), and SafeRx® (Brockway).

Proposed Exemptions for Certain Drugs

Prescription drugs have been proposed for exemption because they had not been involved in serious personal injury or illness among children. The CPSC, in evaluating exemption petitions submitted by pharmaceutical manufacturers on behalf of these products, may find sufficient merit in the petitions to propose for public comment exemption of the subject products. While a number of diverse factors are taken into account in evaluating such petitions, a major consideration is the toxicity of the particular drug product.

Proposed exemptions are not final regulations of the commission. The special packaging requirement for proposed drugs are stayed pending final action by the commission. Drug products may, in the quantities and specific amounts so noted in the exemption proposal, be dispensed in conventional packaging.

Reporting Hazardous Products

A new phone system recently set up by the Consumer Product Safety Commission should make it easier for manufacturers, distributors, and pharmacists to report suspected substantial hazards in consumer products. Callers will now be able to reach CPSC staffers 24 hours a day, seven days a week.

The number for use in the 48 contiguous states is 800-638-2772. The number for use in Alaska, Hawaii, Puerto Rico and the U.S. Virgin Islands is 800-638-8333.

The Consumer Product Safety Act requires manufacturers, distributors and pharmacists to notify the Commission about potentially hazardous products within 24 hours after discovery [9]. In the past, a report of a substantial hazard that came up in the evening or on a weekend had to be submitted by telegram, or by a telephone call registered as a recorded message on the consumer hotline. Under a new arrangement, calls made after regular working hours will automatically be transferred to a CPSC staff member in the Office of Product Defect Identification.

The initial hazard notification must include the identity of the product and the name and address of the person informing CPSC. This may be confirmed within 48 hours by a written report giving detailed information on when the product was manufactured and how widely it was distributed and the nature of potential injuries.

References

1. Public Law 91-601; 15 U.S.C. 1471, et seq; 16 CFR 1700.
2. Public Law 92-573, Sec. 30a.
3. 44 FR 77151, December 31, 1979.
4. 16 CFR 1700.15.
5. 16 CFR 1700.5 (a)(1); Public Law 91-601, Sec. 4(a).
6. 43 FR 11979, March 23, 1978.
7. Public Law 91-601, Sec. 4(b).
8. 16 CFR 1700.15 (2)(c).
9. Public Law 92-573, Sec. 15.

POISON PREVENTION PACKAGING ACT, PART II*

Steven Strauss, Ph.D., R.Ph.

The U.S. Consumer Product Safety Commission (CPSC) is responsible for the implementation

*Reprinted with permission from *U.S. Pharmacist* (September 1983).

of the Poison Prevention Packaging Act of 1970 (PPPA). Since the statute and its regulations have been in effect, there have been remarkable declines in reported ingestions by children of toxic and potentially

toxic household substances [1,2]. Latest figures (1980) from poison control centers showed that accidental ingestions of aspirin had decreased 65 percent; controlled drugs, 58 percent; products containing methyl salicylate 61 percent. In contrast, accidental ingestions of prescription drugs had declined by only 36 percent [1,3].

Some of the reasons for the disparity in reductions among the categories can be attributed to the availability of conventional packaging on request, quality control at the manufacturers' level, misuse or abuse in the home (leaving the container cap off or unsecured, transferring the contents to a non-child-resistant package), and violations of the law by the pharmacist and/or the dispensing physician.

At this point in the program's history, new child-resistant packaging standards are established on a relatively infrequent basis. Requests for exemptions from established standards are far more frequently processed by the CPSC.

An exemption request, in the form of a formal petition, is generally initiated by the manufacturer of a product. By far the majority of such requests are from manufacturers of human oral prescription drugs. Generally such requests seek exemption for a specific package size of drug, normally a package designed for direct dispensing to the consumer after appropriate labeling by the pharmacist.

The petitioner must submit various data relating to the toxicity of the product, and, generally must establish that the amount of product contained within the requested exemption would not be harmful to a child under five years of age. Formal CPSC exemption criteria exist to guide manufacturers in submitting petitions.

Exemption requests are evaluated by CPSC and reviewed by FDA personnel in much the same manner as for the establishment of new child-resistant packaging standards. Should a finding be made by the CPSC that a particular exemption request has merit, a proposal is made in the *Federal Register (FR)*. Following a suitable period for public comment, the issue is reconsidered in light of any such comments, and if no substan-

tial objections are successfully raised, a final order is published by the CPSC. Following publication of the final order in the *FR*, a manufacturer may begin to market the exempt product in a conventional package. On occasion, where the hazard is unquestionably insignificant, the CPSC may waive the requirement for child-resistant packaging at the time the proposal is published in the *FR*.

Recently completed reviews by the FDA's OTC Drug Review Panels have resulted in a number of prescription drugs being released to the OTC market or made available OTC in dosage strengths previously limited to prescription status. It is anticipated that more such releases will occur as the FDA completes its review of panel findings.

The criteria for releasing a drug to OTC status include but are not limited to toxicity; whereas the major consideration in requiring a product to be safety packaged is toxicity. Because the human oral prescription drug standard was established on an "across the board" basis for reasons of convenience and expedience, it follows that some drugs released to the OTC market will, because of their toxicity, merit continued safety packaging while others will not.

In interpreting the Poison Prevention Packaging Act, the Consumer Product Safety Commission has kept before it the concern expressed by the Congress when the legislation was passed: Child-resistant packaging was to be the rule and not the exception. Following are questions most often raised by pharmacists, practicing physicians, and manufacturers regarding child-resistant packaging.

Q. Now that FDA is requiring tamper-resistant packaging for over-the-counter drugs, will this replace the requirement for child-resistant packaging?

A. The two systems are separate. Although there are some child-resistant packages which also are tamper-resistant (blisters, unit-of-use), a child-resistant package is not necessarily tamper-resistant.

The FDA requires that evidence of tampering be visually determined on initial contact whereas child-resistant packages have specific performance standards which must be met. These include maintaining their child-resistance for the number of openings and closings customary for the life of the product.

Q. May an individual request that all of his or her prescriptions be filled in conventional (non-complying) packaging?

A. Yes, the law does not preclude a pharmacist from relying upon a *specific request* from a patient, preferably in writing, *to have all of his or her medications placed in noncomplying packaging, i.e., a blanket waiver.* However, a single request from a patient to dispense a specific prescription in non-child-resistant packaging (CRP) is not a basis for the pharmacist to infer that the patient wants all subsequent prescriptions to be dispensed in non-CRP. Such a request is not a blanket waiver.

A person who previously filed a specific blanket waiver request for non-CRP may later change his or her mind about the use of such packaging because of changing personal circumstances, but the patient may not remember to inform the pharmacist of the change in CRP preference. It would, therefore, be prudent for the dispensing pharmacist to periodically check with all patients who have blanket waiver requests on file to ensure that non-complying packaging continues to be the packaging of choice for the patients' prescription drugs.

Q. Can a state or other political subdivision establish child-resistant packaging regulations which are less or more stringent than those promulgated by the Commission?

A. No, they must be identical. However, a state may require child-resistant packaging on a substance not regulated by CPSC.

Q. How does a pharmacist or physician become aware of those drugs exempted from PPPA standards?

A. This information is available from the Commission or any of its regional offices. Announcements are published in the *Federal Register* and news releases (which may be published in the local press) are issued. In addition, the journals and newsletters of pharmaceutical and medical groups, and the trade press publicize these exemptions.

Q. May I, as a hospital pharmacist, dispense a regulated drug in a conventional package for use by a patient?

A. Yes, provided that the patient is confined in the hospital. Drugs dispensed for outpatient use must be packaged in accordance with the regulations.

Q. Our local hospital sometimes calls upon my pharmacy to provide drugs for patient use within the hospital. Must these drugs be dispensed in child-resistant packaging?

A. No, provided that they are to be used for institutionalized patients. The test is whether the package is likely to enter a home.

Q. I know of several physicians who dispense prescription drugs for a fee. Are they subject to the provisions of the PPPA?

A. Yes. Physicians who dispense drugs (including drug samples), are, and always have been, subject to the regulations under the PPPA. It is important to note, however, that under Section 4(b) of the Act, medical practitioners are given the authority to specify conventional packaging for their patients.

Q. If the pharmacist is aware that one of his patrons prefers conventional packaging for his prescriptions, can the pharmacist make this decision without the patron's specific request?

A. No. The pharmacist may advise his patron that he/she has the option of having the prescription dispensed in non-complying packaging, but the choice must be that of the patron.

Q. Must the patron make the choice for conventional packaging in writing?

A. Although many pharmacists require a written waiver, the law and its regulations neither require nor prohibit a written request. The CPSC has advised, however, that when a blanket waiver is being requested, the pharmacist should get the request in writing.

Q. May a pharmacist or an industrial nurse dispense a prescription drug in a non-complying package in response to a standing order from a physician that it be so dispensed?

A. Only as it applies to refills of a prescription where the physician has prescribed non-complying packaging. However, a drug dispensed to the same person on a different prescription of the same or another prescriber must be dispensed in special packaging unless the prescription directs the use of non-complying packaging or the purchaser requests it.

Q. Who is responsible for determining at the retail level whether or not a prescription drug must be packaged in accordance with PPPA standards.

A. It is the responsibility of the dispensing pharmacist. Unless a prescription drug is expressly exempted from the regulations, or the patron or prescriber requests non-complying packaging, the drug must be dispensed in a child-resistant package.

Q. How does a pharmacist or physician become aware of drugs which are exempted from PPPA standards?

A. This information is available from the CPSC or any of its regional offices. Announcements are published in the *Federal Register,* and news releases (published in the local press) issued. In addition, the journals and newsletters of pharmaceutical organizations, as well as the trade press, publicize these exemptions.

Q. Can a prescriber simply check a box on a prescription blank to indicate to the pharmacist that a drug be dispensed in non-complying packaging?

A. Yes. However, the CPSC seeks to discourage the use by prescribers of prescription blanks having a box to check for non-complying packaging, on the basis that the practice would tend to encourage excessive use of non-complying packaging.

Q. In the case of an antibiotic drug provided by the manufacturer in a granular form to be reconstituted by the pharmacist, who is responsible for providing the child-resistant package, the pharmacist or the manufacturer?

A. Since the product is in the same container intended to be given to the purchaser, the manufacturer and the pharmacist are responsible.

Q. Does this same rule apply to drugs dispensed in dropper bottles?

A. Yes.

Q. In the case of refills, can prescription containers be reused?

A. As a general rule, no. The standards promulgated under the Poison Prevention Packaging Act specifically prohibit the reuse of special packaging in the renewing of prescriptions for drugs subject to the standards. The reason for this prohibition is that plastic closures and containers in which the prescription was originally dispensed to the consumer might well be worn or otherwise damaged within the home to the extent that the original effectiveness specifications might be compromised, but not to the extent that such wear or damage would be noted by the pharmacist or dispensing physician prior to renewing the prescription. While this prohibition is certainly significant in the case of plastic closures fitted on plastic containers, the possibility of wear or undetected damage to glass containers is negligible. Therefore, the reuse of a glass bottle in the renewing of a prescription would not appear to compromise the child-protection embodied in the Poison Prevention Packaging Act. CPSC *would not object to such reuse of glass bottles* in the renewing of prescriptions, provided that a *new plastic closure* meeting the standards would be provided with the renewal [4].

Q. Are prescription drugs intended for topical application to the teeth, or a dosage form intended for inhalation required to be dispensed in child-resistant packaging? (Table 1).

A. No. Such drugs are not intended for oral administration [5].

Q. When the pharmacist dispenses a prescription drug in a child-resistant package, would he/she be in violation of the regulations if he/she included a separate non-complying closure with the package?

A. Although there is no express prohibition to this practice, the CPSC discourages the practice in that it is likely to result in the use of non-complying packaging by those who are able to use child-resistant packaging without difficulty. The potential for children being poisoned thus increases.

Q. Are Investigational New

Table 1
Exempt Drug Products

1. Sublingual dosage forms of nitroglycerin [6].
2. Sublingual and chewable forms of isosorbide dinitrate in strengths of 10 mg or less [7].
3. Liquid and tablet forms of sodium fluoride containing not more than 264 mg of sodium fluoride per package [8].
4. Anhydrous cholestyramine in powder form, e.g., Questran® [9].
5. Methylprednisolone tablets containing not more than 84 mg of the drug, e.g., Medrol® [10].
6. Mebendazole in tablet form containing not more than 600 mg of the drug per package, e.g., Vermox® [11].
7. Betamethasone tablets containing no more than 12.6 mg of the drug, packaged in a child-resistant plastic container that contains twenty-one 0.6 mg tablets that are packaged on a foil backing with a plastic blister covering each tablet, e.g., Celestone® [12].
8. Potassium supplements in unit dose forms, including individually wrapped effervescent tablets, unit dose vials of liquid potassium, and powdered potassium in unit dose packets, containing not more than 50 mEq per unit dose [13].
9. Effervescent tablets or granules containing less than 15% acetaminophen or aspirin, provided the dry tablet or granules have an oral LD_{50} of five (5) grams or more per kilogram of body weight.
10. Unflavored acetaminophen or aspirin-containing preparations in powder form (other than those intended for pediatric use) that are packaged in unit doses providing not more than 13 grains of acetaminophen or 15.4 grains of aspirin per unit dose and which contain no other regulated substance. (The exemption previously was limited to aspirin powders in unit-dose forms containing no more than 13 grains of aspirin) [31].
11. Erythromycin ethylsuccinate granules for oral suspension and oral suspensions in packages containing not more than 8 grams of the equivalent of erythromycin [16].
12. Colestipol in powder form up to five grams in a packet, e.g., Colestid [17].
13. Erythromycin ethylsuccinate tablets in packages containing no more than 16 grams total dosage of the drug [18].
14. Preparations which are packaged in aerosol containers intended for inhalation therapy, and which are not considered to be "oral" dosage forms, e.g., Decadron Turbinaire®, Bronkometer®, Medihalers®, Intal® [19].
15. Pancrelipase preparations in tablet, capsule, or powder form [20].
16. Medically administered oral contraceptives in manufacturer's mnemonic dispenser packages which rely solely upon the activity of one or more of the following progestogen or estrogen substances and provide not more than the indicated amounts per package:
     150.0 mg dimethisterone
     2.2 mg ethinyl estradiol
     21.0 mg ethynodiol diacetate
     6.0 mg mestranol
     200.0 mg norethyndrone
     105.0 mg norethynodrel
     10.5 mg norgestrel
     (A final order exempting these substances has not been issued as of the date of this publication. The requirement to use safety packaging, however, has been waived in the interim) [21].
17. Prednisone in tablet form when dispensed in packages containing not more than 105 mg of the drug [22].
18. Conjugated estrogen tablets in mnemonic packages containing no more than 32 mg total dosage of the drug. [30]
19. Medroxyprogesterone acetate (MPA) tablets [32].
20. Norethindrone acetate tablets in mnemonic dispenser packages containing not more than 50 mg of the drug [33].

Drugs (INDs) subject to the PPPA standards?

A. If the IND is a drug which is for oral administration to humans, can be dispensed only on or by an order of a licensed medical practitioner, and is to be dispensed directly to the patient, it must be packaged in a child-resistant container. A manufacturer must use a child-resistant package if the container is intended to be used for dispensing to the patient in outpatient trials.

Q. Can a pharmacist legally use reversible or other types of dual-purpose packaging for dispensing prescription drugs?

A. As long as the drug is dispensed in a container using the child-resistant mode, the CPSC accepts this type package as meeting PPPA standards. Although this type of packaging is not prohibited, the Commission staff discourages its use because it is likely to result in the use of non child-resistant packaging. This increases the potential for children being poisoned.

Q. Since the pharmacist is responsible for dispensing a prescription drug in a child-resistant package, does the manufacturer have to supply such a package to the pharmacist?

A. If the manufacturer markets the drug in the package intended to be dispensed to the consumer the manufacturer must use child-resistant packaging.

Q. Can the manufacturer supply to the pharmacist one size of a regulated prescription drug in a conventional package in the same manner of supplying a non-complying size for other household substances and over-the-counter drugs?

A. There is no provision in the law for a manufacturer or packager to market a single size non-complying package for a prescription drug as is the case for over-the-counter medications. Every unit of a prescription drug subject to standards which is packaged by the manufacturer in a package intended to be dispensed to a consumer must be in child-resistant

packaging. The only exceptions to the rule for providing child-resistant packaging for prescription drugs are at the dispensing level where the prescriber directs, or the purchaser requests non-complying packaging. The pharmacist would have to repackage with a conventional, non child-resistant package.

Q. Can a supplier of special packaging include an equal number of non-complying closures with each carton of complying packaging?

A. Yes.

Q. What role does the Consumer Product Commission play in informing and educating the public to the use of, and need for, child-resistant packaging?

A. The CPSC has produced and distributed radio and television spot announcements and other audio-visual materials to alert the public, particularly those who are elderly or handicapped, to their options under the law. Considerable emphasis is given to encouraging use of child-resistant packaging. One of the ways this has been done is to point out its effectiveness. For example, seven years after the regulation covering aspirin went into effect, fatalities among children related to this once most-frequently ingested product dropped 83 percent; ingestions declined by 65 percent. Fatalities in children related to all poisonings declined by 64 percent. Declines in reported ingestions of other regulated household products were equally impressive: controlled drugs, 58 percent; methyl salicylate-containing products, 61 percent; lighter fluids, 74 percent; turpentine, 75 percent; lye preparations, 68 percent; ethylene glycol, 61 percent [1].

Q. What role does the CPSC play in the professional education of health care personnel with respect to the child-resistant packaging program?

A. The Commission has been co-sponsoring with pharmaceutical and medical groups symposia and seminars which provide credits

associated with these professions. Commission personnel participate in meetings of these organizations and prepare articles for publications in their journals. The introduction of a teaching unit into the curricula of pharmacy and medical schools is another example of CPSC activity in the professional education of health care personnel. One of the areas where the CPSC has been particularly active has been in encouraging pharmacists to demonstrate to their patrons who need help the proper method of opening and closing a child-resistant package.

Q. Precisely what does the term "special packaging" mean?

A. The term "special packaging" means packaging that is designed or constructed to be significantly difficult for children under five years of age to open or obtain a toxic or harmful amount of the substance within a reasonable time and not difficult for normal adults to use properly, but does not mean packaging which all such children cannot open or obtain a toxic or harmful amount within a reasonable time. Normal adults are regarded as those with no overt physical handicaps which would preclude their manipulating the package. Note that to meet PPPA standards, not all children need to be prevented from gaining access to the regulated product nor need all adults be able to gain entry into the package. These stipulations were included in the legislation so that industrial ingenuity would not be stifled and that the marketplace would provide the key to which type packages would survive. Under all current regulations a package fails if more than 20 percent of a test panel of 200 children are able to gain access (after a visual demonstration of the proper way to open the package, 15% before) or if more than 10 percent of a test panel of 100 adults are unable to open and properly resecure (if appropriate) the test package. Unit dose packaging, popular for many drugs, is evaluated somewhat differently. A test

| Table 2 |
| Products Subject to Safety Packaging Regulations |

- Oral prescription drugs (note exemptions Table 1) [23].
- Controlled Substances in dosage forms intended for oral human administration [24].
- Liquid preparations containing more than 5% by weight of methylsalicylate [25].
- Oral aspirin preparations (note exemptions Table 1) [26].
- Methyl alcohol preparations in concentrations of 4% or more by weight, other than those packaged in pressurized containers [27].
- All drugs and dietary supplements which provide iron for therapeutic or prophylactic purposes, and contain a total amount of elemental iron from any source in a single package that is equivalent to 250 mg or more elemental iron in a concentration of 0.025% or more w/v, and 0.05% or more on w/w for non-liquids [28].
- Oral dosage forms of acetaminophen in containers holding more than one gram [29].
- Ibuprofen in oral dosage forms containing one gram (1,000 mg) or more of the drug in a single package [34].
- Diphenhydramine HCl in oral dosage forms containing more than the equivalent of 66 mg of the diphenhydramine base in a single package [35].
- Loperamide in oral dosage forms containing more than 0.045 mg of the drug in a single package [36].
- Lidocaine—more than 5.0 mg in a single package [37].
- Dibucaine—more than 0.5 mg in a single package [38].
- Ketoprofen—more than 50 mg in each OTC package.
- Naproxen—250 mg or more per retail package [39].
- Mouthwash preparations for human use containing 3 g or more of ethanol in a single package [40].

failure is defined as a child who opens more than eight individual units or the number of units representing a toxic amount, whichever is less.

Q. What is the basis for determining the products which will be covered by the PPPA?

A. A relationship must be established between a particular household substance (because of the way in which it is packaged) and serious personal injury or illness among young children as a result of their having ingested that substance. The potential hazard is also considered. Obviously, there are some substances which do not lend themselves to this requirement. Plants, for example, are involved in ingestions. On the other hand, many of the soaps and detergents are frequently ingested but are not causing serious injury or illness among children.

Q. Suppose a pharmacist dispenses a prescription drug in a conventional package. What is the CPSC's position?

A. The law requires that the pharmacist dispense a regulated prescription drug in a child-resistant package. The only exceptions are those instances when the purchaser or prescriber stipulates that a non-complying package be used. Pharmacists who violate the regulations may be criminally prosecuted.

Q. What is the basis for selecting the non-complying package which the law permits for over-the-counter drugs regulated by the PPPA?

A. The manufacturer may select one of his package sizes as his non-complying package so long as he also supplies the product in popular size packages which comply with the PPPA standards. It is the clear intent of Congress (regarding this provision) that the use of non-complying packaging shall be the exception rather than the rule.

The CPSC may require a manufacturer to use *only* child-resistant packaging if the manufacturer has not supplied the product in popular size packages which comply with the standards and the CPSC finds that the exclusive use of child-resistant packaging is necessary to accomplish the child protection intended by the PPPA.

Q. Now that FDA is requiring tamper-evident packaging for over-the-counter drugs, will this replace the requirement for child-resistant packaging?

A. The two systems are separate. Although there are some child-resistant packages which also are tamper-evident (blisters, unit-of-use) a child-resistant package is not necessarily tamper-evident. The FDA requires that evidence of tampering be visually determined on initial contact whereas child-resistant packages have specific performance standards that must be met. These include maintaining their child-resistance for the number of openings and closings customary for the life of the product.

Q. What types of child-resistant packaging have been approved by the Commission for use with prescription drugs and other regulated household substances?

A. the Commission does not *approve* child-resistant packaging. In fact, the act itself, specifically prohibits the Commission from prescribing specific package designs, product content, package quantity, and, with the exception of appropriate labeling for a single, exempt package size, labeling. The ultimate determination of whether a particular package meets the standards is the responsibility of the manufacturer. The Commission determines compliance, as previously indicated, on the basis of human performance tests.

References

1. Poison Prevention Packaging: A Text for Pharmacists and Physicians. Washington, DC, US Consumer Product Safety Commission, March 1983.

2. Steorts NH: National Poison Prevention Week announcement. Washington, DC, US Consumer Product Safety Commission, Feb 1983.
3. Unintentional Poisoning Among Young Children—Morbidity and Mortality Weekly Report 32(9): 117, March 11, 1983.
4. 16 CFR 1700.15(2)(c); Pharmacy Practice, 16(3):24, March 1981.
5. 21 CFR 295.3(c).
6. 16 CFR 1700.14(a)(10)(i).
7. 16 CFR 1700.14(a)(10)(ii).
8. 16 CFR 1700.14(a)(10)(vii).
9. 16 CFR 1700.14(a)(10)(v).
10. 16 CFR 1700.14(a)(10)(xiv).
11. 16 CFR 1700.14(a)(10)(xiii).
12. 16 CFR 1700.14(a)(10)(viii).
13. 45 FR 64557, September 30, 1980; 47 FR 10201, 10235.
14. 16 CFR 1700.14(a)(16)(i).
15. 16 CFR 1700.14(a)(16)(ii).
16. 16 CFR 1700.14(a)(10)(iii).
17. 16 CFR 1700.14(a)(10)(xv).
18. 16 CFR 1700.14(a)(10)(xvi).
19. 21 CFR 295.3(c).
20. 16 CFR 1700.14(a)(10)(ix).
21. 16 CFR 1700.14(a)(10)(iv).
22. 47 FR 40407, September 14, 1982.
23. 16 CFR 1700.14(a)(10).
24. 16 CFR 1700.14(a)(4).
25. 16 CFR 1700.14(a)(3).
26. 16 CFR 1700.14(a)(1).
27. 16 CFR 1700.14(a)(8).
28. 16 CFR 1700.14(a)(13).
29. 44 FR 51212, August 31, 1979.
30. 53 FR 41159, October 20, 1988.
31. 16 CFR 1700.14(a)(16)(ii).
32. 16 CFR 1700.14(a)(10)(xix).
33. 16 CFR 1700.14(a)(10)(xviii).
34. 16 CFR 1700.14(a)(20).
35. 16 CFR 1700.14(a)(17).
36. 58 FR 38961, August 20, 1993.
37. 61 FR 17992-18005, April 10, 1995
38. 61 FR 17992-18005, April 10, 1995
39. 60 FR 38671-38674, July 28, 1995
40. 60 FR 4536-4541, January 24, 1995

The CPSC has recently acted to increase consumer acceptance of child-resistant packaging by encouraging packaging designs that are both child-resistant and easier for all adults to open and close. Specifically, the agency revised the testing protocol for child-resistant packaging to promote designs that are easier for older persons to open but do not compromise the child-resistant characteristics of current child-resistant packaging.

The revised test protocol applies to products packaged on or after January 21, 1998. It includes a child test to make sure that a large majority of young children are unable to open child-resistant packaging and an adult test to make sure that adults can properly use the packages. The major change is the substitution of 100 older adults, aged 50 to 70 years, for the current adult panel, aged 18 to 45 years. In order for a child-resistant package to pass the revised adult test, at least 90% of the test subjects must be able to open the package twice within allotted test periods. The child test will still require that at least 80% of children are unable to open child-resistant packages during the specified test period.

Child-resistant packaging that passes the new protocol should ultimately lead to reduced child poisonings by increasing the use of more user-friendly child-resistant packaging. The public health community can help achieve this by encouraging all consumers, even older people with limited exposure to young children, to use child-resistant packaging.

QUESTIONS: CHAPTER 5

1. Tamper resistant packaging regulations are enacted by the:

    a. FBI

    b. FDA

    c. FTC

    d. DEA

    e. CPSC

<small>21 CFR 211.132</small>

2. Which one does *not* belong?

    a. Extra Strength Alka-Seltzer

    b. Isordil sublingual tablet

    c. Lomotil tablet

    d. Medihaler-Iso

    e. Cuemid

<small>16 CFR 1700.14(a)(10)</small>

3. Which of the following is exempt from safety closure packaging when dispensed by the pharmacist?

   a. Oral contraceptives
   b. Aspirin
   c. Nitroglycerin
   d. Anhydrous cholestyramine in powder form
   e. Acetaminophen

16 CFR 1700.14(a)(10)

4. Examples of drug products which are not regulated by or are exempt from the prescription drug regulation pertaining to the Poison Prevention Packaging Act are:

   a. NTG sublingual tablets
   b. Hydrocortisone-containing ointments
   c. Seconal capsules
   d. both a. and b.
   e. a., b., and c.

16 CFR 1700.14

5. How many times may the same plastic child-resistant closure container be reused when refilling the same prescription which authorizes refills?

   a. Once
   b. Twice
   c. Five
   d. Not at all
   e. For as many times as refilled in accordance with the refills authorized by the prescriber

16 CFR 1700.15(c)

6. The federal government chose to require that most human oral prescription drugs be dispensed in child-resistant packaging because:

   a. There was concern for the pharmacist's ability to keep track of those prescription drugs which are and are not regulated.
   b. It would be more expeditious to regulate all drugs rather than develop individual regulations for drug categories.
   c. All prescription drugs are inherently toxic.
   d. b. and c.
   e. a. and b.

7. Which sublingual tablet(s) must be dispensed to the patient in its (their) original container by the community pharmacist?

   a. DPX
   b. ISDN
   c. MTX
   d. NTG
   e. NGT

16 CFR 1700.14(a)(10)

8. Which federal government agency is responsible for implementing the Poison Prevention Packaging Act of 1970?

   a. CPSC
   b. FTC
   c. FDA
   d. NIH
   e. NABP

15 U.S.C. 2053(4)

9. What liability do pharmacists assume if they fail to dispense a drug product in a child-resistant container if it is required?

    a. They may be subject to the misbranding provisions of the FDC Act.

    b. They may be accused of adulterating the product.

    c. They may be guilty of negligence.

    d. a., b., and c.

    e. a. and c.

10. A manufacturer may package in conventional packaging a single size of a household product subject to a PPPA regulation, provided:

    a. That the manufacturer label that package to indicate that it should be used in households without young children

    b. That the package chosen to be in conventional packaging is the smallest size marketed

    c. That the manufacturer also supplies that product in packages that are *child-resistant*.

    d. both a. and c.

    e. both b. and c.   16 CFR 1700.5

11. Which federal government agency is responsible for implementing the Poison Prevention Packaging Act of 1970?

    a. Food and Drug Administration

    b. Federal Trade Commission

    c. National Institute of Health

    d. Consumer Product Safety Commission

    e. Federal Poison Prevention Administration   16 CFR 1700.1(a)(2)
                                         15 U.S.C. 2053(4)

12. The Consumer Product Safety Commission is responsible for implementing the:

    a. Poison Prevention Packaging Act

    b. Federal Food, Drug, and Cosmetic Act

    c. Controlled Substances Act

    d. Good Manufacturing Practices (GMPs)

    e. Drug Efficacy Study Implementation (DESI)   15 U.S.C. 2053(4)

13. In order to be exempt from the child-resistant packaging regulations, when dispensed by community pharmacists, isosorbide dinitrate must be:

    a. 5 gr or less

    b. 5 mg or more

    c. 10 gr or less and in chewable or sublingual dosage form

    d. 10 mg or more and in chewable or sublingual dosage form

    e. 10 mg or less and in chewable or sublingual dosage form   16 CFR 1700.14(a)(10)(ii)

14. In order to be exempt from the child-resistant packaging regulations, potassium supplements, when dispensed by community pharmacists in individually packaged effervescent tablet form, must contain no more than what mEq quantity of potassium?

    a. 10

    b. 25

    c. 50

    d. 75

    e. 100   16 CFR 1700.14(a)(10)(vi)

15. **Which one does *not* belong?**

    a. Decadron Turbinaire

    b. Dalmane capsule

    c. Isosorbide dinitrate sublingual tablet 10 mg or less

    d. Sodium fluoride multivitamin drops

    e. Mebendazole in tablet form containing no more than 600 mg of the drug per package

16 CFR 1700.14(a)(10)

16. **Which of the following is exempt from child-resistant packaging when dispensed by the pharmacist?**

    a. Aspirin

    b. Nitroglycerin

    c. Oil of wintergreen

    d. Mebendazole in tablet form in packages containing not more than 500 mg of the drug

    e. Individually packaged effervescent potassium supplement tablets containing not more than 50 mEq of potassium per tablet

16 CFR 1700.14(a)(10)

17. **Which of the following is exempt from safety closure packaging when dispensed by the pharmacist?**

    a. Iron-containing drugs when used for dietary purposes

    b. Betamethasone in tablet form in packages containing not more than 12.6 mg of the drug

    c. Methylprednisolone in tablet form in packages containing not more than 54 mg of the drug

    d. Acetaminophen in unit dose packaging

    e. All controlled substances intended for oral administration

16 CFR 1700.14(a)(10)

18. **Which one does *not* belong?**

    a. Nitroglycerin sublingual tablet

    b. Colestid 5 g

    c. Isosorbide dinitrate chewable tablet 10 mg

    d. Questran powder

    e. Secobarbital capsule

16 CFR 1700.14(a)(10)

19. **Which of the following provides for special packaging to protect young children from serious personal injury or illness that could result from handling, using, or ingesting certain household substances and drugs?**

    a. Controlled Substance Act

    b. Federal Caustic Poison Act

    c. Model Drug Product Selection Act

    d. Poison Prevention Packaging Act

    e. Fair Packaging and Poison/Drug Act

16 CFR 1700.15

20. **The purpose of the Poison Prevention Act is to prevent:**

    a. The pharmacist from dispensing certain prescription drugs

    b. Poisoning of young children

    c. Ingestions of toxic and potentially toxic household substances

    d. The pharmacist from dispensing controlled substances in noncompliant child-resistant containers

    e. The pharmacist from dispensing nitroglycerin sublingual tablets in child-resistant containers

16 CFR 1700.15

21. Which sublingual tablets do not require child-resistant containers when dispensed by the pharmacist?
1) Nitroglycerin
2) Isosorbide dinitrate
3) Isosorbide mononitrate
4) Nitrostat
5) Nitrolingual

   a. 1) and 2) are correct.
   b. 2) and 3) are correct.
   c. 1), 2), and 3) are correct.
   d. 1), 2), 4), and 5) are correct.
   e. 1), 2), and 4) are correct.   16 CFR 1700.14(a)(10)(i)

22. Which of the following are exempt from child-resistant packaging when dispensed by the pharmacist?
1) Nitrostat tablet
2) Imdur tablet
3) Nitrogard tablet
4) Isordil sublingual tablet
5) Sorbitrate tablet 5 mg

   a. 2) and 3) are correct.
   b. 3) and 4) are correct.
   c. 1) and 4) are correct.
   d. 2), 3), and 4) are correct.
   e. 1), 4), and 5) are correct.   16 CFR 1700.14(a)(10)(ii)

23. What is the maximum quantity of Vermox chewable tablets that may be dispensed in a non child-resistant container by the pharmacist?

   a. 100 mg
   b. 200 mg
   c. 300 mg
   d. 500 mg
   e. 600 mg   16 CFR 1700.14(a)(10)(xiii)

CHAPTER 6

Medical Device Law

REGULATION OF MEDICAL DEVICES*

Max Sherman, R.Ph. and Steven Strauss, Ph.D., R.Ph.

Medical devices were not regulated by the Federal government until 1938. At that time, the Federal Food, Drug, and Cosmetic Act (the Act) [1] extended the Food and Drug Administration's (FDA) legal authority to control foods and drugs, and bestowed the agency with new legal powers over cosmetics and medical devices. The Act, however, was limited in scope. Regulatory action against violative devices could be initiated only after a device was introduced into interstate commerce, and only when the device was deemed adulterated or misbranded. (Adulterated devices are those held or packaged under unsanitary conditions and are injurious to health. Misbranded devices contain false or misleading labeling.) The burden was on the government to provide evidence of violation of the Act and to proceed through the Federal court system to prohibit violative products from being marketed in the United States.

Note: There are a number of specific provisions of the Amendments not covered in this review, including establishment registration, device listing, color additives, banned devices, Good Manufacturing Practices, inspections, and exporting provisions. All, of course, are profoundly important to manufacturers, importers, or distributors.

*Reprinted with permission from U.S. Pharmacist (July 1983).

Fraudulent devices, in fact, were the major concern of the Congress in 1938 when it extended FDA's authority.

At the time the 1938 Act was enacted, many of the legitimate medical devices on the market were relatively simple items which applied basic scientific concepts so that experts using them could readily discern whether the device was functioning properly. The major concern with respect to medical devices was to assure truthful labeling. Fraudulent or quack devices were widely in evidence. America's most widely circulated monthly magazines and retail catalogues published advertising with fantastic claims for a host of worthless products.

The 1938 Act could not suppress the marketing of quack medical devices. There was no mechanism to prevent the marketing of the products, and it required considerable legal effort by FDA to remove them from the market after they were introduced. Many gadgeteers took advantage of the agency's limited authority and some of the most notorious medical swindles of all times occurred after 1938. Quackery represented by The Spectrochrome, Z-ray, Ozone Generators, Micro Dynameter, and countless others attests to the law's limitations.

There was also a transformation occurring with legitimate devices. The postwar revolution in biomedical technology resulted in a wide variety of sophisticated devices during the 1950s and 1960s. New developments in the electronic, plastic, metallurgic, and ceramic industries, coupled with progress in design engineering, led to the invention of cardiac pacemakers, kidney dialysis machines, defibrillators, cardiac and renal catheters, surgical implants, artificial vessels and heart valves, and a wide spectrum of other diagnostic and therapeutic devices.

These highly complex devices presented an increased potential for harm, as well as benefits. It became evident that additional legal controls were necessary. The FDA had assumed additional authority for drugs under the Kefauver-Harris Amendments to the Act [2], and the bureau was not averse in regulating products generally regarded as devices as drugs when the need arose. Device manufacturers were fearful that this usurpation or presumption would expand. There was a recognized need for more comprehensive authority to regulate medical devices.

In late 1969, the Secretary of Health, Education, and Welfare convened a medical device study group (Committee), composed of experts in medicine and technology for the best approach to new comprehensive device legislation. The Committee completed its research in mid-1970, and its report was made public in September 1970. For the first time, there was documentation of the problems and hazards directly related to medical devices. An extensive literature search uncovered an alarming 10,000 injuries attributed to medical devices over a ten-year period [3]. More than 700 injuries had proved fatal. The Committee report also emphasized that a predictable increase in the complexity and sophistication of medical devices requires action to prevent the emergence of even more serious and complex problems in the future. In essence, the Committee was convinced of the need for explicit legislation to address existing and potential hazards and the need to assure the reliability and effectiveness of medical devices.

The final congressional bill reflected many of the Committee's recommendations. Members of the public and representatives of the medical device industry also participated in the proposed regulation with members of the House Subcommittee on Health and Environment. The House-Senate conference on the proposed new bill took only two days, and the Medical Device Amendments to the Act [4] were signed into law by President Gerald Ford and became effective on May 28, 1976.

The new law amended the 1938 Act and provides the FDA with significant additional authority concerning the regulation of medical devices. The major purpose of the Amendments is to provide reasonable assurance of the safety and effectiveness of medical devices intended for human use. Fortunately, the Amendments recognized the enormous diversity of medical devices on the market and created a system where all such devices are regulated in proportion to their degree of significance to public health.

Definition

A medical device is defined as "an instrument, apparatus, implement, machine, contrivance, implant, *in vitro* reagent, other similar or related article including any component, part, or accessory which does not achieve any of its principal intended purposes through chemical action within or on the body of man or other animals, and which is not dependent on being metabolized for achievement of its principal intended purpose" [5]. The primary difference between a medical device and a drug and other products appears to be the words "chemical action" and "metabolized."

It is not that simple; a manufacturer still faces a dilemma in determining whether his product is truly "a device." For example, the term "drug" is defined to mean, among other things, "articles intended for use in the diagnosis, cure, mitigation, treatment or prevention of disease and 'articles' (other than food) intended to affect the structure or any function on the body" [6]. The term "articles" appearing in the definition of "drug" is a broad category that contrasts with the list of specific types of products that are devices, appearing in the definition of a "device." Except for body implants and *in vitro* reagents, most items included in the definition of a medical device are mechanical products generally constructed of solid materials, such as metal or plastic. By contrast, a drug is a natural substance or synthetic chemical or a combination of such in liquid, ointment, cream, powder, tablet or other drug dosage form that is inhaled, ingested, injected, or instilled into body orifices, or applied to the body in order to achieve its intended medical purpose. Pursuant to the latter part of the definition for devices, FDA may not regulate as a medical device, an article that achieves any of its principal intended medical purposes through chemical action or by being metabolized. Congress did not, how-

ever, insert any counterpart clause into the definition of "drug" which would make chemical or metabolic action a prerequisite to a product being regulated as a drug. Nor did Congress, in its 1976 revision of the "device" definition, substitute the broader term "article" for the listing of narrower categories of product to be regulated as devices found in the Act since 1938.

There are a number of products that are regulated as "drugs" even though they do not achieve their principal intended purposes through chemical action or by being metabolized. Among these are sun screens, dandruff preparations, and laxative preparations, such as mineral oil and psyllium. If this sounds confusing, consider that Lacrisert® (an ophthalmic preparation intended for dry eye syndrome) was reclassified from a medical device to an approved new drug [7]. The change was made despite the fact that Lacrisert® was subject to the Premarket Approval procedure for a Class III device. Lacrisert® was the first medical device cleared through the 1976 amendments to appear in the prescription department of the pharmacy.

Classification of Devices

Reference to the term "Class III" is important to understanding medical device law. Classification is one key difference between regulating drugs and devices. The law recognizes the enormous diversity among devices on the market and provides a system where all devices are regulated in proportion to their degree of significance to public health. As declared in the Act, all devices intended for human use marketed in the United States must be classified by panels of non-government experts into one of three regulatory classes according to the difficulty in assuring their safety and effectiveness [8]:

Class I, General Controls: General Controls apply to all devices and require truthful labeling, among other provisions, establishment registration, product listing, premarket notification, certain record-keeping requirements, and adherence to Good Manufacturing Practices. Examples include toothbrushes, tongue depressors, manual stethoscopes, eye pads, ice bags, and nasal rubber bulb syringes.

Class II, Performance Standards: Sets performance standards for particular devices to assure safety and effectiveness and are intended for devices for which General Controls alone would not assure safety and effectiveness or for which sufficient knowledge exists to develop such standards. Performance standards may relate to the construction, components, ingredients, and properties of the device. A standard may also provide for devices to be tested to assure that lots or individual products conform to regulatory requirements. Examples include insulin syringes, blood pressure gauges, most diagnostic reagents, electric heating pads, and clinical electronic thermometers.

Class III, Premarket Approval: This is the most restrictive regulation of the three Classes. Where general controls are insufficient to assure safety and effectiveness and there is insufficient evidence available to develop performance standards to assure safety and efficacy, the manufacturer must obtain data and have it reviewed by FDA before the device can be introduced into interstate commerce. Examples of Class III devices include more sophisticated devices, such as heart pacemakers, replacement heart valves, and implanted spinal cord stimulators. Medical devices that were previously regulated by FDA as new drugs—the so-called transitional devices—are automatically placed in Class III [9]. Included would be products such as soft contact lens, cleaning (sterilizing) and wetting agents, injectable silicone, tissue adhesives, and intraocular lens.

Classification has proved the most difficult process for FDA in implementing the Medical Device Amendments. Sixteen panels have proposed classification; only six (anesthesiology, cardiovascular, general hospital and personal use, neurology, Ob/Gyn, hematology and pathology, and microbiology) are classified. There are no performance standards written for products categorized in Class II. Without question, there have been too many devices proposed for Class II and the development of standards is not a trivial undertaking. For example, of 102 neurological devices listed under Part 882, 65 are placed in Class II [10]. The development of a standard can be an extremely costly and time-consuming endeavor. Manufacturers and trade organizations have asked FDA to limit future standards of classification to only those devices which need standards to assure safety and effectiveness. In other words, it appears unreasonable for the FDA to require a performance standard to control alleged risks and hazards for devices that have performed successfully for many years without identifying the problems and without performance standards. Officials at the FDA's National Center for Devices and Radiological Health apparently concur with industry on this matter.

Classification also determines how new devices can be introduced and marketed in the United States and is essential in the FDA response to the manufacturer's Premarket Notification. The Premarket Notification or 510(k) (which refers to that section of the Act added by the amendments) must be submitted by the manufacturer to the FDA at least 90 days before a device is to be introduced into interstate commerce. The 510(k) describes why a new device is substantially equivalent to preenactment devices (those marketed prior to May 28, 1976). If the device is substantially equivalent, the 510(k) notification is approved with the proviso that the device is subject to the General Controls provisions of the Act. The device may be subject to additional controls under Standards or Premarket Approval after final classification.

If the 510(k) does not demonstrate substantial equivalency, the device is classified by statute into Class III (Premarket Approval). The Act requires Class III devices to have an approved Premarket Approval Application (PMA) before they can be legally marketed unless the device has an Investigational Device Exemption (IDE) or unless the device has been reclassified. A Class III device may be distributed only for investigational use. An IDE for devices is synonymous with an Investigational New Drug Application (IND) for drugs.

Investigational Device Exemptions

A manufacturer who wishes to market a Class III device must obtain approval from the FDA pursuant to 21 *CFR* Part 812. This Part provides procedures for the conduct of clinical investigations of devices. An approved IDE permits a device that otherwise would be required to comply with a performance standard or to have premarket approval, to be shipped lawfully for the purpose of conducting investigations of that device. An IDE exempts the device from the requirements of certain sections of the Act including: misbranding, registration, listing, premarket notification, performance standards, premarket approval, Good Manufacturing Practices, banned device regulations, records and reports, and color additive requirements.

Basically, an IDE allows the sponsor to collect safety and effectiveness data for his device. The sponsor must submit a plan to demonstrate: (1) that the testing will be supervised by an Institutional Review Committee; (2) that appropriate patient consent will be provided; and (3) that certain records and reports, such as unanticipated adverse effects or device disposition, will be maintained.

Premarket Approval Applications

Following completion of the clinical study described in the IDE, the manufacturer must submit a Premarket Approval Application (equivalent to a new drug application for drug manufacturers). The PMA is the compilation of data that the manufacturer must submit to the FDA to demonstrate that his device meets the preclearance standards of the Medical Device Amendments. Approval of the PMA depends upon positive recommendations by both the FDA staff and the appropriate classification panel. If the application shows that the medical device is safe and effective for its intended use, that the manufacturers' processes and facilities conform to regulatory requirements, and the device labeling is not misleading, the application will be approved.

A medical device that was in commercial distribution before May 28, 1976, and was placed into Class III later through the classification process, is not required to have an approved PMA until 30 months following publication in the *Federal Register* of the final order classifying the device, or 90 days after publication of a regulation requiring a PMA, whichever is later.

There are distinct similarities between INDs and NDAs needed to market a drug product and IDEs and PMAs required to market a new medical device. The main difference between the two is that the IND/NDA has more specific requirements. Another is that INDs for drugs are all treated in a similar manner. Devices, on the other hand, are separated into two categories: significant risk and insignificant risk. A significant risk device is one that presents a potential for serious risk to health, safety or welfare of a subject. The importance of the distinction of devices based on the level of risk is two-fold: (1) an IDE is not required for nonsignifi-

cant risk devices; and (2) FDA has left the decision as to the level of risk of a given device to the sponsor with concurrence by the Institutional Review Board. Presently, a PMA is reviewed in a more flexible manner in terms of the length of time for review.

Restricted Devices

"Restricted Device" is another term added to the regulatory jargon by the Medical Device Amendments. Pursuant to the authority granted the FDA, a medical device's sale, distribution, or use can be restricted to prescription only if there is potential for harm or if collateral measures are necessary for the proper use of the device [11]. When the Medical Device Amendments were implemented, FDA determined that the category of "restricted" devices included all "prescription" devices defined earlier. The interpretation was challenged in the courts. One manufacturer asked that FDA issue a "restricted device" regulation on a device-by-device basis. The Court of Appeals for the Second Circuit rejected the manufacturer's argument [12]. A subsequent proposed regulation for restricted devices was published in the *Federal Register* [13]. The proposed rule defined types of restricted devices, exclusions, uniform labeling, and advertising requirements. This rule was withdrawn on November 24, 1981 [14]. Still in effect are the original prescription device regulations. Basically, whether a device can be sold directly to consumers without a prescription generally depends on whether adequate directions are provided for safe and effective use of the product by a layman, or whether specialized training or supervision is needed.

The following are examples of devices which are sold without a prescription for patient self care: insulin hypodermic needles and hypodermic syringes, oxygen for emergency use, heating pads, vaporizers, stethoscopes, sphygmomanometers, and clinical ther-

mometers. Prescription devices are to be used only by, or under the supervision of, a health care professional trained to achieve the intended result and able to provide information to the patient about the device, its benefits, and its risks. Diaphragms, antiembolism stockings and TENS units are classified as prescription devices.

Repair, Replacement, or Refund

Under the Medical Device Amendments, manufacturers, importers, and distributors or any combination of them may be required (1) to repair a device so that it doesn't present an unreasonable risk, (2) replace a device not in conformity with applicable requirements of the Act, or (3) refund the purchase price whenever it has been determined that a device presents an unreasonable risk of substantial harm. The repair, replacement, or refund provision was designed to reduce or eliminate risks associated with devices as well as provide an administrative procedure whereby consumers can attain economic redress when they have been sold defective medical devices that present unreasonable risks. The provision also recognizes that some devices present risks that are not unreasonable and thus are not subject to the remedies of refund, replacement, or repair.

Impact on Health Care Professionals

Medical Device Amendments, however, also have an impact on health care professionals. First, so-called "special order" or "custom" devices for individual patients are now only made available by companies on a very limited basis. Second, the use of "prescription devices" may be limited to certain health professionals to assure their safe and effective use. Third, health care professionals must realize that medical devices purchased or used, that violate provisions of the law, may create presumptions of negligence in malpractice suits involving medical devices [15]. Last, and most important, is the significance of device labeling. Health care professionals, such as pharmacists who interact with patients, have received and will be receiving much more information from the FDA and manufacturers about the use, maintenance, installation, and hazards of medical devices. Pharmacists should review this information and, where necessary, disseminate it to the patient. This is particularly important because the patient often plays a major role in determining the success or failure of a medical device.

References

1. 21 U.S.C. 301 et seq.
2. P. L. 87-781; 1962 Drug Amendments, October 10, 1962.
3. Medical Device Amendments of 1976, Report by the Committee on on Interstate and Foreign Commerce. No. 94-853. U.S. Government Printing Office, Washington DC, p. 9, 1976.
4. P. L. 94-295; 15 U.S.C. 55; 21 U.S.C. 321 et seq.
5. 21 U.S.C. 321 (h); FDCA 201 (h).
6. 21 U.S.C. 321 (g)(1); FDCA 201 (g)(1).
7. 47 FR 46139, October 15, 1982.
8. 21 U.S.C. 313; FDCA 513.
9. 42 FR 63472, December 16, 1977.
10. 21 CFR Part 882, 1982.
11. 21 U.S.C. 360j(e); FDCA 520(e).
12. 589 F. (2d Cir. 1978).
13. 45 FR 65619, October 3, 1980.
14. 46 FR 57569, November 24, 1981.
15. Miller MJ: How medical device legislation will affect health care professionals. AAMI News Volume XI(6):9, 1976.

HOW ARE MEDICAL DEVICES REGULATED?*

Thelma C. Holsomback, J.D., R.Ph.

Modern medical devices and surgical instruments have many functions and a diversity of design encompassing the broad sweep of specialized medical practice. This equipment may be as simple as a scalpel, with a basic design that has remained unchanged for centuries, or as complex and progressive as electrosurgical equipment, heart valves, pacemakers, monitoring devices, dialysis machines, intraocular devices, anesthesia machines, and countless other highly specialized devices. Product liability law recognizes this diversity, but also has established basic criteria of safe, non-negligent design and manufacture that all products must satisfy. In addition, medical devices, equipment, and drugs are subject to federal statutory regulation, including the *Food,* *Drug, and Cosmetic Act* [1], the *Medical Devices Act*, the *Medical Device Amendments of 1976* [2], and the *Good Manufacturing Practices (GMP) Regulations of 1978* [3]. If a patient is injured by a device or instrument covered by such a statute, he may bring action for recovery of damages under the statute as well as file suit against the manufacturer for negligence or breach of warranty [4].

The need for minimum standards of quality in this area has been apparent since 1938, when federal authority to regulate medical devices was provided in the *Federal Food, Drug, and Cosmetic Act of 1938*. Under this Act, action could be brought against such products only if a defect were discovered after the product was in use. Premarket approval of medical devices was not required, so there was no way to prevent harmful or ineffective products from getting on the market. Moreover, the FDA bore the burden of proving that a product was, in fact, dangerous or fraudulent, a process that often required extensive research and litigation and considerable expense [5].

The FDA began focusing more attention on the hazards of legitimate medical devices around 1960. The post-war era was characterized by many new medical discoveries and saw the development of a vast array of new and complicated medical equipment, such as intrauterine devices, heart pacemakers, kidney dialysis units, and artificial blood vessels and heart valves. The inadequacy of the 1938 law became a matter of acute concern because of these rapid technological changes. Many devices were so intricate that skilled health professionals were unable to ascertain if they were defective, and increasing numbers of patients would be exposed to serious risks if these were inade-

*Reprinted with permission from *Legal Aspects of Pharmacy Practice* (Oct./Nov. 1982).

quately tested or improperly designed or used. Congress recognized both the potential benefits of these new devices and the need for effective control and regulation to protect the public. It took 19 years from preparation of the first draft bill by the Department of Health, Education, and Welfare until the *Medical Device Amendments of 1976* was enacted. To encourage research and development of medical devices that might improve the health and longevity of the American people and to be sure that the FDA had the proper authority to regulate that process to minimize risk from the use of unsafe and ineffective medical devices, Congress enacted the *Medical Device Amendments of 1976*. Subsequently, the *GMP Regulations of 1978* were accepted by the FDA.

This legislation stated that medical devices must be manufactured, distributed, and labeled in accordance with regulations promulgated by the FDA, and authorized by:

- the *Federal Food, Drug and Cosmetic Act* (FD&C), which includes the *Medical Device Amendments of 1976*
- the *Public Health Service Act* (PHS)
- the *Radiation Control for Health and Safety Act* (RCHS) and
- the *Fair Packaging and Labeling Act*

Certain devices are subject to the regulations of other US government agencies, as well. Atomic pacemakers, for example, are subject to the Nuclear Regulatory Commission's *Atomic Energy Act* [6].

According to the *Medical Device Amendments of 1976*, the FDA must classify all medical devices intended for human use into one of three regulatory classes. These are based upon the extent of control FDA deems necessary to assure their safety and effectiveness.

Class I devices are subject to the following general controls, applicable to all classes of devices:

1. Registration of device manufacturer

2. Listing of devices
3. Premarket review
4. Notification—manufacturers must notify device users of risk; and when notification alone is insufficient to eliminate the risk, they may be required to repair or replace the device or refund its purchase price.
5. Records and reports—manufacturers, distributors, and importers must keep necessary records and make required reports.
6. Good manufacturing practices (GMP)—manufacturers must meet regulations for the manufacture, packing, storage, and installation of devices.
7. Advertising—devices must be labeled properly and advertised truthfully.
8. Ban devices—if a device presents a substantial deception or an unreasonable and substantial risk of illness or injury, it may be banned.
9. Sale, distribution, and use—the FDA may set requirements restricting the sale, distribution, and use of certain devices. Examples of such devices are ice bags, crutches, enema bags, manual blood pressure kits, and otic or nasal rubber bulb syringes.

Class II devices are subject to both general controls and performance standards. Once they have been developed according to procedures required under the FD&C Act, performance standards will be applied. Tampons, disposable hypodermic syringes, electric heating pads, contact lens solutions, and douche bags fall into this category.

Class III devices are subject to both general controls and premarket approval (PMA). Premarket approval requires submission of data proving a device's safety and effectivness before it may be marketed. Devices in this class are "critical"—life-supporting or life-sustaining—and present a potential unreasonable risk of illness or injury. These devices must have FDA-approved premarket applications because there is insufficient information available to assure safety

and effectiveness through general controls and performance standards alone (Classes I and II). Intrauterine devices and their introducers and new pacemakers are Class III devices. Most new items initially are categorized as Class III until they're proved safe and moved to Class II.

Fourteen panels of experts classify devices for regulatory purposes into such categories as: orthopedics, cardiovascular medicine, dentistry, anesthesiology, obstetrics and gynecology, gastroenterology-urology, radiology, neurology, ear-nose-throat, ophthalmology, plastic and general surgery, physical medicine, and general hospital use. A separate panel has been established to recommend regulatory controls for devices used for medical diagnosis rather than treatment [3].

Because experience has demonstrated that a manufacturer cannot rely solely on finished product testing or inspection to assure the safety, efficacy, and high quality of devices, legislation and regulation are vital to the health and welfare of the American public. By complying with the *GMP Regulations of 1978*, a manufacturer of a medical device greatly improves the chances of achieving this quality. FDA inspection and review of more than 14,000 medical devices since 1976 has shown a high level of compliance with the GMP regulations among manufacturers [7].

Patients who use medical devices are sick or injured, and use of a defective device could be catastrophic. Thousands of Americans will have healthier and longer lives because of this legislation.

References

1. *Food, Drug and Cosmetic Act of 1938*, 21 USC §301–392.

2. *Medical Device Amendments of 1976*, 15 USC §55; 21 USC §321, 331, 334, 351, 352, 360, 374, 379, 381.

3. Good Manufacturing Practice for

Medical Devices: General, 43 *Fed Reg* 31508, July 21, 1978.
4. Schwartz EM: Products liability: Manufacturer's responsibility for defective or negligently designed medical and surgical instruments.

DePaul Law Review, Vol. 18, Summer 1969, p. 349.
5. Medical Devices: Strengthening Consumer Protection, *FDA Consumer*, US Dept of Health and Human Services, Oct 1976.

6. US Dept. of Health and Human Services, *SMA Memo*, Vol. 13, Aug. 21, 1981, p 3.
7. US Dept. of Health and Human Services, *SMA Memo*, Vol. 14, Sept 20, 1981, p 2.

A PRIMER ON MEDICAL DEVICE REGULATION*

Glen Drew

Alfred Anyone leaves home for his doctor's office and his regular medical checkup. The checkup is part of the periodic follow-up he receives since the recent implantation of an artificial heart valve and cardiac pacemaker.

At the doctor's office, a nurse checks Mr. A's pulse and temperature with digital recording meters, measures his blood pressure with a sphygmomanometer, records his heart's activity with an electrocardiograph, and monitors the function of his pacemaker with a sensing device placed on his chest. The nurse also tests his reflexes with a reflex hammer and draws blood with a needle for later testing.

The physician then examines Mr. A, looking at his eyes with an ophthalmoscope and his ears with an otoscope, listening to his heart and lungs with a stethoscope, and using a tongue depressor to help look down his throat. The doctor is slightly concerned about Mr. A's convalescence and refers him to other specialists for a chest X-ray and for lung capacity tests on a spirometer, and considers whether magnetic resonance imaging will be needed to evaluate the blood flow pattern of Mr. A's brain.

Meanwhile, at home, Mrs. A puts an adhesive bandage on her daughter's scraped knee, adjusting her eyeglasses to better see the problem. Her son puts in his contact lenses and brushes and flosses his teeth. He admires his appearance, now that his orthodontic braces have been removed.

That little peep into the life of Mr. A and his family reveals the use of no less than 22 medical devices, from the dental floss and toothbrush to the heart valve and X-ray machine.[1] In this highly technological world of ours, Mr. A and his wife and children can hardly be expected to understand all of the devices they encounter. So it falls on the Food and Drug Administration to see to it that those 22 devices and countless others are both safe and effective.

Medical devices are regulated by FDA's Center for Devices and Radiological Health under the 1976 Medical Device Amendments to the Food, Drug, and Cosmetic Act. Devices that emit radiation, such as X-ray machines, are also subject to the Radiation Control for Health and Safety Act of 1968. This act charges FDA with the responsibility for ensuring that radiation-emitting products don't expose people to unnecessary and possibly harmful levels of radiation. The device amendments address not only safety but also effectiveness: whether the device actually does what the manufacturer says it will.

Medical devices first became FDA's responsibility in 1938, when the Food, Drug, and Cosmetic Act became law. Medical devices at that time were mainly simple instruments, such as stethoscopes and scalpels, and any hazards or defects were readily apparent. The major problem then was fraudulent devices, which offered "miracle" cures for a wide range of diseases, but often injured rather than cured. In those days, before FDA could take action against a device, it had to prove that the product was fraudulent or unsafe. There was no way to keep unsafe or ineffective medical devices from reaching the market.

After World War II, the technology boom greatly increased the number and complexity of legiti-

---

[1] The others are: cardiac pacemaker, digital recording pulse meter, digital recording thermometer, sphygmomanometer, electrocardiograph, pacemaker monitor, reflex hammer, needle for blood sampling, ophthalmoscope, otoscope, stethoscope, tongue depressor, spirometer, magnetic resonance imager, adhesive bandage, eyeglasses, contact lenses, and orthodontic braces.

---

*Reprinted with permission from the *FDA Consumer* (May 1986).

mate medical devices, such as heart-lung machines and dialysis equipment. This made it harder for physicians and patients to assess the risks connected with some medical devices and whether the devices were operating properly. It became apparent that new authority was needed to ensure safety and effectiveness before a product was allowed to be sold. The Medical Device Amendments were designed to meet that need.

Today, while fraudulent "miracle cures" continue to demand FDA's attention, it is the number and diversity of legitimate medical devices that present the greatest problems in regulation. There are more than 1,700 types of medical devices; the various models and sizes of each type add up to between 40,000 and 50,000 separate products. The types of devices range from the simplest (such as tongue depressors) to the most complex (such as magnetic resonance imagers), and from the most routine (such as urine collection bottles) to the most critical and life-preserving (such as artificial hearts).

These medical devices are produced by approximately 8,000 firms, many of them small, relatively new enterprises. Over 95 percent have fewer than 500 employees, and half of those have fewer than 50 employees. Many of these small firms are at the leading edge of science and technology, but have relatively little knowledge and experience in meeting regulatory requirements. Because those requirements depend on the nature of the device, rather than the size of the company producing it, small firms may have to spend a larger proportion of their resources for regulatory compliance than larger firms. In recognition of this situation, FDA established the Division of Small Manufacturers Assistance to help small firms cope with the regulations.

Many firms operate in very dynamic, rapidly evolving fields. For instance, the familiar X-ray machine improves continually, and other diagnostic imaging devices now supplement or replace X-rays and film in ever more applications. Images can be generated by high-frequency sound waves (ultrasound), or the reaction of the body's hydrogen atoms to rapidly changing, powerful magnetic fields (magnetic resonance imaging, or MRI). The image may be stored on videotape or computer memory, rather than photographic film. Computer manipulation of such digitized images permits the "removal" of structures such as bones from the image, or creation of three-dimensional models of internal body parts.

Many of the new medical devices permit diagnoses and treatments that previously were impossible. New diagnostic imaging techniques allow study of fetal development or tissue damage caused by blood clots. Fiber optics and lasers are being combined experimentally to clear blocked coronary arteries as a substitute for coronary bypass surgery. The lithotripter (from the Greek for "stone crusher")—approved by FDA in 1985—disintegrates kidney stones by focusing sound waves on the stones through a tank of water in which the patient is immersed. The idea for this device came not from the medical community but from aeronautical engineers studying supersonic flight dynamics. Even more such technological crossovers may be expected in the future.

FDA needs to be current in all areas of medical technology to ensure that these myriad devices are safe and effective. This demands the widest possible range of scientific, engineering and medical expertise.

All medical devices are subject to some level of regulation by FDA, but the nature and amount of that regulation vary. The more hazardous the device, the greater the regulation. The intent is to protect users and patients, while imposing the least possible regulatory burden on producers of devices.

This is accomplished by classifying medical devices into three groups—Class I, Class II, and Class III—with the least hazardous devices in Class I and the most hazardous in Class III. The classification of a device determines which regulatory "channel" it follows.

Class I devices, such as adhesive bandages, toothbrushes, and tongue depressors, present risks that can be managed by "general controls." These "general controls" represent a regulatory baseline, which all manufacturers, importers, and distributors must meet. They include registration of the firm with FDA and periodic listing of all medical devices produced or handled by the firm. Also, whenever a firm intends to introduce a new or significantly modified device to its product line, it must notify FDA at least 90 days before marketing the device.

Other general controls include adequate labeling and good manufacturing practices in producing the devices. There are 460 types of Class I medical devices, 27 percent of the total number of medical device types.

Class II devices, such as cardiac monitors, anesthesia machines and defibrillators, are subject to performance standards in addition to general controls. A performance standard is a set of specifications that the device must meet to be safe and effective. The process of developing a performance standard is long and difficult, and no standards have been put in place yet. Legislation to merge Class I and Class II has been proposed to reduce the ultimate number of standards that will be required. Approximately 1,100 types of devices, or 65 percent of the total, are included in Class II.

Class III devices are those with the greatest risk of injury, or that support or sustain life and have an unknown degree of risk. They include artificial heart valves, heart-lung machines, and the recently approved lithotripter. Class III devices are subject to general controls and pre-market approval. This means that firms must obtain FDA approval before marketing the device. Any devices that were not marketed before the Medical Device Amendments are automatically Class III devices (unless FDA finds that they are substantially equivalent to a Class I or Class II device). Approximately 140 devices are in Class III, or 8 percent of the total.

Pre-market approval depends on the firm showing that the device is safe and effective, based on clinical studies or other clinical experience with the device. In order to develop clinical data for such approval, an investigational device exemption (IDE) must be obtained from FDA. An IDA permits limited distribution under specific conditions for the purpose of studying the device. The IDE provides for the clinical use of devices at a specific number of locations, based on laboratory and animal tests which predict that clinical use in humans will be potentially helpful to patients.

A number of recent groundbreaking medical devices underwent clinical trials under IDEs before they received pre-market approval from FDA. These include the lithotripter, magnetic resonance imagers, and ultrasound devices mentioned above. Cochlear implants, which bring sound perception to some totally deaf persons, and an implantable cardiac defibrillator, which can control overly fast or erratic heart rhythms, are also among the "high-tech" medical devices studied and found safe and effective under investigational device exemptions.

In addition to FDA requirements, clinical studies of medical devices (and drugs, too) also are controlled by institutional review boards at the hospitals or other facilities where the studies are conducted. These boards, composed of medical experts and lay persons, review the patient selection criteria, informed consent obtained from patients, and other aspects of the protection of human subjects who participate in the studies.

A number of regulatory requirements apply to medical device firms after marketing begins. The general controls (including registration, listing, and good manufacturing practices) continue to apply. The Food, Drug, and Cosmetic Act requires that FDA inspect all medical device manufacturers that produce Class II or Class III devices at least once every two years. Companies who make only Class I devices are inspected at least once every four years. FDA may inspect a firm more frequently if problems occur with its products.

A recent addition to the post-marketing requirements is the medical device reporting regulation, which went into effect late in 1984. Under this regulation, medical device firms must report to FDA any death or serious injury that may be related to one of their products, as well as any malfunction that could have caused death or serious injury. The firm must make a telephone report to FDA within five days of first learning of the incident, and it must submit a written report within 15 working days.

If a hazardous device should reach the market, a number of measures are available to protect the public. FDA may ask the firm involved to recall the product. If necessary, FDA can temporarily prevent shipment of the problem devices without waiting for a court order. Seizure of medical devices, injunction against shipment, and criminal prosecution of individuals and firms involved—all through federal court action—are other ways to stop illegal distribution of medical devices.

Marketing approval or an investigational device exemption can be withdrawn if new information indicates a device is unsafe or ineffective. Reclassification of the device or changes in labeling are other means available to deal with problem devices.

The Medical Device Amendments protect consumers in an area where the complexity of the technology prohibits them from personally assessing the safety and efficacy of the products used to prevent, diagnose, or treat their illnesses. However, no regulatory system is foolproof, and no system can protect against all hazards. Consumers and health professionals must still use sense, discretion, and caution with any medical device.

A HISTORY OF GOVERNMENT REGULATION OF ADULTERATION AND MISBRANDING OF MEDICAL DEVICES*

Peter Barton Hutt, Esq.

INTRODUCTION

Although food, drug, and cosmetic products have been articles of commerce and subject to government regulation for centuries [1], medical devices have only recently been recognized as a separate and distinct category of health products and subjected to their own unique form of government regulation. This article traces the history of government concern about the need for regulation of medical devices, their initial regulation under the Federal Food, Drug, and Cosmetic Act of 1938 [2], their more comprehensive regulation under the Medical Device Amendments of 1976 [3], subsequent consideration of refinements in the existing law, and other related legislation that authorizes the Food and Drug Administration (FDA) to regulate medical devices.

THE INITIAL DEVELOPMENT OF MEDICAL DEVICES

Simple medical devices—for example, wooden splints to hold broken bones in place, makeshift crutches, and homemade stretchers to carry the ill—have undoubtedly existed since before recorded history. Evidence of their use has been found at numerous archeological sites. Dental devices, for example, were used by the ancient Egyptians and Etruscans [4].

Perhaps the beginning of the association of exaggerated medical claims with mechanical and electrical devices can be traced to John Graham of England, who promoted a "celestial bed" connected with electric coils as a cure for ste-

*Reprinted with permission from *Food Cosmetic Law Journal*, 44:(2)99–117 (March 1989).

rility in 1745 [5]. But in the 1700s, the best-known medical devices were undoubtedly those used by Franz Anton Mesmer, who arrived in Paris in February 1778 [6]. Mesmer contended that "animal magnetism," the primary "agent of nature," was the source of all health. Those who were sick could be cured by recharging them with animal magnetism through the use of magnets and, later, large tubs in which were placed iron rods connecting patients to specially magnetized jars of water. A Royal Commission convened by the medical establishment, consisting of such prominent scientists as Antoine Lavoisier and Benjamin Franklin, conducted tests and determined in 1784 that Mesmer's treatments were ineffective.

In the United States, the first renowned fraudulent medical device was marketed by Dr. Elisha Perkins in the late 1700s [7]. Perkins developed two rods of brass and iron, about three inches long, called "Perkins' Patent Tractors." He sold them throughout the country and claimed they eliminated disease from the body. Even George Washington purchased a set for his family. After Perkins died in 1799, his son carried on the business. Within ten years, however, it had been exposed as a fraud.

Throughout the 1800s, public and legislative attention in the United States was focused on the need for legislation to control the adulteration and misbranding of food and drugs, but not medical devices [8]. Initially, these laws were enacted at the state and local levels. It was not until the early 1900s that Congress enacted broad nationwide legislation authorizing federal regulation of foods and

drugs, in the form of the Biologics Act of 1902 [9] and the Pure Food and Drugs Act of 1906 [10]. When Congress enacted food and drug legislation for the District of Columbia in 1888 [11] and 1898 [12], for example, it covered only foods, drugs, and cosmetics.

In January 1879, Dr. E. R. Squibb, in an address to the Medical Society of the state of New York, proposed the enactment of a national statute to regulate food and drugs [13]. Ten days later, Representative Wright introduced the first comprehensive legislation in Congress [14]. It took twenty-seven years before such a law ultimately would be enacted by Congress as the Pure Food and Drugs Act of 1906.

In those intervening twenty-seven years, the Division (later the Bureau) of Chemistry in the United States Department of Agriculture (USDA), under the leadership of Dr. Harvey W. Wiley, conducted investigation after investigation, and issued report after report, relating to the adulteration and misbranding of food and drugs. Research has uncovered no USDA report during that era on medical devices. The legislative history of the 1906 Act is, in fact, devoid of any mention of medical devices.

Other sources, however, reveal that the well-publicized problem of exaggerated health claims for patent medicines was beginning to extend to medical devices as well. One of the great crusaders of that era, Samuel Hopkins Adams, wrote a series of articles in *Collier's Weekly* during 1905 and 1906 on nostrums and quackery, which were later reprinted by the American Medical Association [15]. An article on "the specialist humbug" from the September 1, 1906 issue of *Collier's Weekly* describes an "electro-vibration" apparatus for the cure of deafness, "magneto-conservative garments" for the cure of a large number of ailments, and other mechanical "cures" [16]. Nonetheless, the 1906 Act did not cover medical devices.

Following the enactment of the 1906 Act, regulation of fraudulent medical devices, therefore, fell to the United States Post Office under the Postal Fraud Statutes, which provide criminal penalties for mail fraud [17] and state that any mail containing false or fraudulent representations may be declared unmailable by the Postmaster General [18]. The Post Office has enforced these statutes since they were first enacted in 1872 [19], with the assistance of the FDA and its predecessor agencies, and continues to do so to this day. In 1929, for example, the FDA collaborated with the Post Office Department on seventy-three mail order fraud cases, including "a cap device alleged to grow hair, and a supposedly electric belt and insoles for the treatment of rheumatism and kidney ailments" [20].

Throughout this period, fraudulent medical devices flourished. A 1916 report by the American Medical Association solely devoted to "cures" for deafness cited several worthless devices [21]. One of the popular fraudulent devices of this era was the Abrams "dynamizer" machine [22]. By placing a blood sample in the machine, Abrams contended that he could diagnose the precise disease from which the individual was suffering and even the precise spot within the body where the disease had its focus. By the time that Abrams died in 1924, his machine had been exposed as a fraud.

By 1917, it was clear to the FDA that the law should be expanded to include authority over medical devices. In its annual report to Congress that year, the FDA stated that the 1906 Act "has its serious limitations . . . which render it difficult to control . . . fraudulent mechanical devices used for therapeutic

purposes" [23]. Its 1926 annual report described exaggerated therapeutic claims made for products containing radium, including one that consisted of a glass bulb to be hung over the bed to cause the dispersion of "all thoughts and worry about work and troubles and brings contentment, satisfaction, and bodily comfort that soon results in peaceful, restful sleep" [24]. Thus, the FDA monitored these products and assisted the Post Office in its regulatory actions, but could take no action on its own.

THE FEDERAL FOOD, DRUG, AND COSMETIC ACT OF 1938

The Legislative History

In June 1993, as part of the New Deal program, legislation was introduced to modernize and expand the 1906 Act [25]. Five years later, that legislation was enacted as the Federal Food, Drug, and Cosmetic Act of 1938 [26]. As introduced, the legislation covered medical devices as well as foods, drugs, and cosmetics. This was accomplished by defining the term "drug" to include medical devices. The FDA's annual report for 1933 explained the need for this expansion of the law:

> Mechanical devices, represented as helpful in the cure of disease, may be harmful. Many of them serve a useful and definite purpose. The weak and ailing furnish a fertile field, however, for mechanical devices represented as potent in the treatment of many conditions for which there is no effective mechanical cure. The need for legal control of devices of this type is self-evident. Products and devices intended to effect changes in the physical structure of the body not necessarily associated with disease are extremely prevalent and, in some instances, capable of extreme harm. They are at this time almost wholly beyond the control of any Federal statute [27].

In reintroducing the bill in 1934, Senator Royal Copeland, the chief sponsor of the legislation, provided this further explanation:

> The present law defines drugs as substances or mixtures of substances intended to be used for the cure, mitigation, or prevention of disease. This narrow definition permits escape from legal control of all therapeutic or curative devices like electric belts, for example. It also permits the escape of preparations which are intended to alter the structure or some function of the body, as, for example, preparations intended to reduce excessive weight. There are many worthless and some dangerous devices and preparation falling within these classifications. S. 2800 contains ample authority to control them [28].

During the Senate debate on the legislation in April 1935, however, Senator Clark of Missouri contended that it was improper, as a matter of common English language, to classify medical devices as drugs:

> *Mr. CLARK.* Mr. President, I should like to ask the Senator from New York how he can reconcile the language of this section and the language of the amendment with the common, ordinary acceptation of the English language. In other words, here he says it is proper to describe as a drug "all substances, preparations, and devices intended for use in the diagnosis, cure, mitigation, treatment, or prevention of disease in man or other animals." In other words, if a man has invented a shoulder brace, a purely mechanical device, which he claims will straighten a man's shoulders and expand his chest and make for his health, according to the definition contained in this paragraph it has to be described as a drug and treated in law as a drug.
>
> I should like to ask the Senator from New York to justify any such misuse of common, ordinary English terms.
>
> *Mr. COPELAND.* The Senator from New York would have no objection to the proposal about the particular devices mentioned by the Senator. But there are on the market a great many devices which are offered for use, and citizens are exploited, believing that they can be cured of all sorts of ailments by the use of them. For example, there is such a thing as a radium belt carry-

ing a disc alleged to contain radium; it is claimed that if the Senator from Missouri should wear that belt he would never have appendicitis or gall-bladder disease or perhaps any other ailment.

Mr. CLARK. The language the Senator from New York has employed in the bill is broad enough to cover any device of which the Food and Drug Bureau of the Agricultural Department chooses to take jurisdiction. The point I am making is that if the devices ought to be outlawed, they ought to be outlawed, and I have no objection to that; but to maintain that a purely mechanical device is a drug and to be treated as a drug in law and in logic and in lexicography is a palpable absurdity, in my opinion [29].

Senator Clark went on to say that calling a medical device a drug was like "calling a sheep's tail a leg" [30]. Although Senator Copeland continued to defend this choice of language [31], because of continued criticism of the definitional terminology [32], a separate definition of the term "device" was added to the legistliation [33] and later agreed to without further discussion [34].

While the legislation that became the 1938 Act was pending in Congress, four influential books were published that documented some of the more flagrant examples of unproven medical devices: M. Fishbein's *Fads and Quackery in Healing* [35], A. Kallet and F. J. Schlink's *100,000,000 Guinea Pigs* [36], R. Lamb's *American Chamber of Horrors* [37], and A. J. Cramp's *Nostrums and Quackery and Pseudo-Medicine* [38]. These added to the general support for a new medical device law.

Once the definition of "device" was separated from the definition of "drug," the device provisions of the statute paralleled the drug provisions except in one respect. In November 1937, the Massengill Company marketed a new product, Elixir Sulfanilamide, using diethylene glycol as a solvent. During the next several weeks, more than 100 people died of diethylene

glycol poisoning. After a thirty-four page report to Congress by the Secretary of Agriculture [39], Congress added a premarket notification requirement for the safety of new drugs to the pending legislation [40]. There was no comparable provision added, however, for new medical devices. Thus, as the statute was enacted, the provisions relating to the adulteration and misbranding of drugs and devices were basically the same except for the premarket notification provision that applied to new drugs.

The 1938 Act

The 1938 Act provided the FDA with statutory authority to take formal or informal regulatory action against the adulteration or misbranding of medical devices [41]. A device was deemed to be adulterated if it contained any filthy material, was prepared under unsanitary conditions, or differed from the quality represented in its own labeling [42]. A device was deemed to be misbranded if its labeling was false or misleading in any particular; failed to bear a label containing the name and address of the manufacturer, the net quantity of contents, and adequate directions for use and warnings against misuse; or was dangerous to health when used as recommended in its labeling [43]. These provisions were very short and simple. They remain the law today.

Enforcement of the 1938 Act

The FDA enforced the device provisions of the 1938 Act with vigor and determination. Paradoxically, just after the FDA was given adequate statutory authority to police the safety and labeling of devices, a flood of fraudulent devices began to appear on the market. For the next twenty-five years, the FDA's enforcement resources were strained to the limit to handle the regulatory action needed to deal with such widely-distributed quack devices as the Drown Radio-Therapeutic Instrument, the Zerret

Applicator, the Vrilium Tube, the Reich Orgone Accumulator, the Hubbard Electropsychometer (or E-Meter), the Ghadiali Spectrochrome, the Relax-A-Cisor, and the Diapulse devices, to name only a few [44]. These devices were, in fact, the subject of successful regulatory actions by the FDA. These actions consumed such a large amount of the agency's resources, however, that consideration was soon given to enactment of additional legislation to strengthen the FDA's authority.

Consideration of Additional FDA Authority

In response to the need to strengthen the FDA, the Department of Health, Education, and Welfare's (HEW's) Secretary Hobby appointed a Citizens Advisory Committee on the FDA, which issued a sixty-five page report in June 1955 [45]. The Committee recommended "more extensive work on therapeutic devices making false claims of diagnostic and curative properties," while recognizing that additional resources were needed to implement this recommendation [46]. In 1962 a second Citizens Advisory Committee failed to focus specifically on medical devices [47]; however, in 1969 the later Kinslow Report concluded that "FDA has completely inadequate resources and statutory authority to regulate this growing and highly sophisticated industry" and recommended interim measures until "a more comprehensive control system" could be enacted [48].

Beginning in 1959, Senator Estes Kefauver launched an extensive investigation into the FDA's regulation of the drug industry [49]. Following the thalidomide tragedy in 1962 [50], Congress enacted the Drug Amendments of 1962 [51] to strengthen the new drug regulatory system. The 1962 Amendments converted the new drug provisions of the law from premarket notification to premarket approval, and required the FDA to grant explicit approval of the safety and effectiveness of every new drug prior to marketing [52]. While the 1962 Amendments were being considered in Congress, a companion bill was also being considered to require premarket approval of new medical device products under the same type of system as was applied to new drugs [53]. As part of the agreement that resulted in enactment of the 1962 Amendments, however, all provisions relating to medical devices were deleted from the final legislation [54]. It was the understanding, at the time, that Congress would return to the matter of device legislation within a matter of months. In fact, this process consumed another fifteen years.

Although much of the FDA's regulatory activities with respect to regulation of medical devices following the enactment of the 1938 Act involved enforcement action against fraudulent devices, the revolution in biomedical technology following World War II resulted in the introduction of a wide variety of important new lifesaving medical devices that also demanded attention from the agency. Thus, the FDA devoted more and more effort to ensuring the safety and effectiveness of these new devices, as well as to protecting the public against fraudulent devices.

From 1962 to 1969, a wide variety of bills were introduced in Congress to provide the FDA with increased authority over medical devices; these proposals ranged from premarket approval to appointment of a national commission to study the matter. President John F. Kennedy urged enactment of new medical device authority in his consumer message of March 1962 [55]. President Lyndon B. Johnson made the same recommendation in his consumer messages in February 1964 [56], March 1966 [57], and February 1967 [58]. When President Richard M. Nixon assumed office and did not immediately issue a consumer message, the Democratic Study Group Task Force on Consumer Affairs again pushed for new medical device legislation [59].

The February 1967 consumer message of President Johnson contained the most detailed description of proposed legislation:

1. Insuring the safety and effectiveness of medical devices

Under present law, dangerous and worthless devices may be marketed until the Government—sometimes by chance, sometimes by complaint—discovers them and gathers the necessary evidence to establish that they are hazardous or ineffective. This is a laborious process. It requires many months. It is costly.

In the meantime, the elderly and the seriously ill suffer most. Improper treatment with worthless devices can be the cruelest hoax of all.

We want to foster continued research and development of life-saving devices. But we must be sure they have been adequately tested before they are put on the market. We cannot be sure today.

Congressional testimony has revealed that

—Defective nails and screws for bone repair have required repeated operations to correct the damage.

—Some artificial eyes have resulted in serious infection.

—Useless heating and vibrating devices have caused the ill to squander their money and delay the pursuit of effective treatment.

—X-ray machines, which could have been properly safeguarded at little cost, emitted excessive doses of radiation.

I recommend the Medical Device Safety Act of 1967.

Under this Act, the Food and Drug Administration would be required to pre-clear certain therapeutic materials—such as artificial organ transplants—used mainly on or in the body. In addition, the FDA will establish standards to assure the safety and performance of certain classes of widely used devices—bone pins, catheters, x-ray equipment, and diathermy machines.

In every case, the rights of the parties will be protected by fair hearings.

This new law will not apply to simple and ordinary patient care items which have withstood the test of time and are generally recognized as safe and reliable. It will not apply to an item specially ordered or designed by a surgeon or physician. Nor will it inhibit the research and development essential to the advancement of the medical arts. It will, however, protect physican and patient alike from devices which are dangerous and unreliable [60].

Nonetheless, there were no further congressional hearings and, thus, no serious consideration of proposed new device legislation during the 1960s.

The Court Cases and the Cooper Committee

While the legislation was pending, the FDA moved ahead with its routine enforcement activities. As a matter of conscious policy, moreover, the agency sought to classify as drugs, rather than as medical devices, important new products that arguably could be placed under either category in order to achieve maximum regulatory control. Because the definitions of "drug" and "device" in the 1938 Act were virtually identical, and overlapped in many respects, the FDA concluded that there was a strong possibility that the courts would agree with their policy of strengthening regulatory control through this administrative action.

In February 1968, the first of two important court decisions was handed down endorsing the FDA approach. In *AMP Inc. v. Gardner* [61], the United States Court of Appeals for the Second Circuit held that a product consisting of a disposable applicator, a nylon ligature loop, and a nylon locking disc, used to ligate severed blood vessels during surgery, was a drug. The court determined that the product was essentially a suture and, because sutures are listed in official compendia as drugs, the product was properly regarded as a drug. The court gave an expansive interpretation to the statute to be consistent with the congressional purpose "to keep inadequately tested medical and related products which might cause widespread danger to human life out of interstate commerce."

A year later, in April 1969, the Supreme Court held in *United States v. An Article of Drug . . . Bacto Unidisk* [62] that an antibiotic sensitivity disc, used as a laboratory screening test to help determine the proper antibiotic drug to administer to patients, is a drug rather than a device. The Supreme Court decision was based primarily upon public policy grounds. The Court first noted "the well-accepted principle that remedial legislation such as the Food, Drug, and Cosmetic Act is to be given a liberal construction consistent with the Act's overriding purpose to protect the public health" [63] and then concluded that

> [t]he legislative history, read in light of the statute's remedial purpose, directs us to read the classification "drug" broadly, and to confine the device exception as nearly as is possible to the types of items Congress suggested in the debates, such as electric belts, quack diagnostic scales, and therapeutic lamps, as well as bathroom weight scales, shoulder braces, air conditioning units, and crutches [64].

This definitive statement gave the FDA a clear directive to begin to reclassify as drugs a large number of borderline medical products that had previously been regulated as devices.

Thus, the need for legislative resolution of the matter became clear to all interested groups. Indeed, a national conference on the need for new medical device legislation was convened in Washington in September 1969; the results were summarized in the *Journal of the American Medical Association* in December 1969 [65].

In his October 1969 consumer message, President Nixon joined his predecessors in endorsing medical device legislation, but announced that a thorough study would be undertaken before specific legislation was proposed:

> *Another important medical safety problem concerns medical devices—equipment ranging from contact lenses and hearing aids to artificial valves which are implanted in the body. Certain minimum standards should be established for such devices; the government should be given additional authority to require premarket clearance in certain cases. The scope and nature of any legislation in this area must be carefully considered, and the Department of Health, Education, and Welfare is undertaking a thorough study of medical device regulation. I will receive the results of that study early in 1970 [66].*

The Secretary of HEW promptly established a Study Group on Medical Devices, chaired by Dr. Theodore Cooper, then-Director of the National Heart and Lung Institute. The Cooper Committee consisted of ten government officials—two from the FDA, five from various parts of the National Institutes of Health, and three from other parts of HEW. The report, issued in September 1970 [67], concluded that medical devices present entirely different issues from new drugs. It rejected the approach that had been included in most of the pending legislation of applying the new drug provisions of existing law to new medical devices. Instead, the report recommended a different regulatory approach, designed specifically to deal with the breadth and diversity of medical devices.

The Cooper Committee Report recommended two immediate steps: (1) an inventory of all medical devices already on the market and (2) an initial classification of those marketed devices to determine those that should be subject to premarket approval by the FDA, those for which performance standards would be an adequate form of regulation, and those for which neither premarket approval nor standards would be required. Where premarket approval was to be required, the report recommended the establishment of standing advisory review panels as an integral part of the approval system. To implement this broad new concept, the report also recommended a number of specific details, including requirements for records and reports, registration and inspection of establishments, good manufacturing practices, and related provisions.

THE MEDICAL DEVICE AMENDMENTS OF 1976

The Legislative History

Immediately upon receipt of the Cooper Committee Report, both administrative and legislative activity began to take shape. These two independent activities became intertwined during the next six years, culminating in the enactment and implementation of the Medical Device Amendments of 1976 [68].

After receipt of the Cooper Committee Report, the Department of HEW drafted legislation to embody its recommendations and circulated it within the government for comment. It took a full year—largely to accommodate changes demanded by the Department of Commerce and the Department of Defense—before the Administration's bill was introduced in December 1971 [69].

To expedite the legislative process, the FDA undertook administrative action designed to implement the Cooper Committee Report and to prepare for the pending legislation. In 1971, FDA Commissioner Charles C. Edwards transferred the Office of Medical Devices from the Bureau of Drugs to the Office of the Associate Commissioner for Medical Affairs [70]. Following receipt of the Cooper Committee Report, the FDA created a medical device advisory committee, undertook an inventory of existing medical devices on the market, and began the process of classifying medical devices [71]. The FDA had hoped that the pending legislation would be enacted before the final classification process actually began, but Congress did not move quickly enough. Thus, in 1973 the agency began to establish fourteen classification panels of experts and, in May 1975, published a general notice advising device manufacturers about the medical device classification procedures [72]. Classification reports were issued by these panels before the legislation was enacted.

Beginning in 1970, the FDA established its first device performance standard for impact-resistant lenses in eyeglasses and sunglasses [73]. In 1972, the FDA chose to regulate *in vitro* diagnostic products as devices rather than drugs, and to establish a comprehensive system of labeling and performance standards rather than to require new drug applications in reliance upon the pending legislation [74]. Finally, in 1974, FDA Commissioner Alexander M. Schmidt took the Office of Medical Devices out of the Office of the Associate Commissioner for Medical Affairs, and created a new Bureau of Medical Devices and Diagnostic Products [75].

These administrative initiatives by the FDA concerned members of Congress and their staff, who argued that the FDA should have waited for specific statutory authority before acting [76]. Nonetheless, they served a very important function, *i.e.*, keeping pressure on Congress to enact the new legislation.

In the Senate, hearings were held on medical device legislation in September 1973 [77]. S. 2368 was favorably reported on by the Senate Committee on Labor and Public Welfare in January 1974 [78], and was passed in February 1974 [79]. Because the legislation did not pass the House that year, it was again considered by the Senate in the next session of Congress. After hearings on the Dalkon Shield occurred in January 1975 [80], the Senate again favorably reported on device legislation in the form of S. 510 in March 1975 [81]. This bill was passed by the Senate in April 1975 [82].

In the House, hearings were held on intrauterine devices (IUDs) during May and June 1973 [83], and

specifically, in October 1973, on the pending device legislation [84], but no further action was taken on the legislation that year. Thus, by late 1974, the Senate had twice passed the legislation and the FDA had begun to take independent administrative action to force the hand of Congress.

In a marathon series of drafting sessions, four individuals (representing the FDA, the device industry, the House subcommittee, and the House Office of Legislative Counsel) revised the entire legislation during December 1974 and January 1975 to clarify the intended congressional policy. The revised legislation was introduced as H.R. 5545, on which hearings were held in July 1975 [85]. After markup in November 1975, this legislation was reported out of committee in February 1976 [86], and passed the House in March 1976 [87]. The House and Senate conferees met in March 1976 and issued a Conference Report in May 1976 [88]. Both houses concurred, and the bill was signed into law by President Gerald T. Ford on May 28, 1976 [89].

The Provisions of the 1976 Amendments

The final provisions of the 1976 Amendments are remarkably faithful to the Cooper Committee Report. The 1976 Amendments did require an inventory and classification of all medical devices into devices that require general controls (class I), performance standards (class II), and premarket approval (class III) [90]. For all medical devices, the general provisions of the 1938 Act were substantially strengthened. Device manufacturers were required to notify the FDA of every medical device prior to marketing. Devices that were substantially equivalent to pre-1976 devices could be marketed immediately, subject to any existing or future requirements for that type of device [91]. Pre-1976 class III devices could be required to submit proof of safety and effectiveness to

the FDA, but no statutory timetable or deadlines were established for this process [92]. The FDA was authorized to require the development of performance standards for class II devices, but this was not made mandatory and was left to the sole discretion of the FDA according to agency priorities and resources [93]. Registration of device establishments was required [94]. Good manufacturing practice regulations were authorized [95]. The FDA was given authority to deal with the notification, repair, replacement, and refund of defective devices [96], and was authorized to ban any device that presents a substantial deception or substantial unreasonable risk of injury or illness [97]. Thus, the final law greatly strengthened the FDA's authority to regulate medical devices but retained the fundamental concept of the Cooper Committee Report that regulation should be carefully tailored to the type of device involved.

In general, the FDA has implemented the 1976 Amendments efficiently and effectively avoiding both overregulation and underregulation [98]. The agency has, in short, adhered to the Cooper Committee Report and the congressional mandate to regulate medical devices in proportion to the degree of risk presented by each device. There have been no reported medical catastrophes or serious problems caused by devices that can reasonably be attributed to a failure to implement the 1976 Amendments properly. The FDA's approach to medical device regulation has raised the standards of the device industry, and, thus, benefited the public health without imposing unnecessary cost. The kinds of quack medical devices that were still marketed in the 1960s have been eliminated. A 1984 Office of Technology Assessment (OTA) report concluded that "while regulatory costs have been incurred, regulation has generally not had a significant negative impact on the industry" [99]. Thus, the FDA has succeeded in exerting sufficient regulatory control to protect the public health, while at the same time avoiding over-regulation that would discourage medical device innovation and harm the public health.

There has, of course, been criticism of the FDA's regulation of medical devices under the 1976 Amendments. Some members of the device industry have contended that the FDA has stifled innovation, some consumer activists have contended that the FDA has failed to protect the public health, and some members of Congress have contended that the legislation has not been implemented in the way that they would prefer. Much of this criticism, including an adverse congressional report [100], has come from individuals who were not involved with the enactment of the legislation, were not aware of the reasons why the final legislation reflected the policy that it embodies, or simply disagreed with the final version [101]. All of the suggestions for useful administrative changes and legislative clarification of the 1976 Amendments [102] can be accommodated by administrative action taken within the broad discretion and flexibility given to the FDA under the statute. A 1983 General Accounting Office (GAO) report [103] identified a few areas where the FDA could strengthen its administration of the law and suggested some areas where the law itself might be amended. A 1988 GAO report [104] suggested better documentation of "substantial equivalence" decisions under section 510(k). Like the 1984 OTA report, however, these reports did not reflect significant criticism of the FDA's overall approach.

The FDA has responded systematically to these criticisms. In accordance with its Action Plan I [105], ten task forces were established in 1984 from which have emerged a number of important administrative improvements [106] and additional new goals [107]. Not all of the criticisms can or should be accommodated by the

FDA, however, because of resource constraints, priority decisions, and valid policy judgments.

Since 1976, the possibility of revising the Amendments in various different ways has been continuously discussed. Brief House oversight hearings on medical device regulation were held in March 1984 [108] and May 1987 [109]. In December 1987, relatively simple clarifying amendments were proposed by the FDA in S. 1928 [110]. In July 1988, H.R. 4640, the Medical Device Improvements Act of 1988, was reported on [111] and passed by the House [112]. The major provisions in the legislation were designed to require hospitals and other institutional users of medical devices to report serious problems with devices to the FDA or to the manufacturer, extend the requirements of adverse experience reporting to device distributors, make it easier to market generic devices in class III by authorizing the FDA to waive the requirement for safety and effectiveness testing, require the substantial equivalence test in section 510(k) of the Federal Food, Drug, and Cosmetic Act to include evidence that post-1976 devices are at least as safe and effective as the marketed devices, require the FDA to reevaluate the classification of all pre-1976 devices placed in class III and then establish a schedule for requiring premarket approval for all devices that remain in class III after this reevaluation process, simplify the procedure for establishing a performance standard for a class II device, require repair, replacement, or refund for a device if the FDA determines that it was not properly designed and manufactured, require device recalls to be reported to the FDA, clarify that the statute applies to persons who "remanufacture" medical devices by some form of change, and conduct and support public education programs to reduce the risks of devices. The legislation was not the subject of hearings in the House, or of hearings or committee consideration in the Senate. Because it

was controversial, the bill was not enacted and will likely be further considered in future sessions of Congress.

The 1976 Amendments specifically provided that any product that was regulated as a new drug before 1976, but as a device after 1976, was a "transitional" device that would automatically be classified in class III [113]. Although the FDA was authorized to reclassify transitional devices under the same procedures and criteria that apply to all other devices, the agency has not done so largely because of the statutory prohibition against the use of proprietary industry data to support any reclassification. Small contact lens manufacturers have pushed for legislation to open up the soft contact lens market by reclassifying these transitional devices into class II. S. 1808, which was favorably reported out of committee in October 1988 [114], would have required the FDA to review the classification of all transitional devices and, specifically, to reclassify soft contact lenses as class II devices unless the FDA affirmatively retained them in class III. The bill was not enacted and will undoubtedly be considered further by Congress in the future.

ADDITIONAL FDA STATUTORY AUTHORITY RELATING TO MEDICAL DEVICES

The Radiation Control for Health and Safety Act of 1968

In 1968 Congress enacted the Radiation Control for Health and Safety Act [115] to control harmful radiation emissions from electronic products. Responsibility for administration of this statute was delegated to the FDA in 1971 [116]. It was initially administered by the FDA's Bureau of Radiological Health, which was combined with the Bureau of Medical Devices in 1982 to form the current Center for Devices and Radiological Health [117]. Under this statute, the FDA has issued performance standards for X-ray systems, computed tomography (CT) equipment, laser products, sunlamps, ultrasonic therapy products, and other related products [118]. Since 1968, there has been no serious consideration of amending the statute. The Medical Device Improvements Act of 1988 would have transferred the provisions of the 1968 Radiation Control Act from the Public Health Service Act to the Federal Food, Drug, and Cosmetic Act, but would not have made any substantive changes in its provisions.

Drug Price Competition and Patent Term Restoration Act of 1984

In 1984, Congress enacted legislation providing for stronger protection of drug patents, combined with easier entry of generic drugs into the market after the patent and any period of market exclusivity has expired [119]. As part of that legislation, Congress awarded up to five years of patent term restoration for medical devices that are subject to a regulatory review period that would otherwise reduce the effective patent life for the product [120]. Medical devices subject to premarket approval have, in fact, now received patent term restoration under this statute [121].

The Cardiac Pacemaker Registry Act of 1984

As part of the Deficit Reduction Act of 1984, the FDA was required to establish a national registry of all cardiac pacemaker devices and leads implanted or removed, for which Medicare makes payment [122]. The purposes of the registry are to assist the Health Care Financing Administration in determining proper Medicare payments and the FDA in determining the compliance of devices with regulatory requirements. Regulations governing the registry have been promulgated [123].

The Orphan Drug Act

Congress initially enacted the Orphan Drug Act of 1983 [124] to provide additional incentives for industry to make the investment necessary to develop drugs for rare diseases. In 1984, this Act was amended specifically to provide that any drug with a target patient population of fewer than 200,000 people is automatically regarded as an orphan drug [125]. As part of the Orphan Drug Amendments of 1988, medical devices have been added to the provision of the 1988 Act that allows financial assistance to defray the cost of developing products for rare diseases or conditions [126]. The 1988 Amendments also require the Department of Health and Human Services to conduct a study to determine whether the application of the other statutory incentives that apply to orphan drugs should also be applied to orphan medical devices in order to encourage the development of such devices [127]. It is likely that, at some time in the future, all of the provisions that relate to orphan drugs will also be applied to orphan devices.

CONCLUSION

The two major milestones in the FDA's regulation of medical devices occurred when devices are first brought under federal regulatory control in 1938 and when they were first subjected to premarket review in 1976. On both of these occasions, Congress sought to balance the need to protect the public from adulteration and misbranding of medical devices against the need to foster the development of innovative new lifesaving medical devices. The FDA, in turn, has sought to achieve the same balance. Where problems have occurred, the FDA has stepped in to handle them. On the other hand, where major technological advances have become feasible, such as the development of monoclonal anti-bodies for diagnostic use, the FDA has found ways to permit their

marketing with a minimum of regulatory requirements. In this way, Congress and the FDA have forged a unique regulatory system that is truly designed to enhance the public health.

References

1. Hutt & Hutt, *A History of Government Regulation of Adulteration and Misbranding of Food,* 39 Food Drug Cosm. L.J. 2 (1984).
2. Pub. L. No. 75-717, 52 Stat. 1040 (1938), as amended 21 U.S.C. §§ 301-392 (1982).
3. Pub. L. No. 94-295, 90 Stat. 540 (1976).
4. L. Kanner, History of Dentistry: Folklore of the Teeth 205 (1936).
5. M. Fishbein, Fads and Quackery in Healing 5 (1932).
6. R. Darnton, Mesmerism (1968); Janssen, *The Gadgeteers,* in S. Barrett & G. Knight, The Health Robbers ch. 16 (1976); Mesmerism: A Translation of the Original Scientific and Medical Writings of F.A. Mesmer (G. Bolch trans. 1980); R.C. Fuller, Mesmerism and the American Cure of Souls (1982).
7. M. Fishbein, The Medical Follies Ch. II (1925); Fishbein, *supra* note 5, at 9.
8. *See* Hutt & Hutt, *supra* note 1.
9. Pub. L. No. 57-244, 32 Stat. 728 (1902).
10. Pub. L. No. 59-384, 34 Stat. 768 (1906).
11. Public Acts of the Fiftieth Congress, Sess. 1, ch. 1090, 25 Stat. 549 (1888).
12. Public Acts of the Fifty-fifth Congress, Sess. 2, ch. 25, 30 Stat. 246 (1898).
13. E.R. Squibb, Proposed Legislation on the Adulteration of Food and Medicine (Jan. 1879).
14. H.R. 5916, 45th Cong., 3d Sess. (1879).
15. S.H. Adams, The Great American Fraud (various editions, 1905-1912).
16. *Id.*
17. 18 U.S.C. § 1341 (1982).
18. 39 U.S.C. § 3005 (1982). *See also* Hart, *The Postal Fraud Statutes: Their Use and Abuse,* 11 Food Drug Cosm. L.J. 245 (1956); Crumbaugh, *Survey of the Law of Mail Fraud,* 2975 U. Ill. L. Forum 237.

19. J.H. Young, The Medical Messiahs chs. IV, XIII (1967).

20. Food and Drug Admin., Annual Report 17 (1929).

21. American Med. Ass'n, Deafness Cures (1916).

22. Fishbein, *supra* note 7, at ch. VI; Fishbein, *supra* note 5, at ch. X.

23. Food and Drug. Admin., Annual Report 16 (1917).

24. Food and Drug. Admin., Annual Report 26 (1926).

25. S. 1944, 73d Cong., 1st Sess. (1933).

26. Pub. L. No. 75-717, 52 Stat. 1040 (1938), as amended 21 U.S.C. §§ 301-392.

27. Food and Drug Admin., Annual Report 13 (1933).

28. 78 Cong. Rec. 8960 (May 16, 1934).

29. 79 Cong. Rec. 4841 (Apr. 2, 1935).

30. *Id.*

31. *Id.* at 4842.

32. *Id.* at 4842-44.

33. S. Rep. No. 646, 74th Cong., 1st Sess. (1935).

34. 79 Cong. Rec. 8351, 8351-55 (May 28, 1935).

35. Fishbein, *supra* note 5.

36. A. Kallet & F.J. Schlink, 100,000,000 Guinea Pigs: Dangers in Everyday Foods, Drugs, and Cosmetics (1933).

37. R. Lamb, American Chamber of Horrors: The Truth about Food and Drugs (1936).

38. A.J. Cramp, Nostrums and Quackery and Pseudo-Medicine (1936).

39. Elixir Sulfanilamide, S. Doc. No. 124, 75th Cong., 2d Sess. (1937).

40. Pub. L. No. 75-717, § 505, 52 Stat. at 1052, as amended 21 U.S.C. § 355.

41. *Id.* § 304, 52 Stat. at 1044, as amended 21 U.S.C. § 334.

42. *Id.* § 501, 52 Stat. at 1049, as amended 21 U.S.C. § 351.

43. *Id.* § 502, 52 Stat. at 1050, as amended 21 U.S.C. § 352.

44. *See* Janssen, *supra* note 6.

45. Report of the Citizens Advisory Committee on the Food and Drug Administration, H.R. Doc. No. 227, 84th Cong., 1st Sess. (1955).

46. *Id.*

47. Report of the Citizens Advisory Committee on the Food and Drug Administration (1962).

48. Food and Drug Admin., Report from the Study Group on Food and Drug Administration Consumer Protection Objectives and Programs 36, 38 (July 1969).

49. Hutt, *Investigations and Reports Respecting FDA Regulation of New Drugs (Part I)*, 33 Clinical Pharmacology & Therapy 537, 539 (1983).

50. Sherman & Strauss, *Thalidomide: A Twenty-five Year Perspective*, 41 Food Drug Cosm. L.J. 458 (1986).

51. Pub. L. No. 87-781, 76 Stat. 780 (1962) (codified at 21 U.S.C. § 355).

52. *Id. See also* The Food and Drug Law Institute, Seventy-Fifth Anniversary Commemorative Volume of Food and Drug Law 16, 41 (1984) (available from The Food and Drug Law Institute).

53. H.R. 11,582, 87th Cong., 2d Sess. (1962); *Drug Industry Act of 1962: Hearings Before the House Comm. on Interstate and Foreign Commerce*, 87th Cong., 2d Sess. (1962).

54. 108 Cong. Rec. 21,049, 21,058-62 (Sept. 27, 1962).

55. Strengthening of Programs for Protection of Consumer Interests, 108 Cong. Rec. 4167, 4169 (Mar. 15, 1962).

56. Consumer Interests, 110 Cong. Rec. 1958, 1959 (Feb. 5, 1964).

57. Consumer Interests, 2 Weekly Comp. Pres. Doc. 422, 426-27 (Mar. 28, 1966).

58. Protecting the American Consumer, 3 Weekly Comp. Pres. Doc. 261, 263, 267-68 (Feb. 20, 1967).

59. 115 Cong. Rec. 23,149 (Aug. 11, 1969).

60. Protecting the American Consumer, *supra* note 58, at 260.

61. 389 F.2d 825 (2d Cir. 1968).

62. 394 U.S. 784 (1969).

63. *Id.* at 798.

64. *Id.* at 799-800.

65. *Excerpts and Summary of a National Conference on Medical Devices*, 210 J.A.M.A. 1745 (1969).

66. Consumer Protection, 5 Weekly Comp. Pres. Doc. 1516, 1523 (Nov. 3, 1969).

67. Study Group on Med. Devices, Medical Devices: A Legislative Plan (Sept. 1970); *See also* Cooper, *Device Legislation*, 26 Food Drug. Cosm., L.J. 165 (1971).

68. Pub. L. No. 94-295, 90 Stat. 540 (1976).

69. H.R. 12,316, 92d Cong., 1st Sess. (1971).

70. Link & Pilot, *FDA's Medical Device Program*, 6 FDA Papers 24 (1972).

71. Link, *Cooper Committee Report and Its Effect on Current FDA Medical Device Activities*, 27 Food Drug Cosm. L.J. 624 (1972).

72. 40 Fed. Reg. 21,848 (May 19, 1975).

73. 21 C.F.R. § 801.410 (1988).

74. *Id.* pt. 809.

75. 39 Fed. Reg. 5812 (Feb. 15, 1974).

76. Rogers, *Medical Device Law—Intent and Implementation*, 36 Food Drug Cosm. L.J. 4 (1981).

77. *Medical Device Amendments, 1973: Hearings Before the Subcomm. on Health of the Senate Comm. on Labor and Public Welfare*, 93d Cong., 1st Sess. (1973).

78. S. Rep. No. 93-670, 93d Cong., 2d Sess. (1974).

79. 120 Cong. Rec. 1798 (Feb. 1, 1974).

80. *Food and Drug Administration Practice and Procedure, 1975: Joint Hearings Before the Subcomm. on Health of the Comm. on Labor and Public Welfare and the Subcomm. on Administrative Practice and Procedure of the Senate Comm. on the Judiciary*, 94th Cong., 1st Sess. (1975).

81. S. Rep. No. 94-33, 94th Cong., 1st Sess. (1975).

82. 121 Cong. Rec. 10,701 (Apr. 17, 1975).

83. *Regulation of Medical Devices (Intrauterine Contraceptive Devices): Hearings Before a Subcomm. of the House Comm. on Government Operations*, 93d Cong., 1st Sess. (1973).

84. *Medical Devices: Hearings Before the Subcomm. on Public Health and Environment of the House Comm. on Interstate and Foreign Commerce*, 93d Cong., 1st Sess. (1973).

85. *Medical Device Amendments of 1975: Hearings Before the Subcomm. on Health and the Environment of the House Comm. on Interstate and Foreign Commerce*, 94th Cong., 1st Sess. (1975).

86. H. Rep. No. 94-853, 94th Cong., 2d Sess. (1976).

87. 122 Cong. Rec. 5875 (Mar. 9, 1976).

88. H.R. Rep. No. 1090, 94th Cong., 2d Sess. (1976).

89. Pub. L. No. 94-295, 90 Stat. 540 (1976).

90. *Id.* § 513, 90 Stat at 540-46 (codified at 21 U.S.C. § 360c). *See also* Kahan, *Medical Device Reclassification: The Evolution of FDA Policy,* 42 Food Drug Cosm. L.J. 288 (1987).

91. Pub. L. No. 94-295, § 513(f)(1)(A), 90 Stat. at 544-45 (codified at 21 U.S.C. § 360(f)(1)(A)).

92. *Id.* §§ 513(a)(1)(C), 515, 90 Stat. at 540-41, 542-49 (codified at 21 U.S.C. §§ 360c(a)(1)(C), 360e).

93. *Id.* § 514, 90 Stat. at 546-52 (codified at 21 U.S.C. § 360d).

94. *Id.* § 4, 90 Stat. at 579 (codified at 21 U.S.C. § 360).

95. *Id.* § 520(f)(1)(A), 90 Stat. at 567 (codified at 21 U.S.C. § 360j).

96. *Id.* § 518, 90 Stat. at 562-64 (codified at 21 U.S.C. § 360h).

97. *Id.* § 516, 90 Stat. at 560 (codified at 21 U.S.C. § 360f).

98. Hutt, *Medical Device Regulation: Reasonable, Workable,* 3 Legal Times of Washington, May 5, 1980, at 12; Hutt, *Legal Aspects of Introducing New Biomaterials in* Contemporary Biomaterials: Material and Host Response, Clinical Applications, New Technology and Legal Aspects 645 (J.W. Boretos ed. 1984).

99. Office of Technology Assessment, Federal Policies and the Medical Devices Industry, OTA-H-230, at 126 (1984).

100. Staff of Subcomm. on Oversight and Investigations of the House Comm. on Energy and Commerce, 98th Cong., 1st Sess., Report on Medical Device Regulation: The FDA's Neglected Child (Comm. Print 98-F 1983).

101. *See* Adler, *The 1976 Medical Device Amendments: A Step in the Right Direction Needs Another Step in the Right Direction,* 43 Food Drug Cosm. L.J. 511 (1988).

102. Health Indus. Mfrs. Ass'n, Report and Recommendations of the HIMA Device and Diagnostic Product Approval Task Force (Oct. 1985); Kessler, *Federal Regulation of Medical Devices,* 317 New Eng. J. Med. 357 (1987).

103. General Accounting Off., Federal Regulation of Medical Devices—Problems Still to Be Overcome, HRD-83-53 (1983).

104. General Accounting Off., Medical Devices: FDA's 510(k) Operations Could Be Improved, PEMD-88-14 (1988).

105. Food and Drug Admin., A Plan for Action 17-22 (July 1985). *See also* Young, *Remarks on Medical Device Assurance,* 43 Food Drug Cosm. L.J. 719 (1988).

106. Food and Drug Admin., Executive Summary of the Criticisms Task Forces' Reports (1985); Benson, Eccleston & Barnett, *The FDA's Regulation of Medical Devices: A Decade of Change,* 43 Food Drug Cosm. L.J. 495 (1988).

107. Food and Drug Admin., A Plan for Action: Phase II 8-9 (May 1987). *See also* Young, *Strengthening the FDA through Stability, Modernization, and Statesmanship,* 43 Food Drug Cosm. L.J. 447 (1988).

108. *Failed Pacemaker Leads: Hearing Before the Subcomm. on Oversight and Investigations of the House Comm. on Energy and Commerce,* 98th Cong., 2d Sess. (1984).

109. *Medical Devices and Drug Issues: Hearings Before the Subcomm. on Health and the Environment of the House Comm. on Energy and Commerce,* 100th Cong., 1st Sess. 331 (1987).

110. S. 1928, 100th Cong., 1st Sess. (1987).

111. H.R. Rep. No. 100-782, 100th Cong., 2d Sess. (1988).

112. 134 Cong. Rec. H5848 (daily ed. July 26, 1988).

113. Pub. L. No. 94-295, § 513(f), 90 Stat. at 544 (codified at 21 U.S.C., § 360c(f)).

114. S. Rep. No. 100-588, 100th Cong., 2d Sess. (1988).

115. Pub. L. No. 90-602, 82 Stat. 1173 (1968) (codifed at 42 U.S.C. §§ 263b-263n (1982)).

116. 36 Fed. Reg. 12,803 (July 7, 1971).

117. 47 Fed. Reg. 44,614 (Oct. 8, 1982).

118. 21 C.F.R. subch. J.

119. Pub. L. No. 98-417, 98 Stat. 1585 (1984).

120. *Id* § 201, 98 Stat. at 1598-1603 (codified at 35 U.S.C. § 156 (supp. 1985)).

121. 51 Fed. Reg. 34,143 (Sept. 25, 1986).

122. Pub. L. No. 98-369, §2304(c), 98 Stat. 494, 1068 (1984) (codified at 42 U.S.C. §1395y(h) (Supp. 1985)).

123. 52 Fed. Reg. 27,756 (July 23, 1987); 21 C.F.R. pt. 805.

124. Pub. L. No. 97-414, 96 Stat. 2049 (1983).

125. Pub. L. No. 98-551, § 4(a), 98 Stat. at 2815, 2817 (1984).

126. Pub. L. No. 100-290, 102 Stat. 90 (1988).

127. *Id* § 3(c), 102 Stat. at 91.

HIGHLIGHTS OF THE SAFE MEDICAL DEVICES ACT OF 1990 (PUBLIC LAW 101-629)*

Congress has amended the Federal Food, Drug, and Cosmetic (FD&C) Act to add new requirements and provisions concerning the regulation of medical devices.

These requirements are described in the Safe Medical Devices Act (SMDA) of 1990, signed into law by President Bush on November 28, 1990. Some provisions went into effect immediately upon enactment of the SMDA, while others have future effective dates or require implementing regulations.

KEY POINTS OF THE SMDA

• Device problem reporting requirement for user facilities
• Reporting and recordkeeping requirements for distributors of medical devices
• Tracking requirements for certain medical devices
• Additional manufacturer reports, including reporting of product removals and corrective actions
• Postmarket surveillance requirements for certain devices
• Civil penalty provisions
• FDA recall authority
• Temporary suspension of premarket approval (PMA)
• Good Manufacturing Practices (GMP) design validation requirements
• Changes that affect premarket notifications [510(k)s] and premarket approvals (PMAs)
• Changes involving:
   —Preamendment class III devices
   —Transitional devices
   —Reclassification process
   Class II—"Special Controls" provisions
• Humanitarian device exemption provisions

---

*Reprinted from *Public Law,* 101–629, U.S. Dept. of Health and Human Services.

• Clarification of requirements for drug/device/biologic combination products
• New Office of International Relations for medical devices
• Recodification of electronic product radiation safety requirements

IMPORTANT NOTE: User facilities and distributors have reporting obligations to FDA.

NEW REQUIREMENTS IN BRIEF

User Facility Reporting

• Medical device user facilities are required to report incidents that reasonably suggest there is a probability that a medical device caused or contributed to the death of a patient or to a serious injury or serious illness of a patient (Medical Device Reporting reports). The report is due as soon as possible but no later than 10 working days after the user facility becomes aware of the incident.
• "Medical device user facility" includes hospitals, ambulatory surgical facilities, nursing homes, or outpatient treatment facilities that are not a physician's office.
• Reports of deaths must be made to FDA and to the manufacturer if known.
• Reports of serious injuries or illness must be made to the manufacturer or to FDA if the manufacturer is not known.
• User facilities must submit a semiannual report to FDA summarizing the reports.
Effective Date: 12 months after enactment of the SMDA or the promulgation of regulations, whichever occurs first.

Distributor Reports, MDR Reports, and Certification

• FDA must promulgate regula-

tions for distributors requiring them to establish and maintain reports, including Medical Device Reporting (MDR) reports.
• Distributors must submit MDR reports to FDA and to the manufacturer.
• MANUFACTURERS, IMPORTERS, AND DISTRIBUTORS must certify to FDA annually the number of MDR reports they have submitted.
Effective Date: FDA must propose regulations in 9 months and issue final regulations in 18 months, or the proposed regulations become final.

Device Tracking

• Manufacturers must adopt a method of tracking devices, the failure of which would be reasonably likely to have serious adverse health consequences, and that are permanently implanted or are a life-sustaining or a life-supporting device used outside a device user facility.
Effective Date: FDA must propose regulations in 9 months and issue final regulations in 18 months, or the proposed regulations become final.

Reports of Removals and Corrective Actions

• Manufacturers, importers and distributors are required to report to FDA any removals or corrections of a device to:
   —reduce a risk to health posed by the device; or
   —remedy a violation of the FD&C Act caused by the device that may present a risk to health
Note: Routine servicing is not considered a removal or a corrective action.

Effective Date: Upon promulgation of regulations

Postmarket Surveillance

• Manufacturers are required to conduct postmarket surveillance, such as studies to gather data on the safety and effectiveness of a device, for certain devices introduced into interstate commerce after January 1, 1991. This requirement applies to devices that:

— are permanent implants, the failure of which may cause serious adverse health consequences or death;

— are intended for use in supporting or sustaining human life; or

— present a potential serious risk to human health

• FDA may require postmarket surveillance for other devices if deemed necessary to protect the public health.

Within 30 days of introduction of these devices into interstate commerce, manufacturers must submit a postmarket surveillance protocol to FDA for approval.

Effective Date: Immediately

Civil Penalties

• A manufacturer may be liable for a maximum civil penalty of $15,000 per violation of the FD&C Act, and a maximum of $1,000,000 per proceeding before an Administrative Law Judge.

• For GMP violations and MDR violations, civil penalties will not apply unless violations involve a significant or knowing departure from the requirements of the Act or a risk to public health.

• Civil penalties also will not apply for:

— minor violations of requirements concerning tracking and reports of corrections if the person demonstrates substantial compliance; and

— violations concerning devices held under unsanitary conditions unless the devices are defective

• FDA must provide the person

being assessed the opportunity of a hearing.

• Judicial review is available after assessment of penalties.

Effective Date: Immediately

Recall Authority

• After determining that there is a reasonable probability that a device would cause serious adverse health consequences or death, FDA may order a manufacturer or other appropriate firm to:

— begin immediate action to cease distribution of the device; and

— immediately notify health professionals and device user facilities to cease using the device

• The order shall provide the person subject to the order with an opportunity for an informal hearing, to be held not later than 10 days after the date of issuance of the order.

Effective Date: Immediately

Temporary Suspension of Premarket Approval (PMA)

• If, after providing an opportunity for an informal hearing, FDA determines there is a reasonable probability that continued distribution of a PMA-approved device would cause serious adverse health consequences or death, FDA shall by order, temporarily suspend the PMA and proceed expeditiously to withdraw the PMA approval.

Effective Date: Immediately

Design Validation

• The good manufacturing practices (GMP) requirements in section 520(f) of the FD&C Act are amended to include preproduction design validation, including a process to assess the performance of a device but not including an evaluation of the safety and effectiveness of the device.

Effective Date: Upon promulgation of a regulation

New Provisions Related to 510(k)s

• The manufacturer must obtain a substantial equivalence order before beginning commercial distribution of a device for which a premarket notification [510(k)] has been submitted.

• FDA is allowed to make a determination of substantial equivalence to legally marketed predicate devices for which PMAs are not required regardless of the date of introduction of the predicate device.

• Substantial equivalence means that a device has the same intended use and the same technological characteristics as the predicate device, or has the same intended use and different technological characteristics, but it can be demonstrated that the device is as safe and effective as the predicate device and does not raise different questions regarding safety and effectiveness from the predicate device.

• Requires submission to FDA of either (1) a summary of the safety and effectiveness information in the premarket notification submission upon which an equivalence determination could be based, or (2) a statement that safety and effectiveness information will be available to anyone upon request. Depending on the device, this 510(k) summary could be descriptive information about the new and predicate device and about performance or clinical evaluation. This requirement affects all devices that are subject to premarket notification.

• Any 510(k) summaries of information about safety and effectiveness of a device shall be made available by FDA to the public within 30 days of a determination of substantial equivalence.

• Manufacturers who claim that their device is substantially equivalent to a class III preamendments device introduced into interstate commerce before December 1, 1990, and for which a PMA regulation has not been issued, must comply with a class III summary and certification requirement.

They are required to certify that they have conducted a reasonable search of all information known or available about that type of device and to submit a summary to FDA of the type of safety and effectiveness problems associated with the devive being compared and a citation to the information upon which the summary description is based. The summary must be comprehensive and describe the types of problems to which the device is susceptible and the causes of such problems.

Effective Date: Immediately

Use of Premarket Approval (PMA) Data

• Information contained in a PMA application, including clinical and preclinical tests—but excluding descriptions of methods of manufacture and product composition— that demonstrates safety and effectiveness shall be available for use by FDA on year after the approval of the original PMA application for the fourth device of a kind. This information can be used by FDA in approving other PMA applications, establishing a performance standard, or reclassification activities.

• At the time of approval of the fourth PMA application of a kind, FDA shall publish a notice in the *Federal Register* identifying the four devices of a kind and the date on which data will be available for use by the FDA.

• Any challenge to the order authorizing use of PMA data must be made within 30 days after publication of the notice.

Effective Date: The effective dates are complex. Data shall be available for use within one year after publication of the notice, but no sooner than November 15, 1991, for devices for which four of a kind were approved on or before December 31, 1987; and no sooner than November 15, 1992, for devices the fourth of which was approved between December 31, 1987, and November 15, 1991.

Reclassification of Class III Preamendment Devices

• Upon issuance of an order by FDA on or before December 1, 1995, manufacturers of class III preamendment devices shall submit to FDA a summary of and citation to any information known or otherwise available to the manufacturer concerning the device, including adverse safety and effectiveness information. FDA may also require submission of the adverse safety and effectiveness data from which the summary was derived, if available to the manufacturer.

• After reviewing these data, FDA shall determine whether such devices remain in class III or be down-classified into class II or class I, and shall issue proposed regulations concerning such action for comment.

• By December 1, 1995, FDA must issue final regulations for reclassifying class III preamendment devices or retaining them in class III.

• For preamendment devices retained in class III, FDA must, within 12 months after the effective data of the final regulation, establish a schedule for issuance of regulations requiring submission of PMAs.

Transitional Devices

• Before December 1, 1991, FDA shall require manufacturers of class III transitional devices to submit a summary of and citation to any information, including adverse safety and effectiveness information known or available to the manufacturer.

• Before December 1, 1992, FDA shall determine whether class III transitional devices will remain in class III or be down-classified into class I or class II. This period for reclassification can be extended by FDA for 1 year.

• If FDA has not made a determination for daily wear soft or daily wear nonhydrophylic plastic contact lenses within 24 months of

the date of enactment, it must issue an order reclassifying these lenses into class II. This period can be extended by FDA for an additional year.

Class II Redefinition

• Class II has been redefined to include any device for which reasonable assurance of safety and effectiveness can be obtained by application of "Special Controls."

• "Special Controls" may include such controls as performance standards, postmarket surveillance, and patient registries.

• For life-supporting and life-sustaining class II devices, FDA must identify the "Special Controls" necessary to provide adequate assurance of safety and effectiveness and describe how such controls provide such assurance.

• On its own initiative, FDA may reclassify a class III device to class II if it determines that "Special Controls" would provide reasonable assurance of the safety and effectiveness of the device.

Effective Date: Immediately

Performance Standards

• Establishment of mandatory performance standards for class II devices becomes discretionary. See "Class II Redefinition" above.

• Procedures for establishing performance standards are simplified.

Effective Date: Immediately

Humanitarian Device Exemption

• In order to encourage the discovery and use of devices that benefit fewer than 4,000 individuals in the United States, FDA may grant an exemption from the effectiveness requirements of sections 514 (Special Controls) and 515 (Premarket Approval) of the FD&C Act after finding that:

    —the device is designed to treat or diagnose a disease

or condition that affects fewer than 4,000 individuals in the U.S.;

—the device is not available otherwise, and there is no comparable device available to treat or diagnose the disease or condition; and

—the device will not expose patients to unreasonable or significant risk, and the benefits to health from the use outweighs the risks.

• Devices granted an exemption may only be used at facilities that have an established institutional review committee, and the humanitarian use must be approved by the committee before studies begin.

• An exemption is granted for a period of 18 months and may be granted in the 5-year period from the date regulations take effect. The 18-month exemption may be extended.

Effective Date: Upon promulgation of final regulations, which are required within 1 year after enactment of the SMDA.

Combination Products

• FDA will determine the primary mode of action of a combination product.

• After determining the primary mode of action of the product, FDA shall designate the Center within FDA that will have primary jurisdiction of the premarket review of the product.

• For example, if the primary mode of action of a device/drug combination product is attributable to the device component of the product, the Center for Devices and Radiological Health will be responsible for the premarket review.

Effective Date: Regulations to be promulgated within one year after enactment.

Beginning April 11, 1996 hospitals, nursing homes, and other health-care facilities must report medical device-related deaths and serious injuries or illnesses, according to an FDA final rule that also spells out manufacturers' reporting requirements.

The rule requires that medical facilities:

• within 10 days, report deaths to FDA and to the manufacturer

• within 10 days, report serious injuries or illnesses to the manufacturer, or to FDA if the firm's identity is not known

• every six months, send FDA a summary of these reports.

The new criteria, published in the Dec. 11, 1995, *Federal Register,* are part of a universal "alert system," required by the Safe Medical Devices Act of 1990 and the Medical Device Amendments of 1992.

The rule requires that manufacturers:

• within five days, report to FDA any device-related incident requiring immediate action to protect the public health, as well as any incident for which the agency requests a report

• within 30 days, report other device-related deaths, serious injuries, or illnesses, as well as device malfunctions likely to cause or contribute to death, serious injury, or illness

• annually, submit a statement certifying the number of reports filed, or that no reports were filed during the previous 12 months

• report incidents related even to products no longer marketed

The rule helps lower costs by reducing paperwork. Reports can be submitted on the same FDA MED-WATCH form used for reporting drug- and biologics-related adverse events.

QUESTIONS: CHAPTER 6

1. The Medical Device Amendments of 1976:
  a. Established new regulations to decertify antibiotic discs and sutures
  b. Added Section 706 for color additives
  c. Are also known as the Copeland Amendments
  d. Authorized the establishment of three classes of medical devices, based on perceived risks
  e. Provided statutory requirements for marketing medical devices intended for export

2. Adult incontinent products are categorized as medical devices belonging in:
  a. Class I
  b. Class II
  c. Class III
  d. Class IV
  e. Class V

3. A new medical device company need not register with FDA until _____ before it actually starts manufacturing devices:
  a. 30 days
  b. 60 days
  c. 90 days
  d. 180 days
  e. One year

4. The federal government agency primarily responsible for regulating medical device advertising other than labeling is the:
  a. CDRH
  b. FDA
  c. DEA
  d. FTC
  e. CFR

5. Which category of medical devices is subject to premarket approval requirements of Section 515 of the FD&C Act?
  a. Class I
  b. Class II
  c. Class III
  d. Class IV
  e. Class V

6. Pursuant to the FD&C Act manufacturers of medical devices are required to notify FDA at least _____ in advance of their intent to market a device:
  a. 30 days
  b. 60 days
  c. 90 days
  d. 6 months
  e. One year

7. If a manufacturer of a medical device receives no answer within _____ after premarket notification was received by FDA, the manufacturer may proceed to market the device:

   a. 30 days
   b. 60 days
   c. 90 days
   d. 180 days
   e. One year

8. A pre-amendment device is one that was in commercial distribution before _____, the enactment year of the medical device amendments to the FD&C Act:

   a. 1938
   b. 1952
   c. 1962
   d. 1971
   e. 1976

9. Pursuant to the FD&C Act, the FDA has a _____ review period for a premarket approval application for a Class III medical device:

   a. 30 day
   b. 60 day
   c. 90 day
   d. 180 day
   e. One year

10. Which of the following are examples of Class II medical devices?

   a. Insulin syringes, electric heating pads, clinical electric thermometers
   b. Ice bags, eye pads, toothbrushes
   c. Soft contact lenses, intraocular lenses, contact lens wetting agents

11. A medical device is misbranded if it:

   a. Is a banned device
   b. Does not comply with a mandatory performance standard
   c. Is not manufactured in accordance with the GMP requirements
   d. Does not comply with an IDE to which it is subject
   e. None of the above

12. The federal government agency primarily responsible for regulating the truth or falsity of medical device advertising other than labeling is the:

   a. Food and Drug Administration
   b. Federal Trade Commission
   c. Medical Device Enforcement Administration
   d. Bureau of Medical Devices
   e. Center for Devices and Cardiological Health

13. A computer data base that contains reports collected from health care professionals on various problems with medical devices is sometimes referred to by the initials:

   a. DEN
   b. DRP
   c. ADRP
   d. DSMA

14. Which of the following are Class I medical devices?

    a. Sterile gauze bandage, sterile gauze pad, hot water bottle

    b. Vaginal diaphragm, condom, feminine syringe

    c. Vaporizer, humidifier, ice bag

    d. Sanitary napkin or tampon, feminine syringe, hot water bottle

15. A pre-amendment medical device:

    a. Is deemed a *new* device

    b. Is automatically classified as Class I

    c. Is a device in commercial distribution prior to May 28, 1976

    d. Is substantially equivalent to any device marketed after May 28, 1976

    e. Requires a reclassification petition before it can be commercialized

16. A *transitional* device is:

    a. Exempt from the provisions of Good Manufacturing Practices (GMPs)

    b. Automatically classified as Class I

    c. Deemed misbranded under Section 502 of the Act

    d. Exempt from the provisions of 21 CFR 801.109 (Prescription Devices)

    e. A device formerly classified as a *new* drug

17. Failure to comply with Good Manufacturing Practices regulations:

    a. Renders a medical device adulterated under Section 501(h) of the FDA Act

    b. Renders a medical device misbranded under Section 501(h) of the FDA Act

    c. Provides the FDA with authority to recall a medical device

    d. None of the above

18. The Medical Device Amendments of 1976 expanded the definition of *device* to include:

    1) Devices intended for use in the diagnosis of conditions other than disease, such as pregnancy

    2) *In vitro* diagnostic products, including those previously regulated as drugs

    3) Devices intended to affect the structure or any function of the body of man or other animals

    4) Its recognition in the official National Formulary, or the United States Pharmacopeia, or any supplement to them

    5) An intended use in the diagnosis of disease or other conditions, or in the cure, mitigation, treatment, or prevention of disease, in man or other animals

    a. 1) and 2) are correct.

    b. 1), 2), and 3) are correct.

    c. 2) and 3) are correct.

    d. 2), 3), and 4) are correct.

    e. 1), 2), and 5) are correct.

19. A medical device is adulterated if it:

    a. Is a banned device

    b. Does not comply with a mandatory performance standard

    c. Does not comply with an IDE to which it is subject

    d. Is not manufactured in accordance with GMP requirements

    e. All of the above

20. Class III medical devices are:

    a. Exempt from *general controls* and GMPs

    b. Exempt from performance standards and GMPs

    c. *New* or are pre-enactment life-sustaining or life-supporting devices

    d. Banned and subject to recall or seizure

    e. Deemed safe and effective when properly labeled and are suitable for distribution

21. Pursuant to the SMD Act of 1990, device user facilities must report medical device-related deaths to FDA's:

    a. Center for Evaluation and Research
    b. Bureau of Dangerous Medical Devices
    c. Center for Devices and Radiological Health
    d. Center for Medical Devices and Reporting
    e. Office of Compliance and Surveillance

22. What types of reports are required of user facilities pursuant to the SMD Act of 1990?
    1) Reports of deaths
    2) Reports of serious injuries or serious illnesses
    3) Semiannual reports
    4) Biannual reports
    5) Annual reports

    a. 1) and 2) are correct.
    b. 1), 2), and 3) are correct.
    c. 2) and 5) are correct.
    d. 1), 2), and 4) are correct.
    e. 1), 2), and 5) are correct.

23. Which agency within FDA is responsible for protecting the public health in regard to medical devices?

    a. Center for Devices and Radiological Health
    b. Center for Enforcement and Regulatory Affairs
    c. Center for Surveillance, Protection, and Enforcement
    d. Division of Medical Device Compliance
    e. Office of Consumer Affairs

CHAPTER 7

Drug Recalls

DRUG RECALLS*

Steven Strauss, Ph.D., R.Ph.

History and Development

Over the years, product recalls have evolved as the most expeditious and effective method of removing or correcting Food and Drug Administration (FDA) regulated products from the marketplace found to be adulterated, to present a danger to health, to involve gross fraud or deception of consumers, or to be materially misleading to the detriment of consumers' health and welfare [1]. (It must be pointed out that recall procedures are not restricted to drugs, cosmetics, medical devices, and food. A variety of other products which are regulated by different agencies of the federal government are also subject to recalls, such as the Consumer Product Safety Commission [baby pacifiers, children's toys], Food and Drug Administration [radiation leakage from microwave ovens], and National Highway Traffic Safety Commission [automobile tires].)

The use of "recalls" preceded enactment of the Federal Food, Drug and Cosmetic Act of 1938 [2]. One of the worst drug related disasters in the United States, the elixer of sulfanilamide incident of 1937, involved extensive withdrawal of a drug product that caused the deaths of approximately 100 persons. Another nationwide recall occurred in 1941 when FDA inspectors removed from the channels of distribution sulfathiazole tablets that were contaminated with phenobarbital. During the early 1940's, the annual reports of the FDA first mentioned violative product withdrawals, and subsequent reports recorded the number of such actions. The 1947 annual report contained one of the first policy statements concerning recalls. Since then, drug recalls have been accepted by the FDA, the pharmaceutical industry, and the general public as an important means of protecting consumers in a wide variety of circumstances [3].

Public notification of recalls became routine in 1967 through the initiation of the FDA weekly *Enforcement Report* [4]. When this *Report* was published, all product removal actions were considered to be recalls, regardless of the seriousness of the violation or whether a violation actually existed. Consequently, the number of recalls increased greatly, and thus it became increasingly difficult for the FDA to monitor recalls effectively. Even today, the FDA does not generate a computer print-out or analysis that would indicate whether recalled human drugs are generic or brands, type of recalls, level of recalls, etc. Such information can only be obtained and tabulated from the weekly *Enforcement Report*.

Although recalls were initiated approximately 40 years ago, the recall process was developed and gained momentum in the late 1960's and early 1970's when regulations were promulgated to define FDA's policy and authority [5].

Definition

The FDA's guidelines define a recall as "a firm's removal or correction of a marketed product that FDA considers to be in violation of the laws it administers, and against which the agency would initiate legal action, e.g., seizure. 'Recall' does not include a market withdrawal or a stock recovery" [6]. The physical removal of the violative product from the marketplace is not required in order for a recall to be declared. *Stock recoveries* may be instituted in cases where the violative product "has not left the direct control of the firm, i.e., the product is located on premises owned by, or under the control of, the firm and no portion of the lot has been released for sale or use" [6]. *Market withdrawal* refers to the "removal or correction of a distributed product which involves a

*Reprinted with permission from *U.S. Pharmacist* (October 1980).

The Food and Drug Administration becomes aware of potentially violative or violative products from:
- Consumer or professional complaints
- Factory inspections
- Sampling operations
- Notifications from manufacturers, distributors, shippers
- Reports of injury from health officials or agencies
- USP Drug Product Problem Reporting Program

minor violation that would not be subject to legal action by FDA or which involves no violation, e.g., normal stock rotation practices, routine equipment adjustments and repairs, etc." [6].

In order to apply the term *recall* correctly, two distinct but jointly necessary and sufficient criteria must be satisfied. The products must be subject to legal action under FDA's existing compliance policy *and* present any one or more of the following:
- Threat or potential threat to consumer (human or animal) safety or well being;
- Adulteration;
- Misbranding (gross fraud or deception);
- Materially misleading so as to cause injury or damage.

Recalls are divided by the FDA into three major classes to indicate the relative degree of health hazard presented by the product being recalled (Table 1), and the level to which a recall (Table 2) is made is determined by the health hazard involved and the extent of distribution [7].

Although the word *recall* is familiar to many persons, recall procedures, practices and enforcement may not be so well known. Many persons conceive a recall as an action performed by the Food and Drug Administration itself. Product recalls are not government actions.

There are no *specific* provisions in the Federal Food, Drug and Cosmetic Act which describe a recall

Table 1
Types of Recall

Class I
A situation in which there is a reasonable probability that the use of, or exposure to, a violative product will cause serious, adverse health consequences or death, e.g., label mix-up of a potent drug, [or] dangerous insufficiency of a vital nutrient in a hypoallergenic formula for infants.

Class II
A situation in which the use of, or exposure to, a violative product may cause temporary or medically reversible adverse health consequences or where the probability of serious adverse health consequences is remote, e.g., loss of potency, [or] presence of pyrogens.

Class III
A situation in which the use of, or exposure to, a violative product is not likely to cause adverse health consequences, e.g., drug adulterated by extraneous matter, [or] egg shampoo from which the egg has been omitted.

of a violative product from the marketplace as part of the Food and Drug Administration's statutory authority. Therefore, the FDA does not have the authority to *order* a violative product to be recalled. The closest the Act comes to recall

Table 2
Levels of Recall

Consumer or User Level
May vary with product, including any intermediate wholesale or retail level, e.g., consumer (patient), [or] physician.

Retail Level
Recall to the level immediately preceding the consumer or user level, e.g., pharmacies, dispensing physicians, clinics, and nursing homes.

Wholesale Level
All distribution levels between the manufacturer and retailers. This level may not be encountered in every recall situation, e.g., the manufacturer may sell directly to the community pharmacy.

authority are the "three R" (repair, replace, refund) provisions added by the 1976 Medical Device Amendments to the Act, and which only apply to medical devices [8].

The basic enforcement procedures the FDA has against deficient (adulterated, misbranded) products pursuant to the Act are *injunctions* and *seizures* [9]. Injunctions are issued against persons or firms possessing products to prevent further distribution. Under the seizure action, custody of products are taken by U.S. marshals pursuant to a federal district court order, with subsequent legal proceedings to condemn and dispose of them. The disposition of seized goods, if the seizure is uncontested by the owner, is a matter for the court that ordered the seizure to decide. Seizure is generally used *after* distribution has taken place. However, recall is generally more appropriate and affords better protection for consumers when many lots of a product have been widely distributed. Seizure, multiple seizures, or other court action is indicated when a firm refuses to undertake a recall requested by the FDA, or when the agency has reason to believe that a recall would not be effective, determines that a recall is ineffective, or discovers that a violation is continuing.

In addition to seizure action, a recalcitrant manufacturer or distributor faces potential criminal prosecution both on a corporate and on an individual basis (violations of the Act are potentially criminal), and a possible injunction which may cease operations at a manufacturing facility. Furthermore, the FDA is not limited to any *one* of these legal remedies, but may employ whichever combination it deems most suitable under the circumstances/violation [10].

FDA Requested Recalls

Recalls for alleged or supposed violations may be undertaken voluntarily and at any time by manufacturers and distributors, or at the request of the FDA. A request by the FDA that a firm recall a product is reserved for urgent situations and is to be directed to the firm that has the primary responsibility for the manufacture and marketing of the product that is to be recalled.

Thus, where the agency requests a recall, it has no authority to impose or seek sanctions for a firm's refusal to carry out the recall. FDA may, of course, institute legal action respecting the underlying violation that led to the agency's recall request; for example, it may seize an adulterated drug product and/or prosecute those responsible for distributing it.

Recognizing that a recall is to be used only under the most serious situations, past Commissioners of the FDA have ruled that only they or the Associate Commissioner for Regulatory Affairs may authorize a recall request by the FDA. Once a decision is made to initiate such a request, it is generally presented to the manufacturer or distributor through the local FDA regional office where the company is located [11].

Company Initiated Recalls

A firm has the responsibility to manufacture and distribute products that comply with the law. If it is discovered that products are in violation then the firm has the added responsibility of removing or reconditioning that violative product. Therefore, a company may, for a variety of reasons, on its own initiative, without a formal request from FDA, remove, correct, or dispose of an illegal product that it has distributed in commerce. However, the FDA has authority under the Federal Food, Drug and Cosmetic Act and the Public Health Services Act [12], to prescribe mandatory procedures and requirements concerning the conduct of recalls because such procedures and requirements prevent the introduction into commercial channels of adulterated, misbranded, or otherwise violative drugs. Because of this, a company's officials should adhere to FDA's guidelines on how to recall products [13].

Each circumstance necessitating a recall is unique and requires its own recall strategy. FDA reviews and/or recommends the firm's recall strategy, and develops a strategy for its own audit based on the agency's hazard evaluation and other significant factors, such as type of use of the product, distribution pattern, market availability, etc. The need for publicity, the depth of recall, the level of effectiveness and audit checks, and other recall factors are also components of the recall strategy.

After a firm decides to recall its product and notifies the FDA and consignees of its intent, it is the firm's responsibility to monitor the progress of its recall. This is accomplished by "effectiveness checks," the purpose of which is to verify that all consignees at the specified recall depth have received notices of recall and have taken appropriate action (Table 3).

In some cases, a recalling firm may not be able to check the effectiveness of its recall, e.g., when a recall extends to the consumer-user level, when the confidential business records of a company's customers are not accessible, or when wholesalers, distributors, or retailers do not cooperate or because the urgency of the situation requires an all-out effort. In such cases, the FDA will usually assist the recalling firm by seeking assistance from the state and local agencies.

Table 3
Effectiveness
Check Levels [6]

Level A
100 percent of the total number of consignees to be contacted at the specified recall depth.

Level B
Some percentage of the total number of consignees to be contacted, which percentage is to be determined on a case-by-case basis, but is greater than 10 percent and less than 100 percent of the total number of consignees to be contacted.

Level C
10 percent of the total number of consignees to be contacted.

Level D
2 percent of the total number of consignees to be contacted.

Level E
No effectiveness checks.

Project Rx Alert Underway

A project designed to inform pharmacists about drug product recalls as soon as they occur has been initiated by APhA. Project Rx Alert is now undergoing a large-scale test and when instituted on a nationwide basis, will alert pharmacists to drug project recalls before the public is told. The project came about, says APhA, because of pharmacists' complaints that they often are asked about drug recalls by patients who have heard about them from the news media before the pharmacists themselves have been notified in professional publications or by the FDA. The APhA utilizes the latest technology to process this information.

Regardless of whether a company initiates a recall or FDA requests it, the agency monitors a firm's recall to assure that it is conducted promptly and efficiently. If the recall is effective, then FDA will not act to initiate a seizure and/or other measures to affect removal or reconditioning in order to protect the public. The agency also investigates the circumstances and practices in the manufacture and distribution of the product that led to the recall. If it is evident that the violation could continue, the FDA may initiate an injunction against the company.

Recall Communications

A recalling firm is responsible for promptly notifying each of its affected direct accounts about the recall. The purpose of a recall communication is to convey that: a violative product is subject to a recall; further distribution and sale should cease immediately; where appropriate, the direct account should in turn notify its customers who received the product about the recall; instructions regarding what to do with the product.

The method of communicating with consignees may be accomplished by use of sales personnel, telephone, letters, telegrams, Mailgrams, or a combination of these.

FDA guidelines standardize the recall warnings so that physicians, pharmacists and others in the marketing channel can more easily recognize recall notices and thus comply with them. For example, the recall notice written by the manufacturer is to be sent by first-class mail, and the letterhead (Figure 1) and envelope (Figure 2) should be conspicuously and preferably marked in red with "URGENT: DRUG RECALL" for Class I and Class II recalls and, when appropriate, for Class III recalls. This is done to prevent the recall notice from being discarded or mistaken for an advertisement. The recall letter includes a postage-paid, self-addressed postcard (Figure 3)

MODEL DRUG RECALL LETTER

John Doe Laboratories
Somewhere, U.S.A. 12345

Control Division

Date __________

URGENT: DRUG RECALL - ***Nonsterile Injectable***

Re: ***List 1234, Cyanocobalamin Injection, Lot No. 4321***

Recent tests show that the above lot number of this product is not sterile and, therefore, represents a potential public health hazard. Consequently, we are recalling this lot from the market. Other lot numbers are not involved.

Please examine your stocks ***immediately*** to determine if you have any of Lot 4321 on hand. If so, ***discontinue dispensing the lot*** and promptly return via parcel post, to our New York City Plant; ATTENTION: RETURNED GOODS.

> **NOTE:** ***If a sub-recall is indicated in a particular recall situation, the following paragraph should be added:***

"If you have distributed any of lot 4321, please immediately contact your accounts, advise them of the recall situation, and have them return their outstanding recalled stocks to you. Return these stocks as indicated above."

You will be reimbursed by check or credit memo for the returned goods and postage.

Please return the enclosed card immediately providing the requested information.

This recall is being made with the knowledge of the Food and Drug Administration. The FDA has classified this recall as class __________ (if classified).

We appreciate your assistance.

John Doe
President

FIGURE 1. Model drug recall letter.

JOHN
DOE LABORATORIES
Somewhere, U S A 12345

FIRST CLASS MAIL

A. B. C. Pharmacy
Anywhere, U. S. A.

URGENT: DRUG RECALL

FIGURE 2. Model recall envelope.

PLEASE FILL OUT AND RETURN

We do not have any stock of List 1234, Cyanocobalamin injection Lot No. 4321 on hand. ☐

We have requested our accounts to return their stocks of this merchandise to us. ☐

We are returning ______ bottles of List 1234, Lot No. 4321

Name ______________________

Address ______________________

City ____________ State ______ Zip Code ______

First Class
Permit No. 2

BUSINESS REPLY MAIL
No Postage Stamp Necessary if mailed in U.S.A.

Postage will be paid by

JOHN DOE LABORATORIES
Somewhere, U.S.A. 12345

Henry Doe
Director, Quality Control

FIGURE 3. Model recall return postcard.

MODEL RECALL TERMINATION LETTER

Mr. John Doe, President
J.D. Laboratories, Inc.
Somewhere, U.S.A.

Dear Mr. Doe:

The Food and Drug Administration has completed the audit of your firm's actions concerning the recall of ___(product)___, ___(code number(s))___, ___(recall no.(s))___. We conclude that the recall has been completed and there has been proper disposition of the recalled articles. Therefore, FDA considers the recall terminated.

This letter is not intended to imply that the FDA will not recommend civil or criminal legal action related to this matter; nor does it relieve you or your firm from the responsibility of taking all necessary steps to assure compliance with the Food, Drug and Cosmetic Act (or other acts as appropriate) in the future.

Sincerely,

District Director
_________District

FIGURE 4. Model recall termination letter.

which is to be completed by the consignee, e.g., the pharmacist, to indicate the quantity of the recalled drug product in the pharmacy's inventory and its disposition.

A recall communication must contain the name of the drug product and sufficient information to identify the specific batch(es), the name of the manufacturer, the reason for the recall, and disposition instructions. When necessary, follow-up communications are usually sent to those who fail to respond to the initial recall communication.

Termination of a Recall

A recall is *terminated* when the FDA determines through its recall audit checks that all reasonable efforts have been made to remove or correct the violative product, and proper disposition has been made according to the degree of hazard. The method for conducting audit checks may be FDA personnel visits or telephone calls. FDA may be assisted by cooperating federal, state or local officials in such endeavors.

A recall is *completed* when a company has retrieved and impounded all of the violative product that could reasonably be expected to be recovered, or has completed corrections of the product or has destroyed the product in an appropriate manner, usually witnessed by FDA representatives (Figure 4).

Publicizing Recalls

Technically, the Secretary of Health and Human Services is required to disseminate information and publicity pertinent to drugs where the situation involves "imminent danger to health or gross deception of the consumer" [13]. However, in order to accomplish this, the FDA prepares and issues a recall list which is published in the weekly *Enforcement Report.* In addition, the agency makes use of news conferences, briefings for special news media (professional or trade press), communications with specific segments of the population, such as pharmacies, hospitals, physicians and other forms of publicity, such as its *Drug Bulletin.*

The purpose of a public warning is to alert the public that a product being recalled presents a serious hazard to health. It is reserved for urgent situations where other means for preventing use of the violative product appear inadequate. Whenever the FDA publicly announces a recall, it also states the specific action, e.g., removal or correction, the company is to take.

Human Drug Recalls (United States)

Fiscal Year	Number of Recalls
1975	475
1976	525*
1977	350
1985	2085
1987	2398
1989	2183
1990	405
1991	651
1992	524
1993	303**
1994	406

*Includes the 3 month transition period between FY 1976, which ended June 30, 1976, and FY 1977, which began October 1, 1976.
**Up to August 1, 1993.

Source: Food and Drug Administration, Program/Information Analysis Group (301-443-3160)

The FDA, in consultation with the recalling firm, will usually issue such publicity. However, the recalling company that decides to issue its own public warning is requested to submit its proposed public warning and plan for distribution of it for review and comment by the FDA.

Pharmacist Implications

The pharmacist plays a very important role in forestalling the use of violative products when a recall is made to the retail, institutional, or consumer level. The practicing pharmacist, as the last person in the channel of distribution, has the legal, moral and ethical responsibility to dispense only those drug products that are safe and effective to the best of his knowledge and professional training.

Failure to remove a recalled product from inventory to prevent its sale or distribution may result in the dispensing of an adulterated and/or misbranded drug and may result in patient harm, and possible legal action. For example, a pharmacist who dispenses the product after warnings have been issued and recall procedures initiated, may be confronted with alleged product liability and malpractice litigation.

References

1. 21 CFR 3.85.
2. 21 U.S.C.A. 301 et seq.
3. 41 FR 26924, June 30, 1976.
4. Formally titled the "Food and Drug Administration Weekly Report of Seizures, Prosecution, Injunctions, Field Corrections and Recalls."
5. Toffey WV: Are you ready if a recall hits? Product Management 3(2):38, 1974.
6. Food and Drug Administration: Regulatory Procedures Manual, Chapter 5, January 4, 1980.
7. 21 CFR 7.51(a).
8. FDCA Sects. 513–521; 21 U.S.C.A. 360c–360k.
9. FDCA Sects. 302, 304; 21 U.S.C.A. 332, 334.
10. Bozeman DC: The basis of drug recalls, Wisconsin Pharmacy Extension Bulletin 23(9):1, 1979.
11. *Op. Cit.* 6.
12. 42 U.S.C. 262.
13. FDCA Sect. 705(b); 21 U.S.C.A. 375 (b).

RECALLS, THE MEDIA AND MOTHERHOOD*
William Grigg

Catching a moment's leisure over a cup of coffee, Mrs. Loving Motherwell glances over her newspaper. War . . . politics . . . taxes and. . . .

What? Little Phil's fruit juice—the one she bought not more than an hour ago—is being recalled by the manufacturer?

Waving the newspaper, Mrs. Motherwell storms back to the grocery. She pokes the paper and the fruit juice in front of the grocer. "What are you trying to do?" she cries. "Kill my Phil?" The grocer bites his tongue. "Of course not," he says, "but I haven't had a recall notice for that product."

"Notice? Shmotice! Can't you read a newspaper?" Mrs. Motherwell snorts. "Idiot!"

Needless to say, neither she nor the grocer is pleased. The mother has been frightened and the grocer has been shouted at, and it wouldn't be human nature for either to think all is well.

Yet, this is the way the system is supposed to work. Indeed, if it's one of the three or four times a year when the Food and Drug Administration issues a press release announcing a food recall, FDA officials have already decided the urgency of the situation justifies scaring Mrs. Motherwell, and others.

There is no faster way to get notice of a recall to the public—and to food markets—than to distribute it to the nation's wire service and have it announced on the 6 p.m. TV news.

Although there are hundreds of recalls each year by drug manufacturers, food distributors and other firms regulated by FDA, there are only a few in which the agency actively seeks newspaper and radio and TV publicity.

FDA classifies these recalls as Class I because they involve a serious threat to life or health, such as a mix-up in a life-saving drug, a dangerous lack of an important nutrient in infant formula, or cans of mushrooms that contain deadly botulinum toxin.

For less serious situations there are Class II and Class III recalls. Class II recalls involve products that may cause temporary or medically reversible adverse health consequences or involve situations where the probability of serious adverse health consequences are

*Reprinted with permission from the *FDA Consumer* (November 1982).

remote. In a Class III recall, the use of or exposure to the violative product is not likely to cause adverse health consequences.

By seeking publicity in a Class I recall, FDA not only can spread the word fast but also can reach into homes and get consumers to avoid or return already purchased products. This may be inconvenient and even costly to the government and to manufacturers and distributors involved, but in the few cases such an announcement is used, FDA has judged the possible danger to life and health to be worth all the trouble.

Recalls are of two types: those begun by the company on its own and those requested by FDA. When a firm discovers that one of its products is in violation of FDA regulations, that firm may choose to recall the product. Most recalls are of this type.

But when a firm fails to recall a defective product on its own, FDA may request it. Such requests are ordinarily made in urgent situations, and, generally, FDA will have in hand enough evidence to back up its request with a threat of legal action, such as a seizure of products. This gives the agency's request some muscle, even though FDA has no specific

legal authority to *require* a recall.

FDA may portray the alternatives via telephone calls or a visit by a representative from the nearest FDA district office, followed by an electronically delivered letter or telegram.

It remains the firm's responsibility to conduct the recall and to be financially and organizationally prepared to conduct one whenever necessary.

The firm is required to notify each of its affected direct national and foreign accounts promptly about the recall.

The firm should appoint a responsible individual as its recall monitor or coordinator. It is this person's task to coordinate and direct the recall and to establish contact and keep in touch with FDA. The recall coordinator should have company authority to carry the recall to its conclusion.

The company should include in its recall plan a way to check the effectiveness or completeness of the recall, asking consignees if they have complied with the recall instructions. In recalls, it's important to quickly relay the recall message and then monitor it to completion. When there is a health hazard, FDA field offices audit the recalls by checking with a fair percentage

of the consignees to be sure the product has been removed from the market. The consignees may include the nation's 52,000 drugstores or its 165,000 food retailers—or both.

In a recent infant formula recall, FDA decided to check every one of the consignees. Audit checks sometimes can be done by calling a retailer or wholesaler to be sure he received and acted on the recall notice. The infant formula recall check was so urgent that FDA employees were required to dog-sled into remote Alaskan stores where there were no telephones.

When the audits show a product has been completely removed from the market, the recall is terminated.

Attention then can be given to any salvaging and reconditioning operations involving the violative product. A drug that has been improperly labeled can be dangerous but often it can be easily and safely reconditioned just by replacing the label. If a recall was made because a certain number of cans were malformed by a machine that started to function improperly, sometimes the faulty containers can be discovered by inspection and isolated. The others can then be returned to the market.

QUESTIONS: CHAPTER 7

1. "A situation in which the use of, or exposure to, a violative product may cause temporary or medically reversible adverse health consequences is remote." To which class of drug recall does this statement apply?

    a. Class I

    b. Class II

    c. Class III

    d. Class IV

    e. Class V

2. "A situation in which the use of, or exposure to, a violative product is not likely to cause adverse health consequences." To which class of drug recall does this statement apply?

    a. Class I
    b. Class II
    c. Class III
    d. Class IV
    e. Class V

3. "A situation in which there is a reasonable probability that the use of, or exposure to, a violative product will cause serious, adverse health consequences or death." To which class of drug recall does this statement apply?

    a. Class I
    b. Class II
    c. Class III
    d. Class IV
    e. Class V

4. When a marketed drug product violates the Federal Food, Drug and Cosmetic Act, the FDA:

    a. Can initiate a recall
    b. Can initiate a recall only because of the urgency
    c. Can initiate a recall only when it extends to the consumer use level
    d. Can initiate a recall if there is no cooperation from the retailers
    e. Cannot initiate a recall

5. The most effective method to remove a violative drug product from the market is:

    a. Seizure
    b. Recall
    c. Injunction
    d. Administrative action by FDA
    e. Civil action

6. A drug recall constitutes:

    a. Withdrawal of the drug product from the market
    b. Stock recovery
    c. Replacement of the drug product by the marketer
    d. Turnover of the old stock
    e. Withdrawal of the drug product from the market because it violates the FDCA

7. The statement "10% of the total number of consignees to be contacted" best fits what effectiveness check level in case of a drug recall?

    a. Level A
    b. Level B
    c. Level C
    d. Level D
    e. Level E

8. Which of the following is legally mandated to disseminate information and publicize drugs which present "imminent danger to health or gross deception" of the consumer?

    a. Food and Drug Administration
    b. Federal Trade Commission
    c. Secretary of Health and Human Services
    d. Director of the local FDA district
    e. President of the company marketing the violate drug product

9. Which of the following effectiveness check levels best describes the situation where 100% of the total number of consignees receiving a drug are contacted in regard to its recall?

    a. Level A
    b. Level B
    c. Level C
    d. Level D
    e. Level E

10. When a marketer refuses to recall its violative drug product at the request of the FDA, which of the following legal remedies is available to the FDA?

    a. Publicity
    b. Injunction
    c. FDA-initiated recall
    d. Seizure of the product

11. Which class of drug recall is the least serious?

    a. Class I
    b. Class II
    c. Class III
    d. Class IV
    e. Class V

12. Which class of drug recall is the most serious?

    a. Class I
    b. Class II
    c. Class III
    d. Class IV
    e. Class V

13. Which of the following statements regarding drug recalls is *not* true?

    a. A pharmacist who dispenses further amounts of the product after warnings have been issued and recall procedures have been initiated is inviting legal problems.
    b. The need for a recall would exist when a product is misbranded or adulterated within the meaning of the FDC Act.
    c. A priority situation that is possibly or potentially life-threatening is a Class III recall.

14. The purpose of a drug recall communication is to convey:
1) That a violative product is subject to recall
2) That further distribution and sale should not be made
3) That the direct account which received the product should in turn notify its customers about the recall
4) Instructions on what to do with the product

    a. 1) and 2) are correct.
    b. 1), 2), and 3) are correct.
    c. 1), 2), and 4) are correct.
    d. 2) and 4) are correct.
    e. 1), 2), 3), and 4) are correct.

15. Which of the following effectiveness check levels best describes the situation where at least 10% of the total number of consignees receiving a drug are contacted in regard to its recall?

    a. Level A
    b. Level B
    c. Level C
    d. Level D
    e. Level E

CHAPTER 8

Expiration Dating

REGULATIONS PERTAINING TO EXPIRATION DATING OF DRUG PRODUCTS*

Max Sherman, R.Ph. and Steven Strauss, Ph.D., R.Ph.

The Food and Drug Administration (FDA, agency) required all prescription and most over-the-counter (OTC) drug products to bear expiration dates with the promulgation of regulations on September 29, 1978 [1]. This is a relatively recent development when compared to much earlier expiration dating specifications imposed on the manufacturers of insulin, antibiotics and biologicals. Section 507 of the Federal Food, Drug, and Cosmetic Act (the "Act") implemented in 1945 [2] required that all drugs for human use composed wholly or partly of antibiotics be certified and that certification of each batch include a date of expiration. Section 506 of the Act, after which the antibiotic section was patterned, deals with the certification of insulin and contains similar date requirements. The Insulin Amendments were implemented in 1941 [3]. Biological manufacturers have been compelled to provide dating periods for their products since 1919 [4]. Manufacturers filing a New Drug Application also had to comply with 21 CFR 130.4, issued June 1967. This regulation stated that "If no expiration date is proposed, the applicant must justify its absence."

Lack of requirements for expiration dating prior to the 1978 regulation would appear to mean that prescription and OTC drug stability was not a serious problem, at least in terms of safety. With the exception of several reports describing the degradation of tetracycline to epianhydrotetracyline and subsequent toxicity resulting from ingesting outdated products [5–7], there was a paucity of literature describing harmful events. By contrast, the literature in the 1960s was replete with examples of loss of pharmacological activity that occurs during the aging of a drug [8]. This became a significant consideration following enactment of the Kefauver-Harris Amendments in 1962 [9], which intensified control over prescription and investigational drugs. Recognition was given that no drug is truly safe unless it is also effective, and effectiveness was required to be established prior to marketing in the United States. The Amendments also imposed new rules for control procedures used by a manufacturer to conform to "Current Good Manufacturing Practices" (GMP) to assure that drugs meet the requirements of the Act as to safety and have the identity and strength to meet quality and purity characteristics the drug is represented to possess [10].

During the 1960s, there were also new developments for using kinetic and predictive studies to estimate drug stability, and manufacturers began to use computers to process stability data. (Prior to the 1960s, only qualitative or semiqualitative methods and procedures were used in pharmaceutical studies [11].)

The combination, then, of the precedent set by: (1) insulin, antibiotics, and biologicals; (2) literature reports of loss of pharmacological activity; (3) new concerns for efficacy; and (4) increased technology, set the stage for incremental GMP regulations pertaining to expiration dating.

Good Manufacturing Practice Regulations

Expiration dating was originally included in 21 CFR 133.13, under the heading of "Stability," in the initial final regulation entitled Part 133-Drugs: Current Good Manufacturing Practice in Manufacture, Processing, Packing or Holding, published on June 20, 1963. At that time, manufacturers were directed by FDA to provide for suitable expiration dating on the labeling when it was needed to assure that the drug meets appropriate standards of identity, strength, quality and purity at the time of use. In the

*Reprinted with permission from U.S. Pharmacist (April 1985).

next major revision to GMPs published on January 15, 1971, expiration dating appeared under its own heading [12]. The inclusion at that time, despite objections by a number of professional and trade groups, was justified by the Commissioner of Food and Drugs (the Commissioner) who concluded that the interest of consumers must be served by the establishment of valid expiration dates for all drug products. Both Sections 133.13 and 133.14 were changed to set forth basic guidelines for stability studies for all drugs. These changes were intended to allow time for manufacturers to accumulate data to support expiration dating.

The next major change to GMPs came following publication of proposed rules on February 13, 1976 [13]. In a proposed Section 211.137, the 1971 regulation would be revised to require expiration dating for all drug (prescription and OTC) products. This regulation was virtually unchanged when it was published as a final rule on September 29, 1978. The effective date for implementation was March 28, 1979, with the exception of the provision for expiration dating which was extended until September 28, 1979. Extra time was provided to lessen the economic burden on manufacturers who order immediate containers with preprinted labeling well in advance of actual use [14].

The impetus, in part, for the proposed 1976 and final 1978 GMP rule to require expiration dating for all drug products was derived from a conference on dating pharmaceuticals sponsored by the University of Wisconsin in 1969. At that time, several drug manufacturers concluded that drug expiration dating for all pharmaceuticals was desirable, and they voluntarily initiated expiration dating for all of their products. The reasons presented were that: (1) few drug substances or pharmaceutical dosage forms can be compounded so as to completely preclude deterioration for an indefinite time; (2) there was a concern about the appearance of the package and for

repeated use of the closure which may allow excessive moisture to come in contact with the product; and (3) there was a need for proper stock rotation [15]. On the other hand, at least one manufacturer thought that the requirement for dating pharmaceuticals would entail many problems and impose a hardship in a situation where there is serious doubt whether the benefit derived exceeds disadvantages. The manufacturer believed that expiration dating, while understandable in instances of an unstable product, is not needed for dating stable preparations. There was also the thought that dating pharmaceuticals would unduly raise the cost of drugs to the consumer [16].

Maximum Dating

Several major manufacturers represented at the 1969 Conference suggested that a five-year dating period would be appropriate, based on their experiences with respect to the period of time drug products were likely to remain in the distribution system, and as an approximate end point at which stock replacement should be made. In addition, the laboratory space required to develop and maintain data on products beyond five years could be substantial just to hold stability and control samples. When the 1976 proposed rules were announced, the Commissioner stated that, while an arbitrary expiration date of five years for those drug products not requiring a shorter period has been adopted by a number of drug manufacturers, he did not have sufficient information to conclude that setting a specific maximum expiration date period is suitable or even desirable for all drug products. He further stated that there is a paucity of data to support the view that the individual consumer will be better served by a maximum expiration date, such as five years, compared to a longer expiration date that is fully supported by stability data for the special drug product. The Commissioner would not prohibit

individual drug firms from adopting a uniform maximum five-year dating period for their own drug products, providing stability data demonstrates that the five-year dating period is valid. Nor would the Commissioner prohibit individual drug firms from extending the expiration date for their own drug products at any time prior to the original expiration date.

Although it is generally recognized that most manufacturers, if not all, have arbitrarily chosen the five-year date, these manufacturers are free to select any expiration date within the documented stability period. The regulations permit manufacturers to use any expiration date that is supported by appropriate stability data.

Exemptions

Because of the unique nature of homeopathic drugs, they were exempt from the requirements for expiration dating. The Commissioner took into account the imprecise nature of determining extremely low levels of active ingredients for each of a large number of attenuations (dilutions) that may be prepared for each drug substance and the fact that variables, such as potency, absorption, bioavailability and other measures of effectiveness do not appear to be applicable to homeopathic drugs. However, under stability testing in the GMP's (21 *CFR* 211.166), homeopathic drug products must have a written assessment of stability based at least on testing or examination of the drug product for compatibility of the ingredients and based on marketing experience with the drug product to indicate that there is no degradation of the product for the normal or expected period of use. Evaluation of stability shall be based on the same container-closure system in which the drug product is being marketed.

Human OTC drug products are also exempt from the expiration dating regulations if they are stable for at least three years and their labeling does not bear dosage limitations. The FDA recognized that many human OTC drug products are safe and suitable for frequent and often prolonged use. Such drug products are marketed without dosage limitations and typically the contents of the retail package are used in a relatively short time. Examples of such human OTC drug products are: medicated shampoos and topical lotions, creams, ointments, fluoride toothpaste, and rubbing alcohol. The FDA Commissioner believed that given the high market volume of these types of preparations, their safety and their quick rate of consumption, the advantage of expiration dating to the consumer may not be worth the added costs, ultimately borne by the consumer.

The agency also concluded that a few products ordinarily consumed as human foods, but also marketed as drugs, would be more appropriately regulated under good manufacturing practice regulations for foods. Examples of products that the agency believed would be covered by the proposed exemption are: (1) candy cough drops that are formulated entirely of ingredients ordinarily consumed as human foods or ingredients of human food products; and (2) sodium bicarbonate labeled for use as an antacid, but ordinarily used as an ingredient of human foods under the more common "baking soda" label.

Prescription Labels

Of interest to practicing pharmacists is the requirement that expiration dating does not extend to drugs dispensed pursuant to a medication order or prescription from a prescriber. While a number of pharmacists voluntarily indicate an expiration date on the prescription label of a drug container given to a patient, such information is not required by federal law. The regulation of pharmacists' practice rests with the states by virtue of their "police powers."

In one interesting case, the Pharmaceutical Society of the State of New York (PSSNY) objected to a proposed New York state law which would have required the inclusion of an expiration date on drugs dispensed there [17]. In their opinion, a valid expiration date cannot be determined for a drug once it has been removed from the manufacturer's container. The nature of the drug, moisture content, environment, temperature and other factors affect the stability of a drug after it has left the pharmacy. Expiration dates determined by the manufacturer at the time of packaging are not valid after a stock bottle has been opened for dispensing prescriptions. This is substantiated by the current edition of the United States Pharmacopeia, which states that "The manufacturer can guarantee the quality of a product up to the time designated as its expiration date only if the product has been stored in the original container under recommended storage conditions" [18]. The PSSNY also claimed that there is no need to place expiration dates on prescription labels because patients are instructed not to store medications for reuse. With an expiration date on a prescription label, the patient might be misled into taking leftover medication without professional advice. In the rules for GMP implementation dated September 29, 1978 [1], however, the agency sup-

ported legislative proposals to provide expiration dating on all prescription drugs dispensed to consumers.

Storage Conditions

Expiration dates are related to the storage conditions as stated in the labeling which, in turn, is determined by stability studies. The same is true for products reconstituted at the time of dispensing. Labeling must bear information for both the reconstituted and the original drug (unreconstituted) product with appropriate storage conditions. Throughout even the earliest GMP regulations, it was obvious that expiration dating cannot be separated from stability testing requirements. It follows that stability testing has to be related to the labeled storage conditions. Currently, the definitions that are most helpful are those which appear in the *USP's* General Notices [18] (Table 1).

The manufacturer of the drug may specify any storage condition on the label, including a specific temperature range, so long as the expiration date is justified by stability studies reasonably related to those conditions [19]. For establishment of expiration dates, the stability test program should assure not only the chemical integrity of the product (within appropriate limits) but physical and microbiological integrity as well. It should be noted

---

Table 1
USP Storage Temperatures

Cold— Any temperature not exceeding 8 °C (46 °F).
Cool— Any temperature between 8° and 15 °C (46° and 59 °F).
    (An article for which storage in a cool place is directed may,
    alternatively, be stored in a refrigerator, unless otherwise
    specified.)
Room Temperature—The temperature prevailing in a working area.
Controlled Room Temperature—A temperature maintained
    thermostatically between 15° and 30 °C (59° and 86 °F).
Warm—Any temperature between 30° and 40 °C (86° and 104 °F).
Excessive Heat—Any temperature above 40 °C (104 °F).
Refrigerator—A cold place in which the temperature is maintained
    thermostatically between 2° and 8 °C (36° and 46 °F).
Freezer—A cold place in which the temperature is maintained
    thermostatically between −20° and −10 °C (−4° and 14 °F).

Table 2
Factors to Consider in Determining an Expiration Date

- Stability of inactive ingredients
- Interaction between active and inactive ingredients
- Manufacturing processes
- Dosage form
- Container closure system
- Conditions under which the drug product is shipped, stored and handled by wholesalers and retailers
- Length of time between initial manufacture and final use

---

that current regulations do not specify temperature, time interval, or number of tests to be conducted for stability testing. Recently the FDA published a draft guideline for submission of supporting documentation for stability studies on human drugs and biologics [20]. It is important, however, to understand that there are other factors to be considered besides the stability of the active ingredient(s) in determining a suitable expiration date (Table 2).

Unit Dose Repackaging and the FDA

Hospital pharmacists should be aware of the Food and Drug Administration's Compliance Policy Guide No. 7132b.11, dated March 1, 1984. This guide stated that no regulatory action will be initiated against any unit dose repackaging firm, including shared services, or drug product in a unit dose container meeting all other conditions of the FDA's repackaging requirements solely on the basis of the failure of the repackaging firm to have stability studies supporting the expiration dates used. According to the agency, such studies are not always necessary for the protection of health or for assurance of stability of the drug even though current good manufacturing practice regulations require that expiration dates used on unit-dose containers be supported by such tests. To avoid action by the FDA, a unit-dose container must comply with compendial (Class A or B)* standards, and the expiration dating period must not exceed six months. In addition, the six-month period must not exceed 25 percent of the remaining time between the date of repackaging and the expiration date on the original manufacturer's bulk container and the bulk container has not been previously opened. The policy applies only to solid and liquid oral dosage forms in unit containers, not to antibiotics or drugs with well-known stability problems, e.g., nitroglycerin.

With respect to an individual hospital pharmacy's repackaging of drugs into unit dose form, the issue is whether the repackaging constitutes manufacturing or whether it is part of the practice of pharmacy. If it is the latter, then FDA lacks authority; the practice of pharmacy, as mentioned earlier, is regulated by the individual states, not the federal government.

The American Society of Hospital Pharmacists (ASHP) has published guidelines for repackaging oral solids and liquids in single unit and unit-dose packages. These guidelines were developed by ASHP and the American Society of Consulting Pharmacists (ASCP). With regard to expiration dating, the guidelines simply provide that "it is the responsibility of the pharmacist . . . to determine the expiration date to be placed on a package" and that "this date must not be beyond the original package" [22]. FDA has acknowledged the guidelines and has commended ASHP and ASCP for having developed it; it may be that this recommendation derives from FDA's belief that the guidelines are written in the same spirit as the agency's good manufacturing practice regulations.

*Classes relate to the amount of moisture permeation.

Prohibited Acts

Section 301 of the Act establishes that the introduction, delivery or introduction, or receipt in interstate commerce of any drug that is adulterated or misbranded is prohibited.

The FDA considers a drug misbranded when an expiration date is scientifically unsupportable. In such cases, it has charged that pursuant to Section 502(a) of the Act, the product was misbranded in that the labeled expiration date was a false and misleading statement because it implied that the product would be stable for a stated period of time when that claim could not be justified. Under Section 501, a drug is deemed adulterated if it is not manufactured in conformance with current GMP's. Further, Section 502(g) states that a drug is misbranded if it is a compendial drug and is not packaged or labeled as prescribed therein. The expiration date of a drug, when it is required, must appear on the label of the immediate container and also the outer package if any, unless it is easily legible through such outer package, i.e., window cartons. However, when single-dose containers are packed in individual cartons, the expiration date may properly appear on the individual carton instead of the immediate product container [21].

From the standpoint of criminal liability for violation of a statute, the pharmacist is not required to comply with FDA or ASHP's expiration guidelines (see boxed item) because neither has the effect of a law. However, civil liability is another matter. The standard used to determine if a professional has breached his legal duty of care is whether he possessed and exercised skill and knowledge of a member of the profession in good standing in the same or similar community. In determining whether the professional acted reasonably, courts look to existing standards of practice for guidance. Both the FDA and ASHP expiration date guidelines may be considered standards of practice. If so, compliance with those documents would constitute at least *prima facie* evidence of reasonable, prudent conduct on the part of the pharmacist [23].

The pharmacist who dispenses old drugs faces a risk of liability if the product causes an injury or was found to be of diminished strength, quality and purity because of age [24]. In some cases, the pharmacist can determine the date of manufacture of the drug from the lot number [25].

United States Pharmacopeia and National Formulary

While much has already been written with regard to compendial standards and expiration dating, there are few other considerations. For one, the *USP* has required expiration dates on all compendial products since January 1976. As a matter of fact, the requirement for expiration dating was deferred from an earlier date until January 1, 1976, to allow sufficient time for revision of the GMP regulations. *USP VIII*, which became effective in 1906, recognized diphtheria antitoxin, and the monograph on it included the statement that the article "must be labeled with the date beyond which it will not have the strength indicated on the label or statement." This is a first expiry date requirement in either the *USP* or the *NF*. *USP IX*, published ten years later, listed three forms of the diphtheria antitoxin, three forms of tetanus antitoxin, and smallpox vaccine. The monographs for all these products required "a date beyond which the product cannot be expected to yield its specific results."

Each successive Pharmacopeia since 1916 has carried a similar statement for the increasing numbers of products of this kind which are produced under federal license and supervision. (See Table 3 for guidelines for expiration dating). In the current edition of the *USP* there is also a statement that reads "the expiration date identifies the time during which

---

Table 3
USP Expiration Dating

The label of an official drug product shall bear an expiration date. The monographs for some preparations specify the expiration date that shall appear on the label. In the absence of a specific requirement in the individual monograph for a drug product, the label shall bear an expiration date assigned for the particular formulation and package of the article, with the following exception: the label need not show an expiration date in the case of a drug product packaged in a container that is intended for sale without prescription and the labeling of which states no dosage limitations, and which is stable for not less than 3 years when stored under the prescribed conditions.

Where an official article is required to bear an expiration date, such article shall be dispensed solely in, or from, a container labeled with an expiration date, and the date on which the article is dispensed shall be within the labeled expiry period. The expiration date identifies the time during which the article may be expected to meet the requirements of the Pharmacopeial monograph provided it is kept under the prescribed storage conditions. The expiration date limits the time during which the article may be dispensed or used. Where an expiration date is stated only in terms of the month and the year, it is a representation that the intended expiration date is the last day of the stated month.

For articles requiring constitution prior to use, a suitable beyond-use date for the constituted product shall be identified in the labeling.

In determining an appropriate period of time during which a prescription drug may be retained by a patient after its dispensing, the dispenser shall take into account, in addition to any other relevant factors, the nature of the drug; the container in which it was packaged by the manufacturer and the expiration date thereon; the characteristics of the patient's container if the article is repackaged for dispensing; the expected storage conditions to which the article may be exposed; and the expected length of time of the course of therapy. Unless otherwise required, the dispenser may, on taking into account the foregoing, place on the label of a multiple-unit container a suitable beyond-use date to limit the patient's use of the article. Unless otherwise specified in the individual monograph, such beyond-use date shall be not later than (a) the expiration date on the manufacturer's container, or (b) one year from the date the drug is dispensed, whichever is earlier.

Source: United States Pharmacopeia, 22nd revision, 1990, p. 10.

---

the article may be expected to meet the requirements of the Pharmacopeial monograph providing it is kept under the prescribed storage conditions. The expiration date limits the time during which the product may be dispensed or used. Where an expiration date is stated only in terms of the month and the year, it is a representation that the intended expiration date is the last day of the stated month. For articles requiring constitution prior to use, a suitable beyond-use date for the constituted product shall be identified on a labeling.

"In determining an appropriate period of time during which a prescription drug may be retained by a patient after dispensing, the dispenser shall take into account, in addition to any other relevant factors, the nature of the drug; the container in which it was packaged by the manufacturer and the expiration date thereon; the characteristics of the patient's container, if the particle is repackaged for dispensing; the expected storage conditions to which the article may be exposed; and the unexpected length of time of the course of therapy. Unless otherwise required, the dispenser may, on taking into account the foregoing, place on the label of a multiple-unit container a suitable beyond-use date to limit the patient's use of the drug. Unless otherwise specified in the individual monograph, such beyond-use date shall be not later than (a) the expiration date on the manufacturer's container, or (b) one year from the date the drug is dispensed, whichever is earlier" [18].

Of additional importance is the responsibility of the pharmacist. "As a final step in meeting responsibility for the stability of drugs dispensed, the pharmacist is obligated to inform the patient regarding the proper storage conditions (for example, in a cool, dry place—not in the bathroom), for both prescription and nonprescription products, and to suggest a reasonable estimate of time after which the medication should be discarded. Where expiration dates are applied, the pharmacist should emphasize to the patient that the dates are applicable only when proper storage conditions are used. Patients should be encouraged to clean out their drug storage cabinets periodically" [26]. Much of this section relates to expiration dating and stability. For example, the pharmacist is told to dispense oldest stock first and to observe expiration dates. He is also asked to store products under the environmental conditions stated in the individual monographs and/or in the labeling. The pharmacist has the responsibility to observe drug products for evidence of instability and to properly treat and label products when they are repackaged, diluted or mixed with other products. Dispensing the drug in the proper container with the proper closure is an additional consideration. Lastly, the pharmacist has the moral and, in some

states, legal responsibility to inform and educate patients concerning the proper storage and use of products, including the disposition of outdated or excessively aged prescriptions.

References

1. 43 FR 45013-45336, September 29, 1978.
2. 21 U.S.C., 357; FDC Act Sec. 507.
3. Public Law 77-366; 21 U.S.C. 356; FDC Act Sec 506.
4. Regulations for the Sale of Viruses, Serums, Toxins and Analogous Products, U.S. Public Health Service, February 12, 1919.
5. Frimpter GW et al.: Reversible "Fanconi Syndrome" caused by degraded tetracycline. JAMA 154:111, 1963.
6. Gross JM: Fanconi Syndrome (adult type) developing secondary to the ingestion of outdated tetracycline. Ann Int Med 58:523, 1963.
7. Sulkowski SR, Haserick, JR: Simulated systemic lupus erythematosis from degraded tetracycline. JAMA 189:152, 1964.
8. Dearborn EH: The importance of pharmaceutical dating for drug safety. Conference on the Dating of Pharmaceuticals, Univ. Extension, Univ. Wisconsin, Madison WI, 1970, pp. 29–42.
9. Public Law 87-181:76 Stat 780 et seq.
10. 28 FR 6385-6387, June 20, 1963.
11. Lintner CJ: Stability of Pharmaceutical Products. In Osol A, Chase GD, Gennero AR et al. (Eds): Remington's Pharmaceutical Sciences, 16th Ed, Easton PA, Mack Publishing Company, 1980, p. 1419.
12. 36 FR 601-605, January 15, 1971.
13. 41 FR 6878-6894, February 13, 1976.
14. 44 FR 11064-11065, February 27, 1979.
15. Wollish EG: Current experience with drug expiration dating. Conference on the dating of pharmaceuticals. Univ. Extension, Univ. Wisconsin, Madison, WI, 1970, pp. 133–136.
16. Aarons M: Drug dating. Confererence on the dating of pharmaceuticals. Univ. Extension, Univ. Wisconsin, Madison, WI, 1970, pp 116–121.
17. Memorandum in opposition to A-1340 and S-1049, PSSNY, June 1, 1979.
18. The United States Pharmacopeial Convention, Inc.: The United States Pharmacopeia, Twenty-second Revision, Easton PA, Mack Publishing Company, 1990, p. 9.
19. Davis J: Requirements for expiration dating and stability testing in in the United States. Pharm Tech 16:65, 1979.
20. Draft Guideline for Stability Studies for Human Drugs and Biologics, Center for Drugs and Biologics, 5600 Fishers Lane, Rockville, MD, March 1984.
21. 21 CFR 201.17.
22. ASHP Guidelines for repackaging oral solids and liquids in single unit and unit dose packages. Am J Hosp Pharm 36:223, 1979.
23. Vetrano AJ: Expiration dating of drugs repackaged in unit dose form. Am J Hosp Pharm 37:1308, 1980.
24. Greenberg RB: Dispensing drugs that do not have an expiration date. Am J Hosp Pharm 38:1113, 1981.
25. Feldman MJ et al: Determining the date of manufacture of drug products from lot numbers. Am J Hosp Pharm 36:1545, 1979.
26. The United States Pharmacopeial Convention, Inc., *op. cit.*, p. 1347.

When an expiration date of a drug is required, it shall appear on the immediate container and also the outer package, if any, unless it is easily legible through such outer package. However, when single-dose containers are packed in individual cartons, the expiration date may properly appear on the individual carton instead of the immediate product container.

21 CFR 201.17

QUESTIONS: CHAPTER 8

1. If an expiration date for a *USP/NF* drug is stated only in terms of the month and year, what is the effective day of expiration?
   a. First day of the stated month
   b. First day of the stated year
   c. Middle of the stated month—the fifteenth day
   d. Last day of the stated month
   e. Last day of the stated year

   USP XXII, p.10

2. When an expiration date is stated only in terms of the month and year for a compendial drug, the intended date is the _____ day of the stated month:
   a. First
   b. Fifteenth
   c. Last
   d. Thirtieth
   e. Thirty-first

   USP XXII, p.10

3. If the manufacturer does not support the expiration date of a drug product with valid scientific data, according to the FD&C Act the drug product is deemed:
   a. Adulterated
   b. Misbranded
   c. Putrid
   d. Quarantined
   e. Unstable

   21 U.S.C. 352(a)

4. The expiration date for insulin products marketed in the United States is:
   a. 6 months
   b. 12 months
   c. 18 months
   d. 24 months

5. Which of the following are exempt from the federal regulations pertaining to expiration dating?
   a. *U.S. Pharmacopeia* drugs
   b. Drugs listed in the *National Formulary*
   c. Homeopathic drug products
   d. Allergenic extracts
   e. Allopathic medicines

   21 CFR 211.137(e)

6. According to the *USP*, unless otherwise specified in the individual monograph, when a drug is repackaged for dispensing by the pharmacist, the maximum beyond-use date placed on the label shall be:
   a. The first day of the month following the dispensing
   b. The last day of the month following the dispensing
   c. One year from the date of dispensing
   d. The manufacturer's expiration date appearing on the label
   e. The expiration date appearing on the manufacturer's label or one year from the date of dispensing, whichever is earlier

   USP XXII, p.10

7. Factors to consider in determining an expiration date for a drug include:
1) Stability of active ingredients
2) Manufacturing process
3) Container closure system
4) Dosage form
5) Conditions under which the drug is shipped, stored, and handled

    a. 1) and 2) are correct.
    b. 1), 2), and 3) are correct.
    c. 1), 2), 3), and 4) are correct.
    d. 1), 2), 3), and 5) are correct.
    e. 1), 2), 3), 4), and 5) are correct.

21 CFR 211.166
21 CFR 211.137

8. According to compendial requirements, if the label of a compendial drug states "Expires December 1996," it means that:

    a. The drug cannot be dispensed after December 31, 1996.
    b. The drug cannot be used after December 31, 1996.
    c. The drug cannot be dispensed after December 1, 1996.
    d. The drug cannot be dispensed and should not be used after December 31, 1996.
    e. The drug cannot be dispensed and should not be used after December 15, 1996.

USP XXII, p.10

9. Examples of human OTC drug products exempt from FDA's expiration dating regulations include:

    a. Fluoride toothpaste, cough drops
    b. Topical lotions, creams, ointments
    c. Rubbing alcohol, isopropyl alcohol, methyl alcohol
    d. Medicated and nonmedicated shampoos

10. Human OTC drug products are exempt from FDA's expiration dating regulations if:

    a. They are stable for at least five years.
    b. Their labeling bears dosage limitations.
    c. They are safe and effective.
    d. They are safe and suitable for frequent use and often prolonged use.
    e. All of the above

11. According to *USP* standards, a refrigerator is defined as a cold place in which the temperature is maintained between:

    a. 2° and 8°C
    b. 2° and 8°F
    c. 36° and 46°C
    d. −4° and 14°F
    e. −4° and 14°C

12. The *USP* defines a freezer as a cold place in which the temperature is maintained thermostatically between:

    a. −4° and 14°C
    b. 2° and 8°C
    c. 36° and 46°C
    d. −20° and −10°C
    e. 2° and 8°F

CHAPTER 9

Drug Law

PHARMACY . . . AND THE FOOD AND DRUG LAW: A SIGNIFICANT RELATIONSHIP*

Wallace F. Janssen

On June 30, 1906, President Theodore Roosevelt signed the original Pure Food and Drugs Act (often referred to as the Wiley Act).

No single event has had greater significance to the profession of pharmacy. It was not only a victory for scientific pharmacy and medicine but it signaled the beginning of an era of progress in these fields which has had no counterpart in history.

A large book could be written on the subject. And its central figure certainly would be the towering one of Dr. Harvey Washington Wiley, one of the truly great personalities of his time, and the one individual most responsible for the development of food and drug laws in this country. Born October 18, 1844, in a log cabin on a backwoods Indiana farm, Wiley had almost no formal education in his childhood but, fortunately, had a learned father who taught his children Latin and Greek and, around the evening fire, read to them aloud from the Bible, Shakespeare and the *Atlantic Monthly*.

At 19, dressed in a homespun suit and cowhide boots, young Harvey started across the fields to the new Hanover College, five

miles away. Ten years later, this young man had graduated from Hanover, taken his MA degree, graduated from Indiana Medical College, served in the Union Army, and received a Bachelor of Science degree from Harvard University, the latter degree won in 17 days, during which he passed the four-year class examinations with flying colors. Wiley was in residence at Harvard for less than six months. In those six months, however, he attended lectures by such great teaching personalities as Charles Edward Munroe, Louis Agassiz and Charles W. Eliot, and their influence remained with him the rest of his life.

Harvey Wiley then became a teacher, an experience which helped greatly to fit him for the stormy years ahead. He taught chemistry at Indiana Medical College and Butler University—mornings at one and evenings at the other. In 1874, when Purdue University was opened, Wiley was its first professor of chemistry. Later he became state chemist of Indiana. In 1878, he went to Berlin for advanced chemical studies and there became attached to the Imperial Board of Health. Returning from Germany he resumed his post at Purdue, where he received commendation for his teaching, but was formally censured for riding a

high-wheel bicycle and playing baseball with the students. (This bicycle reported is still preserved with other Wiley relics at the University museum.)

In 1883 after nine years at Purdue, Wiley was invited to become chief chemist of the U.S. Department of Agriculture. He remained in this post for 29 years. Early in this period he began his famous crusade to curb the then widespread abuses in the production and sale of foods and drugs.

Conditions Prior to 1906

One of Wiley's first official acts was to expand the studies of food adulteration begun by department chemists in the 1870s. Changes from an agricultural to an industrial economy had made it necessary to provide the rapidly increasing city population with food from distant areas. This led to a boom in commercial food processing. It also led to an extensive use of chemical preservatives such as borax, formaldehyde and salicylates in meats and canned foods. Artificial colors, some of them toxic, were indiscriminately employed. Labeling gave no hint of these deleterious ingredients. While such practices were by no means universal, and many firms were putting out entirely whole-

*Reprinted with permission from *American Pharmacy*, NS21:28–36 (April 1981).

some products, Wiley's chemists had no difficulty finding material for their investigations. The results, reported over a period of 15 years, documented the need for federal controls on the food industry.

In view of Wiley's connection with the Department of Agriculture, it is not surprising that at first he showed little interest in the problems of food and drug adulteration and misbranding. Yet, this was the heyday of "patent medicines" such as Kick-a-poo Indiana Sagwa and Warner's Safe Cure for Diabetes. The existence of thousands of these products reflected both the limited medical knowledge of the period and public acceptance of the doctrine that buyers should look out for themselves. Nostrums were so common that they were largely taken for granted—a part of the normal American scene. Anyone, no matter how ignorant or unqualified, could go into the drug manufacturing business.

Medicines containing such drugs as opium, morphine and cocaine were sold without restriction at almost every crossroads store. Innocuous and inert preparations were labeled for the cure of every disease and symptom. Labels did not declare ingredients, and warnings against misuse were unheard of. What information the public got along these lines came from the physician or pharmacist, from hearsay, or sometimes from bitter experience.

1848—The First Federal Drug Law

Typically, patent medicines were fraudulent and dangerous because of their *misbranding* with false claims. On the other hand, legitimate drugs and drug materials could be just as dangerous, because of widespread *adulteration*. It is hard for us today to realize what a problem this was for 19th century pharmacists and physicians. The United States, lacking laws and regulations of European countries, was the world's dumping ground for substandard and

contaminated drugs. Since there was no mass production of medicines before the Civil War, each physician and pharmacist needed to be a drug inspector as well as a compounder of medicines. In Colonial times the European pharmacopeias were relied on for formulas and methods. The *U.S. Pharmacopeia*, established in 1820, was the first major effort in this country to establish national drug standards. A primary objective of the founders of the first American colleges of pharmacy (Philadelphia in 1829; New York in 1828) was to educate their graduates and the medical profession to cope with the hazards of spurious drugs.

But none of these developments could stop the influx of counterfeit, contaminated, decomposed, and diluted drug materials from overseas. The U.S. had a customs examination, but only to assure correct valuation for duty purposes. Fortunately, however, U.S. Customs had a conscientious and trained examiner at New York, M. J. Bailey, M.D., who used the law as best he could and carried on a campaign through articles and speeches warning physicians and pharmacists to be wary about the quality of drugs.

Bailey's disclosures and statistics eventually reached the U.S. Congress. T. O. Edwards, M.D., an Ohio congressman, who could also present the views of the new American Medical Association, headed the committee which dealt with the matter. Physicians had special reasons to be concerned. Confronted with drugs of unknown, widely varying potency or no potency at all, they could not rely on the official dosages in the *U.S. Pharmacopeia*. Each new shipment, even each patient, was involved, in effect, in a clinical experiment with an unpredictable outcome. Doctors in the frontier states and territories found they had to give heroic doses because the trade practice was to ship the cheapest and worst products "out West." The discrepancies in doses used in different areas perplexed

and alarmed the readers of medical journals.

Rep. Edwards closed his report to the House of Representatives with the shocking statement that disease and death among American soldiers then in Mexico were due in part to fraud in medical supplies bought from the lowest bidders. Heading the list was Peruvian bark for malaria at 5¢ per pound when the market price for the good quality product was 70¢ per pound.

The Import Drugs Act of 1848, our first federal drug law, provided for laboratory inspections at ports of entry, and for detention and destruction or re-export of shipments not meeting pharmacopeial standards.

At first, the approach was successful. It wasn't long, however, before enforcement deteriorated due to lack of support and political interference. In 1850, the New York College of Pharmacy held a meeting with delegates from other colleges to consider the danger of continued adulteration. Another such meeting in 1852 resulted in the establishment of the American Pharmaceutical Association. Thus, professional pharmacy in the United States had its roots in the same problems that led to the establishment of regulatory laws.

Consumer Protection Begins

Before 1906, the only federal law that could have been used against drug misbranding and quackery was the first mail fraud statute, passed in 1872. Yet, for almost 30 years there is no record of its enforcement in the drug area. Postal inspectors were mainly concerned with financial swindles involving investments, mining rights, lotteries, and the like. Then, in 1899, Wiley's Bureau of Chemistry was asked by the Postmaster General for an analysis of some tablets that a postal inspector suspected of being illegally vended through the mails. Wiley's pharmaceutical chemists found that the tablets, represented as a test for kidney disease, contained only methylene blue dye. The seller claimed that, if after taking one tablet at night users found their morning urine blue, they needed a treatment for kidney disease. Noting that the tablets would color anyone's urine, Wiley denounced the scheme as "fraudulent in every particular."

About 1904, when national magazines began to crusade against flagrant social injustice including the exploitation of the ill by patent medicine promoters, the Postal Service began devoting greater efforts to ridding the mails of quack remedies. Wiley was not one to neglect an opportunity. Collaboration with the Postal Service got first priority. Wiley and his staff found flagrant violations in most of the cases. Of nearly 50 postal fraud hearings involving Bureau of Chemistry evidence between 1904 and 1907, almost all resulted in banning the products from the mails, a drastic penalty.

After the new Food and Drugs Act went into effect in January 1907, the two agencies maintained their cooperation. This interagency liaison has continued until the present time—one of the oldest examples of interagency cooperation in federal history.

Tragedy Brings a Law

Drug adulteration is not the kind of problem that disappears; it requires constant vigilance. While leading drug suppliers built successful businesses on reliability, others continued to cheat. In 1902, a group of New York drug manufacturers induced Congress to pass legislation requiring the Secretary of Agriculture to investigate the adulteration of drugs in the United States and its effects on the industry. The legislation was supported at the Senate hearings by a delegation headed by Charles R. Parmele, the manufacturing chemist from New York. This bill became law on June 30, 1902, and a drug laboratory was established in the Bureau of Chemistry to carry on the work.

In the same year, 1902, a drug tragedy caused Congress to pass

the strongest drug control law it has ever enacted: the original Biologics Act. The St. Louis Health Department was making its own diphtheria antitoxin and a tetanus contamination occurred. Twelve children died, ten recoverd. The District of Columbia Medical Society led the effort to secure licensing control over both biological drug laboratories and their products. Administration was assigned to the Public Health Service, then in the Treasury Department. Biologics control, in FDA since 1972, is the nation's oldest drug regulatory program.

From 1879 to 1906, more than 100 food and drug bills were introduced in Congress. The first advocates of such legislation were food industry leaders who were motivated by two problems: cutthroat competition by manufacturers of adulterated products (for example, "lard" made of cottonseed oil) and intolerable variations in state laws. As one food man said: "As it is now, we have to manufacture differently for each state."

From the outset, the pure food and drug movement was supported by state officials, professional groups (especially APhA and AMA) and some members of Congress. But Wiley took his message to the public. He became a popular speaker to women's clubs and business organizations. A group of crusading writers joined in the campaign. *Collier's Weekly*, the *Ladies' Home Journal* and *Good Housekeeping* magazines aroused public opinion with their cartoons, articles and editorials.

Strenuous opposition came from many manufacturers, particularly the whiskey distillers and the makers of patent medicines who were then the largest advertisers in the country. Many of these opponents thought federal legislation would put them out of business.

Beginning in 1902, Wiley captured public attention by establishing a volunteer "poison squad" of young men who agreed to eat only foods treated with measured amounts of chemical preservatives,

with the object of showing their "effects on digestion and health." Even the popular song writers took an interest in these experiments, which continued over a five-year period. For example, Lew Dockstader, the minstrel star, introduced a song dedicated to the "poison squad," with the refrain:

O, they may get over it but they'll never look the same, That kind of bill of fare would drive most men insane. Next week he'll give them mothballs, a la Newburgh or else plain; O, they may get over it but they'll never look the same.

When the final vote came in 1906 on the broad Food and Drugs Act, it was almost unanimous. Wiley had won!

APhA's Role

As we have seen, the American Pharmaceutical Association, from its beginning, had taken an active interest in the problem of drug adulteration. An APhA committee, headed by E. L. Patch of Boston, had made its own study, analyzing samples of various drugs. Reporting at the 50th anniversary APhA convention in Philadelphia in 1902, the committee hailed the establishment of the Washington drug laboratory as "one of the most important events in the history of American pharmacy." An APhA resolution pledged "cordial cooperation" and to use its influence to secure "a reasonable appropriation to properly carry on this work in a systematic and effective manner."

Thus, four years prior to the passage of the 1906 law, APhA had given its official support to Wiley's efforts.

Wiley was present at this 1902 convention. In a brief talk he asked for the Association's help in finding a qualified pharmaceutical chemist to take the new job as chief of the drug laboratory.

The following year Dr. Lyman F. Kebler, previously with Smith Kline and French of Philadelphia, spoke at the opening session of APhA's convention about his first year's work as chief of the new laboratory. That was the beginning of many years of close collaboration between the pharmacy profession and the Bureau of Chemistry, now the Food and Drug Administration.

A Setback for Drug Effectiveness

Everyone thought the 1906 Act would reform patent medicine by outlawing false therapeutic claims. The act, indeed, prohibited adulteration and misbranding, and hundreds of worthless and dangerous products were taken off the market. Many other manufacturers changed their formulas or dropped label claims that could not be sustained in court.

But, in 1911, a serious setback occurred. A divided Supreme Court held that the law did not prohibit false health claims, only false label statements about the identity or ingredients of drugs. Thus, in the case of "Dr. Johnson's Mild Combination Treatment for Cancer," the promoter could not be prosecuted for "mistaken praise," even though the indictment charged that he knew his claims were false.

President Taft at once called on Congress to close this dangerous loophole in the law. Said the president:

"There are none so credulous as sufferers from disease. The need is urgent for legislation that will prevent the raising of false hopes of speedy cures of serious ailments by misstatements of facts as to worthless mixtures on which the sick will rely while their disease progresses unchecked."

In 1912, Congress passed the Sherley Amendment prohibiting false "and fraudulent" label claims of therapeutic effectiveness. Unfortunately, the language required the prosecution to prove that the promoter of a worthless drug had lied deliberately to defraud the public, an impossibility in most cases. For 26 years the "fraud joker" remained in the law, often preventing effective enforcement.

While complying literally with the Sherley Amendment, many drug promoters evaded it by simply transferring the false label claims to their advertising.

The control over narcotics under the 1906 Act was also unsatisfactory. All it required was that drug labels state the quantity of "any alcohol, morphine, opium, heroin, cocaine, alpha or beta eucaine, chloroform, cannabis indica, chloral hydrate, or acetanilide or any derivative" of these. One of the worst abuses of that era was the addition of babies given "soothing syrups" to stop their crying. There were at least a hundred such products on the market containing varying amounts of morphine, opium or heroin.

The *Chicago Tribune* led the fight against the "soothers," calling them "baby killers." The *Ladies Home Journal* and American Medical Association were joined by pharmacists who pledged to stop selling such products without prescription. Public indignation reached the boiling point. The Harrison Narcotic Act (1914) finally established a stricter system of control over all narcotics, a program then administered by the Treasury Department (now under Justice's Drug Enforcement Administration).

1933—Battle for a New Law

The Wiley Act had defined "adulterated" and "misbranded" foods and drugs and prohibited their shipment across state lines. It was a unique and strong law for its times—indeed a milestone in American social history—but the onrush of technological change would soon make it outmoded.

Food adulteration continued to flourish because judges could find no specific authority in the law for the standards of purity and content which the FDA had established. Such products as "fruit" jams made with water, glucose, grass seed, and artificial color undercut the market for honest products.

Economic hardships of the 1930 depression years magnified the many shortcomings of the 1906 act and brought a new consciousness of the needs of the consumer.

The book, *Your Money's Worth*, by Stuart Chase and F. J. Schlink, signaled the start of a new consumer movement, now worldwide.

In 1933, a few days after the inauguration of President Franklin D. Roosevelt, the chief of the Food and Drug Administration, Walter Campbell, seized an opportunity to discuss the weaknesses of the food and drug law with Rexford Tugwell, a member of the president's "brain trust," who had been named Assistant Secretary of Agriculture. The same afternoon Campbell was again called to Tugwell's office. "Mr. Campbell," said Tugwell, "since I saw you this morning I have talked with the president. I repeated our conversation to him, and he has authorized a revision of the Food and Drug Act."

The "Tugwell Bill," introduced in Congress a few weeks later, was a legislative disaster. The opposition of industry and advertising interests to this New Deal legislation was total and overwhelming.

When the smoke cleared away, a new sponsor, Sen. Royal S. Copeland, M.D., of New York, aided by FDA officials, consumer-minded congressmen and staff members, began the laborious process of fashioning a bill that could be enacted, yet would not surrender essential consumer protection.

Five years later, after the deaths of more than 100 people from an "Elixir of Sulfanilamide" containing a poisonous solvent, Congress passed the Federal Food, Drug, and Cosmetic Act which became law on June 30, 1938.

Although many compromises had to be made to secure passage, the new law was a major improvement:

• Proof of fraud was no longer required to stop false claims for drugs.

• Cosmetics and therapeutic devices were regulated for the first time.

• Food standards were required

to set up when needed "to promote honesty and fair dealing in the interest of consumers."

• Addition of poisonous substances to foods was prohibited except where unavoidable or required in production. Safe tolerances were authorized for residues of such substances, for example, pesticides.

• Federal court injunctions against violations were added to previous legal remedies of product seizures and criminal prosecutions.

• Specific authority was provided for factory inspections.

• Drug manufacturers were required to provide scientific proof that new products could be safely used before putting them on the market—the sulfanilamide experience had started what is now the major system of U.S. drug regulation.

Drug Classification— A Matter of Safety

Important pharmaceutical history resulted from the provision (§502(f)) of the 1938 act requiring drug packages to be labeled with adequate warnings and adequate directions for use, with exemptions from the directions requirement where "not necessary for the protection of the public health." A related provision (§502(j)) prohibited traffic in drugs that were dangerous when used as directed in the labeling. Regulations issued in 1939 defined "adequate directions for use" to mean directions under which a lay person can use a drug safely. Drugs labeled for use on the prescription of a physician were exempted from bearing "adequate directions"; these were to be supplied by the prescriber.

Explaining FDA policy, Commissioner Walter G. Campbell's 1939 annual report contained this statement:

Many drugs of great value to the physician are dangerous in the hands of those unskilled in the uses of drugs. The statute obviously was not intended to deprive the medical

profession of potent but valuable medicaments. The administrative conclusion was therefore announced that dangerous drugs like aminopyrine, cinchophen, neocinchophen, sulfanilamide, and related products may not be distributed for unrestricted use by the lay public without violating the statute; to insure compliance with the law, drugs of this character must be labeled with warnings so conspicuous as certainly to arrest attention and in such informative terms as will unfailingly apprise the user of the danger of irreparable injury if the drug is consumed without adequate and continuous medical supervision. Drug distributors have generally acquiesced in this decision, and there is evidence of sincere efforts to comply with its letter and spirit.

This was the rationale of what came to be called the "Rx Legend." From the start most products cleared by FDA as "new drugs" were restricted to prescription because they were considered not safe for lay use. The manufacturer was responsible for deciding which way to label its "not new" drugs, subject, of course, to FDA action if it made the wrong decision. The wording of the legend: "Caution: to be used only by or on the prescription of a _____ (physician, dentist or veterinarian)," was different from what it is now: "Caution: Federal law prohibits dispensing without prescription."

Widespread changes in the labeling and composition of drugs took place during the next five years. Manufacturers scrutinized their labels and voluntarily corrected practices that had previously brought regulatory actions. World War II diverted FDA resources to an important assignment—testing drugs for the armed forces. Penicillin inaugurated a new era in therapeutics.

During this period drug houses which restricted their business to professional channels began the rather widespread practice of labeling all their products for prescription sale. This posed a new problem for FDA: the law required

"adequate directions for use" on all drugs unless exempted by regulations. Using the Rx Legend on over-the-counter drugs defeated the purpose of the act which was to give the consumer essential information about the use of drugs that can be safely and effectively administered without medical supervision. Amended drug labeling regulations issued in 1945 required that:

• Drugs commonly purchased and suitable for use by lay consumers without the intervention of professional guidance shall bear adequate directions for use;

• Drugs dangerous for self-use shall be exempted, since directions for use on the labeling of such drugs are an invitation to the lay public to undertake a dangerous type of self-medication;

• Drugs requiring medical skill for proper use shall also be exempted, even though they are not inherently toxic.

Thus began the distinction, as a matter of federal law, between prescription drugs and nonprescription or over-the-counter drugs.

The main purpose of the 1945 regulations was to prevent the sale for self-medication of potent drugs that were safe for use only under medical supervision. This had already become recognized as a public health problem, particularly in two areas: sale of sulfa drugs and penicillin for self-treatment of VD infections, leading to bacterial resistance; and the growing illicit traffic in barbituates and, later, amphetamines.

FDA was just beginning an all-out effort to prevent the abuse of non-narcotic drugs (a program transferred to the Department of Justice in 1968). Scores of cases had been investigated in which death or serious illness had resulted from unauthorized filling of prescriptions. Criminal prosecutions of pharmacists and doctors involved in illegal sales of dangerous drugs had been sustained by the courts.

Following age-old tradition, physicians still were practicing "mysteriously"; it was thought that patients generally should not be told too much about the drugs prescribed for them. Such was the background for the section of the 1945 regulations that prohibited any indications or directions on manufacturer's packages of prescription drugs—a position that would later be completely reversed.

The Durham-Humphrey Law "Rx vs. OTC"

Pharmacists who sold a "legend" drug without a bonafide prescription were legally liable because they had caused the exemption (from required directions labeling) to be voided—hence, making the product misbranded, a criminal offense. This legally complex approach was cumbersome, confusing and contradictory. Moreover, it was difficult for FDA, on the basis of the law and the 1945 regulations, to enforce the new distinction between prescription and OTC drugs. The same drugs were being labeled with directions by some manufacturers and with the Rx Legend by others, sometimes both ways by the same firm. The law contained no definition of a prescription drug, and FDA had not presumed to provide one. FDA, the courts, the Congress, the medical profession, and pharmacists were all involved in a difficult situation.

On January 19, 1948, the Supreme Court handed down a decision in the Sullivan case, reversing a lower court decision that held that a druggist who sold sulfathiazole OTC could only be prosecuted under state law. And on June 18, 1948, Congress passed the Miller Amendment to the Federal Food, Drug, and Cosmetic Act, extending it to apply to violations in wholesale or retail establishments, making federal protection effective all the way to the ultimate consumer.

Retail pharmacists became concerned over the possibility of being prosecuted for selling legend drugs

over the counter. Their concern became widespread when FDA's Commissioner Paul B. Dunbar made a speech to the 1948 convention of the National Association of Retail Druggists (NARD) in which he compared a prescription to a check that could be cashed only once. Organized pharmacy, with FDA cooperation, went to Congress for clarification of the law. Two prominent pharmacists in Congress, Rep. Carl Durham of North Carolina, and Sen. Hubert Humphrey of Minnesota, sponsored the legislation and took an active role in its development.

The Durham-Humphrey Amendment became law October 26, 1951. It supplied the long-needed definition of the kinds of drugs that must be labeled for prescription use. It prohibited refills without an authorization from the prescriber. It allowed prescriptions and refill authorizations by telephone if recorded in writing. It emphasized the responsibility of the medical profession to prescribe drugs, and the professional service of pharmacists as the licensed and responsible custodians of drugs for the community. In effect, it put the power of federal law behind the ethics of the pharmaceutical profession.

FDA and NARD were the leading proponents of this legislation, with strong help from the two congressional sponsors. There was little public or consumer interest. The lay press gave virtually no coverage. When the bill was debated, the only reference in the *New York Times* was one line in the Washington news index: "House holds routine session." This on legislation affecting every person in the country who might receive a prescription!

At the suggestion of the National Association of Boards of Pharmacy, FDA developed a manual on the new law to aid pharmacists in applying it to situations of doctors and patients. For some years "The Rx Legend" was distributed annually to colleges of pharmacy for their classes in pharmacy law and for all graduating seniors.

Drug Labeling Policy Revised

The Durham-Humphrey law necessitated another revision of the FDA regulations on drug labeling. As previously stated, Rx Legend drugs had been prohibited from bearing directions and, with few exceptions, warning statements were not required. Now, however, there was legal authority to require the prescription drug package to include professional information. One effect was to classify injectables as prescription drugs with directions for use by the medical profession. But FDA medical staff was reluctant to go farther because of their apprehension that physician information in the package could get into the hands of the lay public and encourage dangerous self-treatment. It was thought better to keep technical medical information in professional channels. Besides, it was said, labeling could provide complete information. A condition and justification for omitting such information from the manufacturer's package was that it must be obtainable from "readily available" sources, like text books and journal articles. This presumed, of course, that practitioners keep up to date in their reading.

How and why FDA reversed its policy to bring about the greatest single change in prescription drug labeling was summarized by Dr. Ralph G. Smith, then director of FDA's division of new drugs, in a 1968 paper before the American Society of Hospital Pharmacists. As Smith stated, the rapid increase in the introduction of new drugs which took place in the 1950s had made FDA increasingly aware of a very serious problem:

The drug manufacturers were replacing the medical schools as the principal source of information for physicians in their use of new drugs. The informative labeling worked out by FDA with applicants in the course of processing New Drug Applications, was not reaching physicians. This labeling, in accord with the regulations, was referred to on the drug label as "available to physicians on request." *The pharmaceutical industry, however, was promoting the use of these potent new drugs to physicians by detail men, mailing pieces, medical journal advertising, and reference publications that frequently failed to disclose their hazards. The more informative labeling was usually not part of the drug package and was rarely requested by the physician, nor was there any assurance it would be included in a response to a request for information. As the dangers of this situation were recognized, FDA's division of new drugs increasingly required the informative labeling to be made a part of the prescription drug package. This was not an adequate solution to the problem and in 1961 the so-called "full disclosure" regulations were promulgated.*

Full disclosure was an idea whose time had come. It was clear that the danger of unwise self-treatment resulting from informative labeling of "legend" drugs was far outweighed by the dangers created by the absence of such labeling. Already, the flood of new products had created an "information lag." Promotional practices of the prescription drug industry were examined and condemned in public hearings by Sen. Estes Kefauver's Subcommittee on Antitrust and Monopoly. Legislation was being drafted to make multiple changes in drug regulation. And, as usual, industry representatives were hard at work to reduce the extent of the proposed controls to "something they could live with."

The Lesson of Thalidomide

But, in the early summer of 1962, complacency vanished abruptly as a horrifying story unfolded of the narrow escape of American families from the tragedy of grotesque deformities in babies caused in European countries by a supposedly safe new sleeping pill. Thalidomide did not reach the U.S. market because the new drug safety clearance requirements of 1938 had been applied by an FDA

medical officer, Dr. Frances O. Kelsey, who refused to release the drug on what she believed was inadequate evidence.

Dr. Harry F. Dowling's excellent book, *Medicines for Men*, describes what happened in one sentence:

"The headlines screamed, the public was aroused, the drug manufacturers ran scared, and the opponents of a tough bill jumped for cover."

Thalidomide had been widely distributed to doctors in the U.S. as an investigational drug. As the extent of this distribution was learned, it became apparent that a tightening of controls over investigational drugs was needed. Proposed new regulations were issued; Congress quickened its pace on the pending drug legislation. As statutory gaps in consumer protection came to be interpreted in terms of deformed babies, public clamor arose for strengthening the law in every respect necessary to close those gaps.

Passed unanimously, the Drug Amendments of 1962 contained many important new provisions:

• Drug companies were required to register their establishments with FDA and to be inspected at least once every two years;

• Pertinent records were required to be kept and made available for inspection;

• Reports of adverse effects were required to be promptly transmitted to FDA;

• Regulation of advertising of prescription drugs was transferred from the Federal Trade Commission to FDA and required to include full information on adverse effects and contraindications so as to provide a balanced picture;

• New investigational drug provisions required informed patient consent before trials on human subjects;

• Very importantly, effectiveness as well as safety of new drugs was required to be shown by substantial evidence from controlled studies to obtain FDA approval for marketing.

Extensive litigation followed the 1962 Amendments, and still continues in cases involving the legal status of certain generic drugs. At least a dozen lawsuits by drug companies and associations challenged the effectiveness provisions. Four of these—decided finally by the U.S. Supreme Court in 1973—resulted in opinions that virtually gave the FDA a new charter. With FDA having "primary jurisdiction," as the Court held, the agency can make decisions and regulations with "administrative finality." In short, if FDA's regulations are properly prepared, they have the force of law. The Supreme Court also endorsed regulation-making as the preferred mass approach to compliance, rather than merely prosecuting individuals or firms one by one, a method it described as "inherently unfair" because competitors are left free to keep on violating until the law catches up with them.

For several years after 1962, FDA tried different ways to obtain the "substantial evidence" of drug effectiveness that the law required. Truckloads of data often proved to be mainly opinions and testimonials, not based on valid scientific research.

Then, in 1966, Commissioner James Goddard, M.D., negotiated a unique contract with the National Academy of Sciences and its National Research Council. NAS/NRC established panels of leading experts in therapeutics to review for effectiveness all prescription drugs approved for the U.S. market between 1938 and 1962 based on safety alone. More than 200 representatives of medicine and pharmacy served on these panels. The results have been far-reaching: more than 7,000 prescription drug items have been removed from trade channels because they lacked sufficient evidence of effectiveness, and some 1,500 more have had their labels changed to bring them into line with current medical knowledge.

A somewhat similar mass review of nonprescription drugs has been partially completed and its recommendations are still being reported.

Altogether, FDA's mass review of drugs for compliance with the 1962 Amendments has been a major accomplishment and will be recorded as one of the milestones of medical history.

Not all changes in drug control have resulted from legislation. The progress of science has brought great improvements in research techniques, analytical methods and standards of quality. Computers have changed the methods of management. Compliance has improved, with a new emphasis on preventing violations rather than merely prosecuting them after they occur. Voluntary product recalls have largely replaced court-ordered seizures as a means of consumer protection. Recalls are faster, more efficient and less expensive to the taxpayer than court proceedings. Their success is due to the cooperation of manufacturers and distributors. Pharmacists have played a key role in making drug recalls effective. A new law, the Drug Listing Act of 1972, has made it possible for FDA to keep an up-to-date inventory of the drugs and other health products on the U.S. market.

Not all food and drug laws have been passed because of some publicized catastrophe. Very important amendments have come because far-sighted industry and government leaders saw the need for them. The Humphrey-Durham law has been mentioned. Others include the food safety laws—the Pesticide Amendment of 1954, the Food Additive Amendment of 1958 and the Color Additive Amendment of 1960. The most recent law—the Medical Device Amendments of 1976—was the result of 20 years of discussion and development.

Lawyers and judges have made a tremendous contribution. Little appreciated by FDA critics is the vast experience developed in the "case law" of foods and drugs, which constantly influences policy and action. One cannot really understand FDA without knowledge of the problems presented by actual cases.

Nor can one really understand FDA without knowing something about the industries and professions. Administration of the food and drug law, like the drug industry, is a field requiring professional expertise—not a game of "cops and robbers." The law reflects accepted industry practices. It requires all to come up to levels the leaders have already achieved, thus promoting progress while protecting consumers.

Millions of times a day, people in factories, warehouses, stores (and prescription departments) do things to comply with the food and drug law—yet never give it a thought! Consumer protection happens because so many people do things the right way. But, of course, laws and regulations are needed to provide a basis for corrective action when needed.

Objectives can change greatly. Forty years ago prescription drug labeling regulations prohibited the inclusion of indications and dosages. Pharmacists and physicians had to look elsewhere for information on side effects, collateral measures, counterindications, precautions, and warnings. As time passed and drugs changed greatly, the importance of communicating such information increased.

The neighborhood pharmacy has become a complete library on therapeutics through the literature contained in drug packages. The role of the pharmacist continues to develop in scope and importance. Increasingly, it is recognized that how a drug is dispensed and used, as well as the diagnosis and prescription, are of critical importance to the patient. The patient package insert, now so much in the news, is one more step in the long evolution toward greater safety and effectiveness of drugs.

The relationship of American pharmacy and the U.S. food and drug law is very close. Both have grown from the same seed—the fundamental human need for safe medicines that work. Truly, pharmacy and FDA had grown up together, working at the same job.

1938–1988: THE MAKING OF A MILESTONE IN CONSUMER PROTECTION*

William Grigg

The thirties were years that scarred. Families faced joblessness and hardship, even hunger. Politicians, civil servants, newspaper editors, and manufacturers argued over how to end the downward spiral in jobs, prices and production that was the Great Depression—and, much less urgently, about proposals to revise or replace the 1906 Food and Drugs Act.

The stock market had crashed on Oct. 28, 1929, and the fun and high expectations of the twenties had vanished. Indeed, in the wake of the crash, if you hadn't lost your job or your farm, if you hadn't lost your home to foreclosure, well, then you might consider yourself pretty well off, and lucky, even, if your salary was cut by a third. (Average annual wages dropped from $1,405 in 1929 to $1,091 in 1934 and did not return to their 1929 level until 1941.) There was no unemployment insurance. Once-successful men—stockbrokers, manufacturers, speculators, men who had so recently bought and sold Cadillacs and Packards—now sold apples on the street.

And odds were, according to the muckraking writers of the day, that the apples had arsenic on them! For apples were often sprayed with arsenic-based pesticides, as were many other products: Six people in California were poisoned in 1931 by greens sprayed with lead arsenate. (As if arsenic wasn't bad enough, pesticides also contained lead.) A 4-year-old Philadelphia girl died in 1932 after eating fruit sprayed with such pesticides.

Odds were also that if you couldn't afford a doctor and you bought a patent medicine advertised as a cure, you were going to

*Reprinted from the *FDA Consumer* (October 1988).

spend your money for nothing, for the medicine wouldn't help. Usually, to avoid legal constraints, manufacturers didn't label their nostrums for cancers and arthritis and other problems—but still *advertised* them for these purposes.

The ads appeared, by and large, in the backs of some magazines and newspapers, "back with the truss ads," as disparaging better-educated consumers said. (The larger, more prominent ads were for the new Dodge automobile, which cost $595, for Rinso washing powder, for Heinz Cream of Mushroom Soup, for a machine that dried clothes, for Cameo, "the soap of beautiful women," and for the new Gable-Colbert hit, "It Happened One Night.") Some quack ads also appeared on radio, a medium with such universal appeal that salesmen knew better than to call on a prospect between 7 and 7:15 weeknights, when the "Amos 'n' Andy" program was on. (Television was being developed and would be a curiosity at the 1939 New York World's Fair, but it would be a long time catching on.)

Nevertheless, progress was being made in medicine. Vitamin D was discovered in 1932, leading to the end of rickets and its characteristic bowed legs. World War I had seen the first transfusions of stored blood, and now steps were being taken for the first big blood banks. German and U.S. scientists in 1929 had shared a Nobel Prize for work on estrone, the first of the female hormones to be isolated in pure form. Vaccination for smallpox, tetanus and diphtheria was commonplace. Childbirth was safe, compared to a few generations before. No longer did mothers consider themselves lucky if their children survived infancy. Most now did. (Infant deaths in Massachusetts, for example, had de-

clined nearly two-thirds, from 141 deaths per 1,000 live births in 1900 to 53.9 in 1930. Life expectancy had increased more than 10 years, to 59.7 years.) Surgery, too, was well advanced. And there were some effective drug treatments. Syphilis could be cured with 30 injections of salvarsan (an arsenic compound) alternated with 40 injections of bismuth over a period of many months—a grueling regimen that some refused. Digitalis was used for heart conditions, barbiturates for epilepsy, and gold for rheumatoid arthritis, as they continue to be today. For pain, there were morphine and other narcotics, as well as the old standby, aspirin; nitroglycerin had long been used for angina, but there were no antibiotics, no steroids, no birth control pills, beta and calcium blockers, or polio vaccines. There were no cures for childhood leukemia. A diagnosis of tuberculosis meant months of total rest in a sanatorium.

Yet, to read some of the ads, no further progress in medicine was necessary. B&M External Remedy was advertised as a germicide that could cure grippe, asthma, coughs, colds and blood poisoning—and breast cancer as well, making surgery unnecessary. And, although insulin had been used successfully for diabetes beginning in 1922, dozens of products continued to be advertised as curing diabetes without insulin or a change of diet.

These patent medicines had to list any alcohol or narcotics (such as morphine or cocaine) in them but nothing else, not even such harmful ingredients as arsenic or strychnine. Thus, the years leading up to the passage of the 1938 Food, Drug, and Cosmetic Act were full of paradox. And, as times got worse, desperate people sought cheaper foods and medicines—

and desperate companies were too often ready to peddle worthless or dangerous drugs and diluted and tainted foods.

Consumers—if they read *100,000,000 Guinea Pigs* by Arthur Kallet and F. J. Schlink of the fledgling Consumers' Research organization—learned not only that their apples were likely to be tainted but that their Pebeco toothpaste contained a poison so strong that "a German army officer committed suicide by eating a tubeful."

Nor was arsenic on fresh fruit and vegetables the only food safety problem. The meat preservative sodium sulfite was heavily used by shady operators to restore a fresh red color to meat and destroy the odor of deterioration. The chemical could not only lead you to eat spoiled meat, the Consumers' Research book said, but it also was itself harmful to the kidneys and to digestion, and it was illegal for this use. That didn't stop the processors. As with the arsenic-based pesticides, the profits were too great and the punishments too slight to stop use of the chemical.

And milk? Knowledgeable families insisted on the pasteurized product. Nevertheless, raw milk from tubercular cows was still widely available in some areas—and still responsible for unnecessary illness and as many as 5,000 deaths a year, according to one estimate.

Good mothers forced cod liver oil down protesting youngsters to provide them with vitamin D. But a government report cited by Consumers' Research showed 62 percent of the liquid products were below standard. As for easier-to-take tablets of the stuff, 15 out of 17 brands were deemed "inert and worthless" by the consumer group.

Wallace F. Janssen, FDA's historian, recalls a Brooklyn jam and jelly packer telling him, as prices and wages spiralled lower and lower, "When I come to work I never know how much I have to cut down on the fruit in order to drop my price another 2 cents." Janssen, then a trade journal editor, adds that there were no enforceable federal standards for jams then, and the market was flooded with products diluted with water, pectin, artificial color, "and sometimes even a few grass seeds to create the illusion" of fruit seeds.

Hardly any ingredients in foods or drugs had to be listed on labels. Nor did the Food and Drugs Act of 1906 Known as the Wiley Act for FDA's pioneering early director, Harvey W. Wiley) provide any protection from cosmetics, which by 1930 were a $336-million retail business. The products included an eyelash dye that had blinded some women and a hair remover containing a rat poison, thallium acetate, that had destroyed the nerves and health of others.

Women's magazines like *McCalls, Cosmpolitan* and the *Delineator* carried ads for "safe" laxatives that were really habit-forming cathartics, for freckle creams containing mercury, for Lysol (now, as then, used to clean bathroom floors) as a douche, and for that worthless, though in itself harmless, product for women's ailments, the famous Lydia E. Pinkham's Vegetable Compound.

Good Housekeeping magazine had earned a reputation for policing its ads, but Consumers' Research protested its ads for Pepsodent toothpaste, which had a formula the organization considered too abrasive. Even the *Journal of the American Medical Association* was criticized for carrying a full-page ad for Mercurochrome (a then-popular painless substitute for iodine) one month after its medical pages had reported the product to be a poor germ-killer and toxic to boot.

Consumers' Research *100,000,000 Guinea Pigs* was rough on FDA as well, blaming the agency for lax enforcement of the antiquated 1906 law. The book did note that the agency had a force no larger than the police department of Philadelphia to handle its huge responsibilities.

FDA, however, had already drafted a new omnibus law. It was introduced in Congress in 1933, in the early days of the new Roosevelt administration.

A new law was needed, some said, *to meet the new challenges facing American consumers.*

Humbug and Bolshevism, responded others. *Tougher laws would kill what few businesses and jobs there were left.*

There was grassroots support for legislation from many citizens disturbed by conditions they saw in the marketplace. The militant Consumers' Research organization grew from 1,000 to 45,000 members in the four years after its founding in 1929. And its books—*Eat, Drink and Be Wary* among them—carried its message to many others. The "insider" *Kiplinger Agricultural Letter* predicted that passage of the food, drug and cosmetic legislation was 90 percent sure in 1934.

But it didn't happen. Facing strong business and editorial opposition, the proposal went nowhere. Consumers were to face the likes of Marmola, an over-the-counter thyroid preparation for weight loss, and Radithor, radium water advertised for 160 diseases, for several tough Depression years more.

1938–1988: THE MAKING OF A MILESTONE IN CONSUMER PROTECTION: PART TWO*

William Grigg

"In 1930, when I was 8 and dad was 34," recalls Harold Hopkins, former editorial director of this magazine, "I taught him to walk. He taught me to cuss.

Harold Hopkins' father was trying to reeducate his legs because he was one of 35,000 to 50,000 victims of a toxic substance that was used to adulterate an over-the-counter drug called fluid extract of Jamaica ginger. Properly used, the extract was diluted in water to treat indigestion and stomachaches. But drunk straight, it had a powerful alcoholic kick—and thus, for some years, where Prohibition was enforced, people who were too poor to buy good bootleg drank Jamaica ginger, which they nicknamed Jake.

When a chemical was added in an attempt to produce a cheaper Jake, and more profit, it killed some victims and left others bedridden or on curtches for the rest of their lives. Harold Hopkins' dad was determined, however, to recover his mobility.

"In that summer of 1930 a part of the house was cleared of family clutter to make room for the business of walking," Harold Hopkins recalled. "Dad would get up from his chair, holding onto me for support. As we started across the room he'd let go, wave me away, and start out on his own. In a step or two his legs would crumple under him and he'd sprawl headlong [and] empurple the air with profanity.

"I'd help him up, and we'd try it again across the room, hour upon hour, day afer day."

The older Hopkins did manage to walk again without crutches, but he had a flapping, uncertain gait that people called "Jakeleg."

Two men were eventually

charged in the adulteration under both the National Prohibition Act and the Food and Drugs Act of 1906. Thousands had had their lives taken or blighted. The two men received two years' probation and were fined $1,000 each.

Seeking to research the mass tragedy later for an *FDA Consumer* article ("Blue Language and the Jakewalk Blues," June 1980), Hopkins the son was surprised to find that the Jakeleg epidemic hardly existed in the newspapers of the time—or in histories of the Depression. To Hopkins, the epidemic "showed plainly that legislation was needed to require premarket testing to assure the safety of drugs sold in the United States."

But that was a lesson the nation was not yet ready to learn.

Where Was the Press?

The lack of publicity for Jakeleg may have been because it mostly hit the rural poor—people, in addition, who were violating Prohibition, the 18th amendment to the U.S. Constitution. And investigative journalism, or "muckracking," was more commonly found, during these years, in books, rather than in advertising-dependent newspapers or magazines.

Even objective accounts of the new food, drug and cosmetic proposal ran into trouble. FDA historian Wallace Janssen, then editor of a trade publication called *The Glass Packer*, found that out when he engaged an industry consultant to write a series on the changes the proposed new law might produce. The very first article brought a threat from the *Packer's* major advertiser to cancel its ads. The articles continued—and "the advertising was cancelled, a severe penalty for our small journal," Janssen recalled. But he and publisher

John T. Ogden toughed it out. They believed that their business readers wanted the facts on the legislation—and that many even recognized a need for some reform in the old law.

Other publishers didn't hold firm. And there was considerable pressure. According to *Food and Drug Legislation in the New Deal* by Charles O. Jackson, the Creomulsion Company of Atlanta warned editors of rural papers that passage of the bill would mean "we will be forced to cancel immediately every line of Creomulsion advertising." And the Associated Grocery Manufacturers of America telegraphed newspapers a warning that ad revenues would certainly decline.

The Proprietary Association, a trade group representing drug manufacturers, sent out canned editorials that appeared in the *New York Journal of Commerce*, the *Atlanta Journal*, and the *Houston Post*.

But it wasn't all pressure. Many publishers, like other businessmen, felt uneasy—to put it mildly—when Franklin Delano Roosevelt's inauguration in 1933 brought to the government such left-leaning people as Frances Perkins, Henry Wallace, and the latter's assistant secretary of agriculture, Rexford Tugwell—who had written in *The Industrial Discipline* the shocking view that there was waste in the American system and, further, that most advertising served no useful purpose. Thus, for editorial writers, it was easy to oppose the new proposal as "Tugwellism." As, in a way, it was: FDA was a part of the Department of Agriculture then, and soon after he came to office, Tugwell had an exchange with FDA's chief, Walter Campbell, that led to the drafting of the law.

*Reprinted from the *FDA Consumer* (November 1988).

Horse Liniment for Tuberculosis

Tugwell had objected that an FDA-written letter on pesticides suggested FDA balanced farming economics against consumer safety. According to one recollection, Tugwell wrote a caustic note to Campbell asking why FDA was permitting arsenic residues on vegetables at all, and Campbell stormed over to Tugwell's office to instruct him on FDA's limitations under the out-of-date 1906 law.

Another account makes the exchange a more amicable one concerning only the phraseology of the letter, but both agree that Tugwell, later that day, set FDA to work on a new law. Sen. Royal S. Copeland of New York, a physician and former New York City health commissioner, was persuaded to introduce it on June 12, 1933, though he was not enthusiastic about some of the sweeping authority in that first version.

Hardly a newspaper in the country endorsed it. With thick sarcasm, one rare journalistic supporter, Paul Anderson, wrote in *The Nation*, "The measure frankly challenges the sacred right of freeborn Americans to advertise and sell horse liniment as a remedy for tuberculosis." He added that the legislation raised the kind of ques-

tion "which stirs men to the very depths of their pocket-books."

To combat what he saw as a press blackout, FDA Chief Campbell wrote to his district and station chiefs "to go directly to the people of the nation through the medium of their clubs and other organizations." FDA officials also spoke on the radio and prepared articles in support of the bill. This worked. Stirred up by the popular consumer outrage books—*Counterfeit, Not to Be Broadcast,* and *40,000,000 Guinea Pig Children,* as well as the still-popular *100,000,000 Guinea Pigs*—women's groups lined up in support of new legislation. These included the General Federation of Women's Clubs, the National Consumers' League, the American Association of University Women, the League of Women Voters, the American Home Economics Association, and the National Congress of Parents and Teachers, many of the same groups that had won passage of the 1906 law.

FDA's Chamber of Horrors

To combat hostile Congressional views, FDA Chief Inspector George F. Larrick, who later became commissioner, collected hundreds of products that had injured or

cheated consumers, but which FDA could not control under the old law. After its debut at a Senate hearing, the collection was put on public display. Although no one seemed sure that President Roosevelt himself was strongly committed to the new legislation, Eleanor Roosevelt visited this exhibit—and the press, following her, dubbed it the "Chamber of Horrors."

An aggressively propagandist book of the same name followed, written by FDA information officer Ruth Lamb.

Although the book was privately financed, many of FDA's efforts at "education" were soon criticized as ballyhoo· at public expense— and an illegal use of public funds. Congressmen and the Agriculture Department's solicitor agreed, and FDA was told to limit its promotion of the "Chamber of Horrors" exhibit and halt the radio appearances of officials on the bill's behalf.

Nevertheless, bit by bit, the radical new legislation picked up support. (To be sure, there were also some compromises that made it less drastic.) By 1937, it seemed sure of passage—in some form.

But it would not pass soon enough to save the children from Elixir Sulfanilamide.

1938–1988: THE MAKING OF A MILESTONE IN CONSUMER PROTECTION: PART THREE*

William Grigg

Despite the despair and hard times of the 1930s, there were

*Reprinted from the *FDA Consumer* (December 1988/January 1989).

exciting new products coming onto the market—among them, drugs that actually halted infections.

This progress was used as an

argument against changing the 1906 Food and Drugs Act. People might well hesitate before passing any new law that might hold back such wonder drugs. Look at the

German-developed Prontosyl and the related sulfa drugs that were curing bacterial infections such as pneumonia, blood poisoning, and meningitis.

Sulfanilamide, one of these first sulfa drugs, was effective against gonorrhea and other infections. Too bad this early sulfa drug was hard to swallow as a tablet and hard to dissolve into a liquid medicine.

It was left to a chemist at an old and reputable company called S. E. Massengill of Bristol, Tenn., to find a way to dissolve it into a liquid product, easier for children to swallow. The company, confident in the solvent as well as the active ingredient, put the liquid on the market without safety testing.

It was Oct. 11, 1937, when the American Medical Association received reports from physicians in Tulsa, Okla., of six deaths from this new elixir of sulfanilamide. And in New Orleans, one doctor alone had six patients die, one of them his best friend. ("Nobody but Almighty God and I can know what I have been through these past few days," he wrote in a letter. "I have spent hours on my knees . . . I have known hours when death for me would be a welcome relief from this agony.")

The solvent that had liquified the sulfa had proved to be poison. As a result, children who may have been treated for an infected and sore throat suffered intense pain with stoppage of urine, vomiting and ultimately convulsions, stupor and death. Mrs. Maise Nidiffer of Tulsa wrote President Roosevelt that even the memory of her daughter Joan is cruel because "we can see her little body tossing to and fro and hear that little voice screaming with pain [until] it seems as though it would drive me insane." The 6-year-old had been in this condition for nine days before dying.

Most physicians went to great lengths to track down patients given the medicine to try to stop them from taking it. One postponed his wedding in order to help

FDA's inspector track down a 3-year-old mountain boy.

However, another physician apparently sought to avoid any possible responsibility by denying he had prescribed the drug It was a practice in that part of the South to leave personal effects on a grave, and an FDA inspector found a partly empty bottle of the elixir on the grave of the denying doctor's child-patient.

Only six gallons of Elixir Sulfanilamide killed 107 people, mostly children. The Associated Press reported "a nationwide race with death" as every agent of the FDA scoured the country for the 700 remaining pints of the deadly drug. Amazingly, 99.2 percent of this remaining supply was rounded up.

One inspector spent four days trying to track down a bottle, knowing only that it was purchased by a member of a family named Long. He traveled through several small towns in Arkansas, finally reaching the right Long family—as a funeral for their 7-year-old daughter, who had taken the medicine, got under way.

Sulfa was such a new drug that no one was sure whether it was the active ingredient or the solvent that was killing people, Dr. Frances Kelsey recalls. As a graduate student at the University of Chicago, she helped with one of several studies conducted to find the answer. It proved to be the solvent, diethylene glycol, similar to a substance used as an antifreeze. (See "Taste of Raspberries, Taste of Death: The 1937 Elixir Sulfanilamide Incident" in the June 1981 *FDA Consumer.*)

(A Canadian, Dr. Kelsey later became an FDA employee—and prevented another drug catastrophe, birth defects from thalidomide, by blocking that drug's sale here.)

The tragedy of sulfanilamide led to the suicide of Massengill's, chemist, although he was charged with no crime, and to a fine of only $26,000 for the company—the highest possible under the old law.

Public outrage led swiftly to passage of the 1938 Food, Drug, and Cosmetic Act with a provision requiring drugs to be cleared for safety before they go on the market.

The law was no longer derided as the "Tugwell bill." In truth, many changes had been made. As modified, the legislation was now called the Copeland bill after Senator-physician Royal S. Copeland of New York, who had labored over it, improving it, compromising, modifying. The struggle hastened his death. He collapsed on the Senate floor and died soon after the bill's passage.

The grieving Mrs. Nidiffer, after describing her daughter Joan's death, had asked President Roosevelt, "as you enjoy your grandchildren of whom we read about, it is my plea that you will take steps to prevent such sales of drugs that will take little lives and leave such suffering behind."

President Roosevelt signed the bill into law on June 25, 1938. By that time, many newspapers, many businesses, much of the advertising trade, and various professional associations had lined up with the consumer groups in favor of it.

None of these, probably, could foresee all that the new law would mean. In retrospect, however, it is clear that the law significantly shifted the burden of proof: No longer was consumer protection to rely only on a small band of federal cops chasing food and drug violators after the fact. From then on, particularly as a result of changes made in response to the sulfanilamide disaster, the law sought to prevent problems by establishing a product's safety *before* it got on the market.

Although some predicted that the 1938 Food, Drug, and Cosmetic Act would stifle research, FDA historian Wallace Janssen says the reverse has been true: The research required by the law has stimulated medical progress.

Certainly, the law and subsequent amendments (as well as the science of the day) have increased the chance that sick patients will get good drug therapy. Fifty years ago, although the American Medical Association provided guidance, doctors and, particularly, patients often played a roulette game—hoping that the medicine they chose from the many with miraculous claims was at least safe. And most devices "quacked" when you started them up. Today, patients and physicians are assured of drugs and devices that have been demonstrated to be not only safe but effective—from antibiotics, agents to lower blood pressure or cholesterol, and emergency heart attack treatments to contact lenses and artificial knees and hip joints.

Most people will credit science for the progress, and certainly science and support for science have been crucial. But the law helps make good science possible and profitable—by making good scientific work necessary to get a drug or device on the market, and by eliminating the undermining competition of unproved and quack products.

From our morning OJ and cornflakes to our evening dessert of kiwi fruit or apple pie, today's foods meet high standards of quality, as well as manufacturing and storage standards. Where secrecy about the contents of a product was the norm before 1938, consumers now read labels that tell the ingredients and whether there are artificial colors, flavors or preservatives. Where nutrients have been added, nutrition labeling is provided.

Although an occasional problem still occurs, pesticides today are far safer than the lead arsenates of the past. The Environmental Protection Agency now approves pesticides for safety for the farm worker as well as the consumer, and FDA checks foods for residues—which, despite polls that show consumers remain concerned about them, are very low and well within international safety standards.

Our cosmetic powders and paints no longer contain chemicals that blind and poison. (They may not always live up to their exaggerated promises of youth and beauty, but that's another story.)

And when you read the directions on your nonprescription headache tablet or antacid, remember when no directions were required and, in fact, the labels didn't list the same uses claimed in the advertising.

Perhaps in no area does the consumer find more change than in the contents of today's nonprescription products. As a result of a retrospective review carried out under the law (with the cooperation of the same Proprietary Association that had once opposed the law) today's consumers need not fear dangerous ingredients in nonprescription products. Indeed the review is ensuring that our cold medicines, sleep aids, digestive medications, athlete's foot cures, and other remedies actually work. That seems a simple change, but it's a radical departure from the world as it existed 50 years ago.

For the first time, the 1938 law provided specific authority for factory inspections. In 1962, by law, and in 1969, by regulatory interpretation, this authority was extended to require that drug and food manufacturers follow good manufacturing practices designed to ensure that filth, error and accident are unlikely—and to keep records that would enable FDA inspectors to determine not only what was happening at the moment of inspection but for months before.

FDA was authorized to go to court to obtain injunctions against false claims or unsafe products, and to issue warnings about products, as well as to seize them in the marketplace. The law did not give FDA authority to recall products—but recalls have evolved as a way to avoid these more drastic and reputation-damaging actions.

The 1938 law had many very specific provisions. It required that products sold as "antiseptics" actually have germicidal powers, for example, and barred the inclusion of metallic trinkets and other inedible substances in candies. It specified that packages be reasonably full—and not deceptive as to content. It required that medical devices have directions for safe use.

But beyond the specifics and beyond the new authority was a shift in philosophy. No longer was the law to be a primarily criminal statute aimed at punishing manufacturers and distributors after death, disability, fraud or illness occurred.

The emphasis was changed toward prevention, toward standards that would head off problems before they occurred. Instead of picking up filthy products after they were on the market, FDA would now inspect canneries, granaries and warehouses so that there was less opportunity for filth to contaminate a product.

Instead of only acting on a drug after children died or poor people were crippled, FDA would now require testing before a product was sold.

Manufacturers complained of red tape, of delays, and of intrusion on their rights and property. They still do. Years of research may be required before a company can show a drug is safe and effective—and ready for market. FDA's review of these data, which for a single drug may fill the bookcases lining a small room, can take three months to three years or more. And there are still lapses and failures—tamperings, the Dalkon Shield, *Listeria* contamination of soft cheeses, and unexpected side effects such as those with the hormone DES.

But manufacturers and consumers both benefit today from safe and effective medical products and clean and wholesome foods—all sold with honest claims in protective and informative packaging.

We are the inheritors and beneficiaries of a great law.

HOW THE LAW CHANGED IN 1938*

Wallace Janssen

Comparing the Federal Food, Drug, and Cosmetic Act with the original Food and Drugs Act of 1906 shows fundamental and revolutionary differences. Whereas the 7-page "Wiley Act" was designed to deter widespread abuses through court proceedings and punishments, the 22-page 1938 law closed many loopholes and added specific requirements that were explanatory and preventive in character. A digest of the legislation, issued by FDA soon after its passage, listed fewer than 38 "principal changes." Looking at the most significant of these, half a century later, shows the beginning of an evolution of consumer protection that is still going on.

Cosmetics

The new law gave to FDA, for the first time, authority to regulate cosmetics, especially those harmful to users. Blindness and death had been caused by an eyelash dye called "Lash-Lure," one of the "horrors" that spurred Congress to pass the law. Soap got an exemption.

Medical Devices

Control was also extended to medical devices, made subject to the same misbranding and adulteration provisions as drugs. Widespread quackery in the promotion of worthless health gadgets was the principal problem; highly sophisticated medical equipment such as heart pacemakers had not yet been invented.

Diet Aids

Deadly nostrums for weight reduction, another of the pre-1938 horrors, could not be stopped by

---

*Reprinted from the *FDA Consumer* (December 1988/January 1989).

the 1906 law because they were not legally "drugs." Drugs were defined as treatments for disease, and obesity was not recognized as a disease. So the definition of drugs was broadened to include products "intended to affect the structure or any function of the body." Also included as drugs were products used for diagnosing disease.

Labeling

Truth in labeling was a major objective of the 1906 law, perhaps its greatest. Products could be seized for misbranding; their shippers sent to jail. But there were hardly any requirements as to what labels should tell. Important provisions of the 1938 law aimed at giving vitally needed information to consumers—information now taken for granted. Drug labels, for example, were required to include directions for use and warnings against misuse that could endanger health. Telling consumers on the label what they were buying and eating was another radical change. Among the new requirements was declaration on food labels of artificial colors, flavors, or chemical preservatives (but butter, cheese and ice cream were exempt from having to declare colors). Other new provisions required ingredient labeling for foods and drugs not subject to official standards.

Fraud

One of the greatest improvements was to eliminate a so-called "fraud joker" in a 1912 amendment intended to prohibit false claims for drugs. Because the amendment outlawed claims that were "false *and fraudulent*" the government had to prove that the promoter intended to cheat his customers—an impossibility in most cases. Promoters who

claimed to believe in their fake products could easily escape conviction, as many did.

Vitamins

Vitamins were very new and popular in 1938, and the public needed information to make intelligent choices. Under the new law, labels of foods for special dietary uses were required to inform purchasers fully as to vitamin, mineral and other dietary properties.

Colors

FDA had been testing artificial colors used in foods, drugs and cosmetics since 1910, but this was a voluntary arrangement and done at the request of the manufacturers. The new law made illegal the use of any artificial color not tested and certified by the agency. Color certification was the first FDA program for pre-market research, testing and approval.

Unavoidable Contaminants

Injurious food was prohibited by the 1906 law only if a poisonous substance had been added. The 1938 law eliminated this dangerous limitation, but provided for safe tolerances to be set for otherwise toxic ingredients that are required in production or are unavoidable in food manufacturing practices.

Dangerous Drugs

The fact that a drug was dangerous to health when used as directed by its label did not make it illegal under the 1906 law. The deadly Elixir Sulfanilamide was not "adulterated" under the law. It was "misbranded," but only because of a technical error in its label—an elixir was required to be made with alcohol. If poisonous solvent diethylene glycol had been declared on the elixir's label, it would have been a legal product. And there were others on the market that, though dangerous or deadly, escaped control because they were neither misbranded nor adulterated under the limited scope of the 1906 law. The 1938 law made two major changes. First, drugs were misbranded if "dangerous to health when used in the dosage or manner, or with the frequency or duration prescribed, recommended or suggested in the labeling thereof." Second, interstate traffic in new drugs was prohibited unless they are adequately tested to show that they are safe for use under the conditions prescribed in their labeling, with the exception of drugs intended solely for investigational use by qualified scientific experts. Evolving from this new requirement, in the ensuing half century, has come the world's most extensive, effective and productive system of drug research and regulation.

Injunctions

Enforcement was greatly strengthened by authorizing the federal courts to restrain violators by issuing injunctions. The 1906 law had been enforced largely by seizure of illegal products, and to a lesser extent by prosecuting shippers, who could be fined or imprisoned. Injunctions are court orders to not only stop violating the law but also to take whatever steps are needed to ensure compliance. Also, the penalties for violating a court order are virtually unlimited—much greater than those prescribed for violating the law. A judge, for example, can order a plant shut down if a court order is not obeyed.

Inspections

FDA inspectors had been visiting food and drug establishments from the beginning of enforcement in 1907, but without specific legal authorization to do so. Tact and diplomacy on the part of inspectors, and the willingness of firms to undergo inspection enabled FDA to enter most regulated establishments, but there were many situations where analysis of samples was the only way to get evidence of violations. This, of course, was little protection against insanitary conditions or loose practices in food and drug plants. The 1938 law made two important changes: Inspection of establishments producing food, drugs, devices and cosmetics for interstate shipment was specifically authorized, along with procurement of transportation records and other documents needed to establish federal jurisdiction, and products from insanitary facilities were automatically considered adulterated.

Food Standards

Very frustrating for FDA, food processors, and consumers was the failure of efforts to set legally effective standards for food products. The need for standards—to prevent fraud and ensure fair competition—had been realized long before 1906. But FDA continued to lose its court cases against such frauds as "strawberry jam" made with pectin, water, grass seeds, and a few berries.

The 1938 law allows FDA to establish a food standard whenever one is needed "to promote honesty and fair dealing in the interest of consumers."

These important changes in food and drug law came about through the nation's struggling for more than a generation with the weakness of the 1906 act. They show that it's not always true that we learn little from experience.

AMENDMENTS TO THE FEDERAL FOOD, DRUG, AND COSMETIC ACT*

Max Sherman, R.Ph. and Steven Strauss, Ph.D., R.Ph.

The Federal Food, Drug, and Cosmetic Act [1] (the Act), signed into law by Franklin D.

*Reprinted with permission from *U.S. Pharmacist* (August 1984).

Roosevelt on June 25, 1938, becoming effective one year later, may be ranked as the *commercial law* of greatest social and economic importance in the United States because it regulates two of the most vital commodities—food and drugs.

While the Act enhanced the cause of food and drug law, it proved inadequate over time to deal with expanded scientific developments. The Act has therefore undergone evolutionary changes with a goal of continuing protection. Fortunately, Congress has wisely enacted strengthening amendments to keep pace with evolving technology. The amendments have operated effectively through the years to fulfill the Act's basic purpose of assuring the American public with safe and effective drugs, cosmetics, biologics, medical devices, and foods. Many of these amendments pertain to, or directly concern, the pharmacist.

Insulin Amendment

The first amendment to the Act added new standards to ensure the purity, quality, strength, and identity of insulin products [2]. This added section required that every drug composed in whole or in part of insulin be certified before the drug was placed on the market [3]. The reason for this was that early insulin preparations, although life saving, were relatively crude, contained unknown impurities, were inconvenient to use and required several injections daily. Recognizing the importance of a standard potency if insulin were to be manufactured commercially, the University of Toronto (where insulin was discovered) patented the product and its process of manufacture. An Insulin Committee was created to administer a licensing program and to establish a laboratory to test each batch of finished product. Through its licensing arrangements with manufacturers in the United States, the Committee was able to maintain standards by requiring that the manufacturers first assay or standardize each batch of insulin and insulin product and then submit a sample to the laboratory in Toronto which also assayed the finished product to confirm the reference standards of the Committee prior to approval for marketing.

This protection ceased December 24, 1941 when the patent expired. Continued surveillance was essential to assure that each dose of insulin administered to a diabetic was of uniform potency. This need was answered by the enactment of the Insulin Amendment on December 22, 1941. Regulations to control the manufacture of insulin are found in 21 CFR part 429.

Part 429 has also been revised over the years. Revisions were necessary, in view of technological changes in the development and manufacture of insulin products. For example, until recently, insulin for use by humans was obtained from beef and pork pancreata. Firms preparing such products have developed manufacturing procedures capable of producing insulins that are highly purified. To distinguish these insulins from less purified insulins, manufacturers have been permitted to label these products as purified insulin. Although standards for these purified insulins are set forth in individual new drug applications, regulations for certification of these products also must be revised to include appropriate standards for quality and purity. The Food and Drug Administration (FDA) has recently approved a new source of insulin called "human" insulin. Beef and pork insulin are obtained from pancreatic glands of beef and swine, respectively. Human insulin, however, is not obtained from the pancreatic glands of humans but is produced by means of recombinant DNA technology or by enzymatic modification of pork insulin. All products identified as "human" insulin have the same molecular structure as the insulin produced by the human body. However, because these insulins are produced by different methods, the certification standards in effect earlier now must be revised to set forth standards of quality and purity depending upon the method of production. The FDA has recently announced its intention to review its existing regulations of insulin and to propose appropriate changes in the regulations [4].

Antibiotic Amendment

On July 6, 1945, new certification standards were added to ensure the safety and efficacy of penicillin [5]. Rigid control was necessary because of the uncertainties in production technologies experienced by early penicillin manufacturers. There were problems with stability and the potency varied from batch to batch.

The original penicillin substance was impure, noncrystalline, and highly unstable. Its physical and chemical properties, and particularly its compatibility with additive materials used in compounding dosage forms, were a mystery to most of the industry.

During the first few years during World War II, the United States Armed Forces received all the penicillin that was produced. Recognizing the difficulties of production and assay, the War Production Board requested the FDA to create specifications for the drug, and to review each batch manufactured against those specifications. The FDA established laboratories for this purpose during 1942 and 1943. By 1945, it was apparent that supplies of penicillin would soon suffice for civilians as well as military demands.

The July 6, 1945 Amendment directed the administrator of the Federal Security Agency (now Secretary of Health and Human Services) to provide for the certification of drugs composed wholly or partly of any type of penicillin.

The Act authorized the administrator to set up such standards of identity, strength, quality, and purity as necessary to adequately ensure the safety and efficacy of use. The certification procedure meant that the FDA would examine each batch of the drug produced against the standards before it could be shipped in interstate commerce. This certification of penicillin and products containing penicillin established a precedent for similar drugs [6]. The 1962 amendments to the Act [7], which became effective May 1, 1963, extended the requirements of certification to "any other antibiotic drug or any derivative thereof." The revised definition added 28 groups of antibiotic drugs to the five groups already requiring certification. These amendments at the same time further defined an "antibiotic" drug as "any drug intended for use by man containing any quantity of any chemical substance which is produced by a microorganism and which had the capacity to inhibit or destroy microorganisms in dilute solution (including the chemically synthesized equivalent of such substance)" [8]. Prior to the enactment of the Kefauver-Harris Amendment, the Act required that each batch of a drug composed wholly or partly of bacitracin, chloramphenicol, chlortetracycline, penicillin, and streptomycin, or any derivative thereof, be certified by the Secretary of Health, Education and Welfare, unless he has exempted such drugs from such requirements. Scientific proof of safety and efficacy was required.

In 1982 the FDA reached a decision to exempt antibiotic products from the certification program [9]. FDA's conclusion that antibiotic drug products no longer present the quality problems that justified establishment of the certification program provides an example of how federal government involvement may successfully address an important problem, to such an extent, in fact, that the need for the program ceases.

Durham-Humphrey Amendments

Of particular major interest to the pharmacist are the Durham-Humphrey Amendments, which became the law on October 26, 1951 [10]. The Amendments, sometimes referred to as the "prescription drug amendments," provide for a statutory scheme for distinguishing between prescription and non-prescription drugs (over-the-counter drugs), and prohibit refills of prescriptions without the express consent of the prescriber. The

Durham-Humphrey Amendments make it illegal to dispense a prescription drug without prescription order or to refill a prescription without the authorization of the prescriber. Thus, the Amendments carried out the principle that the prescriber should control the amount of medication dispensed to a patient. Prescription restricted drugs are required by law to be labeled with the legend "Caution: Federal Law Prohibits Dispensing Without Prescription," and it is illegal to place this legend on drugs that are not so restricted. The fundamental purpose of Congress in enacting the Durham-Humphrey Amendments was to provide the pharmacist with fair guidance as to which drugs may not be sold without a prescription or be refilled without the prescriber's authorization, as distinguished from those that can be sold to a layman for self-medication. To dispense drugs legally, the pharmacist was guided by the Rx legend on the label. There were three categories of prescription drugs in the Durham-Humphrey Amendments:

1. Hypnotic or habit-forming drugs and their derivatives that are specifically named in the law unless specifically exempted by regulations.

2. A drug which is not safe for self-medication "because of its toxicity or potentiality for harmful effect, or the method of its use, or the collateral measures necessary to its use."

3. "New drug" which has not been shown to be safe for its use in self-medication and which under the terms of an effective new drug application is limited to prescription use.

The Amendments also gave guidance to the pharmacist as to what minimal information must be included on the prescription label. The prescription container must bear a label with the name and address of the dispenser (pharmacy), the serial number of the prescription, the date of its filling, the name of the prescriber, the name of the patient, the directions for use,

and cautionary statements, if any, contained in such prescription.

Color Additive Amendments

The Color Additive Amendments were enacted on July 12, 1960, to authorize the FDA to establish, by regulation, the conditions of use of color additives in foods, drugs, and cosmetics, and to require manufacturers to perform the necessary scientific investigations to establish safety for their intended uses [11]. The Amendments provide for the separate listing and certification of batches of color additives, unless exempted by regulation. The 1960 Amendments require premarket safety testing and FDA approval of all color additives. The manufacturer or would-be user of a color additive may petition the agency for the issuance of a regulation permitting the color to be used. Before it may approve, or "list" the color additive, FDA must find with reasonable certainty that the additive poses no risk to human health; that it accomplishes the intended effect; and that its use will not result in deception of consumers. The FDA is authorized to impose restrictions on the use of color to assure that these criteria are satisfied. These restrictions may include limitations on levels of use, a requirement that individual batches of color be certified by FDA to assure that the color actually used is identical to the substance shown in experiments to be safe, and specifications of the products in which a color may be used. The Color Additive Amendments culminate the federal government's concern for the safety of color additives which have emerged in the United States following the enactment of the original 1906 Pure Food and Drugs Act [12].

Kefauver-Harris Amendments

Possibly the most significant change in the Act occurred on October 10, 1962 with the enactment of the Kefauver-Harris Amendments [7]. These Amendments intensified control over prescription drugs, new drugs and investigational drugs. It was recognized that no drug is truly safe unless it is also effective, and effectiveness was required to be established prior to marketing in the United States. Controls were added to simplify drug nomenclature, to improve factory inspections, and to regulate prescription drug advertising. Specifically, the Amendments:

1. Transferred jurisdiction over medical advertising of Rx products from FTC to FDA, and required that the label of each drug bear:
   • The tradename and the established or generic name
   • A list of active ingredients

2. FDA's inspection authority over establishments in which Rx drugs are manufactured, processed, packed or held was broadened to include records, files, papers, processes, controls, and facilities.

3. Require registration and periodic inspections (at least once every two years) of all drug manufacturing establishments, regardless of whether they are engaged in interstate or intrastate commerce.

4. Require that facilities, methods, and control procedures used by a manufacturer conform to "current good manufacturing practices." Drugs which fail to meet requirements are "adulterated."

5. More extensive control over clinical investigations.

6. Full certification of each batch of antibiotic, with some exemptions.

7. Strengthened the federal government's authority over clinical (human) testing of new drugs by:
   • Providing added safeguards for those on whom drugs are tested
   • Improving reports by drug investigators
   • Establishing investigative procedures to supply substantial evidence that a drug is safe *and* effective

The Kefauver-Harris Amendments also emphasized the key role of the pharmacist in terms of

medical information [13]. Another intent of the Amendments was to legally require manufacturers and distributors to readily provide full information about their drug products to the medical profession. Under the "full disclosure" requirements, the most vital, up-to-date and reliable information about a drug was required to be included in its labeling, in the form of a package insert.

The Amendments were the result of more than 17 months of hearings by Senator Estes Kefauver and his senate subcommittee on Antitrust and Monopoly—variously described as "the drug industry's trial by publicity."

The new regulations, which went into effect February 7, 1963, stipulated that a firm planning to undertake a clinical investigation had to inform FDA of its plans, including information concerning the preclinical studies, the numbers and qualifications of the investigators, and the nature of the study. The firm had to monitor the progress of the studies and periodically report its findings to the FDA. All investigators had to sign a statement affirming that they understood the conditions applying to the use of investigational drugs, which included keeping adequate records and receipts and names of persons to whom the drug was administered. The FDA by virtue of the Amendments was given the power to terminate the investigation on numerous grounds, such as evidence that the drug was being commercialized, substantial evidence that the drug was unsafe, or evidence that the sponsor of the program failed to submit progress reports.

The furor caused by the thalidomide scare helped to revive Senator Kefauver's initial inquisition of the pharmaceutical industry. It is interesting that as originally introduced, the Kefauver bill only tangentially touched on the safety question as related to prescription drugs [14]. But in response to the obvious need to tighten control at the level of clinical investigation,

the Drug Amendments of 1962 considerably strengthened FDA's control of experimentation at the human level.

Drug Abuse Control Amendments of 1965 and 1970

The Drug Abuse Control Amendments (DACA) enacted July 15, 1965, were intended to eliminate illicit traffic in depressant, stimulant and other drugs which were determined to have a potential for abuse [15]. The Amendments increased recordkeeping and inspection requirements providing control of interstate commerce in these drugs, and made possession of them illegal under certain specified conditions. For the convenience of the pharmacists, the law required manufacturers to identify DACA drugs with certain prescribed symbols.

On October 27, 1970, President Nixon signed into law the Comprehensive Drug Abuse Prevention and Control Act of 1970 [16]; this Act repealed the Drug Abuse Control Amendments of 1965 and created new control measures. The 1970 Act also repealed the 1916 Harrison Narcotic Act. This latter Act, limited to narcotic drugs, was a tax law enforced by the Treasury Department that stipulated that narcotics could only be legally sold if they had a stamp procured by its manufacturer by paying the appropriate tax.

The Comprehensive Drug Abuse Prevention and Control Act amended the Public Health Service's Act and the other laws to increase research into, and prevention of, drug abuse and drug dependent persons; and to strengthen existing law enforcement authority in the field of drug abuse. The Act was divided into four titles dealing with the following subjects: Title 1—Rehabilitation Programs Relating to Drug Abuse, Title 2—Control and Enforcement, Title 3—Importation and Exportation; Amendments and Repeals of Revenue Laws, Title 4—Report of Advisory Councils.

The 1970 law was based on Congressional authority to regulate interstate commerce, rather than on the power to levy taxes. It extended a uniform system of regulation of all drugs with a potential for abuse and conferred such broad authority on the U.S. Attorney General as Congress felt necessary for efficient enforcement of the law.

Regulation of the distribution of "controlled" drugs is accomplished through registration and recordkeeping requirements, sufficiently detailed to yield an accurate accounting of the distribution of drugs by any particular registrant. The law authorizes administrative inspections of any "controlled premises" and specifies penalties for failure to register or maintain required records.

Medical Device Amendments

The Medical Device Amendments, signed into law on May 28, 1976, by President Nixon, brought new controls and added responsibilities to manufacturers of medical devices [17]. Prior to enactment of the Medical Device Amendments, manufacturers of medical devices could never be sure what their legal obligations were under existing laws. The public knew that the government was unable to maintain control over the safety and efficacy of numerous health care products and their daily use. And the FDA knew its authority to monitor and regulate the flow of medical devices was limited when it was ambiguous and constantly subject to legal attack. Until 1976, the FDA had no distinct authority to regulate the entry of medical devices in interstate commerce. The agency was authorized to enjoin the further sale of adulterated or misbranded devices and to remove them from the market through its seizure powers [18]. But it could not take steps to ensure the devices were safe and effective before they were marketed except in circumstances where the agency was prepared to convince a court that the device was a drug within the

meaning of the Act. The Medical Device Amendments had a significant effect on manufacturers; however, they also had an impact on health care professionals. The use of "prescription devices" under the Medical Device Amendments may be limited to certain health care professionals to ensure their safe and effective use. Health care professionals must realize that medical devices purchased or used that violate provisions of the law may create presumptions of negligence in malpractice suits involving medical devices [19]. Perhaps most important is the significance of device labeling. Health care professionals, such as pharmacists, who interact with patients, have and will be receiving much more information from the FDA and manufacturers about the use, maintenance, installation, and hazards of medical devices.

Orphan Drug Act

On July 4, 1983, President Reagan signed into law the Orphan Drug Act [20]. The legislation is based on a finding that adequate drugs for some rare diseases are not being researched and developed and that some of these "orphan" drugs will not be marketed in the United States unless changes are made in applicable federal laws.

The Orphan Drug Act creates a comprehensive scheme to assist sponsors to develop such drugs. The Orphan Drug Act amends the Act by adding sections 525, 526, 527, 528.

The Orphan Drug Act was amended in 1984, 1985 and 1988. In the 10 years prior to passage of the act, 12 products were approved that would have been designated orphan products. Since that time, 112 orphan products have been approved.

Orphan drug products receive seven years of marketing exclusivity. In addition, sponsors of orphan products receive clinical research tax credits. Requests for orphan drug designation are filed

in confidence with the Office of Orphan Drug Development (OOPD) whose staff reviews the request and determines its validity. Safety and efficacy data on the product are not reviewed by the OOPD, but by the appropriate review division. To receive orphan designation, the prevalence of the targeted condition in the U.S. population must be under 200,000. The only exception to this requirement is if it can be demonstrated that U.S. R&D costs cannot be recovered.

Orphan product designations are saleable intellectual property, and thus can be transferred to a different sponsor with FDA consent. Requests for orphan status must be made prior to filing of the NDA or PLA. The designation of a product as an orphan drug by OOPD does not have to occur before the regulatory filing. Only drugs and biologics can be granted orphan status. This option is not available for medical devices, foods or veterinary drugs.

Other Amendments

While some of the aforementioned amendments strengthened the authority of the FDA, it should be known that there have been efforts to the contrary.

The Proxmire Amendment of 1976 [21] curtailed FDA's authority to regulate vitamins and prohibited FDA from establishing maximum limits on potency of any synthetic or natural vitamin or mineral except foods for special dietary use. In addition, this Amendment specified that FDA may not classify any natural or synthetic vitamin or mineral or combination thereof as a drug solely because it exceeds the level of potency which FDA determines is nutritionally rational or useful. The agency may also not limit the combination or number of any synthetic or natural vitamin, or other ingredient of food, except for special dietary use and the FDA cannot ban nutritionally worthless ingredients from dietary supplements of vitamins or minerals.

Lastly, FDA cannot establish standards for permissible combination of vitamins or minerals. The Proxmire Amendment, however, does not affect FDA's existing authority to act against any vitamin or mineral product whose labeling is false or misleading, nor does it affect FDA's authority to classify and regulate vitamins or minerals as drugs if they are represented for use in the diagnosis, cure, mitigation, treatment, or prevention of disease in man or animal.

The Federal Food and Cosmetic Act and its amendments have effectively served the cause of the American public health. Significant amendments have been added since 1938. The structure of legislation of laws designed to protect the American public may be far from perfect, but the present day consumer is at least better protected than ever before.

References

1. 21 U.S.C. 301 et seq.
2. Public Law 77-366; 21 U.S.C. 356; FDC Act Sec 506.
3. 21 U.S.C. 356.
4. 48 FR 16704, April 19, 1983.
5. 21 U.S.C. 357; FDC Act Sec 507.
6. FDA Compliance Program Guidance Manual, No. 7356-13, October 18, 1977.
7. Public Law 87-181; 76 Stat. 780 et seq.
8. 21 U.S.C. 357(a); FDC Sec 507(a); Further amended by Sec 105(b) of Public Law 90-399.
9. 47 FR 39155, September 7, 1982.
10. Public Law 82-215.
11. Public Law 86-618.
12. Act of June 30, 1906, Ch. 3915, 34 Stat. 768.
13. Cohen WJ: Our objectives in the field of health. JAPhA NS5(6):306, 1965.
14. McFadyen RE: Thalidomide in America: A brush with tragedy. Clio Medica, 11(2):79, 1976.
15. Public Law 89-74; 79 Stat 226.
16. Public Law 91-513.
17. Public Law 94-295; 21 U.S.C. 360; FDC Act Sec 513–521.
18. FDC Act Sec 304.
19. Miller MJ: How medical device legislation will affect health care professionals. AAMI News, XI(6):9, 1976.
20. Public Law 97-414.
21. Public Law 94-278.

A CAPSULED HISTORY OF DRUG LAW IN THE U.S.*

Max Sherman, R.Ph. and Steven Strauss, Ph.D., R.Ph.

The Federal Food, Drug, and Cosmetic Act (FDCA) enacted in 1938 [1] is the basic food and drug law in the United States. With its numerous amendments, it is the most extensive law of its kind in the world. From the perspective of the pharmacist, the law is intended to assure the consumer that foods, drugs, medical devices, cosmetics, and biologicals are safe and effective for their intended use and that all labeling is truthful, informative and not deceptive. In terms of time, however, the FDCA was passed almost one hundred years after the first efforts by the federal government to control quality and the federal law was antedated by private standards promulgated by the United States Pharmacopoeia, in 1820.

From a historical perspective, the current law was spawned by increased public interest and the spirit of reform which swept the United States during the "New Deal" era of the 1930s. The FDCA, itself, required a national disaster, more than 100 deaths from elixir of sulfanilamide, to assure its enactment. A chronology and synopsis of past drug laws, court cases, administrative and personnel changes will provide the pharmacist with a capsuled history and a greater interpretation as to the reasons why our current law has made the present-day consumer better protected than ever before.

*Reprinted with permission from *U.S. Pharmacist* (November 1985).

1848 The IMPORT DRUGS ACT—first Federal statute to ensure the quality of drugs was enacted when quinine, used by American troops in Mexico against malaria, was found to be adulterated.

1879 Chief Chemist PETER COLLIER, Bureau of Chemistry, U.S. Department of Agriculture (USDA), began investigating food and drug adulteration. The following year he recommended enactment of a national food and drug law. In the next 25 years more than 100 food and drug bills were introduced in Congress.

1883 DR. HARVEY W. WILEY became Chief Chemist of the Bureau of Chemistry. He immediately assigned some members of his staff to study the problems of food and drug adulteration.

1902 Congress enacted the BIOLOGICS CONTROL ACT to license and regulate interstate sale of serums, vaccines, etc., used to prevent or treat diseases in humans.

1906 The original PURE FOOD AND DRUGS ACT of 1906 [2] passed Congress and was signed by President Theodore Roosevelt. The Act prohibited interstate commerce of misbranded and adulterated foods, drinks and drugs.

1907 The BUREAU OF CHEMISTRY of the USDA, headed by Dr. Harvey W. Wiley, began administering the Food and Drug Act.

1911 U.S. v. JOHNSON [3]. The Supreme Court ruled that the 1906 Act did not prohibit false therapeutic claims, but prohibited only false and misleading claims as to the identity of the drug

SHERLEY AMENDMENT [4] enacted to overcome ruling in U.S. v. Johnson. It prohibited labeling medicines with false therapeutic claims intended to defraud the purchaser (but government had to prove this).

1914 U.S. v. LEXINGTON MILL AND ELEVATOR CO. [5]: The Supreme Court ruled that USDA is not required to establish that articles containing poisonous or deleterious substances will affect the public health, but only that they may do so.

1927 A separate law enforcement agency was formed, first known as the Food, Drug, and Insecticide Administration and then, in 1931, as the FOOD AND DRUG ADMINISTRATION (FDA).

CAUSTIC POISON ACT [6] provided for warning labels and antidotes on 10 dangerous or corrosive substances packed in containers for household use.

1933 FDA expressed the need for a complete revision of the basic 1906 Act. First bill was introduced into the Senate, launching a 5-year legislative battle.

1937 ELIXIR OF SULFANILAMIDE killed 107 persons, showing need to establish drug safety before marketing and to enact the pending 1938 food and drug law.

1938 THE FEDERAL FOOD, DRUG, AND COSMETIC ACT of 1938 (FDCA) was enacted, and contained these new provisions:
- Extended coverage to cosmetics and devices.
- Required predistribution clearance for safety of new drugs that an approved New Drug Application (NDA) was mandated before a manufacturer could commercially distribute a new drug.
- Eliminated Sherley Amendment requirement to prove intent to defraud in drug misbranding cases.
- Provided for tolerances for unavoidable poisonous substances.
- Authorized standards of identity, quality, and fill of container for foods.
- Authorized factory inspections.
- Added the remedy of court injunction to previous remedies of seizure and prosecution.

1940 FDA TRANSFERRED from the Department of Agriculture to the Federal Security Agency.

1941 FDCA AMENDED to require certification of the safety and efficacy of insulin [7].

1943 FEDERAL SECURITY ADMINISTRATOR v. QUAKER OATS COMPANY [8]. The U.S. Supreme Court ruled that the FDCA authorized the Administrator to use his judgment, based on "substantial evidence," to promulgate definitions and standards of identity for certain products where truthful labeling is not adequate to maintain their integrity. The courts, in reviewing the administrator's decision, will not substitute their judgment for his.

U.S. v. DOTTERWEICH [9]. The Supreme Court ruled that the responsible officials of a business, such as a corporation, as well as the business itself, may be prosecuted for violations of the FDCA.

1945 The FDCA was amended [10] on June 6th to require certification of the safety and efficacy of penicillin because of the uncertainties in production technologies experienced by the early penicillin manufacturers. Subsequent amendments [11] which became effective on May 1st, 1963 extended certification to any other antibiotic drug or any derivative thereof.

1950 ALBERTY FOOD PRODUCTS CO. v. U.S. [12]. The U.S. Court of Appeals held that the directions for use on a drug label must include the purpose for which the drug is offered. Therefore, a worthless remedy cannot escape the FDC Act by not stating the condition the drug is supposed to treat.

1951 DURHAM-HUMPHREY AMENDMENTS [13] to the FDCA specifically required that drugs which cannot be safely used without medical supervision must be dispensed only by prescription of a licensed practitioner, and prohibits refills of prescriptions without the express consent of the prescriber. The Amendments also gave guidance to the pharmacist as to what minimal information must be included on the prescription label.

1953 FEDERAL SECURITY AGENCY became the Department of Health, Education, and Welfare (DHEW). (Currently, it is the Department of Health and Human Services DHHS.)

FACTORY INSPECTION AMENDMENTS [14] clarified previous law and required FDA to give manufacturers written reports on inspections and analyses of factory samples.

1957 U.S. v. ADOLPHUS HOHENSEE [15]. The U.S. Court of Appeals held that oral representations may be used to show the intended purpose of a drug to establish that it is misbranded.

1960 COLOR ADDITIVE AMENDMENTS [16] to the FDCA were enacted to allow FDA to establish, by regulation, the conditions of safe use for color additives in foods, drugs, and cosmetics, and to require manufacturers to perform the necessary scientific investigations to establish safety for their intended uses.

1962 NEWS REPORTS on the role of Dr. Frances O. Kelsey, FDA Medical Officer, in keeping thalidomide off the American market aroused public interest in drug regulation. The drug had been associated with the birth of thousands of malformed babies (phocomelia) in western Europe.

The KEFAUVER-HARRIS DRUG AMENDMENTS [17] to the FDCA passed October 10th to assure a greater degree of safety and to strengthen new drug clearance procedures. For the first time, drug manufacturers were required to prove to FDA the effectiveness of their products before marketing them. In addition, the Amendments:

- Transferred jurisdiction over medical advertising of prescription products from the FTC to FDA;
- Extended FDA's inspection authority over establishments in which Rx drugs are manufactured, processed, packed or held to include records, files, papers, controls, and facilities;
- Required that facilities, methods, and control procedures used by manufacturers conform to "current good manufacturing practices";
- Established "full disclosure" under which the most vital, up-to-date and reliable information about an Rx drug was required in its labeling, in the form of a package insert;
- Added more extensive control for clinical investigations by strengthening FDA's authority governing human testing of new drugs.

1965 DRUG ABUSE CONTROL AMENDMENTS [18] (DACA) were enacted to deal with problems caused by abuse of three groups of dangerous drugs: depressants, stimulants, and hallucinogens.

1966 FDA contracted with the National Academy of Sciences/National Research Council to evaluate the effectiveness of 4,000 drugs approved on the basis of safety alone between 1938 and 1962 (DESI Review).

FAIR PACKAGING AND LABELING ACT [19] enacted to require that consumer products in interstate commerce be honestly and informatively labeled. FDA to enforce provisions which affect foods, drugs, cosmetics, and medical devices.

1968 FDA BUREAU OF DRUG ABUSE CONTROL was transferred to the new Bureau of Narcotics and Dangerous Drugs (BNDD) in Department of Justice, to consolidate policing of illegal drug traffic.

1969 Expanded FDA begins administration of programs transferred from other units of the Public Health Service, for milk, food service, shellfish, and interstate travel sanitation; and poisoning and accident prevention.

1970 UPJOHN v. FINCH [20]. The U.S. Court of Appeals made possible the enforcement of the 1962 Drug Effectiveness Amendments by holding that commercial success of a drug alone does not constitute substantial evidence of safety and efficacy, and that hearings will be held only if issues of fact exist.

DRUG ABUSE CONTROL AMENDMENTS of 1965 were repealed [21] with the enactment of the Comprehensive Drug Abuse Prevention and Control Act of 1970 [22]. BNDD becomes Drug Enforcement Administration (DEA).

THE POISON PREVENTION PACKAGING ACT [23] became effective December 30th. Its basic purpose was to provide special packaging to protect children from serious personal injury or illness that could result from handling, using, or ingesting certain toxic or harmful household substances and certain OTC and Rx drug products.

1972 FDA embarked on a long-range regulatory program to apply the Drug Efficacy Amendments to drugs sold over-the-counter (OTC Drug Review).

REGULATION OF BIOLOGICS (serums, vaccines, etc.), begun in 1902, was transferred to FDA.

DRUG LISTING ACT [24] amended the FDCA to provide the FDA with a continuous current list, by pharmacological category, of human and veterinary drug products, blood and blood products, biologicals, and *in-vitro* diagnostic products in commercial distribution in the United States. Required all manufacturers of such products to register annually with the FDA.

1973 THE SUPREME COURT, on June 18, upheld FDA in four drug effectiveness cases and gave the FDA a new charter to control entire classes of products by regulations rather than through time-consuming litigation. The Court held that enforcement limited to acting case-by-case against individual products is "inherently unfair because it requires compliance by one manufacturer while his competitors marketing similar products remain free to violate the Act."

1976 MEDICAL DEVICE AMENDMENTS [25] to the FDCA passed May 28th to (1) assure safety and effectiveness of medical devices, including certain diagnostic and laboratory products, and (2) upgrade the regulatory authority over such devices. In addition, the amendments required:
- Classification of all devices with graded regulatory requirements;
- Establishment registration;
- Device listing;
- Premarket approval;
- Investigational device (IDE) exemptions;
- Good Manufacturing Practice (GMP) regulations;
- Records and reporting requirements;
- Preemption of state and local regulation of devices;
- Performance standards

1980 INFANT FORMULA ACT [26] amended the FDCA to require that all infant formulas contain minimum amounts of nutrients essential for normal growth and development, and quality control procedures to be used during the manufacturing process. The Act was signed into law on September 26th.

TAMPER RESISTANT PACKAGING [27] regulations were enacted to require packaging of certain drugs, cosmetics, and medical devices in such a manner that any product tampering will be visibly evident to the consumer-purchaser.

1983 ORPHAN DRUG ACT [28] amended the FDCA to provide incentives for manufacturers to develop and market drugs or biological products intended for a rare disease or medical condition occurring in the United States. The Act was signed into law on January 4th. Products are termed "orphans" because commercial markets sufficient to cover the cost of development do not exist.

FEDERAL ANTI-TAMPERING ACT [29] amended the U.S. Code to establish penalties for threatening to tamper or tampering with an article subject to the FDCA in a manner to create a risk of death or bodily injury.

1984 DRUG PRICE COMPETITION AND PATENT ACT [30] (Waxman-Hatch Amendments) was signed into law on September 24th. There are two titles which concern new drugs. Title 1, which amended Section 505 of the Federal Food, Drug, and Cosmetic Act, codifies FDA's authority to accept abbreviated new drug applications (ANDAs) for generic versions of drug products first approved *after 1962*. Prior to Title I, ANDAs were only permitted under FDA regulations for generic versions of drug products first approved *between 1938 and 1962*. (The FDA can approve ANDAs for drugs without the submission of safety and effectiveness data if they are generically equivalent to brand name drugs already proved to be safe and effective.) Title II requires FDA's involvement in the process to allow holders of patents for drugs, biologics, medical devices, food, and color additives to obtain up to five years of patent life lost during FDA's regulatory review of a product. (Patent protection ordinarily lasts 17 years, but some of this time is often lost while products are evaluated prior to approval. Title II permits up to five years of this time to be restored but limits the total time to no more than 14 years.)

MEDICAL DEVICE REPORTING RULE [31], which became effective December 13th, requires manufacturers and importers of medical devices to report within five days to the FDA information that suggests that one of their devices has (1) caused or contributed to a death or serious injury, or (2) has malfunctioned and that device would be likely to cause or contribute to a death or serious injury if the malfunction were to recur.

1985 The FDA revised its regulations governing the approval for marketing of new drugs and antibiotic drugs for human use to improve the efficiency of the agency's approval process and

to improve the surveillance of marketed drugs. The major provisions pertain to:
- Application format
- Safety up-date reports
- Case reports and data tabulations
- Foreign clinical data
- Action letters

The regulations became effective May 23rd.

References

1. P.L. 75-717; 52 Stat. 1040; 21 U.S.C. 301 et seq.
2. 34 Stat. 768.
3. 221 US 488 (1911): 31 SCt 627.
4. Chapt 352, 37 Stat. 416.
5. 232 U.S. 399 (1914); 34 SCt 337.
6. 44 Stat. 1406; 15 U.S.C. 401.
7. P.L. 7-366; 21 U.S.C. 356.
8. 318 U.S. 218: 63 SCt 589.
9. 320 U.S. 277 (1943).
10. 21 U.S.C. 357.
11. P.L. 87-181: 76 Stat. 780.
12. 185 F. 2nd 321.
13. P.L. 82-215: 65 Stat. 648.
14. P.L. 83-217.
15. 243 F. 2nd 367.
16. P.L. 86-618.
17. P.L. 87-781: 76 Stat. 780.
18. P.L. 89-74: 79 Stat. 226.
19. 15 U.S.C. 1451.
20. 422 F. 2nd 944 (CA-6, 1970).
21. P.L. 91-513, Sect. 701.
22. P.L. 91-513; 84 Stat. 1242; 21 U.S.C. 801.
23. P.L. 91-601; 15 U.S.C. 1471.
24. P.L. 92-387; 86 Stat. 559.
25. P.L. 94-295; 21 U.S.C. 360.
26. P.L. 96-259.
27. 21 CFR 211, 314, 700.
28. P.L. 97-414; 96 Stat. 2049; 21 U.S.C. 360.
29. P.L. 98-127.
30. P.L. 98-417; 98 Stat. 1585.
31. 49 FR 36326, September 14, 1984.

FD&C Act

The purpose of the ACT is to safeguard the consumer by applying its requirements to articles from the moment of their conception all the way through the process of their use.

NEW DRUG DEVELOPMENTS IN THE U.S.*

Jack M. Rosenberg, Pharm.D., Ph.D. and Nicholas LaBella, Jr., R.Ph.

The long and complex process involved in the development of a new prescription product may begin at many places, including a pharmaceutical manufacturer's or university's laboratory, contract research service, or from research at a government facility, such as the National Institutes of Health. Before the drug is marketed, it is carefully studied in animals and man

*Reprinted with permission from *U.S. Pharmacist* (September 1980).

and the prescribing information needed by practitioners to utilize the drug correctly must be approved. The intent of this article is to provide an overview for the practicing pharmacist of the regulations pertinent to the development of a new drug including the clinical testing procedures involved in this process. [The Food and Drug Administration (FDA) is responsible for approving new drugs to be marketed in the United States and for monitoring their use

once they become available.] It emphasizes the "IND," three phases of clinical investigation, and the "NDA." Figure 1 provides a flow-chart outlining the steps from synthesis of a new chemical entity to its appearance on the pharmacy's shelf.

Background and Definitions

The 1962 Kefauver-Harris Amendment to the 1938 Food, Drug, and Cosmetic Act requires

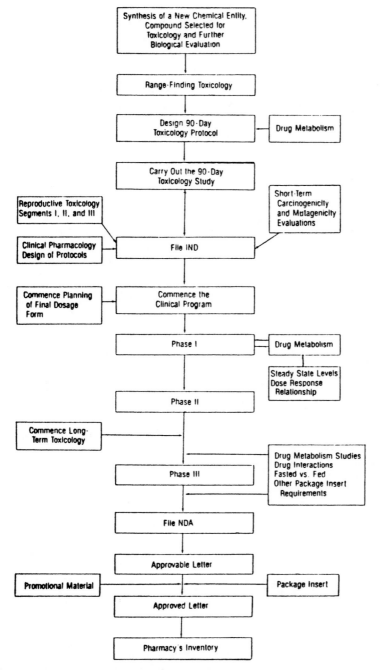

FIGURE 1. This flow-chart outlines the steps from synthesis of a new chemical entity to the marketing stage.

that a "new drug" demonstrate substantial evidence of safety and efficacy through adequate studies [1]. This is in contrast to the original Act, which only required proven safety.

A "new drug" is a drug not generally recognized by qualified experts as safe and effective for the use proposed [2]. The concept includes seeking approval for a new indication or even a new dosage form of an already marketed drug. The "new drug" cannot be distributed interstate for use in humans without FDA approval [3] and an exemption is required from the FDA in order to permit its clinical investigation. This is sought by the "sponsor"—usually a pharmaceutical company—but sometimes a private investigator filing a Notice of Claimed Investigational Exemption for a New Drug (IND). In order to gain approval to market a drug, a manufacturer files a New Drug Application (NDA) [5]. A Supplemental New Drug Application (SNDA) is submitted whenever a company wants to change any part of the procedures used in formulating a product that has an approved NDA or altering its labeling or packaging. An Abbreviated New Drug Application (ANDA) is utilized to market a "me too" drug and requires less information than was supplied by the original sponsor.

The IND

As stated, before a new drug can be tested in humans, the sponsor must file an IND. Among other things, it must contain results of previous pre-clinical investigations for which standards are prescribed under the FDA's Good Laboratory Practices Regulations. Such investigations are designed to indicate the drug's safety [6,7]. The drug should not appear to represent an unusual hazard for human use. Acute toxicity data, which is a prerequisite to more definitive tests, is derived from studies which last from two to four weeks in at least two species of animals. This includes determination of the LD_{50} (lethal dose for 50 percent of the experimental population), ED_{50} (effective dose for 50 percent of the experimental population) and therapeutic ratio (LD_{50}/ED_{50}).

Next, 90-day toxicity studies utilizing low, medium and high doses of the compound are conducted. The high dose is the highest that animals will tolerate during the 90-day study, without excessive mortality. The low dose is chosen to correspond with the range of the intended clinical dosage while the medium dose is between the two. Animals are then sacrificed and histopathological studies are performed on various tissues.

Other subacute toxicity data from animal trials as well as adverse effects on the kidney, liver, and bone marrow, when available, are to be included. However, the data are not limited to those organ systems, and other organ systems should be included if available. Also desirable, but not required at time of filing, is data from metabolic studies, designed to determine the drug's mechanism of action and its fate in animals. Frequently, additional animal experiments are necessary which are conducted concurrently with human trials.

The IND also includes information about the drug, its source and how it is manufactured [8]. Also needed is a description of the investigation, the training and experience of the investigators, the facilities where the drug will be utilized and the observations to be recorded. Copies of material supplied to each investigator are included with the IND. The sponsor also agrees to notify the FDA and all investigators of adverse effects that may arise during the human and animal studies and that "informed consent" will be obtained from subjects receiving the drug. The sponsor must agree to submit an annual progress report.

An investigator, such as a physician, may wish to sponsor an early clinical investigation of a drug which appears to possess therapeutic or diagnostic potential [8]. This may be the case when no pharmaceutical manufacturer is interested in doing so. A simpler abbreviated form of an IND is acceptable, and the investigator works directly with the FDA. Although a practitioner may legally use an approved drug for a non-approved indication without submitting an IND, he may assume additional responsibilities under civil law for consequences that may arise [3,4]. The FDA encourages voluntary submission of an IND from the practitioner in order to accumulate data concerning safety and efficacy under such circumstances.

After filing the IND, the sponsor must wait 30 days, unless extended by the FDA, before starting human trials [5]. This period is utilized to review the information and determine if subjects will be exposed to unnecessary risks. An investigation may be terminated at any time if a drug is found to represent excessive hazard, is ineffective, or the sponsor has not complied with any of the FDA regulations.

Clinical Investigation

There are three phases of human investigation (designated Phase I, II and III) utilized as part of the IND procedure. The first phase emphasizes definition of the drug's clinical pharmacology; Phase II continues this as well as focusing on the safety and effectiveness of the drug in treating a specific disease; Phase III is concerned with wide-spread clinical use to further assess effectiveness and most desirable dosage range.

Phase I trials are conducted to determine the drug's human pharmacological actions including absorption, metabolism and elimination [6]. It emphasizes determination of the safe dosage range and toxic manifestations of the agent. The investigators must have clinical pharmacology training and the proposed clinical plan permits considerable flexibility on their part. A small number of healthy volunteers, usually 15 to 30, are studied under carefully controlled circumstances, usually one at a time, to minimize the risks to them. Subjects may be utilized more than once after sufficient time has elapsed to insure no interference from the previous drug exposure [9]. To determine the minimal and optimal effective dose, the drug is initiated at a level thought to have no pharmacological action as extrapolated from the animal studies. It is then increased until evidence of activity is observed. Many times in normal, healthy volunteers it may not be possible to observe activity for certain types of drugs, for example an analgesic

agent. The drug in a radiolabeled form may be utilized *in vivo* to help elucidate pharmacological effects. The drug's activity is studied on different organ systems as well as an evaluation of its safety after single and multiple dosage regimens. Individual studies in this phase usually last no longer than two weeks, but may be more extensive if dealing with a unique entity.

Phase II trials may be initiated after completion of Phase I but these can overlap. This phase is primarily concerned with determining the usefulness of the drug in preventing or treating the disease for which it is intended [8]. For this reason, the physician-investigator must be knowledgeable about the treatment and evaluation of that disease process. Studies are first conducted on a small number of afflicted individuals, usually three to six, to determine safety and efficacy. In this phase, as well as in Phase I, experiments are performed concurrently in animals to indicate the drug's safety for extension of the Phase II investigation. Rodent and non-rodent animal species are utilized for these toxicity studies [7]. Special studies are initiated in animals to determine any effect of the drug on the reproductive and fertility processes as well as its potential for inducing abnormalities (teratogenicity) in the developing fetus. During Phase I and most of Phase II, women of childbearing potential are not permitted to participate in clinical trials until at least three segments of the reproductive studies are completed. Pregnant women and fetuses are also protected as no studies can be initiated involving them without completion of appropriate tests on animals and non-pregnant women unless the agent poses minimal risks and meets a specific health need of an individual [11].

Carcinogenic testing is also initiated at this time. A two-year (lifetime) study in rats is required in order to prove a compound is not carcinogenic. Often lifetime feeding in a second species, e.g., mouse, for eighteen months, is requested, or chronic feeding for one year in a nonrodent species. If a compound does prove to be carcinogenic, the manufacturer may be required to provide lifetime follow-up data on all patients exposed to that agent. Additionally, further metabolic and behavioral studies are conducted for at least 13 weeks in animals while they receive the drug. These animals are then sacrificed for gross and microscopic examinations. If warranted, the Phase II studies are expanded to a population of between 100 to 200.

Phase III studies are implemented after successful completion of the earlier phases and there is reasonable assurance of the drug's safety and efficacy or that its potential value outweighs the risks. This phase is intended to assess, in carefully monitored and controlled trials, the drug's effectiveness and most desirable dosage range in treating a large number of patients with the specific disease for which the drug is intended [10]. It offers the opportunity to obtain data from extensive use of the drug in controlled clinical settings. The medication is supplied in the dosage form the sponsor desires to market, and the investigators follow approved administration protocols.

In addition to work by experienced investigators, Phase III studies may involve, where practical, clinical trials initiated by physicians whose training and experience in drug evaluation has been less and whose facilities may not be so elaborate [6]. In either case, the studies are carefully monitored by the sponsor. Since the clinical trials are extensive and patients may suffer from more than one disease state, the introduction of many variables necessitates use of the control groups. These control groups may receive placebo or recognized drugs for the treatment of the specific disease. The control permits assessment of whether the new drug produced the desired effect rather than chance or other

variables. The active treatment control group(s) also allow comparison of the new drug to the standard(s) utilized in the treatment of that disease.

The NDA

After human pharmacological and clinical testing studies have been completed, and the sponsor is convinced that the new drug is safe and effective, an NDA is filed. The NDA, that is the request for approval for marketing, is submitted with supportive data and proposed labeling to show that "it could be fairly and responsibly considered by qualified experts that the drug is safe and will have the effects it purports or is represented to have under conditions of use prescribed, recommended or suggested in the proposed labeling" [6]. The NDA must contain all information generated concerning the drug product. This includes full reports of investigations, components used in its manufacturing, a statement of composition of the product, description of facilities and methods used in manufacturing, processing and packaging, a sample of the drug product if required, and examples of the proposed label and labeling. The summary alone may be as long as 4,000 to 5,000 pages, while the total package may run between 50,000 and 100,000 pages. By this time the drug was studied in several hundred to several thousand patients and a wide variety of animal testing performed. Each subject's case report in the clinical studies is included. It is a truly formidable document.

The information is reviewed by one of the six reviewing divisions of the FDA Bureau of Drugs: anti-infective, cardiorenal, surgical-dental, metabolic and endocrine, neuropharmacological, or oncological and radiopharmaceutical [5]. The review is conducted by physicians, pharmacists, chemists, and other health professionals experienced in evaluating that category of drug. It includes a deter-

mination of whether the drug's quality is assured, appropriate studies conducted to define its potential toxicity, and is it truthfully and thoroughly labeled. One of the most difficult tasks involves the determination of risks versus benefits of the new drug. This involves medical and social implications for no drug is completely free from side effects. The FDA is required to act on the application within 180 days [12]. If an application is incomplete, it may be completed by supplying the lacking data, with an additional 180 days again allowed to the FDA.

The potential importance of the drug has an effect on the length of time involved in the approval process. A recent analysis by the FDA's Bureau of Drugs indicated that the average time from when an NDA is received until it is approved was 32 months [13]. The same analysis showed that drugs that offer a therapeutic advantage over products currently marketed required approximately 22 months for approval. Thus, potentially important new drugs get priority "fast track" treatment, while those of lesser importance must wait their turn. Under the priority classification system, new drugs are classified according to chemical type and therapeutic potential (Table 1) [14]. These ratings are assigned by FDA reviewers at the time the drug is first submitted to the agency, during either the IND or NDA stage of development, and are subject to change. A final classification is assigned at time of approval of the NDA.

Bioavailability and Bioequivalence as Related to the NDA

The FDA has regulations for both *in vitro* and *in vivo* testing of bioequivalence and bioavailability of selected pharmaceuticals [15]. Bioavailability is defined to mean the rate and extent of absorption of the active drug or therapeutic moiety along with its availability at the site of action. NDAs and Sup-

Table 1
FDA Rating and Classification System for New Drugs

Chemical Type

Number	Classification
1	**New molecular entity**
	The active moiety is not yet marketed in the U.S. by any drug manufacturer either as a single entity or part of a new combination product.
2	**New salt**
	The active moiety in the U.S. by the same or another manufacturer but the particular salt, ester, or derivative is not yet marketed in the U.S. by any drug manufacturer either as a single entity or as part of a combination product.
3	**New formulation**
	The compound is marketed in the U.S. by the same or another manufacturer, but the particular dosage form or formulation is not.

Number	Classification
4	**New combination**
	Contains two or more compounds which have not previously been marketed together in a drug product by any manufacturer in the U.S.
5	**Already marketed drug product**
	The product duplicates a drug product (the same active moiety, same salt, same formulation, or same combination) already marketed in the U.S. by another firm.
6	**Already marketed drug product by the same firm**
	Used primarily for new indications for marketed drugs.

Therapeutic Potential

Type	Classification
A	**Important therapeutic gain.**
	Drug may provide effective therapy or diagnosis (by virtue of greatly increased effectiveness or safety) for a disease not adequately treated for diagnosed by any marketed drug, or provide improved treatment of a disease through improved effectiveness or safety (including decreased abuse potential).
B	**Modest therapeutic gain.**
	Drug has a modest, but real potential over other available marketed drugs—i.e., greater patient convenience, elimination of an annoying but not dangerous adverse reaction, potential for large cost reduction, less frequent dosage schedule, useful in specific sub-population of those with disease (i.e., those allergic to other available drugs), etc.
C	**Little or no therapeutic gain.**
	Drug essentially duplicates in medical importance and therapeutic usage one or more already marketed drugs.

Type	Classification
M	**Drug already marketed in a** foreign country.
R	**Drug is subject to specific unique** conditions of approval (i.e., additional studies) outlined in appropriate or approval letter for NDA.
T	**Important problem in toxicity,** i.e., carcinogenic in animals.
U	**Drug is likely to be used in** children.
D	**Special stiuation. Drug has de-**creased safety or effectiveness compared with alternative marketed drugs, but also has some compensating virtue (i.e., provides treatment for patients who do not respond to or are intolerant of alternative drugs).
P	**A very important feature of** application is the packaging or container, not the drug itself.
S	**Application is sensitive by virtue** of wide publicity, congressional interest, unusual request from firm, etc.

plemental NDAs must be submitted with evidence *in vivo* bioavailability. This requirement may be waived if the drug meets certain criteria.

Bioequivalence is defined as either equivalent or alternative drugs whose rate and extent of absorption do not differ significantly when administered in the same dose. Any drug may have a bioequivalence requirement placed on it if there is evidence from well-controlled clinical trials that the agent does not give a comparable therapeutic effect, has a narrow margin of safety, is not bioequivalent, or shows significant differences in physiochemical parameters.

Post Marketing Surveillance ("Phase IV")

After a new drug is marketed, the manufacturer's responsibilities do not end [16]. They must supply periodic reports as specified in the FDA's regulations, including information concerning current clinical studies, quantity of drugs distributed and copies of mailing pieces, labeling, and advertising. Since many useful drugs have subsequently been found to have serious side effects associated with their general use that were not recognized or detected during clinical testing, prompt reports are required of unexpected side effect, injury, toxicity or sensitivity reactions made known to the manufacturer. It also involves following up on adverse reactions. Failure of the drug to exert an expected pharmacological effect must also be reported. Immediate reports are required in case of drug mixups or evidence of contamination. Post marketing surveillance may include initiating studies to substantiate or rule out suspected toxicity, as will as extending claims of safety and efficacy where indicated. This phase allows for perspective studies of the drug using placebo or standard therapy as control. An excellent example of Phase IV post market surveillance was seen recently in the voluntary withdrawal of ticrynafen (Selacryn) by its manufacturer after it was shown to produce hepatocellular damage [17].

Withdrawing NDA Approval

If an approved drug is not as safe or effective as anticipated, the FDA can withdraw approval. Although a firm is given an opportunity to present its view, the FDA is the final judge concerning the drug's safety and efficacy. An example of

an NDA withdrawal involved the drug phenformin [18]. In July, 1977, phenformin's NDA was suspended by the FDA based on the high incidence of lactic acidosis associated with its use. Since the drug's withdrawal in October of 1977, the FDA has recognized that phenformin may be useful in certain instances, and has made it available for limited use under an IND exemption.

References

1. Anello C: FDA principles on clinical investigation. FDA Papers 4(5): 14, 1970.
2. Anon: Drugs for human use, requirements of laws and regulations enforced by the U.S. food and drug administration. DHEW publication No. (FDA) 79-1042, pp 38–39.
3. Gyarfas WJ, Welch A: The IND procedure: assuring safe and effective drugs. FDA Papers 3(7):27, 1969.
4. Fink JL: Dispensing FDA approved drugs for non-approved uses. US Pharm 2(9) 24, 1977.
5. Pines WL: A primer on new drug development. FDA Consumer 8(1): 12, 1974.
6. Anon: Clinical testing: synopsis of the new drug regulations. FDA Papers 1(2):21, 1967.

7. Swinyard EA: Introduction of new drugs. In Hoover JE (ED.): Remington's Pharmaceutical Sciences, 15th Ed., Easton, PA, Mack Publishing Company, 1975, pp 1301–1304.
8. Anon: Clinical testing for safe and effective drugs. FDA Papers 1(2):21, 1967.
9. 21 CFR 312.1.
10. Martz BL, Kiplinger FG: Investigational drugs and clinical research. Blissit CW, Webb OL, Stanaszek WF (Eds.): In Clinical Pharmacy Practice, Philadelphia PA, Lea & Febiger, 1972, pp 414–421.
11. 45 CFR 46, 103.
12. FDCA Sect. 505(c); 21 U.S.C. 300 et seq.
13. Anon: Providing a breakthrough for drugs with a promise FDA Consumer 13(6):25, 1979.
14. Schneiweiss, F: Understanding the FDA's guarded system for classifying new drugs. Hosp Form 14:262, 1979.
15. 21 CFR 320 et seq.
16. DeHaan RM: Clinical Studies to evaluate safety and efficacy in phase IV investigations. Drug Inf Bull 2:84, 1968.
17. Hospital pharmacy letter, urgent: drug recall. Smith, Kline and French, January 16, 1980.
18. FDA Drug Bulletin, August 1977, p. 14.

HOW NEW DRUGS WIN FDA APPROVAL*

William M. Troetel, Ph.D., R.Ph.

Development of a new drug product for marketing in the United States is an extremely complicated process. It is the Food & Drug Administration's (FDA) responsibility to assure that all

*Reprinted with permission from *U.S. Pharmacist* (November 1986).

marketed drugs are both safe and effective.

Prior to 1938, it was not necessary for a manufacturer to submit to the Federal government any evidence of safety or efficacy of a new drug product before marketing it. In 1938, a tragic incident occurred in which more than 100 children

died because a toxic solvent, ethylene glycol, was used to solubilize a sulfa drug product. Congress reacted almost immediately and passed the Federal Food, Drug, and Cosmetic Act of 1938.

This act required that any new drug placed on the market must first be evaluated by the manufacturer for safety. Surprisingly, it was not until 1962 that the Kefauver-Harris Amendments were passed so that in addition to requiring safety, all drug products also had to be proven effective for the labeled indication before being granted approval by FDA for marketing in the United States. Thus we have the two requirements today of demonstrating safety and efficacy for a new chemical entity.

What Are INDs?

It is not possible to test a new drug in the United States without first filing a document that is officially entitled a Notice of Claimed Investigational Exemption for a New Drug. This document title is frequently abbreviated to the more common term "Investigational New Drug Application," or more simply, IND. The reason that an IND must be submitted prior to the evaluation of an unapproved new drug entity is that there is no provision in the Food, Drug and Cosmetic Act that allows an unapproved new drug to be shipped in interstate commerce.

As a result, the IND is really an exemption from the Food & Drug legislation that allows an unapproved drug to be shipped for clinical research purposes in interstate commerce.

Before FDA allows such shipment of a new drug, the IND must be filed with the FDA by the sponsor. An initial filing of an IND contains results of pharmacological and toxicological evaluations, chemistry and pharmaceutical manufacturing and controls data, a clinical plan for the development of the new drug product, and a specific protocol for the initial clinical trial proposed to be conducted.

Table 1 shows the 16 basic elements that constitute an IND filing. The pharmacology data generally lends support for the intended indication for the drug under investigation. In addition, the drug is evaluated pharmacologically to determine its effects on various bio-

Table 1—IND Items

Items 1–5	Chemistry of Product
	Manufacturing Methods
	Quality Control Testing
Item 6	Statement of Relative Safety
	Pertinent Pre-Clinical and Clinical Data
Item 7	Informational Material for Investigator
Item 8	Investigator Qualifications
Item 9	Identity of Investigators and Monitor and Their Qualifications
Item 10	Outline of Clinical Investigational Protocol
	Case Report Form
Item 11	Agreement to Notify FDA if Discontinued
Item 12	Agreement to Notify Investigator if NDA Approved/Studies Discontinued
Item 13	Avoid Commercialization
Item 14	30-Day Delay
Item 15	Environmental Impact Analysis
Item 16	Good Laboratory Practices Statements

Items 1–5 are discussed in the text. Item 6 is summary of the pre-clinical data plus any clinical data that may also exist on the new drug substance, for example if it is marketed in Europe. Item 7 is the investigator drug brochure that summarizes and details information found in item 6. Item 9 indicates the location for the filing of the identity of the investigator and monitoring staff and item 10 is the section in which the complete protocol is provided as well as a specimen of the case report form and the outline of the clinical investigations. The other items in the IND are statements in which it is agreed that certain items will be followed with regard to the filing of an IND. For example, item 13 means that commercialization of the IND product will be avoided and item 14 is an agreement that a clinical trial will not begin until 30 days have elapsed from the time of filing.

logical systems such as the central nervous system, the cardiovascular system and the autonomic nervous system. With regard to toxicology, FDA generally requires at least three acute toxicity studies in which the LD50 has been determined in several animal species by various routes of administration, and specifically by the route of administration that is to be studied clinically in humans.

Also contained in the initial IND filing are at least two subacute toxicity studies (generally conducted in the rat and dog). The subacute studies may span 30–90 days of drug administration with the animals randomized into low, middle, and high dose groups, as well as a control group. Parameters evaluated include clinical chemistries, urinalyses, behavioral observations, ophthalmological examinations and macroscopic and microscopic histopathological examinations following terminal sacrifice. All of these preclinical data are contained in item 6 of the IND application.

The chemistry and the pharmaceutical manufacturing and con-

trols data provide the FDA with information relating to the sites of manufacture and the quality control practices employed in the production of the active drug substance and the dosage form.

This includes detailed information on the preparation and the synthesis of the active drug substance as well as on the formulated dosage form. Stability data as well as packaging information of the active drug substance, in addition to the formulated dosage form, must also be provided.

The chemistry and pharmacy information contained within the IND are provided in items one through five. Item 4 is generally the information that describes the required data on the active drug substance, and item 5 will provide FDA with all of the required data on the dosage form itself including placebos if these are to be used in comparison with the active ingredient in a clinical trial program.

The clinical section of the IND provides the protocol which is usually a phase I study designed to examine the effects of increasing doses of the new drug in normal male volunteers. Information identifying the investigator who will conduct the study and information relating to the qualifications of the sponsor's staff who will monitor the study to assure that the concepts of good clinical practices are being followed are also a part of the IND.

Three-Phase Program

The initial protocol that is submitted in an IND is usually a phase I study (Table 2). Clinical research programs are divided into three phases. Phase I represents an assessment of the dose tolerance and the safety, bioavailability and general metabolic and elimination pattern of the drug substance.

These studies are usually conducted in healthy, normal male volunteers. The phase I program may utilize between 50 and 70 volunteer subjects. Once the dose tolerance has been established, phase II clinical trials may be initiated.

The phase II studies are designed to assess the safety and efficacy of the drug for the first time in patients who have the disease or condition that the drug is intended to treat, and it may include up to a total of 200 patients.

The initial part of phase II studies are generally conducted in male patients or in females of non-child bearing potential. Once the FDA has reviewed and accepted the required level of preclinical fertility and reproductive studies generally conducted in rats and rabbits on the new drug, permission is granted by FDA to include women of all ages into the late phase II studies so long as they are not pregnant.

Providing the data appear promising and continue to demonstrate a good risk to benefit ratio with regard to safety and efficacy, clinical trials extend into the phase III long-term program.

The phase III program, in which well controlled trials continue to provide data on safety and efficacy may include upwards of 1000 or more patients depending on the indication for the drug.

It is frequently asked how much time is required for complete drug development programs. That includes the pre-clinical data, pharmaceutical and manufacturing and controls data, as well as the com-

---

Table 2—Drug Approval Process

Phase 1 Study
1. Normal or Disease Population Patients
2. 20–80 Patients
3. Open Study

Phase 1 Study—Objectives
Determination of:
1. Safety
2. Dose and Schedule
3. Pharmacokinetics
4. Pharmacological Actions
5. Enough Information to Permit Design of Well-Controlled Scientifically Valid Phase 2 study

Phase 1 Study—General Information
1. Provides Rationale and Toxicological Information on Dose and Schedule
2. Number of Subjects Sufficient to Detect Frequency of Dose-Related Toxicities
3. Conduct Dose Escalation and Monitor Toxicity
4. Early Information on Safety and Effectiveness
5. Single Dose–Multiple Dose
6. Various Doses

Phase 2 Study
1. Patients with Disease
2. 100–200 Patients
3. Controlled Study—Randomized—Multicenter

Phase 2 Study Objectives
Determination of:
1. Safety and Effectiveness
2. Dose, Route, and Schedule
3. Toxicity Profile
4. Clinical Endpoints
5. Dose-Response Curve

6. Short-Term Adverse Effects
7. Reasons for Non-Response
8. Possible Drug Interactions
9. Pharmacological Effects
10. Pharmacokinetics of Drug

Phase 2 Study—General Information
1. Controlled Studies
2. First Indication of Effectiveness
3. Additional Safety Information
4. Determine Final Formulation
5. Enough Information to Permit Design of Well-Controlled Scientifically Valid Phase 3 Studies (Pivotal Studies)

Phase 3 Study
1. Patients with Disease
2. 200–(?) Patients
3. Controlled Study—Randomized—Multicenter

Phase 3 Study—Objectives
Determination of:
1. Safety and Effectiveness in a Large Population
2. Patient Population
3. Product Claims
4. Final Formulation
5. Product Stability and Storage Conditions
6. Drug-Related Adverse Effects

Phase 3 Study—General Information
• Phase 3 Study Conducted on Larger Varied Population so as to Obtain Additional Information about Safety and Effectiveness That Is Needed to Evaluate the Overall Benefit-Risk Relationship of Drug and to Provide an Adequate Basis for Labeling.

plete clinical trials program ranging from phase I, II, and through phase III. Generally, an IND developmental program can last anywhere from 2½ years (very optimistically) to six or more years. At the conclusion of this time period, when all of the studies are completed and all of the safety and efficacy data have been analyzed, a new drug application is prepared and submitted to the FDA.

The NDA Process

The new drug application, or NDA, is an assembly of all information that has been obtained regarding the new drug product during the IND program (Table 3). In addition to providing all of the pre-clinical studies including pharmacology and toxicology reports, there is a complete section on manufacturing and controls in which the complete synthesis of the chemical substance is characterized, including all impurities and synthetic byproducts. The formulation is provided in detail, stability data are presented for both the active drug substance as well as the formulated dosage form, and information relating to packaging and labeling is provided. The clinical section is perhaps the most lengthy section of the new drug application since it provides full reports of clinical and statistical analyses of data relating to safety and efficacy in all volunteers and patients studied with the new drug product.

The total NDA may, therefore, contain details and reports on treatment of over 1200 patients with the new drug substance. Table 3 shows that the NDA is subdivided into five or six technical sections which include the chemistry, manufacturing and controls technical section, a section on nonclinical pharmacology and toxicology data, a section on human pharmacokinetics and bioavailability, a very lengthy section on clinical data, and a technical section on the statistical analyses. The microbiological section is only applicable in the event that one is filing an NDA for an antibiotic drug substance or a drug that requires some significant microbiological testing.

Each of these technical sections requires FDA review by an expert in the specific scientific discipline. The FDA reviewers, therefore, include chemists, pharmacists, pharmacologists, physicians, pharmacokineticists, statisticians and microbiologists.

Once the NDA is filed, the average review time may range from 18 months to three years for approval. Therefore, from the time an IND is filed to the time an NDA is approved, the average amount of time that could elapse is anywhere from 4–10 years. Typically, a new drug developmental program requires an average of approximately 7–8 years from start to end and costs upwards of $50–60 million. Once the NDA is approved, the company has legal authorization to sell the drug product in interstate commerce. A new drug product cannot be sold in the United States without an appropriate registration document having been reviewed and approved by the FDA. As long as the research and development or innovator company, as it is frequently called, has a patent that protects the exclusivity of the drug, no other company is entitled to sell this product.

The ANDA

Once the patent has expired, however, it is possible for a generic pharmaceutical company to submit a document to the FDA that will allow that generic firm to also enter the market with a drug product that the FDA has determined is therapeutically equivalent to the innovator's drug product. The document that must be submitted by a generic pharmaceutical manufacturer is called an "Abbreviated New Drug Application," or more simply, an ANDA.

With one exception, the ANDA does not contain any biological data. Therefore, an ANDA is not required to contain any pharmacological or toxicological studies and an ANDA is also not required to contain any studies of a clinical research nature. Provided that the generic drug sponsor of an ANDA plans to sell a drug that is identical in potency, dosage form, and product labeling, the FDA does not require any preclinical or clinical testing.

The one exception to this requirement is that almost all solid dosage forms are required to be proven to be bioequivalent to the innovator's drug product. Therefore, almost every generic sponsor of an ANDA is required to conduct one bioequivalency study in which the formulation of the generic sponsor is compared with the formulation of the innovator firm.

Bioequivalence

A typical bioequivalency study may involve 18–24 normal, healthy male volunteers (Table 4). In a randomized fashion, half receive the innovator's formulation and half the generic formulation. Blood samples are collected at different time intervals from prior to drug administration, usually up to 24 hours after a single oral dose.

The times for blood collections are chosen so that an assessment can be made regarding the rate of absorption, the time when the peak plasma concentration is at-

---

Table 3—New Drug Application Technical Sections

Chemistry, Manufacturing and Controls
Non-Clinical Pharmacology/Toxicology
Human Pharmacokinetics and Bioavailability
Clinical Data
Statistical
Microbiology (if Applicable)

Table 4—Bioequivalency Studies

Innovator's Formulation *versus* Generic Manufacturer's Formulation
18 to 24 Normal Healthy Male Volunteers
Randomized
Typical Sample Times:
    Prior to Drug Administration and
    0.5, 1, 2, 3, 4, 6, 8, 12, 24 Hours Post Administration
Parameters Evaluated:
    Area Under Curve
    Half-Life
    Time to Peak Plasma Concentration
    Value of Peak Plasma Concentration

tained and the value of that peak plasma concentration.

The last time point generally represents a very low or nondetectable blood level. Therefore, the area under the blood concentration time curve can be calculated as well as the half-life for the drug.

Following a suitable interval, generally one to two weeks, the groups are crossed over so that the group that initially received the innovator's formulation will now receive the generic formulation and vice versa. Blood samples are collected at the same time intervals, and the pharmacokinetic parameters of area under the curve, maximum plasma concentration, time to peak plasma concentration, and plasma half-life are calculated.

The general FDA guideline for bioequivalence is that the bioavailability of the generic product should not differ from that of the innovator's product by more than 20 percent with regard to the mean extent of absorption which is generally a reflection of the area under the curve.

The generic product must also have the same rate of bioavailability as measured by a method that shows the average maximum and minimum concentrations, that these will not differ from those of the innovator's product by more than 20 percent, and that the times for the two products to reach their maximum concentrations do not differ significantly.

Statistical methods are also used to insure that the generic product is not excessively variable from dose to dose within subjects. A few drugs cannot meet the statistical criteria due to an inherent variability of both the innovator's and generic products, in which case the 75/25 rule is used.

This requires that at least 75 percent of the people tested do not show a variation of more than 25 percent between the innovator's and the generic product. For one class of drugs, the psychotropic phenothiazines, the criterion has been expanded to allow 70 percent of the people tested to show a variation of 30 percent or less between the two products. In a very recent public letter from FDA, the FDA claims that no product had been approved by the agency for which a 30 percent variation in the extent of absorption has been permitted.

In summary, the information that is required of a generic drug manufacturer in an ANDA filing is complete pharmaceutical and manufacturing controls information about the dosage form and the results of one bioequivalency study.

The cost of a typical bioequivalency study is largely dependent on the number of subject volunteers that are required and the ease or difficulty associated with the specific assay of the drug in the blood. Typically, however, a bioequivalence study can be conducted in the price range of $40,000 to $150,000.

The passage of the Waxman-Hatch Amendment to the Food, Drug & Cosmetic Act significantly increased the ability of generic pharmaceutical manufacturers to enter the U.S. market. Prior to the passage of the Waxman-Hatch Amendment, the only drug products for which the FDA could accept an abbreviated new drug application were products that were approved by the FDA between 1938 and 1962.

All drugs approved after 1962, regardless of patent status, required a full new drug application filing. This meant that complete pharmacology and toxicology data and complete clinical research programs were necessary even though the drug was intended to be used for the same indication as the original innovator product and that the dosage form and potencies to be offered by the generic drug manufacturer were the same as the innovator's drug product.

The Complex Waxman-Hatch Amendment

The Waxman-Hatch Amendment is an extremely complicated law. In addition to permitting the filing of abbreviated new drug applications for post-1962 drugs once the patent of the innovator has expired, the amendment is also coupled with a patent restoration bill.

The purpose of the patent restoration portion of this legislation is to provide the innovator with additional patent time to compensate for some of the patent time that is lost during the FDA review period of the NDA.

Therefore, the patent restoration act allows the FDA to add the NDA review time on to the original expiration date of the patent. This can frequently add two to three years of patent life to the innovator's product. With regard to the ANDA portion of the Waxman-Hatch Amendment, the innovator is granted a period of five years' exclusivity on every NDA that is approved by the FDA. Therefore, regardless of how much patent life remains on a given product, the innovator firm will be guaranteed at least five years of exclusivity.

For many years, generic companies attempted to convince the FDA that once the patent of an innovator's product had expired, there was no reason why they should have to duplicate research programs for drugs that had already been proven to be safe and effective since they were approved by the FDA after 1962 or after the Kefauver-Harris Amendment.

For a time the FDA agreed with this logic and developed the paper NDA concept. The paper NDA was essentially an abbreviated new drug application, except that the FDA had no authority to waive the requirements for a full new drug application. Therefore, they adopted a program that permitted the generic industry to file a paper NDA which contained full manufacturing and controls data, a bioequivalence study (previously described), and the summary of literature supporting the safety and efficacy of the drug product being submitted as a paper NDA.

The term "paper" obviously refers to medical and scientific literature sources for both preclinical and clinical data that support the safety and effectiveness of the drug. Many drug products were approved under the paper NDA system. However, as a result of the passage of the Waxman-Hatch Amendment, the paper NDA has fallen by the wayside since the Waxman-Hatch Amendment permits any generic pharmaceutical manufacturer to file an abbreviated new drug application on drugs now referred to as post-1962 drugs . . . providing that the patent has expired and therefore the need to search the literature for supportive safety and efficacy data has been eliminated.

By the time the NDA is filed, a new drug candidate may have been evaluated in four or five species for as long as two years and has been evaluated as a potential carcinogen, a potential mutagen and teratogen (Table 5). Its patterns of absorption, distribution, metabolism, and excretion have all been assessed. The toxicity of the drug

Table 5—Minimal Animal Toxicity Requirements

Acute Toxicity (LD_{50})	—3 or 4 Species
Subacute Toxicity	—2 Species, 3 Months
	—2 Species, 6 Months
Chronic Toxicity	—2 Species, 12 Months (Rat)
	12 Months (Dog)
	—Carcinogenicity, 2 Years Rat
	18 Months (Mouse)
Fertility and Reproduction	—Segment I (Fertility)
	—Segment II (Teratology)
	—Segment III (Peri- and Post-Natal)
	2 Species, Rat and Rabbits
Mutagenicity	

on target organs, other organ systems, the blood and the eye has also been evaluated. All of these are requirements just in the preclinical area for the innovator firm on a new drug substance.

In humans, the drug has initially been given to upwards of 70 normal, healthy male volunteers to assess its safety, dose tolerance and bioavailability in this population. Following this stage, patients are treated very carefully in well controlled trials so that a dose response pattern can be predicted and an appropriate dosage regimen determined.

This phase II clinical program may include 200 patients. The expanded clinical program or phase III may add an additional 800 to 1000 patients so that the firm may continue to assess safety and efficacy of the new drug. The phase III program itself may last as long as three or more years.

With this level of research activity it is not difficult to comprehend that the total time and cost leading to an NDA filing are estimated at between seven and 10 years and $50–60 million.

Another significant risk is that a very large percentage of drug candidates never pass beyond the phase II programs for reasons related to possible lack of safety or efficacy, yet millions of dollars and several years of research effort must be expended before such a "no go" decision can be reached.

A generic pharmaceutical manufacturer can be granted ANDA approval by filing pharmaceutical, manufacturing, and controls data and at least one bioequivalency study. A bioequivalency study may cost upwards of $150,000 and take six months to complete. The cost of the trial essentially depends on two factors: the number of volunteers required, and the complexity of the chemical assay of the drug in the blood. The study may require six months from the time of initiation to the generation of the final clinical and statistical report.

The majority of the time required for a bioequivalency study is not in the dosing phase but in the blood analysis and statistical evaluation portion of the study.

The time required for ANDA approval can vary from approximately nine months to two years. The approval time for an ANDA is dependent upon the workload within the FDA's Division of Generic Drug Monographs, the ability of the Biopharmaceutics Division of the FDA to assess the bioequivalency study, and of course, on the quality of the chemistry and manufacturing and controls data that comprise the nucleus of the ANDA.

Many months of delay will be incurred if the FDA raises questions relating to any of the data contained within the ANDA submission. There is very little difference with regard to the data required for manufacturing and controls between a brand name and a generic drug manufacturer. The FDA requires as much detail as possible about the preparation of the active drug substance, complete information relating to the impurities and degradation products of the active drug substance, information on the formulation, its dissolution and disintegration profiles, its packaging and container and closure systems, and its labeling, as well as complete reports on the stability of the product that will assure a proper expiration date.

All analytical methodology that is used to determine the potency for release of the drug or to determine the drug's stability profile must be properly validated to demonstrate to the FDA that the assay procedure is specific, sensitive, linear and reproducible.

Therefore, the key differences between the generic pharmaceutical company and a research and development oriented pharmaceutical company prior to approval for sale of a new drug are not represented in terms of the quality of the manufacturing process or the quantity of the required chemistry and manufacturing and controls data, but actually in the quantity and quality of basic research data that are required in the areas of pharmacology, toxicology, clinical research and statistical analyses.

New Drug

- Meets "drug" definition of Federal Food, Drug and Cosmetic Act, and
- Not generally recognized by experts as safe and effective for the indicated use

Product new drug if:
- Product in existence but never approved in USA
- Approved drug—new indications
- Approved drug—new dosage form
- Approved drug—new route of administration
- Approved drug—new dose schedule
- Other significant clinical differences from those approved

DRUG MASTER FILES*

M. Douglas Winship and Steven Strauss, Ph.D., R.Ph.

A Drug Master File (DMF) is a confidential reference source, not available to the public at large under the Freedom of Information Act (FoIA) [1]. The DMF provides detailed information about a specific facility, process, article, or ingredient used in the manufacture, processing, packaging, or holding of a substance which is the subject of an investigational new drug application (IND) [2], a new drug application (NDA) [3], an abbreviated new drug application (ANDA) [4], or an Antibiotic Form 5 or Form 6 [5,6]. A drug master file is *not* a

substitute for any of these applications or forms.

Drug master files are subject to certain regulatory provisions of Title 21, Part 314.11 of the *Code of Federal Regulations*, which make reference to Sections 505(b), 507, and 301(j) of the Federal Food, Drug, and Cosmetic Act (FDCA) [7].

Section 505(b) of the FDCA provides that any person may file with the Secretary of Health and Human Services (HHS) an application with respect to a new drug, which shall include, among other things, a full list of components and a full statement of the composition of such drug. These requirements ap-

ply to all components of a new drug, whether or not they are therapeutically active. Fulfillment of these requirements may be met by submitting a full statement including the chemical, common or usual name, and the quantity of each component of the drug. Furthermore, a full description of the method used in, and the facilities and controls used for, the manufacture, processing, and packaging of such drug shall also be included. Such requirements may also be met through the inclusion in the new drug application of properly authorized reference to a previous application or other Food and Drug Administration (FDA) file

---

*Reprinted with permission from *U.S. Pharmacist* (July 1982).

containing the relevant information.

Section 507 of the FDCA contains requirements for certification of antibiotics and products containing antibiotics. Regulations providing for such certifications include but are not limited to provisions for: standards of identity, potency, quality, and purity; tests and methods of assay to determine compliance; packaging and labeling; and the establishment and maintenance of records.

Drug master files should always be identified as such to distinguish them from master files pertaining to foods, medical devices, or cosmetics (Figure 1).

History

Drug master files came into being on March 10, 1943 with the submission of documentation for *Lethane* to support its application pursuant to Section 505(b) of the FDCA. Since the Rohm and Haas Company had no intention of expanding its activities into pharmaceutical marketing, the company established the file as a confidential reference to be used by its customers in support of applications filed with the FDA. Manufacturers of raw materials and basic components sometimes submit data to the FDA in the form of master files for the purpose of establishing the safety of ingredients that may be used in new drug products and of authorizing specified applicants to incorporate by reference such data in support of their applications (Figure 1).

The growth in the use of DMFs for filing supporting information is demonstrated by the assignment of their document control (file) number. For example, 23 years elapsed from the first filing in 1943 before file number 1,000 was assigned; six years later the number 2,000 was assigned. In July, 1977, the number 3,000 was assigned [8]. And, as of December 31st, 1981 there were 4,385 drug master files in the possession of FDA's Scientific Information Officer, Department of New Drug Evaluations, Bureau of Drugs [9].

Confidentiality

The confidentiality of data in a drug master file is determined in accordance with FDA's implementing regulations in 21 CFR 20 and the provisions of the Freedom of Information Act [10]. To a large extent, the disclosure of industry information and data under FDA's control is restricted by the exemptions in Subsection (e) of the FoIA. Of the nine exemptions, (2) through (7) are most pertinent to FDA, with exemptions (3) and (4) applicable to DMFs.

Exemption (3) exempts from disclosure matters which are specifically exempted from disclosure by statute. This exemption includes Section 301(j) of the FDCA, which prohibits the use by any person to his own advantage, or revealing, other than to the Secretary or employees of the Department (HHS) or to the courts when relevant in any judicial proceeding, any information acquired under the Authority of Sections 505, 506, 507, 704 or 706 concerning any method or process which as a trade secret is entitled to protection. Therefore, for example, any method or process which is a trade secret submitted in an NDA under Section 505 cannot be disclosed under FoIA. And, the same applies to a trade secret obtained during the course of an inspection under Section 704 of the FDCA.

Closely related to exemption (3) is exemption (4), which exempts from disclosure trade secrets and commercial information deemed to be privileged or confidential. Exemption (4) would include any trade secrets obtained by FDA through other means than those cited in Section 301(j). This exemption would assure the confidentiality of information obtained by the government through questionnaires or through materials submitted and disclosures made in proceedings.

Generally, the existence of a DMF is acknowledged by the FDA and the identity of the submitter and descriptive title of the DMF will be disclosed. However, data and information contained in the DMF have the same status that they would have in investigational drug

---

Department of Health, Education and Welfare
Food and Drug Administration
Bureau of Drugs
5600 Fishers Lane
Rockville, MD 20857

Attn: Mrs. Rita Pessoti
      Product Coordination Staff (HFD-105)

Re: Drug Master File #   for   Corporation.

Dear Mrs. Pessoti:

We hereby authorize the incorporation by reference of any
information contained in the above Drug Master File
(DMF #   ) by   Corporation, New Jersey
in support of the Supplement to the New Drug Application
for   and
NDA #   being filed by this firm whereby
Corporation will be listed as an alternative site of
manufacturing for   and

It is understood that the information contained in our Drug
Master File #   will be treated with confidentiality as
provided in Section 314.11 of the Code of Federal Regulations.

Would you please acknowledge receipt of this authorization.

Very truly yours,

FIGURE 1.

and pre-market approval applications, and are treated in accordance with the confidentiality provisions set forth in 21 CFR 314.14. One of the advantages of the DMF here is that its confidentiality is maintained, while the contents of an IND will be released under the FoIA if an IND is abandoned.

Once established, the DMF is reviewed by the Bureau of Drugs only when the holder of the DMF authorizes the FDA to refer to the DMF on behalf of an applicant/ sponsor. Acknowledgement of receipt of a DMF and an assignment of a document control number to it does not constitute any legal approval or disapproval of the document by the FDA. However, if the FDA reviewer of a formal NDA, IND, ANDA, or Supplemental Application, in referring to the DMF, finds the file deficient in the information he/she deems necessary to complete the review, he/she will cite these deficiencies and both the sponsor of the application and the holder of the DMF will be informed of said shortcomings. The holder of the DMF will have an opportunity to rectify it by amendment or file a completely new one to negate the cited deficiencies. Additional information may be added to a DMF at any time. In recognition of the FDA's agreement to maintain the DMF service, it is advantageous for a company with a DMF to annually inform the FDA, in writing, that the information in the DMF is current and correct. Any alteration, deletion, or addition should properly identify the DMF by number, and the page number to which it pertains. Any DMF not annually up-dated is placed in "dead storage" by the FDA, thus delaying retrieval for review purposes and thus approval of the application it purports to support.

Types of Drug Master Files

There are five types of drug master files [11]. Each can be identified by the information it contains:
• Type I pertains to facilities, personnel, and general operating procedures.
• Type II contains information about specific drug substances (other than antibiotics which should be submitted on Form 6), intermediates, or dosage forms.
• Type III includes detailed supporting information in regard to packaging materials, such as immediate containers, and their component parts.
• Type IV includes supporting information about colorants, flavors, essences, capsule shells, and other additives used in drug dosage forms.
• Type V pertains to results of animal and clinical studies.

It is essential that the DMF holder also include a statement that all materials and services performed are pursuant to the Good Manufacturing Practices (GMPs) [12] or Good Laboratory Practices (GLPs) [13] regulations. In addition, an Environmental Impact [14] statement should be added, if applicable.

Conclusion

A drug master file is used when the DMF holder wants to incorporate by reference the contents of the DMF to support a current application, or when a drug applicant/sponsor who is not the DMF holder receives proper authorization from the holder to incorporate by reference the contents of the holder's DMF to support an application, notice, or Form.

Because the information contained in a DMF may be used to support various submissions, a DMF must be well organized and coherent [15].

Drug master files are a convenient means of filing with FDA routine information concerning manufacturing, processing, pre-clinical and clinical information on drug substances and components, dosage form excipients, the dosage forms themselves, and packaging materials. Such filings permit the DMF holder to maintain confidentiality pursuant to regulations and statute, while affording the FDA opportunity to review such information in the context of the submissions it is intended to support.

References

1. P.L. 89-487.
2. Investigational new drug regulations are included in 21 CFR 312 as they pertain to Section 505(i) of the FDCA. These regulations also apply to insulin for investigational use. The investigational use of antibiotics is covered in 21 CFR 433.17 as they pertain to Section 507(d) of the FDCA.
3. New drug regulations are included in 21 CFR 314 as they pertain to Section 505(b) of the FDCA. Insulin is also subject to this section.
4. Abbreviated new drug regulations can be found in 21 CFR 314 as they pertain to Section 505(b) of the FDCA.
5. Requirements for application for *new* antibiotics or antibiotic-containing products (Form 5) are included in 21 CFR 431.17 as they pertain to Section 507 of the FDCA.
6. Requirements for application for antibiotics or antibiotic-containing products already covered by certification monographs (Form 6) are included in 21 CFR 431.1(b) as they pertain to Section 507 of the FDCA.
7. U.S.C. 301 et seq.
8. Zinsitz FA: Drug Master Files and Their Significance in the Support of Submissions to the FDA. Presented at the Spring Symposium of the Regulatory Affairs Professional Society, April 10, 1979.
9. Personal communication.
10. Pursuant to 21 CFR 20.61, a trade secret may consist of any formula, pattern, device, or compilation of information that is used in a person's business and gives the owner an opportunity to obtain an advantage over competitors who do not know or use it.
11. United States Department of Health, Education and Welfare, Public Health Service, Food and Drug Administration. Guidelines for Drug Master Files, HEW (FDA) 79-3072. Washington, DC, US Government Printing Office, November, 1978.
12. 21 CFR 210–211.
13. 21 CFR 3(e).
14. 21 CFR 25.
15. 44 FR 29161, May 18, 1979.

THE LEGAL ASPECTS OF THE MANUFACTURE, CERTIFICATION, AND MARKETING OF INSULIN PRODUCTS IN THE UNITED STATES*

Steven Strauss, Ph.D., R.Ph.

The discovery of insulin in December, 1921, is usually credited to two researchers at the University of Toronto (Canada), Frederick G. Banting and Charles H. Best, who extracted the active principle from animal pancreas and proved its therapeutic effects in diabetic dogs and humans [1].

Early insulin preparations, although life-saving, were relatively crude, contained unknown impurities, were inconvenient to use and required several injections daily. Recognizing the importance of a standardized potency if insulin were to be manufactured commercially, the University of Toronto patented the product and its process of manufacture. An Insulin Committee was created to administer a licensing program and to establish a laboratory to test each batch of a finished product. Through its licensing arrangements with manufacturers in the United States, the Committee was able to maintain standards by requiring that the manufacturers first assay and standardize each batch of insulin and insulin product, and then submit a sample to the laboratory in Toronto, which also assayed the finished product to confirm the reference standards of the Commitee prior to approval for marketing.

This protection ceased December 24, 1941, through the expiration of the patents. Continued surveillance was essential to assure that each dose of insulin administered to a diabetic was of uniform potency. A product that was either subpotent or too strong could have led to serious immunological consequences for diabetics dependent on a specific titrated dose of insulin. Because of the growing concern with this problem in the United States, Congress enacted the Insulin Amendment [2] to the Federal Food, Drug and Cosmetic Act (FDCA) [3] on December 22nd, 1941 (just two days before the expiration of the patents) [4]. The Amendment categorized insulin as a drug and decreed that every batch of insulin and products composed wholly or partly of insulin manufactured in or imported into the United States must be certified as meeting standards of purity, quality, strength, and identity in accordance with regulations promulgated by the Food and Drug Administration (FDA) in order to ensure safety and efficacy of use. It is interesting to note that this safety and efficacy factor written into the Amendment predates the 1962 Kefauver-Harris Amendments to the FDCA.

The precedent for certification was established with the provisions of the FDCA prohibiting the use of coal-tar colors in foods, drugs, and cosmetics unless such colors were from batches previously certified by the FDA as harmless and suitable for such use [5].

Five American companies (Burroughs Wellcome, Eli Lilly and Company, Merck Sharp & Dohme, E.R. Squibb & Sons, and Winthrop-Stearns) marketed insulin preparations in the United States until the latter part of the 1940s and the early part of the 1950s. Today, Lilly, Squibb, Nordisk, and Novo Laboratories are the only ones marketing insulin products in the United States. (The last two named are subsidiaries of Danish companies.)

Definition

The term "insulin," as defined in the *Code of Federal Regulations* *(CFR)*, means the "active principle of pancreas which affects the metabolism of carbohydrate in the animal body and which is of value in the treatment of diabetes mellitus" [6].

The United States Pharmacopeia defines insulin as a "protein, obtained from the pancreas of healthy bovine or porcine animals used for food by man, that affects the metabolism of glucose" [7].

Insulin must not be confused with the various products composed wholly or partly of insulin which are administered by injection, with or without other substances, such as protamine sulfate or zinc chloride.

There are seven types of insulin preparations listed in the *USP.* These differ mainly in the time their effect begins after injection, and in the length of time their action lasts. Not all companies market all of the *USP* preparations.

Unit of Insulin

Insulin is measured in units. A unit of insulin is always constant because it measures a specific amount of activity. The unit is the same for every insulin product. One unit of U-40 insulin is exactly the same and performs the same work as one unit of U-100 insulin or any other strength of insulin. The only difference among the three strengths available is the volume of liquid containing the insulin. For example, because U-100 is more concentrated than the U-40, a smaller volume of U-100 is needed to deliver the same dose.

One of the tasks confronting the researchers in the development of insulin was that of establishing a reference standard for determining its potency. The first standards were based on the hypoglycemic

Reprinted with permission from U.S. Pharmacist (May 1982).

effect of insulin on rabbits. However, with improved techniques of extraction and manufacture, the potency of the insulin solutions became greater, and this resulted in increasing variations in the value of the unit in terms of actual hypoglycemic activity. To insure uniformity, several insulin manufacturers and researchers joined efforts in preparing insulin in a dry, stable form. With this material, the unit was carefully determined with respect to the standard preparation and redefined in terms of exact weight [8].

The first reference standard for insulin contained 8 u/mg [9]. The present *USP* Standard is not less than 26.0 *USP* Insulin Units per mg, based on an absolute dry weight of insulin prepared from a crystalline composite sample [10].

Concentration of Insulin

The first commercially sold insulin product in the United States contained about 3 u/ml. As manufacturing technology improved and as the purity of insulin increased, the concentration of the marketed products progressively increased to 10, 20, 40, 80, and 500 u/ml, the latter three being the most often used.

In far too many instances, patients confused the quantity or concentration of insulin or the correctly calibrated insulin syringe to be used, and injected themselves with incorrect doses of the insulin product. In order to minimize the potential for patient dosage errors, the American Diabetes Association (ADA) in 1971 proposed that only one concentration of insulin product be marketed to diabetics in the United States. The proposal would leave U-100 insulin as the single available concentration (with the exception of the low-potency U-40 and the high-potency U-500). This was agreed upon by the FDA, ADA, the Juvenile Diabetes Foundation, and the manufacturers of insulin products, based on 1) the trend toward adoption of the metric system in the United States,

2) the desirability of reducing the volumes of the injectable, and 3) the availability of U-100 insulin syringes capable of delivering small doses of the new concentrated insulin.

The first U-100 insulin was marketed in early 1973 by Eli Lilly and Company. As of March 24, 1980, the FDA no longer accepted U-80 insulin preparations for certification [11]. However, U-80 products in the channel of distribution could be sold until their expiration dates.

The U-40 potency has been retained to satisfy the pediatric market and those diabetics who require small doses of insulin. This segment of the diabetic market accounts for approximately six percent of total insulin product sales, and the FDA is currently evaluating whether there is a continuing need for a low-strength insulin.

The use of the U-500 insulin is limited to insulin coma therapy and diabetic patients with marked insulin resistance whose daily requirements exceed 200 units. Lilly is the only company which markets the U-500 potency product in the United States.

Certification

The first certificate for insulin was issued in February, 1942, to Eli Lilly and Company.

A drug composed partly or wholly of insulin is misbranded unless it is from a batch that has been certified in accordance with Section 506(a) of the Federal Food, Drug, and Cosmetic Act [12].

Regulations providing for such certification shall contain provisions as are necessary to carry out the purposes of Section 506, including provisions prescribing:

a) Standards of identity, strength, quality, and purity;

b) Tests and methods of assay to determine compliance with such standards;

c) Effective periods for certificates, and other conditions under which they shall cease to be effective as to certified batches;

d) Administration and procedure;

e) Such fees, specified in such regulations, as are necessary to provide, equip, and maintain an adequate certification service [13].

Such regulations shall prescribe no standard of identity or of strength, quality, or purity for any drug different from the standards set forth for such drug in the official compendium.

When the FDA believes that the tests and methods of assay pursuant to regulations under Section 506(b) have not been prescribed in or differ from those in the official compendium, it will serve notice on the *USP.* If the *USP* fails within a reasonable period of time to mandate satisfactory tests and methods of assay, the FDA will promulgate regulations to that effect in accordance with Section 501(b) of the FDCA.

The formal rulemaking provisions of the FDCA provide for hearings prior to the issuance, amendment, or repeal of certain regulations [14], and for judicial review of any order issued by the FDA [15], as applicable to the portion of the regulations prescribing tests and methods of assay which differ from those in the compendium [16].

Section 502(k) of the FDCA implements the basic provisions for the certification of insulin and products composed wholly or partly of insulin so that compliance with Section 506 can be enforced under the civil and criminal provisions of the FDCA [17].

To date, the *USP* has not established standards for the new purified insulins. It is worthy of note that the FDA has approved the marketing of these products not through the certification process that the Congress established, but through the New Drug Application (NDA) procedures.

The initial request for certification must be accompanied or preceded by a full statement of the facilities and controls used to maintain the identity, strength, quality, and purity of each batch of the drug. Also required is a description of the equipment, methods, and processes used in diluting master lots, and in maintaining the identity, strength, quality, and purity of master lots and their dilutions. In addition, tests and assays made on master lots, and their dilutions and batches, and the ingredients used, must be described [18].

The party requesting initial certification of a batch, must submit representative samples for which there are specific regulatory requirements [19].

If the FDA's Certification Services Branch, Bureau of Drugs, finds that the required information contains no untrue statements and that the submitted batch conforms to standards, regulations and the FDCA, a certificate will be issued attesting to its safety and effectiveness.

A person to whom a certificate is issued must maintain records pertaining to shipments for two years as set forth in the regulations [20].

A certificate will not be granted or will be suspended if fraud, misrepresentation, or concealment of facts, or falsified records have been submitted in connection with the certification process [21].

The schedule of fees for assaying, testing, and certifying individual batches, and methods of payment of fees are set forth in the regulations. These fees are borne entirely by the manufacturers of insulin and insulin products [22].

In a recent memorandum to the Federal Accounting Office, the FDA reiterated that it will continue to test and certify insulin and insulin products batch by batch until new technologies for insulin production have been proven to meet applicable standards consistently [23].

Packaging

Specific requirements for insulin state that each batch of drug shall be packaged in immediate containers of colorless transparent glass. Such containers must be closed with a substance through which successive doses may be withdrawn by hypodermic needle without removing the closure or destroying its effectiveness. In addition, the containers and closures shall be sterile at the time the containers are filled and closed.

The composition of the containers and closures must be such that neither will cause any change in the strength, quality, or purity of the insulin products. Any change beyond the prescribed limits is subject to a finding of adulteration [24].

Other specific requirements pertain to the shapes of the containers. All must be cylindrical. In addition, isophane insulin preparations containing less than 100 u/ml must be marketed in rounded square containers, while the zinc insulin products (except protamine zinc) containing less than 100 u/ml must be contained in hexagonal shaped containers [25].

Furthermore, containers holding the U-40 and U-100 insulin products must have a capacity of no less than 10 ml, and the container for the U-500 must not contain less than 20 ml of the product [26]. An insulin product is misbranded if it is packaged in a container that is made or filled in a misleading manner [27].

The pharmacist must dispense (sell) insulin products in unopened, original containers. The U-40 and U-100 preparations are marketed over-the-counter, while the U-500 product requires a prescription prior to sale in the United States [28].

Labeling

The regulations require that the batch mark, the potency of the drug in terms of *USP* Insulin Units per milliliter, a "shake well" legend, and the expiration date, appear on the outside wrapper or container *and* the immediate container of a retail package of a certified batch of insulin preparation [29].

The regulations do not include expiration dates for specific types of insulins; the USP does. For example, all insulin products have an expiration date of 24 months [30].

In addition to the preceding, the legend "Keep in a cold place, avoid freezing" must appear on the outside container or wrapper of the retail package [31].

Since U-500 insulin injection requires a prescription prior to dispensing, the *"Caution: Federal law prohibits dispensing without a prescription"* statement must appear on the outside wrapper or container and the label [32]. The words "Warning—High potency—Not for ordinary use" must also be included [33]. Even though the U-500 requires a prescription, *all* insulin preparations should be used pursuant to the directions of a physician.

Furthermore, the labeling of each product must contain: specific instructions to the patient on how to withdraw insulin from the vial; an explanation of hypoglycemia; a statement explaining the meaning of the volume markings on the hypodermic syringe used to withdraw insulin from the vial; an explanation of the different insulin products and their effectiveness; an explanation of the different insulin products local reactions; cautionary statements on when not to use an insulin product; and, warning statements regarding the mixing of the different insulin injections. The species of animal(s) from which the insulin was obtained must also be indicated on the label and on the package.

Insulin preparations are misbranded if their labeling is false or misleading, if they are not prominently labeled with the required warnings and other necessary information enumerated above or if they do not comply with any applicable packaging and labeling regulations or special standards.

Legal actions that may be taken when insulin products are found to be adulterated or misbranded include seizure by order of a federal court [34], injunctions [35], or prosecution of the manufacturer or distributor.

Misleading representations may include not only implied or stated inaccuracies about the product itself but also failure to state with sufficient prominence any required information concerning the nature of the insulin preparation.

Further, the FDA has the authority to require that warning statements appear on the immediate label of a product rather than on the product's labeling or packaging [36].

Insulin preparations are exempt from the Fair Packaging and Labeling Act [37].

Packaging Colors [38]

Prior to the current regulations, as an added precaution against inadvertent use of the incorrect potency and type of insulin injection, the outside wrapper or container, and the label on the immediate container of the U-40, U-80, and U-500 preparations were color coded to identify the potency and the type of insulin. This color coding has been retained for the U-40 and U-500 insulins. For example, all U-40 products have red in their package design.

Special color coding was not invoked for the U-100 potency because colors are not as important as is the potency and the type of insulin in identifying the correct product to be used. Further, the elimination of colors also serves to wean the diabetic patient from reliance on colors to relying more on reading the label.

Different companies are using different colored closures for their products. However, this is not a legal requirement and is merely for aesthetic purposes.

References

1. Larner J, Haynes RC Jr: Insulin and oral hypoglycemic drugs; glucagon. in Goodman LS, Gilman A (Ed.): The Pharmacological Basis of Therapeutics 5th Ed., New York, NY. Macmillan Publishing Company, Inc. 1975, pp. 1507–1508.
2. Public Law 77-366.
3. 21 U.S.C. 301 et seq.
4. Hecht A: Insulin standards: Precision with a purpose. FDA Consumer 11(3):10, 1977.
5. Public Law 76-61.
6. 21 CFR 429.3(g).
7. United States Pharmacopeia 20th Revision. Rockville MD, United States Pharmacopeial Convention, Inc., 1980, p. 401.
8. Waife SO (Ed.): Diabetes Mellitus 7th Ed., Indianapolis IN, Eli Lilly and Company, 1973, p 44.
9. Ibid.
10. United States Pharmacopeia 20th Revision, Op. Cit. p 401.
11. 44 FR 55169, September 25, 1979.
12. 21 U.S.C. 356(a); FDCA Section 506(a).
13. 21 U.S.C. 356(b): FDCA Section 506(b).
14. 21 U.S.C. 371(e); FDCA Section 701(e).
15. 21 U.S.C. 371(f); FDCA Section 701(f).
16. 21 U.S.C. 356(c); FDCA Section 506(c).
17. 21 U.S.C. 352(k); FDCA Section 502(k).
18. 21 CFR 429.40(b).
19. 21 CFR 429.40(d).
20. 21 CFR 429.60.
21. 21 CFR 429.47.
22. 21 CFR 429.55.
23. F-D-C Reports, "The Pink Sheet," December 21, 1981, p. 14.
24. 21 U.S.C. 351(a) (3); FDCA Section 501(a)(3).
25. 21 CFR 429.10.
26. United States Pharmacopeia 20th Revision. Op. Cit. p 401.
27. 21 U.S.C. 352(i)(1); FDCA Section 502(i)(1).
28. 21 CFR 429.11(h)(1).
29. 21 CFR 429.11(a) (1) (2) (3).
30. United States Pharmacopeia 20th Revision, Op. Cit. pp 401–405.
31. 21 CFR 429.11(b).
32. 21 CFR 429.11(h)(1).
33. 21 CFR 429.11(h)(2).
34. 21 U.S.C. 334; FDCA Section 304.
35. 21 U.S.C. 332; FDCA Section 302.
36. Cosmetic, Toiletry and Fragrance Association v. Schmidt, (DC D.C. 1976) 409 F. Supp 57.
37. 15 U.S.C. 1451–1461; Public Law 89-755.
38. 21 CFR 429.12.

- The certification requirements for insulin and insulin products pursuant to the FDCA have been repealed.
- Insulin products are the only injectables sold in the United States that do not require a prescription.
- Humalog™ is the only insulin product that requires a prescription.

A LONG REACH BACK TO ASSURE DRUG QUALITY*
Annabel Hecht

Say "DESI" to most consumers and you'll likely be greeted with blank stares. What they don't real-

*Reprinted with permission from the FDA Consumer (January 1985).

ize is that these four letters have had a major impact on the quality of the medicines they take. The acronym stands for Drug Efficacy Study Implementation, an FDA program considered the most far-reaching evaluation of the effectiveness of prescription drugs in the history of drug relation worldwide.

Virtually finished in September 1984, the multi-million-dollar project involved the review of more than 3,400 prescription drugs with more than 16,000 therapeutic claims. The end result:

• 1,099 drugs were found to be ineffective and were taken off the market.

• 2,302 were found effective, with any questionable claims removed from the label.

• About 7,000 drugs identical or similar to the drugs under review were relabeled or withdrawn from the market.

The DESI project was mandated by the 1962 Kefauver-Harris Amendments to the Food, Drug, and Cosmetic Act, which required manufacturers to prove that their products were effective—that is, that the drugs did what they were supposed to do. (Proof of safety had been required since 1938.) The new amendments were to be applied to all new drugs and, retrospectively, to those approved by FDA in the years between 1938 and 1962.

Such a retrospective review was a huge order, not only because of the sheer numbers—a total of 3,443 prescription and 532 nonprescription drug products—but also because most of these drugs had several intended uses. In fact, on the average, the manufacturers claimed their products could be used for as many as five conditions. Each claim had to be evaluated. In addition, for every drug initially sold between 1938 and 1962 with FDA approval, five others were on the market without approval. Many were copies of or closely related to previously approved drugs. Others were combinations of approved ingredients. Altogether, the study covered 80 percent of the prescription drugs sold in the United States.

Because of limited resources, FDA asked the National Academy of Sciences/National Research Council (NAS/NRC) to conduct the first phase of the review. The study was conducted by 30 panels, each composed of six medical experts. Each panel was assigned to a different category of drugs—antibiotics, heart drugs and so forth.

The NAS/NRC panels evaluated evidence of effectiveness from material submitted by the manufacturers, information in FDA's files, and a review of medical literature. Each claimed use for each drug was rated as:

• *Effective*—The evidence was adequate to justify the claim.

• *Probably effective*—More evidence was needed to support the claim, or some clarification or change in the labeling was needed.

• *Possibly effective*—The claim needed substantial research to provide evidence of effectiveness.

• *Ineffective*—There was no scientific evidence to support the claim.

• *Ineffective as a fixed combination*—Although each of the ingredients in a combination might be effective, combining them did not make the drug any more useful than if one or more were used separately.

The initial phase of the review began in 1966. By late 1967 the NAS/NRC reports started coming in, and by mid-1969 all were completed. The panels found that the drugs could not be considered effective for about 60 percent of the claimed uses made by the manufacturers, although 60 percent of the products they reviewed had at least one effective use. Only 12 percent of all products reviewed were effective for all of the claimed uses.

The discovery that only 25 percent of the nonprescription drugs were effective led to the FDA's massive review of all nonprescription, or over-the-counter, drugs, which started in 1972 and is still going on.

FDA's implementation of the panels' findings—the DESI part of the evaluation—began in 1968. The NAS/NRC recommendations were published in the *Federal Register* between 1968 and 1974. Manufacturers were given time to submit further data on disputed claims. Manufacturers also had the opportunity for a hearing before an administrative law judge.

Despite hearings and several protracted legal challenges, including several cases ultimately reviewed by the Supreme Court, the review process was completed on Sept. 17, 1984, for all but 37 of the DESI drugs. Still in the pipeline are five drugs designated as medically necessary. Because of a compelling justification of the medical need for these drugs, they have been allowed to remain on the market pending the completion of scientific studies to determine their effectiveness. Complicating the analysis of these studies is the fact that some deal with combination products. Nevertheless, final action is expected on these drugs in early 1985.

In addition, FDA announced its intention to remove 32 other products from the market and gave manufacturers the opportunity to request a hearing. In all cases, the manufacturers of the 32 DESI drugs and other, related drugs requested a hearing. Most of these products are combination drugs in which one or two ingredients are considered effective, but the remainder do not contribute to the desired effect.

FOOD, DRUG AND COSMETIC ACT
Summary of Important Points

It is designed to protect public health by requiring that:
(1) Only safe, effective, and properly labeled drugs be introduced into interstate commerce
(2) The food and cosmetic preparations subject to the Act be safe and properly labeled
(3) Medical devices be safe and effective and conform to government standards or, before marketing, have government approval
(4) The manufacturing, processing, packaging, and holding of drugs comply with the Current Good Manufacturing Practices (CGMP), set by the Federal Food and Drug Administration (FDA)
(5) The FDA enforce it
(6) Over-the-counter [OTC] (nonprescription) drugs be labeled for safe use by consumers in self-medication
(7) Prescription or "legend" drugs be dispensed to an individual only pursuant to a prescription or administered directly by the physician or other prescriber
(8) Drug prescriptions be refilled only as authorized by a physician or other prescriber
(9) Specific labeling be used for both prescription and nonprescription drugs
(10) Dispensing a drug for distribution in violation of the Act's labeling requirements is "misbranding" the drug.
(11) Drugs containing filthy, putrid, and decomposed substances and drugs packed and held under unsanitary conditions be deemed "adulterated"
(12) Seizures of misbranded or adulterated drugs be made by the FDA
(13) A first offense committed under the Act is a misdemeanor unless it is committed with the intention to defraud or mislead. A second offense carries a felony penalty.
(14) Interpretations of the Act show that lack of knowledge or lack of criminal intent will not excuse a violation.
(15) An employer or other responsible person to be prosecuted for violations of the Act committed by an employee
(16) FDA have broad inspection powers over factories, warehouses, and establishments where drugs, food, medical devices, and cosmetics are made or processed
(17) The FDA be authorized to perform limited inspection of pharmacies in certain circumstances
(18) Manufacturers or processors of drugs must register with the FDA

Adulteration

An adulteration occurs when something affects the quality or purity of the product; i.e., something is actually wrong with the product or that a situation exists where there is a strong likelihood that the quality or purity could be affected.
Section 501 of the Federal Food Drug and Cosmetic Act (the Act) defines adulteration to include situations where
• The product contains filthy, putrid, or decomposed substances.
• The product is prepared or packaged under unsanitary conditions.
• The product was manufactured in a manner inconsistent with good manufacturing practices.
• The product is a compendial (USP/NF) product and does not meet compendial standards.
• The product differs in strength, quality, or purity from that represented.

Misbranding

A misbranding is a violation of Section 502 of the Act that does not affect the integrity of the product itself—that is the defect is not in the product but is due to some other factor. Misbrandings include situations where
• The label is false or misleading in any way.
• The label fails to contain the required information.
• The label information is incorrect.
• The label fails to include adequate directions for use.
• The product is packaged improperly.
• The accompanying labeling or advertising is false and/or misleading.
• The product was produced in an unregistered establishment.
• The product is not packaged in accord with the Poison Prevention Packaging Act.
• The packaging is false or misleading.
• The label lacks the necessary conspicuousness for required information.
• The product is represented as a compendial product but is not packaged and labeled in accord with compendial standards.

QUESTIONS: CHAPTER 9

1. A drug may be considered *new* if changes occur in which of the following?
    a. Indication for use
    b. Dosage form
    c. Duration of action
    d. Route of administration
    e. All of the above

2. Which of the following amendments to the FD&C Act required that a drug be effective as well as safe before it could be marketed in the U.S.A.?
    a. Durham-Humphrey
    b. Kefauver-Harris
    c. Proxmire Amendment of 1976
    d. DACA of 1970
    e. Drug Price Competition and Patent Term Restoration Act (DPCPTRA)

3. Pursuant to the FD&C Act, for which of the following reasons is a drug considered adulterated?
    a. Methods used in the manufacture do not conform to GMPs
    b. Does not meet compendial standards
    c. Is stored under unsanitary conditions
    d. Contains any filthy or putrid substance
    e. All of the above

4. The reporting to FDA of any developments that may affect the safety and effectiveness of a drug product is known as:
    a. Medical Device Reporting Rule
    b. Good Manufacturing Practices Reports
    c. Adverse Reaction Reports
    d. Drug Experience Reports
    e. Drug Products Problem Reporting Program

5. Which amendments to the Federal Food, Drug, and Cosmetic Act established the legal difference between prescription and nonprescription drugs?
    a. Kefauver-Harris
    b. Wheeler-Lea
    c. Harrison-Ford
    d. Carter-Mondale
    e. Durham-Humphrey

6. Which of the following is a component of the definition for *drug*?
    a. Soap
    b. Articles that are manufactured, packed, and distributed for the purpose of inducing a cure in man or animals
    c. Likely to be destructive to adult human life in quantities of 60 grains or less
    d. Articles intended for use in the diagnosis, cure, mitigation, treatment, or prevention of disease in man or animals
    e. Articles intended to be rubbed, poured, sprinkled, sprayed on, introduced into, or otherwise applied to the human body or any part thereof for cleansing, beautifying, promoting attractiveness, or altering the appearance of

7. Which of the following is an example of a drug?

    a. Mouthwash

    b. Toothpaste

    c. Deodorant

    d. Antiperspirant

    e. Vaginal douche

8. The advertising of OTC drug products is regulated by the:

    a. FDA

    b. HHS

    c. FTC

    d. NDA

    e. USP

9. Which of the following amendments to the Federal Food, Drug, and Cosmetic Act established the Rx and OTC categories of drugs?

    a. Kefauver-Harris

    b. Truman-Eisenhower

    c. Wheeler-Lea

    d. Durham-Humphrey

    e. Delaney-Humphrey

10. The federal agency having jurisdiction over the sale of all OTC medications on the basis of safety, effectiveness, and proper labeling is:

    a. DESI

    b. FTC

    c. HHS

    d. DEA

    e. FDA

11. The federal government has the authority to oversee the development of new drugs in the United States based on the:

    a. Federal Food, Drug, and Cosmetic Act

    b. Kefauver-Harris Amendments

    c. Waxman-Hatch Amendments

    d. The Pure Food and Drugs Act

    e. Harrison-Ford Amendments

12. The advertising of prescription drugs is regulated by the:

    a. FDA

    b. HHS

    c. FTC

    d. DHEW

    e. DEA

13. Certain types of prescription drug advertising are exempt by the FDA from fully disclosing prescribing information about the advertised Rx drug product. Such ads are referred to as:

    a. Abridged ads

    b. Abstracts

    c. Abbreviated ads

    d. Reminder ads

    e. Partial ads

14. A pharmaceutical firm that does not have an IND filed for a new chemical entity may not:

   a. Study the toxicology of the new drug in monkeys.
   b. Evaluate the safety of low doses in normal males.
   c. Develop a pharmaceutical dosage form.
   d. Determine if the drug is mutagenic.

15. The initial filing of an IND would generally not contain:

   a. Subacute toxicity information
   b. A Phase III clinical protocol
   c. Information on the synthesis of the new drug substance
   d. Data on the stability of the dosage form

16. An abbreviated new drug application (ANDA) must contain:

   a. Statistically valid clinical data to support safety and efficacy
   b. A carcinogenicity study conducted in the rat
   c. Validated analytical methodology to analyze the drug in the dosage form
   d. At least two LD_{50} studies

17. A new drug application will not contain:

   a. A proposed package insert
   b. Data from the Phase II clinical program
   c. U.S. marketing data on the drug
   d. Results of pharmacological investigations

18. When a drug's patent expires:

   a. The innovator company must give permission to a generic drug company to file an ANDA
   b. The innovator company may petition the patent office for an extension of the expiration date of the patent
   c. FDA notifies all registered generic drug manufacturers
   d. A generic drug manufacturer may file an abbreviated new drug application

19. An ANDA need not contain:

   a. The proposed labeling
   b. A proposed expiration date for the product
   c. The name of the supplier of the active drug substance
   d. A study to determine effects of the drug on the cardiovascular system

20. Which statement is false?

   a. An NDA implies that a drug product is safe and effective.
   b. An NDA is necessary for marketing a drug product in the United States.
   c. Generic drug products require FDA approval prior to marketing in the U.S.
   d. Generic drug products must have exactly the same formulation as the innovator drug product.

21. A *paper* NDA:

   a. Allows generic manufacturers to bypass the Kefauver-Harris Amendments
   b. Eliminates the need for manufacturing and controls data
   c. Relies heavily on the scientific literature to support safety and efficacy of a drug
   d. Is now illegal

22. A typical bioequivalency study does not evaluate:

    a. The maximum plasma concentration

    b. The time to achieve the maximum plasma concentration

    c. The extent of absorption of a drug

    d. The rate of dissolution of a drug

23. The 75/25 guideline means:

    a. 75 of every 100 patients demonstrate a bioequivalency.

    b. A generic drug product is 75 percent as good as the innovator drug.

    c. 75 percent of subjects show bioequivalency to within 25 percent of the innovator's drug product.

    d. For every 75 mg of drug administered, 25 mg need not be metabolized.

24. Which of the following best describes postmarketing surveillance and perspective studies of prescription drugs in the United States?

    a. Phase I

    b. Phase II

    c. Phase III

    d. Phase IV

    e. Postmarketing NDA phase

25. The greatest number of patients are treated in:

    a. Phase I

    b. Phase II

    c. Phase III

    d. Bioequivalency studies

26. Preclinical testing does not imply:

    a. Acute toxicology evaluations

    b. Subacute toxicology evaluations

    c. Fertility and reproductive testing

    d. Bioequivalency testing

27. A Phase II study:

    a. May only be conducted in males

    b. Is not concerned with efficacy, but only with safety

    c. Is conducted in patients with the disease intended to be treated

    d. Is only required for parenterally-administered drug products

28. Which of the following best describes expanded controlled and uncontrolled large-scale clinical studies of prescription drugs in patients in the United States?

    a. Phase I

    b. Phase II

    c. Phase III

    d. Phase IV

    e. Postmarketing NDA phase

29. The term that best describes the rate *and* extent of absorption of a drug is:

    a. Bioequivalence

    b. Area under the curve

    c. Clinical equivalence

    d. Bioavailability

    e. Therapeutic equivalence

30. A substance that does not achieve any of its intended purposes by being metabolized or by chemical action in or on the body is a:

    a. Food
    b. Biologic
    c. Cosmetic
    d. Drug
    e. Medical device

31. The Drug Price Competition and Patent Term Restoration Act is also known as the:

    a. Wiley Act
    b. Sherley Amendment
    c. Durham-Humphrey Amendments
    d. Waxman-Hatch Amendments
    e. Copeland Amendment

32. A published clinical/medical study submitted to the FDA as the main supporting documentation for the safety and effectiveness of a drug is known as a(n):

    a. NDA
    b. ANDA
    c. IND
    d. GMP
    e. Paper NDA

33. Applications for which the clinical investigations relied upon by the applicant to show safety and efficacy were not conducted by or for the applicant, and for which the applicant has not obtained a right of reference or use from the person who conducted the studies or for whom the studies were conducted are referred to as:

    a. NDAs
    b. ANDAs
    c. INDs
    d. Paper NDAs
    e. GMPAs

34. Expanded clinical studies of a drug in multiple locations used to validate safety and efficacy in large patient populations and to explore such issues as drug interactions are referred to as _____ studies:

    a. Phase I
    b. Phase II
    c. Phase III
    d. Phase IV

35. The rigidly controlled clinical trials that explore the safety and efficacy of a drug are referred to as _____ studies:

    a. Phase I
    b. Phase II
    c. Phase III
    d. Phase IV

36. A double blind study refers to one in which:

    a. Only the physician/investigator knows what is being administered.
    b. The patient nor the physician/investigator knows what is being administered.
    c. The patient is blind in each eye and knows what is being administered.
    d. The physician/investigator does not know what is being administered.
    e. No one knows what is being administered to the patient in the study.

37. The term that best describes the measure of the extent of absorption of a drug is:

    a. Bioequivalence

    b. Area under the curve (AUC)

    c. Clinical equivalence

    d. Bioavailability

    e. Therapeutic equivalence

38. The standards of ethics that guide physicians in biomedical research involving human subjects and that have been accepted worldwide are referred to as the:

    a. Declaration of Independence

    b. Treaty of Versailles

    c. Agreement of Chateaubriand

    d. Declaration of Helsinki

    e. Brussels Accords

39. Studies which provide the primary documentation of the safety and efficacy of the drug and which will be used to describe the conditions of safety and efficacy for proposed labeling may be referred to as:

    a. Equivalence

    b. Discovery

    c. Development

    d. Validation

    e. Coordinating studies

40. The unanimous U.S. Supreme Court decision which held that generic drugs cannot be sold in the United States without FDA approval, even though their active ingredients are the same as found in drug products which have been approved by FDA, may be referred to as:

    a. *U.S. v. Lannett*

    b. *U.S. v. Premo*

    c. *U.S. v. Generix*

    d. *U.S. v. Pharmadyne*

    e. *U.S. v. Hohensee*

41. The landmark legal decision which best demonstrates that individuals with responsible positions within, say, a multinational pharmaceutical manufacturing corporation may be held accountable for violations of the FD&C Act is known by its legal citation as:

    a. *United States v. Hohensee*

    b. *United States v. Park*

    c. *United States v. Dotterweich*

    d. *United States v. Wiley*

    e. *Alberty v. United States*

42. The amendments to the FD&C Act that granted authority to the FDA to issue regulations with the force and effect of law are known by the name of:

    a. Kefauver-Harris

    b. Durham-Humphrey

    c. Truman-Eisenhower

    d. Wheeler-Lea

    e. Delaney

43. The original 1938 Federal Food, Drug, and Cosmetic Act:

    a. May also be referred to as the Wiley Act

    b. For the first time included misbranding and adulteration provisions for drugs

    c. Provided new requirements for the manufacture and marketing of medical devices

    d. Discontinued the authorization provision dealing with factory inspections

    e. Established the Food and Drug Administration as a distinct agency of the federal government

44. The *established* name of a drug is its:

    a. Brand name

    b. Trademark name

    c. Proprietary name

    d. Generic name

    e. International chemical name by which it is recognized throughout the world

45. The section of the FD&C Act which pertains to the FDA's authority to enter and inspect a pharmacuetical manufacturing facility is:

    a. Section 303

    b. Section 305

    c. Section 505

    d. Section 510

    e. Section 704

46. A *notice of adverse finding letter* to a pharmaceutical manufacturer generally requests the firm to respond to FDA within:

    a. 7 working days

    b. 10 days

    c. 30 calendar days

    d. 3 months

    e. 60 days

47. Section 305 of the Federal Food, Drug, and Cosmetic Act provides for:

    a. Seizure

    b. Injunction

    c. Seizure and injunction

    d. Prosecution

    e. Informal hearings in cases of violation of the act

48. The reference source which identifies current and retrospective names of drugs marketed in the United States is the:

    a. Federal Food, Drug and Cosmetic Act

    b. *The United States Dispensatory*

    c. *Martindale's Extra Pharmacopoeia*

    d. *USAN and the USP Dictionary of Drug Names*

    e. *The American Heritage Dictionary of Drug Names*

49. A *regulatory letter* from the FDA to a manufacturer of a drug generally requests that the firm respond within:

    a. 7 working days

    b. 10 days

    c. 30 calendar days

    d. One month

    e. 60 days

50. The Waxman-Hatch Amendments to the Federal Food, Drug, and Cosmetic Act:

    a. Permits the marketing of inferior drug products

    b. Discourages new drug research in the United States

    c. Permits marketing of off-patent post-1962 drugs in the United States

    d. Decreases the role of FDA in the new drug approval process

51. The Waxman-Hatch Amendments to the FD&C Act:

    a. Includes patent extension for innovator drug companies

    b. Eliminates the safety and efficacy requirements for ANDAs

    c. Excludes phenothiazines from ANDA approval if they do not meet the 75/25 rule

    d. Makes the Kefauver-Harris Amendments null and void

52. Batch certification of human antibiotics was granted to the FDA as a result of the _____ Amendments to the FD&C Act:

    a. Kefauver-Harris

    b. Waxman-Hatch

    c. Durham-Humphrey

    d. Wheeler-Lea

    e. Delaney

53. Which of the following must be tested batch-by-batch prior to certification by the FDA?

    a. Insulin, insulin products

    b. Insulin, insulin products, human antibiotics

    c. Insulin, insulin products, human antibiotics, animal antibiotics

    d. Insulin, human antibiotics, veterinary antibiotics

    e. Insulin, insulin products, veterinary antibiotics

54. The organization responsible for setting standards for human antibiotics is:

    a. FTC

    b. FDA

    c. USP

    d. DEA

    e. DHA

55. Pursuant to Section 508 of the FD&C Act, the person who is authorized to designate an official name for any drug in the United States is the:

    a. Commissioner of FDA

    b. Secretary of HHS

    c. Executive secretary of the United States Pharmacopoeial Convention, Inc.

    d. Either a. or b.

56. A drug with a potential therapeutic value and a limited market which discourages private investment in its research and development, testing, and marketing is known as a(n):

    a. New drug

    b. Generic drug

    c. Me-too product

    d. Orphan drug

    e. Limited market product

57. Which one of the following requires that the FDA be provided a current list of drugs marketed by a particular company in the United States?

    a. Federal Drug Regulatory Act of 1972

    b. CGMP Act

    c. Drug Listing Act of 1972

    d. Annual Drug Reporting Program

    e. Annual Drug Marketing Act of 1970

58. An innovator drug manufacturer in the United States:

    a. Need not file an ANDA

    b. May spend $60 million to develop a new drug

    c. Follows different Good Manufacturing Practice regulations (GMPs) than a manufacturer of generic drugs

    d. Need not comply with the Waxman-Hatch Amendments to the FD&C Act

59. A confidential reference that contains detailed information about a specific pharmaceutical manufacturing facility, process, article, or ingredient used in the manufacture of a substance which is the subject of an IND may be referred to as a:

    a. Confidential Manufacturing Protocol

    b. Company Formulary

    c. New Drug Application

    d. Good Manufacturing Practices

    e. Drug Master File

60. A single standard system which identifies each drug product and which promotes economy and efficiency in drug distribution is known by which one of the following initials?

    a. DRLS

    b. FDCA

    c. UPC

    d. NBC

    e. NDC

CHAPTER 10

National Drug Code

THE NATIONAL DRUG CODE*

David C. Oppenheimer, R.Ph.

The last two decades witnessed the tremendous growth of government-sponsored and privately insured medical insurance programs which include payment for health related items, primarily prescription drugs. The proliferation of these programs has created the need for an effective automated system to deal with drug products through their normal manufacturer-through-consumer cycle. In the traditional cycle, payment is made by the patient. However, under third-party programs, payment is a subsequent and final step, usually occurring well after the prescription product has been consumed. Hence, paper work must be generated by the dispensing pharmacist to the insurer, or third-party payer, who will eventually reimburse the pharmacist. To provide efficiency and accuracy, a single standard coding system to identify each drug product was required. From this basic need was born the National Drug Code (NDC). This article will describe the NDC's development and current use, and, more importantly, will relate observations and perceptions of the NDC system by those involved with it: community

*Reprinted with permission from *U.S. Pharmacist* (May 1981).

pharmacists, hospital pharmacists, and third-party insurers.

The National Drug Code

By 1969, the then Department of Health, Education, and Welfare's (DHEW) expanding health care programs anticipated federal coverage of out-patient prescriptions as part of a National Health Insurance (NHI) scheme. Congress, however, has never passed NHI; out-patient prescription reimbursement is currently included in the majority of the states' medicaid programs.

Regardless of whether federal or state money reimbursed these prescription costs, identifying the individual drugs was a major administrative challenge. The Secretary of DHEW's Task Force Committee on Nomenclature and Coding[1] developed a nine-character NDC, which was announced by the Secretary who said that, "the National Drug Code will provide the needed common language in which to communicate rapidly and accurately essential information

[1]This *ad hoc* committee included significant involvement from industry and government, viz., the Pharmaceutical Manufacturers Association, National Pharmaceutical Council, National Wholesale Druggists Association, American Society of Hospital Pharmacists, National Drug Trade Council, Social Security Administration, and the FDA [1].

about drugs. It will play a significant role not only in promoting economy and efficiency in drug distribution but in improving the quality of health care" [2]. DHEW delegated to the Food and Drug Administration (FDA) the task of developing and operating the NDC, since the FDA's responsibilities include the collection, processing, and regulation of information concerning new drug products vis-a-vis its role in the protection of the consumer's health.

Thus, the then FDA Commissioner published the Notice in the *Federal Register* concerning the NDC system, requesting that drug firms apply for labeler identity code designations [3], this being the first part of the NDC. This Notice stated that the NDC would provide an identification system in computer language to permit automated processing of drug data by government agencies, drug manufacturers and distributors, hospitals, and insurance companies. The original NDC was nine-character numeric or alpha-numeric, made up of three segments, in a 3-4-2 configuration: the first three characters were the labeler identity code (now simply "labeler code"), assigned by the FDA to each manufacturer. The next four characters, the second segment, identified the drug product itself, including its strength and dosage form. The remaining two characters (the third segment) identified the trade package, e.g., 50's, 100's, 100 ml.

The latter two segments are assigned by the drug firms, and originally took advantage of the alpha-numeric option in cases where such product identity systems were already in use in 1969, e.g., Lilly's "Identi-Code." (Lilly has retained its "Identi-Code" and, in addition, now uses all-numeric NDC numbers). Currently, newly assigned NDC's are all-numeric, to facilitate keyboard transcription and to provide compatibility with the Universal Product Code (UPC), which will be mentioned later.

The FDA published its first edition of the NDC Directory in 1969; the same information is available on magnetic computer tape (from the Department of Commerce, National Technical Information Service, Springfield, VA 22161).

Early in the 1970s, the NDC was changed to the present ten-digit all-numeric structure. The three segments and their identities remain as originally developed, i.e., the labeler, the drug product, and the trade package. The FDA now assigns five-digit labeler codes; firms in the original program may retain the four-digit labeler segment, depending on whether they utilize five or six digits for their product-plus-package identification. Thus, three alternate configurations for the NDC number are in use:

Labeler		Product		Package
4	—	4	—	2
5	—	4	—	1
5	—	3	—	2

It is anticipated that there is sufficient growth space for the ten-digit system to remain adequate for some time.

The NDC Directory (Fifth Edition, 1976) is limited to human prescription drugs, and selected OTC drugs often prescribed by physicians, e.g., insulin. Some 60,000 human prescription drug products are now listed with the FDA [4].

The Drug Listing Act of 1972 (DLA) [5] amended the Federal Food, Drug, and Cosmetic Act (FD&C Act) to require that an NDC be assigned to all drugs covered by the FD&C Act. Imprinting the NDC on product labels remains voluntary; most firms however do include the NDC on their labels. In addition, the DLA also requires drug manufacturers, packagers, and distributors to register their establishments (FDA's form FDA 2656) and to list all their drug products individually with the FDA. Each NDC must be entered on each drug listing form (form FDA 2657), and this information must be updated semi-annually. This provides the input for the FDA's massive computer program, the Drug Registration and Listing System (DRLS), which enables the FDA to know what drug products are being marketed, who makes them, and how they are labeled. The DRLS consists primarily of two linked modules. One module contains data on establishments, and the other contains drug product data. The DRLS establishment module includes over 18,000 drug firms which must register as drug processors (and be subject to the mandatory periodic good manufacturing practices inspections by the FDA's field force). The product module of the DRLS contains information on over 250,000 drug products, almost half of which are marketed by distributors [6]. The law and the implementing regulations

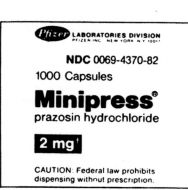

Above
The drug industry NDC code must be placed in the top third of the container of wrapper label. The NDC is preceded by "NDC" or "N."

for the DRLS, including the NDC system, are in the FD&C Act [7] and the Code of Federal Regulations [8].

As mentioned, the NDC is *requested* (not required) by FDA to appear on all drug product labels and labeling. When it is used, it must be placed in the top third of the principal display panel of the immediate container label and of any outside container or wrapper label. The exception is that the NDC may be used as part of and contiguous to the UPC symbol, provided such symbol is displayed prominently and in a conspicuous location other than the natural bottom of the immediate drug product package. The NDC is preceded by "NDC" or "N." Many firms make an important additional use of the NDC for product identification: the product identity segment (the middle three or four digits) is imprinted on solid dosage forms, together with the manufacturer's (labeler's) name or identifying logo. This is helpful in identifying stray tablets or capsules, particularly prescription drugs, which a patient might be using or which might have been used in an overdose situation. Thus, for example,

• Terramycin capsules 250 mg = "PFIZER 073"
• HydroDIURIL tablets 50 mg = "MSD 105"

Whenever a material change to a drug product occurs (active ingredient, strength/concentration, dosage form, route of administration if accompanied by a formulation change), or a significant label change is instituted, a new NDC number must be assigned, i.e., the product identity segment is changed (as is the trade package segment, if appropriate) [9]. The manufacturer initiates the revising during the semi-annual drug listing (June and December). When a drug product has been discontinued, its NDC number may be reassigned to another drug product five years after the expiration date of the discontinued product, or, if there is no expiration date, five years after the last shipment of the discontinued product into commercial distribution [10].

The Universal Product Code

In 1973, the grocery manufacturing and distribution industry created the UPC: that now-familiar vertically elongated "keyboard" of varied-width linear bars. Immediately underneath this machine-readable symbol are ten digits: the first five identify the manufacturer (or distributor) and the second five digits represent the product-package. The UPC system was designed to allow simpler and more accurate product identification as goods move from manufacturer to wholesaler to retailer, and to allow the use of scanner-equipped checkstands in supermarkets and other retail outlets which, in turn, speed customer checkout operations and allow the collection of complete and accurate information on all aspects of the transaction [11].

For OTC drug products, manufacturers may use their NDC number as the UPC number (underneath the UPC symbol), e.g., Bufferin Tablets = N-19810-0057-7; Dristan Tablets = N-0573-1241-30; or they may use an independent UPC number, e.g., Ben-Gay Ointment = 74300-00062; Alka-Seltzer = 16500-04012.

The NDC and Third-Party Payments

Probably the most significant present use and greatest potential for NDC numbers on prescription drug products' labels is in the processing of third-party prescription drug reimbursement claims. One of the original intents of the NDC was to eliminate the laborious, error-prone filling out of these reimbursement forms: writing out the product name, strength, dosage form, and sales code number was to be replaced by simply writing the ten-digit NDC on the form. In theory, this was great; in practice, use (or lack of use) of the NDC varies, as will be seen shortly.

Consonant with the third-party payment issue for prescription drugs was the idea of the universal claim (reimbursement) form. Conceptually, this single form would have satisfied the government agencies involved as well as the private insurers. And what a blessing this would have been to the dispensers of the drugs: *the community and hospital pharmacists* so often neglected by government (and industry) when these schemes, with which pharmacists are so intimately involved, are developed.

Even though these universal claim forms are not yet widely used, it must be kept in mind that the NDC is one of the most important elements in the use of these forms. It is the FDA's responsibility to maintain the accurate registry of the NDC numbers and to ensure its accessibility to the public.

Most private and government-sponsored third-party insurers require the NDC numbers on their reimbursement forms. The federal government, for example, could probably not cope with its drug reimbursement responsibilities without the common language of the all-numeric NDC. Intimately involved in this area is the National Council for Prescription Drug Programs (NCPDP), an *ad hoc* group which includes government (Health Care Financing Administration), industry, insurers, dispensers (National Association of Retail Druggists and National Association of Chain Drug Stores), and other professional and trade representation. One of the NCPDP's goals is the acceptance of general use of the universal claim form which they developed with the NDC number as the key element.

The NDC and Pharmacists

Observation of pharmacists' prescription drug stocks demonstrates that practically all[2] responsible

[2]The qualifying word "practically" can probably be omitted: the writer was unable to find a current Rx drug product label without an NDC number.

firms include the NDC on labels. This is a commendable effort, as the inclusion of the number on labels is voluntary. Further, the majority of these manufacturers also imprint the significant portion of the product identification segment of the NDC on solid dosage forms. For OTC drug products, however, the NDC situation varies. The NDC may be printed as such on the packaging, or it may be printed as the numerical part of the UPC. Other firms elect not to use the NDC in any form on OTC drug products.

Community pharmacists report that the NDC is a valuable tool in product identification, both as it appears on the label, and as the product identity imprint on solid dosage forms.

Use of different labeler codes (the NDC's first segment) by ostensibly the same firm can be puzzling. This is explained by the fact that many firms have facilities located in Puerto Rico. As such, and to be regarded as an "arm's length relationship" corporation as specified by the Internal Revenue Service vis-a-vis Puerto Rico's particular tax situation, the firm located on the island must be a separate corporation. Thus, the labeler code for Searle-U.S. is 0025, for Searle-P.R. is 0014; Endo-U.S. is 0056, while Endo-P.R. is 0600. To further complicate labeler codes, each marketer (vendor) generally operates individually. For example, Pfizer Laboratories, Roerig, and Pfipharmecs marketing divisions each has a unique labeler code. Bristol Laboratories is labeler code 0015, while Bristol Myers for its OTC products uses a UPC vendor number. (For Rx vs. OTC drug products, some firms use the identical NDC labeler code for prescription drugs and use the UPC manufacturer identification number for their OTC drug products.)

Suggestions from community pharmacists include enlarging the NDC's print size, and consideration of the concept of a standardized trade package segment for NDC's, e.g., "-05" = 50's; "-01" =

100's; "-50" = 500's; "-10" = 1000's. This latter could be considered if the NDC were starting anew, although it would probably be impossible for the firms using the 5-4-1 NDC configuration. Another suggestion was for a standardized middle segment, i.e., the product identification. Thus, all digoxin tablets 0.25 mg, for example, would have identical codes. While an excellent idea, this met with resistance from the drug manufacturers [12], again probably because of the variation in ongoing identification systems; formulation differences between firms were no doubt part of the problem.

To aid the dispensing pharmacist, a few companies are providing small tear-off labels with their prescription drug trade packages. These labels include the drug's NDC, lot number, and expiration date, and are intended to be affixed to both the customer's individual prescription vial and simultaneously to the prescription itself for future reference. Examples of this include Smith Kline's Dyazide and Sandoz's Cafergot. Pharmacists would welcome the expansion of this concept.

Concerning the NDC's use with third-party payers' reimbursement forms, pharmacists find it becoming as ubiquitous as one's social security number. In fact, the New York State plan for city and county workers requires only the NDC of the prescription drug and the physician's name on its claim form. Many other forms do include the name of the drug product. Problems can arise with claim forms using only the NDC: some of the more recent generic drug manufacturers are not yet on the third-party master lists. In such cases, the insurer may return the reimbursement form to the pharmacist, to be resubmitted with the manufacturer's name and product dispensed included thereon.

In private hospitals, the pharmacists generally make no more use of the NDC system than do community pharmacists, viz., product identification and reimbursement forms. Some hospitals include NDC's in their product inventory control and purchasing systems. A suggestion that the entire NDC be placed on tablets and capsules is mechanically impractical; several firms, however, now imprint the actual product name, e.g., Inderal, Keflex, Vibramycin, Valium, in addition to the product strength and/or identification number. Hospitals with poison control centers find the solid dosage form identification numbers valuable in overdose and other abuse situations and for physician inquiries.

State and federal government hospitals use the NDC when ordering from drug manufacturers. The NDC number on a label provides an effective double-check, especially for non-professional people handling certain aspects of inventory control. Thus, once again, a practical aspect of the NDC system is demonstrated by its product identification use. Pharmacists note, too, the value of having NDC's included with individual product entries in pricing catalogs.

Since the NDC numbers are critical to efficient prescription drug reimbursement by third-party payers, it behooves the FDA to provide current, accurate data. Toward this end, the FDA had anticipated a new NDC Directory by October 1980; it is expected soon. The FDA also anticipates that a new computer tape of the NDC numbers will be available and will be updated quarterly [13]. Beyond this, the FDA's future plans call for a directory of NDC numbers for over-the-counter drugs and, eventually, perhaps even one for veterinary drugs (which, incidentally, are covered by the DLA, but are not included in the NDC Directory). These, however, are only in the initial planning stages and will depend upon future allotments of dollar and personnel resources.

Future plans notwithstanding, a very real problem exists for community pharmacists: the FDA's failure to keep the NDC Directory current, even though monthly updates are published. Some third-party payers do not refer to these updates, or do not put the new information into their computers, and thus can delay reimbursing pharmacists' claims until manual checks confirm new NDC numbers. Such delays are quite troublesome to the dispensing pharmacists and can cause financial hardship; significant staff reductions at the FDA's Drug Listing Branch (which deals with the NDC's) have contributed to this situation [14].

The practical values of the National Drug Code to practicing pharmacists, then, appear to be with the NDC numbers themselves: their use in drug product identification, for simpler and faster third-party reimbursement of prescription drug claims, and, to some extent, with certain inventory control functions.

References

1. Taubman AH, McEvilla JD: The utilization of the national drug code in drug information systems. The Apothecary 88:6, 1974.
2. Slavin M: The origin, development and application of the national drug code. Presentation to Academy of General Practice APhA, Montreal, Canada 1969.
3. FR 34:11157, 1969.
4. Yellin AK: Drug registration and listing system. Presentation to Southeastern Regional Symposium on Pharmacy Information Systems, Auburn, Alabama 1977.
5. Public Law No. 92-387, 92nd Congress.
6. Cobb W: Drug listing act and the national drug code. Presentation to the NACDS Pharmaceutical Conference, Marco Island, Florida 1976.
7. Federal Food, Drug & Cosmetic Act, as Amended, Section 510, 1980.
8. 21 CFR Part 207; revised in FR 45:30842, 1980.
9. Ibid, Section 207.35 (b) (4) (i).
10. Op. cit. Note 8, Section 207.35 (b) (4) (ii).
11. Uniform Product Code Council Inc: About the universal product code, 1978.
12. Slavin M: NDC/UPC compatibility and its potential in drug product packaging and marketing. Presentation to the Second National Packaging Regulations and Legislation Conference, Washington DC, 1975.
13. FDC Reports 42:T&G 13, June 9, 1980.
14. FDA staff cut increases Rx claim rejects. Drug Topics 123:14, 1979.

NDC System

1. Tracking drugs listed with FDA
2. Emergency use
3. Distribution use

NATIONAL DRUG CODE (NDC)—UPDATE*

J. L. Fink, K. W. Marquardt, and L. M. Simonsmeier

The NDC system facilitates automated processing of drug data by government agencies, drug manufacturers and wholesalers, fiscal intermediaries for Medicare and Medicaid, private insurance companies and drug providers.

The NDC number consists of at least ten characters. The code is divided into three segments: A labeler code, a drug product code, and a package code. Formerly, a nine-character code was used, but the FDA has added a lead zero to the code for all of the drugs listed under the older code. Therefore, drug products coded in the older editions of the NDC system will have the ten-character code broken down into a four-character labeler part, a four-character drug identity part, and a two-character package segment. Although the older drug code may have alphanumerical characters, the FDA permits changeover to all numerical digits, as it used in the new drug code.

New participants in the NDC system will have a ten-digit code assigned to drug products, the first five digits of which identify a drug manufacturer or distributor; the last five digits identify the drug name, package size, and type of drug. An eleven-digit code will be used when the available five-digit labeler portions of the code have been exhausted.

Drug manufacturers or distributors must register with the FDA submitting form FD-2656; they must submit a list of their drug products on form FD-2657. From these drug lists, a national drug code directory is prepared.

To obtain a copy of the National Drug Code Directory, write to the Superintendent of Documents, U.S. Government Printing Office, Washington, DC 20402. This information is also available on magnetic tape from the Technical Information Service, U.S. Department of Commerce, Springfield, VA 22151.

The National Drug Code (NDC) number is requested but not required to appear on all drug labels and in all drug labeling, including the label of any prescription drug container furnished to a consumer. If the NDC number is shown on a drug label, it shall be displayed as required in §207.35(b)(3).

The existence of an NDC number on the label of a drug product does not necessarily mean that the product has an approved New Drug Application. There is no relationship between the NDC number and the NDA. The NDC number is simply a number assigned for data processing purposes.

*Reprinted with permission from J. L. Fink, K. W. Marquardt, and L. M. Simonsmeier, *Pharmacy Law Digest*, St. Louis, MO: J. B. Lippincott Co. (1986).

QUESTIONS: CHAPTER 10

1. How many numerals are there in the NDC?

    a. Four

    b. Five

    c. Ten

    d. Twelve

2. Into how many segments is the NDC divided?

    a. Two

    b. Three

    c. Four

    d. Five

3. Which federal government agency compiles the *National Drug Code Directory?*

    a. Drug Enforcement Administration

    b. United States Department of Commerce

    c. U.S. Government Printing Office

    d. Food and Drug Administration

4. The first five digits of the NDC identify the _____ of the drug:

    a. Dosage form

    b. Name

    c. Manufacturer or distributor

    d. Package size

    e. Potency

5. The second segment of numerals of the NDC identify the _____ of the drug:

    a. Name

    b. Dosage form

    c. Package size

    d. Manufacturer or distributor

    e. Potency

6. The third segment of digits of the NDC identify the _____ of the drug:

    a. Potency

    b. Package size

    c. Manufacturer or distributor

    d. Dosage form

    e. Name

7. Which one of the following federal statutes created the NDC?

    a. Prescription Drug Marketing Act

    b. Generic Drug Enforcement Act

    c. Poison Prevention Packaging Act

    d. Fair Packaging and Labeling Act

    e. Drug Listing Act

8. Which one of the following is similar to the NDC?

    a. ICU

    b. UPC

    c. UPS

    d. CCU

9. The National Drug Code (NDC):

    1) Enhances third party reimbursement for pharmaceutical services

    2) Aids in identifying drug products

    3) Promotes economy

    4) Encourages efficient drug distribution

    5) Facilitates automated processing of drug product data

    a. 1), 3), and 5) are correct.

    b. 2), 3), and 4) are correct.

    c. 1), 2), 4), and 5) are correct.

    d. 1), 2), 3), 4), and 5) are correct.

10. The *new* NDC consists of _____ numerals:

    a. Five

    b. Seven

    c. Ten

    d. Fifteen

11. Into how many segments is the *new* NDC divided?

    a. Two

    b. Three

    c. Four

    d. Five

12. What do the first five numerals of a *new* NDC identify?

    a. Name of the drug product

    b. Package size and type of drug

    c. Manufacturer or distributor

    d. Dosage form and potency

13. What do the last five digits of a *new* NDC identify?

    a. Manufacturer or distributor

    b. Type of drug and dosage form

    c. Dosage form, name of drug, manufacturer/distributor

    d. Drug name, package size, type of drug

CHAPTER 11

U.S. Postal Regulations

POSTAL SERVICES MAILING REQUIREMENTS FOR CONTROLLED SUBSTANCES

The following are the mailing rules as set forth in the *U.S. Postal Service Domestic Mail Manual*, 11-1-81, Issue 7.

124.364 Controlled Substances (18 *U.S.C.* 1716)

.364 Controlled Substances

a. A controlled substance is any narcotic, hallucinogenic, stimulant or depressant drug in Schedules I through V of the *Controlled Substances Act* (Public Law 91-513), 21 *U.S.C.* 801, et seq., and the regulations thereunder, 21 *CFR* 1300, et seq.

b. Narcotic drugs, as defined in the Controlled Substances Act, include opium, cocaine and opiates (synthetic narcotics) and the derivatives thereof.

c. Controlled substances are, by reason of their addictive nature or capacity for abuse, hereby declared to be articles, compositions, or materials which may kill or injure another within the intent and meaning of 18 *U.S.C.* 1716.

d. Except under the conditions specified in 124.365, controlled substances are nonmailable matter and must not be conveyed in the mails or delivered from any post, branch or station thereof nor by any letter carrier.

.365 Mailing Requirements

a. **Authorized Mailings.** Controlled substances may be transmitted in the mails between persons registered with the Drug Enforcement Administration or between persons who are exempted from registration such as military, law enforcement, and civil defense personnel in the performance of their official duties. Prescription medicines containing nonnarcotic controlled substances may be mailed from a registered practitioner or dispenser to an ultimate user. Prescription medicines containing narcotic drugs may be mailed only by Veterans Administration medical facilities to certain veterans. Parcels containing controlled substances must be prepared and packaged for mailing in accordance with the requirements of 124.365b.

b. **Preparation and Packing.**
1. The inner container or any parcel containing controlled substances must be marked and sealed in accordance with the applicable provisions of the Controlled Substances Act, 21 *U.S.C.* 801, and the regulations promulgated thereunder, 21 *CFR* 1300, et seq.
2. The inner container of prescription medicines containing controlled substances must, in addition to the marketing and sealing requirements set forth in 124.365b, be labeled to show the name and address of the practitioner, or the name and address of the pharmacy or other person dispensing the prescription (if other than the practitioner), and the prescription number.
3. Every parcel containing controlled substances must be

Note

There is nothing in federal law which prohibits the use of delivery services, e.g., Federal Express, United Parcel Service, DHL Worldwide, for shipping narcotic and non-narcotic controlled substances or any other prescription drugs, i.e., pharmacist to patient, manufacturer to pharmacy.

placed in a plain outer container or securely over-wrapped in plain paper.

4. No markings of any kind which would indicate the nature of the contents shall be placed on the outside wrapper or container of any parcel containing controlled substances.

c. Exempt Shipments. Small quantities of unknown matter suspected of containing controlled substances may be sent by regular mail without regard to the other provisions of 124.364 only when addressed to a Federal, State, or local law enforcement agency for law enforcement purposes. Such mailings must comply with 124.365b (3) and (4).

.366 Violations

Violations of this section must be referred to the Inspection Service.

Note

The U.S. Postal Service issued a final rule, effective October 5, 1994, which amended its Domestic Mail Manual, to remove postal regulations which restricted the use of mail to transport prescription medicine containing narcotic drugs. As a result, use of the mail by dispensers (pharmacists) of such medicine is allowed to the same extent that distribution via any carrier is permitted pursuant to the federal Controlled Substances Act and implementing regulations.

QUESTIONS: CHAPTER 11

1. Which of the following can be mailed to the ultimate user by the pharmacist?
1) Schedule III Controlled Substances
2) Schedule IV Controlled Substances
3) Schedule II narcotic drugs
4) Schedule II non-narcotic drugs
5) Schedule V OTC drugs

    a. 1), 2), and 3) are correct.
    b. 1), 2), 3), 4), and 5) are correct.
    c. 3), 4), and 5) are correct.
    d. 3) is correct.
    e. 3) and 4) are correct.

2. Mr. Tom Jones, a patient known in the pharmacy where you are employed in New York, is going on a business trip and will be based in Chicago for three months. He asks you to mail to him Noctec Capsule 500 mg., #30, for which you have a written prescription on file. What should you do to comply with U.S. postal regulations?

    a. Send it by regular mail.
    b. Send it by registered mail, unless Mr. Jones requests otherwise.
    c. Refuse to mail it because it is a C-II controlled substance.
    d. Refuse to mail it because it is a narcotic.
    e. Refuse to mail it because a New York prescription is not valid in Illinois.   39 CFR 124.365(a)

3. Which of the following can be mailed from a registered practitioner/dispenser to an ultimate user?
1) Schedule II narcotic drugs
2) Schedule II non-narcotic drugs
3) Schedule III narcotic drugs
4) Schedule IV drugs
5) Schedule V drugs

    a. 1), 2), and 3) are correct.

    b. 1) and 2) are correct.

    c. 1) and 3) are correct.

    d. 1), 2), 3), and 4) are correct.

    e. 1), 2), 3), 4), and 5) are correct.   39 CFR 124.365(a)

4. Dr. A. Sicko, a clinical psychiatrist practicing at the local VA hospital, issues a written prescription for one of his patients. The prescription is for twenty-four tablets of Tylenol w/Codeine No. 3. The prescriber requests that you, the pharmacist at the hospital, mail the medication to the patient, a veteran, who is too ill to come to the pharmacy for it. Which of the following is *not* correct?

    a. Send the prescription by Federal Express.

    b. Mail the prescription by certified mail, return receipt requested.

    c. You cannot mail the medication because the prescription is not a valid Rx.

    d. You can mail the Rx because it is a non-narcotic C-III substance.   39 CFR 124.365(a)

5. Which of the following statements are correct?
1) Every parcel containing controlled substances must be placed in a plain outer container or securely wrapped in plain paper.
2) No markings of any kind which would indicate the nature of the contents should be placed on the outside wrapper or container of any parcel containing controlled substances.
3) Registered or certified mail must be used whenever mailing any controlled substance.
4) Regular mail is permitted for mailing controlled substances between DEA registrants.
5) Controlled substances listed in Schedules III, IV, and V in amount not exceeding a 100-day supply or 300 dosage units, whichever is less, can be sent by regular mail to the ultimate user.

    a. 1) and 2) are correct.

    b. 1), 2), and 3) are correct.

    c. 1), 2), and 4) are correct.

    d. 3) and 5) are correct.

    e. 3), 4), and 5) are correct.   39 CFR 124.365(b)

CHAPTER 12

Cosmetics

WHEN DOES A COSMETIC BECOME A DRUG?*

Steven Strauss, Ph.D., R.Ph.

What's the difference between a cosmetic and a drug, and is the difference really important?

Why does the Food and Drug Administration (FDA) sometimes decide that an article sold for years as a cosmetic must at some time be classified as a drug, or both a cosmetic and a drug, even though there may have been no change at all in its formulation, or physical or chemical composition?

When *does* a cosmetic become a drug?

Drugs are expected to improve health or treat disease, and cosmetics are expected to enhance personal attractiveness and physical appearance, two entirely different uses. However, it is a known fact that: 1) the toothpaste you may be using to clean your teeth and prevent tooth cavities is a drug; 2) a "suntan" product providing "protection from sunburn" is a drug subject to the FDA's Good Manufacturing Practice (GMP) drug regulations [1]; 3) a shampoo represented to contain an active ingredient that prevents the formation of dandruff is regulated as a drug; and 4) antiperspirants are considered drugs because they alter a body function.

*Reprinted with permission from *U.S. Pharmacist* (August 1983).

Definition

When a drug is a drug and a cosmetic a cosmetic is best appreciated by reviewing the definitions for these two categories of products in the Federal Food, Drug, and Cosmetic Act (FDCA) [2].

The term "cosmetic" means "1) articles intended to be rubbed, poured, sprinkled, or sprayed on, introduced into, or otherwise applied to the human body or any part thereof for cleansing, beautifying, promoting attractiveness, or altering the appearance, and 2) articles intended for use as a component of any such articles; except that such term shall not include soap" [3].

The term "drug", in pertinent part, means ". . . articles intended for use in the diagnosis, cure, mitigation, treatment, or prevention of disease in man . . . and . . . articles (other than food) intended to affect the structure or any function of the body of man . . . and . . . articles for use as a component of any such articles . . ." [4].

There are three important points to remember with respect to these definitions:

1) These are terms of the art, written by lawyers. Common consumer understanding of the terms "cosmetic" and "drug", or common commercial usage, is not con-

trolling. In determining whether an article is a cosmetic or a drug, the FDA has utilized these definitions and none other.

2) As a rule, it is not the ingredients in a formulation, but the claims made in the labeling or advertising, that determine whether an article will be deemed to be a cosmetic or drug. The FDA generally has taken the position that the intended use of an article is demonstrated by the claims for it, by its manufacturer or distributor, in labeling or advertising.

3) These definitions are not mutually exclusive; an article may be both a cosmetic and a drug.

There is an additional definition of drug that warrants mention. The opening statement of the FDCA definition also recognizes a drug as "articles recognized in the official *United States Pharmacopeia,* or official *National Formulary,* or any supplements to any of them." The inter-relationship of the compendial definitions that hinge on intent is open to question. Does inclusion of an article's ingredient in the compendia designate an article as a drug for regulatory purposes, despite labeling limited to cosmetic claims?

Court cases addressing the cosmetic-drug issue have arisen most frequently in the context of products claiming dubious therapeutic effects. The courts thus have been able to hold the product to be a drug by reference to the product's intended use without facing the hard question of whether or not the fact of compendial listing alone would change the status from drug to cosmetic. The courts may have a good reason for skirting the issue. Reference to the compendia, which are periodically revised, can be seen as a delegation of law-making authority to a private organization, i.e., the editors or committees on revision of the compendia who periodically revise the listings [5].

Reference to the compendia for resolution of the question: "Is it a drug?" also seems inappropriate in view of the compendia's functions. The focus of the compendia is on the quality, purity, strength, labeling and packaging specifications of drugs, and not on any distinction between drugs and non-drugs i.e., cosmetics [6].

Although the judicial record is sparse on the question of when a cosmetic may also be a drug, the three decisions on point, or so-called wrinkle lotion cases [7], are generally consistent in affirming that promotional claims may bring a cosmetic under the definition for a drug. A commentator has summarized well the essence of these cases in noting that a "cosmetic intended to improve the appearance is also a drug if its claimed effect on the structure or function of the body relates to health; it is not a drug, despite a minor, actual and claimed structural or function effect, if the claims relate to beauty and not health; if the incidental claimed effect on the structure or function is substantial, and not minor, then the product may be a drug [8].

Legal Significances/Differences

Whether an article is considered a drug or a cosmetic is a question of considerable significance because drugs must be manufactured pursuant to the Good Manufacturing Practices. In addition, the man-

ufacturer of drugs bears a heavier regulatory burden with additional labeling, registration, reports, the OTC Drug Review, and pre-clearance formalities pertaining to safety and efficacy, just to name a few pertinent regulatory requirements.

The following is a review of some of the basic regulatory differences between a drug and a cosmetic:

Labeling—A cosmetic product is required to have a list of all its ingredients in descending order of predominance except that fragrances or flavors may be listed as such [9]; a drug is required to list only its active ingredient(s) [10]. In this respect, cosmetics bear more informative labeling for consumers than any other article regulated by the FDA. Consumers can use cosmetic ingredient labeling to compare products and to avoid substances to which they may be allergic. If an article is both a cosmetic and a drug, it must list the active drug ingredient(s) first pursuant to section 502(e) of the Federal Food, Drug, and Cosmetic Act, followed by the cosmetic ingredients in descending order of predominance [11].

A cosmetic is required to declare the ingredients on the outside of the container or wrapping seen by the consumer at the point of purchase [12]. A drug is required to declare its active ingredient(s) both on the outside of the container or wrapper and on the label affixed to the immediate container [13]. If an article is both a cosmetic and a drug, all active ingredients first, followed by other ingredients, must appear on the outside of the container or wrapper, while the active ingredient only must appear on the label of the immediate container [14].

The exemption from ingredient labeling for cosmetics intended for use solely in beauty salons applies only to the Fair Packaging and Labeling Act cosmetic ingredient labeling regulations [15]; the exemption does not apply to drug labeling required by the

FDCA. Thus, a drug intended for use in a beauty salon is required to list its active ingredients. Ingredients of cosmetics must be listed by uniform (generic) names established especially for ingredient labeling. This rule is intended to prevent consumers from being confused or misled by the use of different names for the same ingredient.

Registration—Manufacturers of drugs are required to register themselves and their products with the FDA, pursuant to the drug registration provisions of the FDCA [16]. Firms that manufacture and package cosmetics are requested but are not required to register with the FDA [17]. However, in recent years, some cosmetic manufacturers have voluntarily registered their firms and products with the FDA and have voluntarily made available to the agency product experience reports, i.e., adverse effects caused by their products [18].

Drug GMPs—The FDA has published regulations estalishing GMP regulations for drugs [19]. There are no GMPs for cosmetics. However, the Cosmetic, Toiletry and Fragrance Association, a leading trade organization in the United States, has petitioned the FDA to establish appropriate GMPs for cosmetics.

New Drug Application—"New drugs" may not be marketed in the United States until a new drug application, the so-called NDA, has been approved by the FDA [20]. By contrast, the FDA has no statutory authority to require pre-market testing of cosmetics for safety or efficacy, potency or purity. The agency can take legal action to have a cosmetic removed from the market if it proves to be a health hazard, is adulterated or misbranded.

If the safety of any cosmetic product or ingredient has not been adequately substantiated by the manufacturer prior to marketing, regulations require that the label includes the statement: "Warning—The safety of this product has not been determined." However, a cosmetic manufacturer need not submit safety data to the FDA [21]. Although most cosmetic manufacturers test their products for safety before marketing them, the law does not require such tests.

OTC Drug Review—The FDA has established "monographs" for many categories of over-the-counter drugs [22]. There is no similar review for cosmetics. However, five of the monographs have some bearing to varying degrees on the cosmetic versus drug controversy. The five monographs are: topical antimicrobial products [23], skin protectant drug products [24], sunscreen drug products [25], antiperspirant drug products [26], and skin bleaching creams [27].

Inspections—Drug manufacturing establishments must be inspected at least once every two years [28]. Cosmetic manufacturing establishments need not be inspected within such time period.

Furthermore, the FDA does not have the legal authority to inspect and review manufacturing records and complaint files for cosmetics, as it does for drugs, inspection of which is authorized by the FDCA [29].

Conclusion

Historically, the FDA has provided guidance to the cosmetic industry by using trade correspondence (TC) pertaining to the drug versus cosmetic issue. Thus came determinations that such products as baby oil, deodorant powder, cuticle remover, and products "that soften lips, hands, rough skin" are cosmetics and not drugs [30]. Such TCs formed the basis for regulating products in this gray area.

More recently, the FDA confirmed its traditional approach in determining whether an article is a cosmetic or a drug when it stated that "the distinction between a drug and a cosmetic rests upon the intended use of the article. We would have to approach the problem of whether a particular ingredient is a drug on a case by case basis. In each case we would have to look at all the facts to determine if we can prove that the product was intended for use as a cosmetic or as a drug" [31].

Despite the apparent differences in the definitions and the regulations, historically it has been recognized that there can be similarities and that, indeed, formulations, and particularly labeling claims, may cause a cosmetic to become a drug.

The basic test of determining which characterization is appropriate has remained largely unchanged, namely, evaluating the representation or claims made for a product by its vendor [32]. Cosmetics thus displayed on the same shelf may be legally classified as cosmetics only, as drugs only, or they may be both cosmetics and drugs. Although you probably won't see the identifying words "cosmetic" or "drug" or "cosmetic-drug" on the package, the claims made for them will give you a clue to their legal classification. By reading these claims carefully you should be able to judge which is which, and whether the difference is really of any importance to you.

References

1. 21 CFR 210, 211.
2. 21 U.S.C. 301 et seq.
3. 21 U.S.C. 321 (i); FDCA 201 (i).
4. 21 U.S.C. 321 (g)(1); FDCA 201 (g)(1).
5. Hartnett PL: Implications of the drug vs. cosmetic question. Drug & Cosm Ind, 128 (4): 36, 1980.
6. Valentino JG: The compendia and their role in drug regulation. Pharm Tech, 5 (4): 45, 1980.
7. Adams LJ, Jr: Cosmetic or drug? FDA's OTC drug review provides some answers and raises new questions. Food, Drug, Cosm Law J., 35 (2): 98, 1980.
8. Quoted in *Ibid*, p. 102.
9. 21 CFR 701.3(a), (f).
10. 21 U.S.C. 352(e)(1).
11. 21 CFR 701.3(d).
12. 15 U.S.C. 1454(c)(3), 1459 (b).
13. 21 U.S.C. 321(k), 352(e)(1).
14. 15 U.S.C. 1454(c)(3), 1459 (b), 21 U.S.C. 321(k), 352(e)(1).
15. P L. 89-755; this law applies only to consumer commodities, i.e., products customarily distributed for retail sale for consumption by individuals for personal care in the home. Products used in commercial establishments are not required to bear an ingredient statement.
16. 21 U.S.C. 360; FDCA 510.
17. 21 CFR 710.
18. 21 CFR 730.
19. Op. Cit. Ref. 1.
20. 21 U.S.C. 321 (p), 355; FDCA 201 (p), 505.
21. 21 CFR 740.10.
22. 21 CFR 330.10.
23. 43 FR 1209, Jan 6, 1978; 44 FR 13041, Mar 9, 1979.
24. 43 FR 34627, Aug 4, 1978.
25. 43 FR 38205, Aug 25, 1978.
26. 43 FR 46693, Oct 10, 1978.
27. 43 FR 51546, Nov 3, 1978.
28. 21 U.S.C. 360 (h); FDCA 510 (h).
29. 21 U.S.C. 374 (a); FDCA 704 (a).
30. FDA Trade Correspondence 42, 1940 in Kleinfeld V. and Dunn C: Federal Food Drug and Cosmetic Act, 1938–1949, pp. 561–572.
31. Comments of the DHEW reproduced in the Comptroller General's Report to the Congress Concerning Cosmetics, HRD, 78-139, p. 132 (August 8, 1978).
32. Op. Cit. Ref. 7.

COSMETICS*

Cosmetics marketed in the United States, whether made here or imported, must comply with the Federal Food, Drug, and Cosmetic Act, the Fair Packaging and Labeling Act, and the regulations issued under the authority of these laws. The regulations applicable to cosmetics are in the *Code of Federal Regulations*, Title 21, Parts 700 to 740. The color additive regulations applicable to cosmetics are in 21 *CFR* Parts 73, 74, 81 and 82.

The FD&C Act (Sec. 201 (i)(1)) defines cosmetics as articles intended to be applied to the human body for cleansing, beautifying, promoting attractiveness, or altering the appearance without affecting the body's structure or functions. Included in this definition are products such as skin creams, lotions, perfumes, lipsticks, fingernail polishes, eye and facial make-up preparations, shampoos, permanent waves, hair colors, toothpastes, deodorants, and any ingredient intended for use as a component of a cosmetic product. Soap products consisting primarily of an alkali salt of fatty acid and making no label claim other than cleansing of the human body are not considered cosmetics under the law.

Cosmetics That Are Also Drugs

Products that are cosmetics but are also intended to treat or prevent disease, or affect the structure or functions of the human body, are considered drugs and cosmetics, and must comply with both the drug and cosmetic provisions of the law. Examples include "fluoride" toothpaste, hormone

creams, suntanning preparations intended to protect against sunburn, antiperspirants that are also deodorants, and anti-dandruff shampoos. Most cosmetics which are also drugs are over-the-counter drugs. Some are new drugs for which safety and effectiveness had to be proved to the FDA before they could be marketed. The requirements for drugs are more extensive than those for cosmetics. For example, the Federal Food, Drug, and Cosmetic Act requires that drug manufacturers register every year with the FDA and update their lists of all manufactured drugs twice annually. Additionally, drugs must be manufactured in accordance with current Good Manufacturing Practice regulations as codified in 21 *CFR* 210 and 211.

Adulterated or Misbranded Cosmetics

The Federal Food, Drug, and Cosmetic Act prohibits the distribution of cosmetics which are adulterated or misbranded. A cosmetic is considered adulterated if it contains a substance which may make it harmful to consumers under customary conditions of use; if it contains a filthy, putrid, or decomposed substance; if its container is composed of a harmful substance; if it is manufactured or held under insanitary conditions whereby it may have become contaminated with filth, or may have become harmful to consumers; or if it contains a non-permitted color and is not a hair dye. Coal-tar hair dyes labeled with the caution statement prescribed by law (Sec. 601(a)) and "patch-test" instructions are exempted from the adulteration provision even if they are irritating to the skin or otherwise harmful. Eyelash and eyebrow dyes are not included in this exemption. All dyes used in eye-

lash and eyebrow dye products must be approved by the FDA for such use.

A cosmetic is misbranded if its labeling is false or misleading, if it does not bear the required labeling information, or if the container is made or filled in a deceptive manner (Sec. 602).

Cosmetic Safety

Although the Federal Food, Drug, and Cosmetic Act does not require that cosmetic manufacturers or marketers test their products for safety, the FDA strongly urges cosmetic manufacturers to conduct whatever toxicological or other tests are appropriate to substantiate the safety of the cosmetics. If the safety of a cosmetic is not adequately substantiated, the product may be considered misbranded and may be subject to regulatory action unless the label bears the following statement: *Warning—The safety of this product has not been determined* (21 *CFR* 740.10).

With the exception of color additives and a few prohibited ingredients, a cosmetic manufacturer may, on his own responsibility, use essentially any raw material as a cosmetic ingredient and market the product without approval. The law requires that color additives used in food, drugs, and cosmetics must be tested for safety and approved by FDA for their intended uses. A cosmetic containing an unlisted color additive (i.e., one not approved by FDA for its intended use) is considered adulterated and subject to regulatory action. The colors approved for use in cosmetics are listed in 21 *CFR* 73, 74, 81 and 82.

The use of the following ingredients is either restricted or prohibited in cosmetics: bithionol, mercury compounds, vinyl chloride,

*Reprinted with permission from *Requirements of Laws and Regulations Enforced by the U.S. Food and Drug Administration.* DHHS Publication No. (FDA) 89-1115.

halogenated salicylanilides, zirconium complexes in aerosol cosmetics, chloroform, chlorofluorocarbon propellants, and hexachlorophene (21 *CFR* 700.11 to 700.23 and 250.250). FDA also considers adulterated cosmetic nail products containing methyl methacrylate monomer or those containing more than 5 percent formaldehyde.

Voluntary Registration

Although the Federal Food, Drug, and Cosmetic Act does not require cosmetic firms to register their establishments or formulas with FDA or make available safety data or other information before a product is marketed in the United States, the manufacturers or distributors may submit this information voluntarily. Voluntary registration and assignment of a registration number by the FDA does not denote approval of a firm, raw material, or product by FDA. Any use of a registration number in labeling must be accompanied by a conspicuous disclaimer phrase as prescribed by regulation (21 *CFR* 710, 720 and 730).

Cosmetic Labeling

Cosmetics distributed in the United States must comply with the labeling regulations published by FDA under the Federal Food, Drug, and Cosmetic Act and the Fair Packaging and Labeling Act. Labeling means all labels and other written, printed, or graphic matter on or accompanying a product. The label statements required by the Federal Food, Drug, and Cosmetic Act must appear on the inside as well as any outside container or wrapper. Fair Packaging and Labeling Act requirements (e.g., ingredient labeling) only apply to the label of the outer container. The labeling requirements are codified at 21 *CFR* 701 and 740. Cosmetics bearing false or misleading label statements or otherwise not labeled in accordance with these requirements may be considered misbranded

and may be subject to regulatory action.

The principal display panel—i.e., the part of the label most likely displayed or examined under customary conditions of display for sale (21 *CFR* 701.10)—must state the name of the product, identify by descriptive name or illustration the nature or use of the product, and bear an accurate statement of the net quantity of contents of the cosmetic in the package in terms of weight, measure, numerical count, or a combination of numerical count and weight or measure. The declaration must be distinct, placed in the bottom area of the panel in line generally parallel to the base on which the package rests, and in a type size commensurate with the size of the container as prescribed by regulation. The net quantity of contents statement of a solid, semisolid or viscous cosmetic must be in terms of the avoirdupois pound and ounce, and a statement of liquid measure must be in terms of the U.S. gallon of 231 cubic inches and the quart, pint, and fluid ounce subdivisions thereof. If the net quantity of contents is one pound or one pint or more, it must be expressed in ounces, followed in parenthesis ( ) by a declaration of the largest whole units (i.e., pounds and ounces or quarts and pints and ounces). The net quantity of contents may also be stated in terms of the U.S. system and the metric system of weights or measures.

The name and place of business of the firm marketing the product must be stated on an information panel of the label (21 *CFR* 701.12). The address must state the street address, city, state, and zip code. If a domestic firm is listed in a current city or telephone directory, the street address may be omitted. If the distributor is not the manufacturer or packer, this fact must be stated on the label by the qualifying phrase "Manufactured for * * *" or "Distributed by * * *" or similar appropriate wording. A firm located outside of the

United States may omit the zip code.

The Tariff Act of 1930 requires that all imported articles state on the label the English name of the country of origin.

Declaration of Ingredients

Cosmetics produced or distributed for retail sale to consumers for their personal care are required to bear an ingredient declaration (21 *CFR* 701.3). Cosmetics not customarily distributed for retail sale—e.g., hair preparations or make-up products used by professionals on customers at their establishments and skin cleansing or emollient creams used by persons at their places of work—are exempt from this requirement provided these products are not also sold to consumers at professional establishments or workplaces for consumption at home.

The ingredient declaration must be conspicuous so that it is likely to be read at the time of purchase. It may appear on any information panel of the package—i.e., the folding carton, box or wrapping if the immediate container is so packaged—and may also appear on a firmly affixed tag, tape, or card. The letters must not be less than 1/16 of an inch in height (21 *CFR* 701.3(b)). If the total package surface available to bear labeling is less than 12 square inches, the letters must not be less than 1/32 of an inch in height (21 *CFR* 701.3(p)). Off-package ingredient labeling is permitted if the cosmetic is held in tightly compartmented trays or racks, it is not enclosed in a folding carton, and the package surface area is less than 12 square inches (21 *CFR* 701.3(i)).

The ingredients must be declared in descending order of predominance. Color additives (21 *CFR* 701.3(f)(3)) and ingredients present at one percent or less (21 *CFR* 701.3(f)(2)) may be declared without regard for predominance. The ingredients must be identified by the names established or adopted by regulation (21 *CFR*

701.3(c)); those accepted by FDA as exempt from public disclosure may be stated as "and other ingredients" (21 CFR 701.3(a)).

Cosmetics which are also drugs must first identify the drug ingredient(s) as "active ingredient(s)" before listing the cosmetic ingredients (21 CFR 701.3(d)).

All label statements required by regulation must be in the English language and must be placed on the label or labeling with such prominence and conspicuousness that they are readily noticed and understood by consumers under customary conditions of purchase (21 CFR 701.2).

Label Warnings

Cosmetics which may be hazardous to consumers when misused must bear appropriate label warnings and adequate directions for safe use. The statements must be prominent and conspicuous. Some cosmetics must bear label warnings or cautions prescribed by regulation (21 CFR 740). Cosmetics in self-pressurized containers (aerosol products), feminine deo-dorant sprays, and children's bubble bath products are examples of products requiring such statements.

Tamper-Resistant Packaging

Liquid oral hygiene products (e.g., mouthwashes, fresheners) and all cosmetic vaginal products (e.g., douches, tablets) must be packaged in tamper-resistant packages when sold at retail. A package is considered tamper-resistant if it has an indicator or barrier to entry (e.g., shrink or tape seal, sealed carton, tube or pouch, aerosol container) which, if breached or missing, alerts a consumer that tampering has occurred. The indicator must be distinctive by design (breakable cap, blister) or appearance (logo, vignette, other illustration) to preclude substitution. The tamper-resistant feature may involve the immediate or outer container or both. The package must also bear a prominently placed statement alerting the consumer to the tamper-resistant feature. This statement must remain unaffected if the tamper-resistant feature is breached or missing (21 CFR 700.25).

Enforcement Authority

For enforcement of the law, FDA may conduct examinations and investigations of products, inspect establishments in which products are manufactured or held, and seize adulterated (harmful) or misbranded (incorrectly or deceptively labeled or filled) cosmetics. Adulterated or misbranded foreign products may be refused entry into the United States. To prevent further shipment of an adulterated or misbranded product, the Agency may request a Federal district court to issue a restraining order against the manufacturer or distributor of the violative cosmetic. FDA may also initiate criminal action against a person violating the law. Examples of products seized in recent years are nail preparations containing methyl methacrylate and formaldehyde, various eyebrow and eyelash dye products containing prohibited coal-tar dyes, and products contaminated with harmful microorganisms.

PRACTICAL AND THEORETICAL DISTINCTIONS BETWEEN DRUGS AND COSMETICS*

C. L. Hagenbush, Associate Counsel, S. C. Johnson & Son

Differences between theory and practice always hold the attention of serious students of the relevant discipline. These differences are most interesting when they are most pronounced. In the area of

*Reprinted with permission from Drug Information Journal, 21:403–408 (1987).

drug/cosmetic classification, the differences are at once very obvious and very significant. The factual and legal subtleties of the theory as distinguished from the practice of drug/cosmetic classification are, at the same time, so complex as to render them almost mystical. Of course, the difference

between drugs and cosmetics is important, particularly to the cosmetic manufacturer who intends to market a product in compliance with a regulatory scheme that does not require, among other restrictions, the agreement of the Food and Drug Administration (FDA) as to the safety and efficiency of the product prior to marketing. (Compare §§201(p), 505, 601, 602 and 603 of the Federal Food, Drug, and Cosmetic Act.)

This article deals with the theory as expressed in the statute and scant case law on the subject. It discusses the practicalities for the regulatory and legal professional attempting to understand where the problems exist in the cosmetic/drug classification area. Also discussed will be the practical limitations of regulation as expressed by the FDA enforcement activities. Unfortunately, the reader may be left with more questions than answers. This confusion results as much from the differences between what the FDA says and what it does in regulating industry as it does from the complexity of the topic.

First, an attempt should be made to define terms. The term "drug" is defined at §201(g)(1) of the Federal Food, Drug, and Cosmetic Act. That definition includes:

(A) articles recognized in the official United States Pharmacopeia, official Homeopathic Pharmacopeia of the United States, or official National Formulary, or any supplement to any of them; and (B) articles intended for use in the diagnosis, cure, mitigation, treatment, or prevention of disease in man or other animals; and (C) articles (other than food) intended to affect the structure or any function of the body of man or other animals; and (D) articles intended for use as a component of any articles specified in clause (A), (B), or (C); but does not include devices or their components, parts, or accessories.

Cosmetics are defined at §201(i) of the Act.

(i) The term "cosmetic" means (1) articles intended to be rubbed, poured, sprinkled, or sprayed on, introduced into, or otherwise applied to the human body or any part thereof for cleansing, beautifying, promoting attractiveness, or altering the appearance, and (2) articles intended for use as a component of any such articles; except that such term shall not include soap.

These definitions say that a "drug" is a substance officially recognized as such, intended to deal in some beneficial way with disease in man or animal, intended to affect the structure or function of the body of man or animal or which is used as a component of the previously mentioned substances. "Cosmetics," on the other hand, are substances applied to the body in some manner which are intended to beneficially affect appearance or which are components of such substances. "Food" is excluded from the "drug" definition. "Soap" is excluded from the "cosmetic" definition.

While the rules seem clear, it takes only a little thought to discover that they are not. Almost every cosmetic is intended to affect the structure or function of the human body in some manner. To conclude that every such cosmetic is also a drug is to completely frustrate the intent of Congress in setting up different structures to deal with the two classes of products. A better working definition is required.

The cases are one potential source of clarification. Unfortunately, there have been only three reported cases on the precise question of drug/cosmetic classification. The so-called "wrinkle remover" cases actually cause more confusion than clarification. Several points of well-settled food and drug law are established by the cases.

1. The intended use or effect of the product determines its status.

2. Products can have dual identities.

3. Promotional materials of all kinds can be used as evidence of the intended use of the product.

4. The question of drug/cosmetic status is highly fact sensitive.

The fourth point is perhaps the most important in understanding practice and theory in drug/cosmetic classification. Even though factual differences have been given great weight, it is difficult to explain today's marketplace in a manner that would give even mini-

mal significance to the "wrinkle remover" cases. A brief discussion of the cases follows:

US v Sudden Change, (1969), 409 F2d 734. The government seized 216 bottles of a cosmetic containing bovine albumin sold by the Hazel Bishop Company, which was called "Sudden Change." At the trial, the government prevailed by claiming the product to be a drug because certain statements made in labeling and advertising showed that the product was intended to affect the structure or function of the body of man.

On appeal, the Second Circuit Court of Appeals upheld the District Court finding of drug status for Sudden Change.

The court said, in effect, that claims that appear to a credulous and unthinking consumer to have a medical or physiological flavor would cause a cosmetic to also be considered a drug. It attached controlling significance to claims such as gives "a facelift without surgery" and "lift out puffs." It distinguished such claims from those regarding the cosmetic's ability "merely" to alter the appearance.

In this dissent, Judge Mansfield strongly criticized the majority.

To summarize my position, unless a product is in fact a "drug" as defined in the Food, Drug and Cosmetic Act or a reasonable person would conclude from a reading of the label and enclosure as a whole that it is intended to possess the properties of a drug as so defined, I would not classify it as such merely because one or two phrases, taken out of context, imply possible drug properties. The effort of such a course is to draw a line between permissible and impermissible description of cosmetics that is altogether too illusory and shadowy to permit a workable standard, with the result that most cosmetics must be classified as drugs. [emphasis added] id, at 744-5.

US v Line Away, (1969), 415 F2d 369. In the Line Away case the Third Circuit Court of Appeals also upheld the lower court's finding of drug status of another bovine albumin product. This product was said to temporarily alter the appearance of the skin by physically changing its contours. The rationale for the Court's decision is unclear from the opinion. The most that can be said is that the court found what it called "strong therapeutic implications," which caused it to believe that the product was a drug. These implications arose from promotional phrases such as "tingling sensation," "amazing protein lotion," and "packed under biologically aseptic conditions."

US v Helene Curtis Magic Secret, (1971), 331 F Supp 912. The District Court in the final case reached a different result. The Maryland District Court found that a third bovine albumin wrinkle remover was not a "drug" as defined by the Act.

The Maryland District Court claimed to follow the earlier Second and Third Circuit holdings but found controlling factual differences in the cases. Promotional materials for Magic Secret, it said, made only two statements that were therapeutic or medical in nature. Promotional claims such as "tightens tired skin," "soothes away wrinkles in minutes," and "has dramatic power to smooth away crowsfeet, puffy undereye circles, laugh, frown, and throat lines in just minutes," which were so troublesome to the earlier courts, were ignored by the Maryland District Court. It considered claims of "pure protein" and "astringent sensation" to be potentially troublesome, but dismissed these as "less exaggerated than those reported" in the other two cases.

Such fine-spun factual distinctions are so confusing and sensitive as to render the theoretical rule unworkable. Taken literally, the cases allow one court to conclude that a product promising an "astringent sensation" is a cosmetic, while a different court finds a product that offers a "tingling sensation" to be a drug. A cosmetic may be composed of "pure protein," which "smooths away laugh lines, crowsfeet, and puffy undereye circles" in one jurisdiction, but could not be "pure natural protein to smooth away crowsfeet, laugh and frown lines, even undereye puffiness," in another, unless it is first subjected to the new drug approval process. Such a scheme gives effect to Judge Mansfield's concern expressed in dissent in the "Sudden Change" case.

No cases have appeared since to reverse the case law established by these three decisions, and there has been no amendment to the Federal Food Drug and Cosmetic Act. Accordingly, it could be expected that prudent business people promoting cosmetics would avoid therapeutic, medicinal, or physiological claims.

Current promotional activities for cosmetic products sold today demonstrate a difference between the rules that are practiced and those that are written.

The most effective anti-aging breakthrough that has hit the market in recent months . . . [R]esearchers worked for five years on developing the final formulation which includes nature's 18 most effective anti-aging ingredients.

Efficiency testing was then conducted at a renowned Paris Hospital using the rigorous Marschall Method of measuring results. These tests confirmed after 15 days application, a noticeable improvement in firmer facial features, better elasticity and minimized lines/ wrinkles.

Formulated with gentle, natural plant extracts, they work to desensitize tempermental skin. . . . Provide relief from irritation with this intensive treatment. Lavender and soya extracts combine to soothe, soften and help restructure the epidermis. Elasticity is improved and moisture balance restored—so skin looks and feels better. . . . Concentrated licorice extracts, Vitamins A and E, help to rebuild skin defenses.

Extensive research led . . . cosmetic chemists to an unprecedented discovery to help aid in the prevention and reversal of the aging process.

[Neutralize] free radicals [which can] weaken cell structure . . . [P]revent visible signs of aging.

Serum, Prescriptives, Clinique and many other names with a therapeutic meaning can be found in the cosmetic marketplace. Factual analysis that was so important in deciding the old wrinkle remover cases now apparently is simply not material to the drug/cosmetic definition.

After some discussion of the cases and the law, as contrasted with the current flavor of promotional activities in the cosmetic area, it should be clear that there are discrepancies between theory and practice. The industry has come a long way from the era of the wrinkle remover cases.

In such a day and age, how can a cosmetic manufacturer effectively compete without serious risk of regulatory action by FDA or others? The following guidelines may be helpful.

1. It is most important that the product sold be safe and wholesome. A cosmetic product that is not safe or that has not been carefully tested to evaluate its safety and toxicity will expose the seller to several risks. FDA may allow many potentially difficult issues to pass unregulated, but a true safety problem is the most certain cause of regulatory activity by the agency. In addition, an inadequate or improper safety analysis can result in product liability exposure.

2. If the "intended to affect on the structure or function of the body of man" portion of the definition has life, it is being enforced in certain areas that are rather well understood. Dandruff control products, baldness cures, antibacterials, sunscreens, antiperspirants, and anticaries products have been historically classified as drugs. Indeed, most recent cosmetic enforcement activity has taken place in the sunscreen and hair restoration categories. Consider, for example, Clarins, Estee Lauder, and Givaudan regulatory letters issued

in 1985 and 1986 and the multiple seizures of Rivixil in recent months.

3. Statements informing consumers of the benefits of cosmetic products should be supported by strong scientific evidence. Whether FDA decides to attempt to assert drug status for your product may depend on the support that can be shown for the claims. A cosmetic manufacturer with the weight of the scientific evidence in its favor is more likely to prevail. Of course, any product promising to cure a frank disease condition is likely to be regulated as a drug. Any such product sold as a cosmetic is at risk irrespective of its efficacy and safety.

4. Followers often fare better than leaders in the regulatory arena. Put another way, it is better for others to risk exposure first. The more bold the claim, the higher the risk of regulatory action.

5. A cosmetic that can also function as a drug may change the nature of claims that can safely be made. For example, petrolatum is recognized as an effective drug at a certain level for certain indications. It is also an effective component of moisturizing cosmetics. Fluoride is an effective anticaries agent. No cosmetic use for fluoride is currently recognized, other than its ability to promote attractiveness by preventing ugly cavities. If a cosmetic product offers a fluoride product for cosmetic use in the mouth, it is likely that FDA will not accept the use as appropriate for cosmetic regulation. Knowledge of the science and regulations in both the drug and the cosmetic area will help avoid such problems.

6. In other countries, antiperspirants, sunscreens, antibacterial products, and dandruff treatments are regulated differently than in the United States. Such products are often cosmetics (many EC countries) or quasi-drugs (Japan). New foreign companies must be aware of these kinds of distinctions and prepare accordingly.

7. It may be unnecessary to say that the answers to product classification question change with different enforcement policy and advances in science. A recent example involves FDA's Tentative Final Monograph for OTC dandruff products. Dandruff treatment products have historically been viewed by the agency as drugs. However, in July of 1986, the FDA sought to establish a dandruff claim that could be made without imposing drug status on products making such claims. The Proprietary Association disagreed with the agency, responding with data to support the view that consumers understood the FDA cosmetic labeling as promising drug efficacy. More than 75% of the consumers interviewed interpreted the "cosmetic phrase" to promise dandruff control. Nearly half said the product labeled with the FDA language as a cosmetic would prevent dandruff.

Firm conclusions about theory and practice in the drug/cosmetic classification analysis are not easily drawn. It is difficult to pin down a number of theoretical points with precision. Most perplexing is exactly where the theoretical safe harbor for cosmetics exists. If it is true that any article intended to affect the structure or function of the body is technically a drug, then it seems there are no cosmetics. Yet, even restrictive interpretations are imposed, as in the wrinkle remover cases, with some intuitive respect for the existence of functional cosmetics. The technical definitional problem obviously continues to elude precise description.

If the theoretical problem is difficult, the practical one approaches the impossible. Analysis of the precise point at which FDA will take regulatory action against products crossing the drug/cosmetic line presumes that such a line is understood and identified by that institution. Recent history suggests that no practical concensus on this point exists at the agency. Selling a sunscreen as a cosmetic has been strictly prohibited in recent months. Offering cosmetic baldness cures is, at times, acceptable and at other times forbidden. Almost anything can be said about cosmetic dentifrices and their ability to treat, cure, prevent, or mitigate a host of oral cavity diseases without fear of FDA regulatory action, according to recent activity in that area. Of course, the combination of a Category I anticaries ingredient with a Category III tooth desensitizer has resulted in multiple seizures and a protracted legal battle over the product's new drug status.

Clearly, the only guidance about agency policy that can be gathered from recent history is that decisions are made largely on an ad hoc basis. The decision to act may be based as much on the likelihood of quick victory as on any predetermined and consistent policy.

The reasons for deciding *not* to take enforcement action are often more obvious. Budgetary constraints, a climate of "deregulation," a broadening respect for the judgment of consumers, First Amendment issues, changes in management at the FDA, and a host of other practical factors more often than not can be used to justify lack of enforcement activity.

It is clear that no consistent general rule has evolved to predict which products and promotions will trigger an unfavorable agency response. Nonetheless, the practical guidelines mentioned above can be useful. In addition, it should be said that there is great potential for products to accurately claim their intended effects on the body so long as those effects do not explicitly involve treatment or prevention of disease. The only recent consistently applied exception to this view has involved the agency's tenacious campaign against cosmetic sunscreens. Most any other statement about a cosmetic's ability to improve or change the user's appearance through an effect on the body should not expose the seller to regulatory action by FDA, so long as no safety issues arise.

LEGAL PERSPECTIVE—OTC DRUGS AND COSMETICS*

Ann H. Wion, Associate Chief Counsel for Drugs and Biologics, Office of General Counsel, Food and Drug Administration

Many consumers might be surprised to learn that the toothpastes, antiperspirants, or sunscreen lotions they use are legally classified as "drugs." But manufacturers of such products are well aware that their products may be subject to regulation by the Food and Drug Administration (FDA) not only as "cosmetics" but also as "drugs." Although the Federal Food, Drug, and Cosmetic Act includes definitions and regulatory schemes for both "drugs" and "cosmetics," it can be an interesting challenge to determine the proper classification for a particular product.

The Statutory Definitions

Section 201(g) of the Act defines the term "drug" as (A) articles recognized in certain official compendia, (B) articles "intended for use in the diagnosis, cure, mitigation, treatment, or prevention of disease . . .", (C) "articles (other than food) intended to affect the structure or any function of the body . . .", or (D) articles intended for use as a component of any of the articles listed above [21 USC §321(g)].

"Cosmetic" is defined in §201(i) as (1) "articles intended to be rubbed, poured, sprinkled, or sprayed on, introduced into, or otherwise applied to the human body . . . for cleansing, beautifying, promoting attractiveness, or altering the appearance," and (2) articles intended for use as a component of such articles. Soap is specifically excluded from the definition [21 USC §321(i)].

It is clear from the statute that a product can be both a cosmetic and a drug. Section 509 was added to the act to specify that the 1962

*Reprinted with permission from *Drug Information Journal,* 21:409–416 (1987).

drug amendments do not apply to any cosmetic unless the cosmetic is also a drug or device [21 USC §359]. Even before 1962 it was evident from the legislative history of the 1938 act that the definitions of "drug" and "cosmetic" were not to be construed as mutually exclusive [1].

When FDA promulgated its regulations on voluntary registration of cosmetic product establishments and voluntary filing of cosmetic product ingredient statements, the agency proposed to identify categories of cosmetics that would also be regarded as drugs [2]. The list of such products included eye lotions, nail hardeners, douches, depilatories, hormones, tanning products, wrinkle removers, and a few others. However, in response to comments, the agency deleted the illustrative list and substituted the general statement that "Any cosmetic product which is also a drug or device or component thereof is also subject to the requirements of Chapter V of the Act" [3] [21 CFR §700.3(b)]. Consequently, the regulations are not particularly helpful in making drug/cosmetic determinations.

The Legal Consequences of Drug/Cosmetic Classification

Before focusing more directly on approaches to classifying products as cosmetics, drugs, or both, it may be useful to describe the legal consequences of such classification. The legal consequences lead to the practical effects of drug/cosmetic classification for the manufacturer or consumer of these products.

More restrictions and requirements attach to products classified as drugs than to products classified solely as cosmetics. A drug that meets the statutory definition of "new drug" may not be introduced into interstate commerce unless a new drug application

(NDA) for the product has been approved by FDA [21 USC §355]. A "new drug" is defined as a drug that is not generally recognized by qualified experts as safe and effective for use under the conditions prescribed, recommended, or suggested in the labeling [21 USC §321(p)(1)]. A drug may also be a "new drug" if it has not been used to a material extent or for a material time under such conditions [21 USC §321(p)(2)].

The Act requires evidence of safety and effectiveness for all drugs. Safety must be demonstrated through "adequate tests by all methods reasonably applicable" to show whether or not the drug is safe. There must also be evidence from adequate and well-controlled clinical investigations to show that the drug will have the effect claimed in the labeling [4] [21 USC §355(d)].

FDA's over-the-counter (OTC) drug review was established in 1972 essentially to make determinations about which OTC drugs could be considered generally recognized as safe and effective and could, therefore, be marketed without prior approval of an NDA [5]. OTC drug products that do not conform to applicable final monographs developed through the OTC review rulemakings will be liable to regulatory action [21 CFR §330.10(b)]. In short, an OTC drug product will either have to meet the terms of the monograph for its category of drug or be the subject of an approved NDA.

There is no statutory premarket approval scheme for cosmetics [6]. Although there is no premarket approval of the safety of cosmetics, FDA regulations do require that each ingredient used in a cosmetic product either be adequately substantiated for safety prior to marketing or carry a warning that the safety of the product has not been determined [21 *CFR* §740.10].

Sections 601 and 602 of the Act describe when cosmetics will be deemed to be adulterated and misbranded; sections 501 and 502 are the comparable drug provisions. There are similar statutory provisions for cosmetics and drugs concerning adulteration from poisonous or deleterious substances, from filth, or from preparation under insanitary conditions [cf 21 *USC* §361(a)-(e) and 21 *USC* §351(a)(1), (2)(A), (3), (4)(A)]. However, §501(a)(2)(B) of the Act requires that current good manufacturing practice (GMP) methods be used in drug manufacture to assure that safety and related requirements are met [21 *USC* §351(a)(2)(B)]. FDA has promulgated extensive regulations detailing drug GMP requirements concerning methods, facilities, equipment, and records [21 *CFR* Parts 210 and 211]. There are no comparable GMP requirements for cosmetic product manufacture.

Misbranding provisions quite similar to those in §602 governing cosmetics are included in the drug misbranding provisions of §502 [cf 21 *USC* §362(a)-(f) with 21 *USC* §352(a), (b), (c), (i), (m), (p)]. The statutory prohibitions against false or misleading labeling and against misleading containers as well as the requirements for including manufacturer, packer, or distributor information and quantity of contents in the labeling are essentially the same for drugs and cosmetics [cf 21 *USC* §362(a)-(f) with 21 *USC* §352(a)-(c), (i), (m), (p)]. However, the drug misbranding provisions go further in requiring adequate directions for use, adequate warnings against unsafe use, and packaging and labeling restrictions related to official compendia [21 *USC* §352(e)-(h)]. Among other things, the drug misbranding provisions also prohibit the imitation of another drug and include requirements for specified drugs, such as those that are habit-forming [21 *USC* §352(i)(2), (d)].

Although the statutory drug misbranding provisions are more ex-

tensive, FDA regulations make cosmetic labeling requirements more demanding than drug labeling requirements in at least one respect. That is, the label of a cosmetic product must bear the name of each ingredient in descending order of predominance, except that fragrance or flavor may be listed as fragrance or flavor and trade secret ingredients need not be listed [21 *CFR* §701.3(a)]. The Act requires that the established name of each active ingredient in a drug be listed [21 *USC* §352(e)]. FDA has not required that the inactive ingredients of OTC drugs or of oral prescription drugs be listed on the label [7]. If a product is both a cosmetic and a drug, FDA regulations require that the label first declare the active drug ingredients, then declare the cosmetic ingredients [21 *CFR* §701.3(d)].

Unapproved new drugs may be exported only to certain countries under specified circumstances [See 21 *USC* §382]. The Act does not restrict the export of cosmetics that are not adulterated or misbranded. Even cosmetics and drugs that would be misbranded or adulterated for domestic use may be exported to any country, so long as they comply with the laws of the country to which they are being exported and meet certain other requirements of §801(d) of the Act [21 *USC* §381(d)(1)].

Another difference between the regulatory requirements for drugs and those for cosmetics concerns registration requirements. Under section 510 of the Act every drug manufacturer must register the establishment and provide FDA a list of drugs being manufactured for commercial distribution [21 *USC* §360; 21 *CFR* Part 207]. In contrast, FDA regulations request voluntary registration of cosmetic product establishments and voluntary filing of cosmetic product ingredient statements [21 *CFR* Parts 710, 720]. Similarly, FDA requires manufacturers of new drugs to submit reports of adverse drug experiences, whereas FDA requests manufacturers of cosmetics to submit

analogous information voluntarily [21 *USC* §355(k); 21 *CFR* §314.80; 21 *CFR* Part 730]. Finally, most OTC drug products, with a few exceptions, are subject to requirements for tamper-resistant packaging [21 *CFR* §211.132]. Only liquid oral hygiene and vaginal cosmetic products must meet tamper-resistant packaging requirements [21 *CFR* §700.25].

Judicial and Administrative Interpretations of the Drug/Cosmetic Definitions

It should be evident from this discussion why some manufacturers might prefer that their cosmetic products not also be considered drug products, as well as why some consumer protection advocates would favor drug classification for such products. As would be expected, most of the legal controversy has involved the limits of the drug definition, not the limits of the cosmetic definition. However, at least one shampoo manufacturer has tried, unsuccessfully, to take advantage of the "soap" exception to escape cosmetic status for his product [8]. Consistent with the legislative history, FDA has defined "soap" narrowly, to include only alkali-fatty acid products labeled solely as soap [9] [21 *CFR* §701.20].

The limits of the drug definition have been tested more frequently. The two leading cases concerning cosmetics that may also be drugs continue to be the 1969 cases involving the facial skin lotions "Sudden Change" and "Line Away" [10]. These and other litigated cases focusing on the drug definition help us to develop an approach for discerning when a cosmetic has crossed over the drug line.

The concept of "intended use" is important to both cosmetic and drug definitions. Summarizing the "cosmetic" definition, the term covers articles "intended to be" applied in or on the body for "cleansing, beautifying, promoting attractiveness, or altering the appearance" [21 *USC* §321(i)]. The first part of the drug definition, subsection A, does not depend on intended use, but includes articles recognized in the *USP, Homeopathic Pharmacopeia,* or *National Formulary.* Although several cases have relied on inclusion in an official compendium as a basis for considering the product a drug [11], reliance on this factor as the sole basis for drug classification has been called into question. In suits brought by the National Nutritional Foods Association, the Second Circuit concluded, based on FDA's treatment of vitamins and minerals in promulgated regulations, that inclusion in the *USP* or *NF* would not automatically establish that classification of such an article as a drug would be reasonable [12]. On the other hand, lack of inclusion of an article in an official compendium does not necessarily mean it is not a drug [13]. Therefore, although inclusion in the *USP* or *NF* is a factor to be considered, in making the "drug" determination one should usually also examine the potential applicability of other parts of the definition.

Subsections (B) and (C) of §201(g) focus essentially on whether the articles are intended for use related to disease or intended to affect the structure or function of the body. The Second Circuit, in the *Sudden Change* case, pointed out that "It is well settled that the intended use of a product may be determined from its label, accompanying labeling, promotional material, advertising and any other relevant source" [14]. For example, statements made in lectures, in magazine testimonials, and in radio programs have been used to prove intended drug use, as well as more traditional labeling sources [15].

FDA's regulation on the meaning of "intended uses" [21 *CFR* §201.128] states that the phrase refers to "the objective intent of the persons legally responsible for the labeling of drugs." This intent "is determined by such persons' expressions or may be shown by the circumstances surrounding the distribution" of the product [21 *CFR* §201.128]. The intended use may change after the product has left the manufacturer's hands. For example, a distributor or seller may intend a different use [*Id*].

As the court again pointed out in *Sudden Change,* "regardless of the actual physical effect of a product, it will be deemed a drug . . . where the labeling and promotional claims show intended uses that bring it within the drug definition" [16]. Although this approach makes it clear that a product may be a drug even if it has no effect on the body, it leaves unanswered the question of whether a product may be a drug if it has an effect but no claims for the effect are made [17]. It can quite reasonably be argued that simply by including in a product an ingredient known to have an effect on the structure or function of the body or known to have a therapeutic effect, the manufacturer intends that effect. For example, in 1976 the FDA's Associate Commissioner for Compliance took the position that products containing sunscreen ingredients are drugs even though they make only tanning claims [18]. On the other hand, the agency has taken the position that a soap containing an antimicrobial ingredient may be either a drug or a cosmetic, depending on the claims made [19].

The question of whether consumer intent can be relevant to the drug determination was addressed by the Court of Appeals for the DC Circuit in *Action on Smoking and Health v Harris,* a case involving whether cigarettes are drugs [20]. The Court discussed the legislative history of the drug definition and concluded, as had the Second Circuit in one of the vitamin cases, that " '[t]he vendors' intent in selling the product to the public is the key element in this statutory definition' " [21]. This does not mean, however, that consumer intent is necessarily irrelevant. As the DC Circuit put it, "[w]hether evidence of consumer intent is a 'relevant source' for these purposes depends on whether such evidence is strong enough to justify an inference as to the vendors' intent" [22]. Judge Friendly had stated in one of the vitamin cases that "a fact finder should be free to pierce all of a manufacturer's subjective claims of intent" to find actual therapeutic intent on the basis of objective intent [23]. The DC Circuit concluded that "consumers must use the product predominantly—and in fact nearly exclusively—with the appropriate intent before the requisite statutory intent can be inferred" [24]. The Court concluded that the plaintiffs had not established the nearly exclusive use of cigarettes by consumers with the intent to affect the structure or function of the body. Similarly, with respect to vitamins A and D, the Second Circuit concluded that the record did not show that the therapeutic use of the vitamins by consumers so far outweighed their use as dietary supplements as to show an objective intent that the products were used in the mitigation and cure of disease [25]. Consequently, it seems clear from the case law that reliance on consumer intent alone would require a very strong showing to trigger drug classification. However, evidence of consumer intent is one element of the circumstances surrounding commercial distribution that may be considered in making the drug classification.

With respect to the promotional claims that are made for a product, the question of the standard to use in evaluating the claims also arises. In addressing this question, the Second Circuit, again in the *Sudden Change* case, determined that the legislative history reveals the purpose of the Act to be not only protection of the public health but also protection of the consumer's economic interests [26]. The Court concluded that to achieve these purposes of the Act the product claims should be evaluated by how they might be understood by the "ignorant, unthinking, or credulous" consumer [27]. The Court did make an exception for claims that are so associated with the familiar exaggerations of cosmetics advertising that virtually everyone can be assumed to recognize them as puffery [28].

Using this standard, the Court found the claims "lift out puffs" and "face lift without surgery" to carry physiological connotations suggesting that the product would affect the structure of the body in a way other than merely temporarily altering the appearance [28]. In the *Line Away* case, the Court of Appeals for the Third Circuit considered statements that the product was made in a "pharmaceutical laboratory" and packaged under "biologically aseptic conditions" to imply that the product is a pharmaceutical [29]. That Court also noted that describing the product as an "amazing protein lotion" suggests that the lotion nourishes the skin. Furthermore, phrases describing the lotion as "super-active" and "amazing," creating a "tingling sensation" when "at work," "tightening" the skin, and "discouraging new wrinkles from forming" were found to reinforce the impression that it was a therapeutic product, the protein content of which had a physiological effect on the skin [29]. On the other hand, when the District Court of Maryland reviewed the claims for another skin lotion, "Magic Secret," the court concluded that the drug line had not been crossed [30]. There the court found that even the "ignorant, unthinking and credulous" consumer would not be led by the claims " 'a pure protein' which causes an 'astringent sensation' " to think the product would do anything other than alter the appearance [31].

An Approach to Making Drug/Cosmetic Determinations

With this background in mind, it is possible to develop a general approach to making difficult drug/cosmetic classifications. It may be useful to look first at the ingredients in the product. If the prod-

uct contains an ingredient listed in the *USP, Homeopathic Pharmacopeia*, or *NF*, it may be a drug. If an ingredient, at the concentration present in the product, has a drug effect, it may be a drug. "Drug effect" in this sense means affects the structure or function of the body or cures, mitigates, treats, or prevents disease.

If the ingredient has a cosmetic effect, it may be a cosmetic. "Cosmetic effect" means cleanses, beautifies, promotes attractiveness, or alters the appearance. A product that has both a drug effect and a cosmetic effect may be both a drug and a cosmetic or the labeling and other claims may be determinative. For example, one might argue that a douche containing water and vinegar is a drug because the vinegar changes the pH of the body. The product may also be considered a cosmetic because it has a cleansing effect. If vinegar adds nothing to the effect of the product other than to change the body's pH, then the objective intent of including the ingredient in the product is to have a drug effect. If vinegar has a cleansing effect apart from the pH action, a manufacturer could argue that the product is solely a cosmetic.

Another complication in considering the ingredients in the product is whether the ingredient has a cosmetic effect, such as beautifying, through affecting the structure or function of the body. Antiperspirants may be considered drugs as well as cosmetics even if promoting attractiveness is both the manufacturer's and the consumer's goal because the ingredients achieve their goal by affecting a function of the body. Deodorants containing ingredients that do not impede perspiration, but simply perfume the smell could escape drug status. Consumer perception of the effect of the ingredients may also be relevant to the determination.

Having considered the actual and perceived effects of the ingredients of the product, one should then also examine the claims. It is

clear that even in the absence of an actual drug effect, claims of a drug effect will make the product a drug. Determining whether a claim implies the requisite association with disease or implies that the product affects the structure or function of the body can be complicated. For example, a claim that a mouthwash "kills germs in the throat" seems to imply prevention or treatment of sore throats, a drug effect, whereas "kills germs that cause bad breath" seems to imply only a cosmetic effect. The more ambiguous phrase "kills germs," because of the absence of a limiting phrase, can be interpreted fairly to imply a drug effect. A claim that suggests beautification through affecting the structure or function of the body would logically make the product both a cosmetic and a drug.

Again, consumer perception of the meaning of a claim may be important. If the "ignorant, unthinking, and credulous" consumer would perceive a drug effect from the claim, then the product would be a drug. Product names or the characterization of ingredients on the label may suffice to cross the drug line. For example, listing something as an "active ingredient" can imply a drug effect. Just as in the *Line Away* case the phrase "protein lotion" was found to suggest a drug effect, so might using a term such as "hormone" to describe an ingredient imply an effect on the function of the body.

Some of the drug/cosmetic distinctions will be addressed by the FDA in the course of the OTC review rulemakings. Questions have arisen in the course of the review concerning the drug/cosmetic status of antimicrobial soaps, skin protectants, skin bleaching agents, sunscreens, antiperspirants, shampoos, mouthwashes, hormone-containing products, and vaginal products. FDA's interpretations of the Act, including the construction of terms such as "drug" and "cosmetic," are given substantial deference by the courts [32]. Although this does not mean the agency's interpretation necessarily prevails in court [33], it does suggest that those concerned about the outcome of a drug/cosmetic classification should participate in the administrative process and present their views to the agency. Although it is not always easy to make drug/cosmetic determinations, nevertheless, a manufacturer is obligated to obey the law and to formulate, market, and promote products accordingly. Erring on the side of the public health is ultimately in everyone's best interest.

References

1. S. Rep. No. 361, 74th Cong., 1st Sess. (1935), reprinted in Dunn, *Federal Food, Drug, and Cosmetic Act* 239–240 (1938); *United States v An Article . . . Sudden Change,* 409 F2d 734, 739 (2d Cir 1969).

2. *Federal Register* 1971; 36 (Aug 26): 16934.

3. *Federal Register* 1972; 37 (Apr 11): 7151–7152.

4. See 21 CFR Part 330; *Federal Register* 1972; 37 (May 11): 9464. Misbranding determinations are also made in OTC review rulemakings.

5. The criteria for evidence of safety and effectiveness set forth in §505(d) must also be met for drugs to meet the general recognition requirements of §201(p) and escape new drug status. *Weinberger v Hynson, Westcott & Dunning, Inc,* 412 US 609, 629–30, 632 (1973); 21 CFR §330.10(a)(4)(ii).

6. *Toilet Goods Ass'n v Finch,* 419 F2d 21 (2d Cir 1969).

7. 21 CFR §201.100(b)(5).

8. *United States v An Article of Cosmetic . . . Beacon Castile Shampoo,* No. C71-53 (ND Ohio, Nov 6, 1973), reprinted in Kleinfeld et al., *Federal Food, Drug, and Cosmetic Act Judicial Record 1969–1974* at 149.

9. Dunn, *supra* n1, at 239.

10. *United States v An Article . . . Sudden Change,* 409 F2d 734 (2d Cir 1969); *United States v An Article of Drug . . "Line Away",* 415 F2d 369 (3d Cir 1969).

11. *AMP, Inc v Gardner,* 389 F2d 825 (2d Cir), *cert. denied,* 393 US 825 (1968); *United States v Dianovin Pharmaceuticals, Inc.,* 342 F Supp 724 (D.P.R. 1972), *aff'd,* 475 F2d 100 (1st Cir), *cert. denied,* 414 US 830 (1973); *United States v Articles of Drug,* 263 F Supp 212 (D Neb 1967); *United States v 39 Cases,* 192 F Supp. 51 (ED Mich 1961).

12. *National Nutritional Foods Ass'n v Mathews,* 557 F2d 325, 337–38 (2d Cir 1977); *National Nutritional Foods Ass'n v FDA,* 504 F2d 761, 788–89 (2d Cir 1974), *cert. denied,* 420 US 946 (1975).

13. *United States v 48 Dozen Packages,* 94 F2d 641 (2d Cir 1938).

14. 409 F2d at 739.

15. *United States v Articles of Drug . . . Foods Plus, Inc.,* 362 F2d 923, 926 (3d Cir 1966); *United States v Millpax, Inc.,* 313 F2d 152, 154 (7th Cir), *cert. denied,* 373 US 903 (1963); *Nature Food Centres, Inc. v United States,* 310 F2d 67, 69 (1st Cir 1962), *cert. denied,* 371 US 968 (1963); *United States v Hohensee,* 243 F2d 367, 370 (3d Cir), *cert. denied,* 353 US 976 (1957).

16. 409 F2d at 739.

17. The District Court in *Sudden Change* had concluded that the product did not affect the structure of the body. The appellate court found it "unnecessary to reach the issue of actual physical effect." 409 F2d at 739 n2.

18. Letter dated June 17, 1976, from Sam D. Fine to Richard F. Kingham.

19. Letter dated November 22, 1982, from Richard J. Ronk to Robert S. McQuate.

20. 655 F2d 236 (DC Cir) (1980).

21. 655 F2d at 239, quoting *National Nutritional Foods Ass'n v Matthews,* 557 F2d 325, 333 (2d Cir 1977).

22. 655 F2d at 239.

23. 504 F2d at 789.

24. 655 F2d at 240.

25. 557 F2d at 336. For discussions of the "food"/"drug" distinction in the context of 21 USC §321(g)(1)(C), see *Nutrilab, Inc. v. Schweiker,* 713 F2d 335 (7th Cir 1983) and *American Health Products Co. v Hayes,* 574 F Supp 1498 (SDNY 1983), *aff'd,* 744 F2d 912 (2d Cir 1984).

26. 409 F2d at 740.

27. 409 F2d at 741–42.

28. 409 F2d at 741.

29. 415 F2d at 372.

30. *United States v An Article of Drug . . . "Helene Curtis Magic Secret",* 331 F Supp 912 (D Md 1971).

31. 331 F Supp at 917.

32. *Action on Smoking and Health v Harris,* 655 F2d at 237–38.

33. *"Magic Secret",* 331 F Supp 912 (D Md 1971).

QUESTIONS: CHAPTER 12

1. According to the FD&C Act, a cosmetic is considered adulterated if:
1) It is harmful to consumers under customary conditions of use.
2) It is manufactured or held under unsanitary conditions.
3) It does not bear the required labeling information.
4) It contains a filthy, putrid, or decomposed substance.
5) The container is filled in a deceptive manner.

    a. 1), 2), and 3) are correct.
    b. 1), 3), and 5) are correct.
    c. 2), 3), and 5) are correct.
    d. 1), 2), and 4) are correct.
    e. 3) and 5) are correct.

2. Which is an example of a cosmetic that may also be a drug?

    a. Antiperspirant
    b. Toothpaste
    c. Suntanning product
    d. Cold cream

3. Which is an example of a cosmetic that may also be a drug?

    a. Deodorant
    b. Antidandruff shampoo
    c. Suntanning product
    d. Toothpaste

4. Pursuant to the FD&C Act, a cosmetic is deemed to be misbranded if:
1) Its labeling is false or misleading.
2) Its container is composed of a harmful substance.
3) It does not bear the required labeling information.
4) The container is made in a deceptive manner.
5) It contains a nonpermitted color and is not a hair dye.

    a. 1), 3), and 5) are correct.
    b. 1), 2), and 4) are correct.
    c. 2), 3), and 4) are correct.
    d. 1), 3), and 4) are correct.
    e. 2) and 4) are correct.

5. Federal law requires that cosmetics marketed in the United States:
1) Be safe and effective
2) Have a label which lists major ingredients in descending order of predominance
3) Be packaged in tamper-resistant packages when sold at retail
4) Need not include on the label names of specific fragrances
5) Have a label which lists major ingredients by generic name

    a. 1), 3), and 5) are correct.
    b. 2), 3), and 5) are correct.
    c. 2), 4), and 5) are correct.
    d. 2), 3), and 4) are correct.
    e. 1), 2), and 4) are correct.

CHAPTER 13

Anabolic Steroids

Anabolic steroids are defined as synthetic derivatives of the male hormone testosterone, having pronounced anabolic properties and relatively weak androgenic properties (i.e., producing masculine characteristics), which are used clinically mainly to promote growth and to repair body tissue in senility, debilitating illness, and convalescence. Anabolic steroids may also be referred to as *androgenic-anabolic steroids.*

FDA has approved a relatively small number of anabolic steroids as prescription drugs, which may be prescribed only by licensed practitioners for legitimate medical purposes. Such uses include the treatment of anemias, hereditary angioedema, and metastatic breast cancer in females.

Unfortunately, anabolic steroids have been and are being primary used/abused for non-therapeutic purposes. According to a number of published reports, the first such use occurred during World War II when German combat troops were given anabolic steroids to increase their aggressiveness. Anecdotal reports indicate that the Russians initiated their use in athletics in 1954. Since that time the use of anabolic steroids has increased dramatically with an "abuse explosion" occurring in the 1980s. Abuse of these potent drugs has spread to professional, college, and high school sports.

The primary source of the anabolic steroids abused by body-builders and others seeking muscle bulk, such as football players, is the black market. The sources of these drugs are: (1) legitimate drugs manufactured in the U.S. and diverted to illegal use; (2) foreign-manufactured drugs smuggled into the U.S. from Mexico, South America, the Bahamas, and Europe (primarily Germany and The Netherlands); and (3) clandestine laboratories.

On November 29, 1990, the Congress enacted and President George H. W. Bush signed into law the Anabolic Steroids Control Act (the ASCA) as Title XIX of the Crime Control Act of 1990 (P.L. 101-647), which became effective February 27, 1991. The intent of the ASCA is to minimize (or eliminate) the use of anabolic steroids for non-medical purposes. Prior to the ASCA, anabolic steroids were regulated as drugs pursuant to the Federal Food, Drug, and Cosmetic Act.

The Drug Enforcement Administration (DEA) has classified anabolic steroids as Schedule III controlled substances pursuant to 21 *CFR* 1308.13. However, certain products which are considered to have no significant potential for abuse because of their concentration, preparation, mixture, or delivery system, are exempt from being classified as controlled substances (Table 3).

In addition, the classification does not include anabolic steroids expressly intended for administration through implants to cattle or other non-human species and which are approved by the U.S. Food and Drug Administration. However, prescribing, dispensing or distributing such substances for other than implantation in cattle and other non-human species is a violation of law.

Any material, compound, mixture or preparation which contains any amount of the following substances is considered to be an anabolic steroid (Table 1).

Table 1

Generic Name	Trade Name
Boldenone undecyclamate	
Chorionic gonadotrophin	
Clostebol	
Dehydrochlormethyltestosterone	
Ethylestrenol	Maxibolin
Fluoxymesterone	Halotestin, Ora-Testryl
Mesterolone	
Mentenolone	
Methandienone	
Methandrostenolone	
Methyltestosterone	Oreton Methyl
Nandrolone decanoate	Deca-Durabolin
Nandrolone phenpropionate	Durabolin
Norethandrolone	
Oxandrolone	Anavar
Oxymesterone	
Oxymetholone	Anadrol-50
Stanozolol	Winstrol
Testosterone propionate	
Testosterone-like related compounds	
Testosterone (patch)	Androderm, Testoderm

Table 2
"Anabolic Steroids" Encountered in the Black-Market

Anabolicum	Halotestin	Permastril
Anadrol	Halostein	pizotyline
Anatrofin	Hombreol	Primobolone/Primobolan depot
Anavar	Iontanyl	Primotestin/Primotestin depot
Androxon	Laurabolin	Proviron
Andriol	Lipodex	Quinalone
Android	Maxibolin	Quinbolone
bolandiol	mesterolone	Restandol
bolasterone	metanabol	silandrone
boldenone	methenolone acetate	Sostanon
boldenone undecylenate	methenolone enanthate	Spectriol
bolenol	methandienone	stanolone
Bolfortan	methandranone	stanozolol
bolmantalate	methandriol	stenbolone acetate
Cheque	methandrostenolone	Stromba
chlorotestosterone	methyltestosterone	Sustanon
clostebol	mibolerone	Tes-10
Deca Durabolin	Myagen	Tes-20
dehydrochlormethyltestosterone	Nandrolin	Tes-30
Delatestyl	nandrolone	Teslac
Dianabol	nandrolone decanoate	testolactone
Dihydrolone	nandrolone cyclotate	testosterone
dihydrotestosterone	nandrolone phenpropionate	testosterone cypionate
dimethazine	Nelavar	testosterone enanthate
Drive	Nerobol	testosterone ketolaurate
Drolban	Nilevar	testosterone phenylacetate
drostanolone	nisterime acetate	testosterone propionate
Durabolin	Norbolethone	testosterone undecanoate
Durateston	Nor-Diethylin	Testred
Equipoise	norethandrolone	Thiomucase
Esiclene	Normethazine	tibolone
ethylestrenol	Omnifin	trenbolone
Exoboline	oxandrolone	trenbolone acetate
Finaject	oxymesterone	trestolone acetate
fluoxymesterone	oxymetholone	Trophobolene
formebolone	Parabolan	Winstrol

Note: Brand name products begin with capital letters; generic drug names are in lowercase.

Table 3
Some Exempt Anabolic Steroid Products
Androgyn L.A. injection (Forest)
Estratest tablet (Solvay)
Estratest HS tablet (Solvay)
Premarin w/methyltestosterone tablet (Wyeth/Ayerst)
Test-Estro injection (Rugby)
Testosterone cypionate injection (Steris)
Testosterone enanthate injection (Steris)

Source: 21 CFR 1308.34.

QUESTIONS: CHAPTER 13

1. Which one of the following trade name products is an anabolic steroid?

   a. Anavar
   b. Deltasone
   c. Sterobol
   d. Synalar
   e. Anabol

2. Which one of the following is an anabolic steroid?

   a. Nadolol
   b. Betaxolol
   c. Stanozolol
   d. Penbutolol
   e. Atenolol

3. Which one of the following is an anabolic steroid?

   a. Anabol
   b. Oreton Methyl
   c. Deltasone
   d. Muscletone
   e. Sterosterone

4. Which one of the following does *not* require a federal triplicate order form?

   a. Codeine sulfate powder
   b. Seconal Pulvule 100 mg
   c. Demerol tablet 100 mg
   d. Opium tincture
   e. Halotestin tablet

5. Which one of the following is an anabolic steroid?

   a. Betaxolol
   b. Acebutolol
   c. Cyclopentol
   d. Ethylestrenol
   e. Dehydrochloranol

6. A practitioner may prescribe and a pharmacist may dispense anabolic steroids for the treatment of:

    a. Angioedema or MDD

    b. Panic disorders or narcolepsy

    c. Metastatic breast cancer in males

    d. Convulsive disorders or narcolepsy

    e. Anemia or angioedema

7. How are anabolic steroids classified according to federal law?

    a. Schedule I

    b. Schedule II

    c. Schedule III

    d. Schedule IV

    e. Schedule V

8. Which one of the following is an exempt anabolic steroid product?

    a. Android

    b. Boldenone

    c. Chlorotestosterone

    d. Durabolin

    e. Estratest

9. Which one of the following is *not* common with the others?

    a. Estratest tablet

    b. Estratest HS tablet

    c. Premarin w/methyltestosterone tablet

    d. Winstrol tablet

10. Which agency of the federal government has primary enforcement jurisdiction over anabolic steroids?

    a. FBI

    b. BPA

    c. CPSC

    d. DEA

    e. EPA

11. What is the maximum number of times, if any, and within what period of time may refills be authorized for anabolic steroids for therapeutic purposes by a medical practitioner?

    a. 5× within 6 months

    b. 6× within 5 months

    c. 5× within 6 months from date of issue of prescription

    d. 6× within 5 months from date of issue of prescription

    e. Prescriptions for anabolic steroids cannot be refilled

12. What is the most number of refills, if any, that the pharmacist may dispense pursuant to a written prescription for an anabolic steroid?

    a. 3

    b. 5

    c. 6

    d. As many refills as authorized by the prescriber

    e. Prescriptions for anabolic steroids may not be refilled

13. According to federal law, which one of the following statements is required as part of the prescription label when dispensing an anabolic steroid?

    a. Controlled Substance, Dangerous Unless Used As Directed

    b. Caution: Federal Law Prohibits Dispensing Without A Prescription

    c. Caution: Federal law prohibits the transfer of this drug to any person other than the patient for whom it was prescribed

    d. Federal law has classified this drug as a Schedule III Controlled Substance

    e. Beware: This drug may be dangerous to your health and should only be used on the advice of your physician

14. Which president of the United States signed the Anabolic Steroids Control Act into law?

    a. William Clinton

    b. George Bush

    c. Ronald Reagan

    d. Jimmy Carter

    e. Gerald Ford

CHAPTER 14

Prescription Drug Marketing Act of 1987

The Prescription Drug Marketing Act (the Act) of 1987 (P.L. 100-293) was signed into law on April 22, 1988 by President Ronald Reagan, and became effective July 21, 1988. The Act may be referred to as the "Dingell Bill" or "drug diversion law," in honor of Representative John D. Dingell (D-MI) who introduced the Act.

The intent of the statute is to maintain the integrity of the distribution system for marketed prescription drugs by eliminating the wholesale submarket, or "diversion market," to prevent adulterated, misbranded, subpotent, or expired drugs from being sold to the American consumer.

Also, to investigate and take corrective action against prescription drug products that have been diverted from normal channels of commerce, or have traveled outside of domestic channels of commerce, and may have become substandard or ineffective and therefore unfit for sale.

An additional intent is to investigate and take corrective action against individuals or parties who may divert, or contribute to the diversion of, prescription drug products and prescription drug samples.

The Act amends several sections of the *Federal Food, Drug, and Cosmetic Act* by prohibiting the reimportation of drugs produced in the United States, to place restrictions on the distribution of drug samples, to ban certain resales of drugs by hospitals and other health care facilities, and for other purposes.

The effective date for most provisions was July 22, 1988, except that the sample distribution requirements became effective October 20, 1988, and the requirement for state licensing of wholesale distributors became effective September 14, 1992, two years after the FDA published a final rule establishing minimum guidelines for state licensing of wholesale distributors engaged in interstate commerce.

Specifically, the *Act:*

- Prohibits the reimportation of exported U.S. produced pharmaceuticals except by the original manufacturer.
- Prohibits the sale, purchase or trade or the offer to sell, purchase or trade any drug sample or coupon redeemable for a drug product. A drug sample is a dosage unit intended to promote sale, rather than be sold, and a coupon is a form that may be redeemed at no cost or reduced cost for drugs. Counterfeiting of drug coupons is also prohibited.
- Prohibits the sale, purchase or trade or offer to sell purchase or trade drug:
  —which was purchased by a public or private hospital or other health care entity or
  —which was donated or supplied at reduced price to a charitable organization.
- Establishes controls on wholesale distribution:
  —sales information requirements for wholesalers who are not authorized distributors for such drugs.
  —requires licensure by the state.
  —requires the Secretary of HHS to issue guidelines establishing minimum standards, terms and conditions for licensure including requirements for storage and handling of drugs and maintenance of records of drug distribution.
- Provides for strict controls on prescription drug sampling by the sales representative and by mail:
  —only practitioners licensed to prescribe such drugs may be provided samples.
  —requires written request and written receipt.
  —requires establishment of strict accountability of samples delivered by sales representatives.

—requires annual inventory and balancing of sales representatives' sample inventories.

—requires written receipt of samples delivered by mail or common carrier and a system to detect patterns of non-return.

—requires reporting of significant losses or any theft of drug samples to the federal authority.

• Establishes penalties for violations.

The law does not allow pharmacists to request drug product samples.

Upon receipt of specific form, manufacturers or distributors may distribute samples to "licensed practitioners," who are defined as any person authorized by state law to prescribe prescription drugs. The legislation requires that practitioners requesting samples must submit their DEA and state license numbers and mandates that this information be stored by the pharmaceutical manufacturer for at least three years. In addition to the annual reports, the records are to be made available to the FDA upon request.

Pharmacies can receive, store and handle samples only when requested to do so by a licensed practitioner, and licensed practitioners who designate a pharmacy to store and handle their samples must submit a document attesting to this relationship with the FDA. The name and address of the intended recipient at the "pharmacy or health care entity" must be given on the request form. If the sample is to be delivered by common carrier, the FDA has required the name and address of the "responsible party who will sign the delivery receipt." Those failing to execute a receipt for delivery will be barred from receiving additional samples.

Since the law requires drug wholesalers to be registered by states according to federal guidelines, it is important to note that the transfer of prescription drugs by retail pharmacy to another retail pharmacy in order to alleviate a temporary shortage will not be interpreted to be a "wholesale distribution," and is allowed.

The PDMA State Licensing Requirement

PDMA amended the *Federal Food, Drug, and Cosmetic Act* (the *Act*), 21 *U.S.C.* 301 et seq., to regulate certain aspects of the marketing of prescription human drugs. Among other things, PDMA requires, section 503(e)(2)(A), that any person who engages in wholesale distribution of prescription drugs must be licensed by the state in accordance with federal guidelines issued through notice and comment rulemaking. PDMA prohibits interstate wholesale distribution of prescription human drugs by persons who are not licensed by the state in accordance with these guidelines.

The federal guidelines that were necessary to implement this requirement, the guidelines for state licensing of wholesale drug distributors, were published as

---

FDA Interprets PDMA Requirements: Drug Samples in Hospital Pharmacies

In hospitals where the pharmacy is located in a clinic that serves both outpatient and retail customers, drug samples are permissible if the following stipulations are achieved:

a) All drug samples must go to the pharmacy pursuant to an agreement with the practitioner.

b) The pharmacy must keep copies of a practitioner's written request for drug samples.

c) Drug samples must be stored separately from the rest of the pharmacy stock.

d) The accountability and recordkeeping of the pharmacy's outpatient and retail services must be kept separate.

e) There must be a written contractual agreement between the pharmacy and the health care entity.

f) The original packaging for the drug sample must be used for dispensing.

g) The drug sample cannot be purchased by any individual or cannot be offered for sale by the pharmacy.

---

a final rule on September 14, 1990 (55 *FR* 38012). The guidelines, which include minimum standards for storage, handling, and recordkeeping, are codified in [21 *CFR* 205]. The PDMA state licensing requirement for wholesalers became effective on September 15, 1992.

Licensing Requirement Changes under the Amendments

The Amendments modify section 503(e) of the *Act* (21 *U.S.C.* 353(e)) to establish a temporary alternative federal wholesale distributor registration procedure. The temporary alternative federal wholesale distributor registration procedure covers wholesale drug distributors in those states that do not have a licensing program that meets the federal guidelines. Under the Amendments, after September 14, 1992, any person engaging in the interstate wholesale distribution of human prescription drugs must be licensed by the state, except for wholesalers in those states that do not have a licensing program that meets the federal guidelines, who must be registered in accordance with the Amendments.

Registration by a wholesale distributor under the temporary alternative federal wholesale distributor registration procedure does not relieve a wholesale distributor from any licensing or registration requirement that may be imposed by state law, even if that program does not conform to the federal minimum guidelines. The wholesale distributor shall immediately apply for and obtain a state license in accordance with section 503(e)(2)(A) when the state in which the wholesaler is located establishes a licensing program that meets the federal guidelines.

Under section 303(b)(1) of the *Act*, knowing failure to comply with section 503(e)(2)(A) can result in imprisonment for no more than 10 years, a fine of no more than $250,000, or both.

Persons currently registered in accordance with other registration requirements under the *Act* and regulations (e.g., section 510 of the *Act*, or 21 *CFR* 207) are not exempt from registering in accordance with the Amendments for the purposes of satisfying section 503(e)(2)(C) of the *Act*. Registration under the temporary alternative federal wholesale distributor registration procedure does not in any way denote approval of a firm or its products.

Effective Dates and Duration

The Amendments are effective immediately and the temporary alternative federal wholesale distributor registration procedure expires September 14, 1994. After September 14, 1994, all persons engaged in the wholesale distribution of prescription human drugs in interstate commerce must be licensed by the state in which they are located.

Temporary Registration Procedure Requirements

The Amendments require, at amended section 503(e)(3), that any person who engages in the wholesale distribution in interstate commerce of prescription human drugs in a state that does not have a licensing program that meets the federal guidelines shall register with the Secretary of the Department of Health and Human Services the following information:
1. The person's name and place of business; and
2. The name of each establishment the person owns or operates that is engaged in the wholesale distribution of drugs in a state which does not have a conforming program.

Guidance for Registration under the Temporary Program

FDA encourages wholesale distributors in states

without licensing programs that meet the federal guidelines who register under the temporary alternative federal wholesale distributor registration procedure to comply with the minimum storage, handling, and recordkeeping requirements in 21 *CFR* 205.

FDA requests that the required registration information and any subsequent changes thereto be submitted on company letterhead, if available, to the appropriate FDA District Office (District Director) (see 21 *CFR* 5.115), with the following information:
1. The address of each establishment listed;
2. The dated signature of the registrant; and
3. The name, address, and telephone number of a contract person in case further information is needed.

The FDA district office will note the date and time of receipt on a copy of the submission, and return a copy of the submission with the acknowledgment of receipt on it to the sender. The District Office will return illegible or incomplete submissions to the sender without an acknowledgment of receipt. If a copy of the submission with the acknowledgment of receipt is not received within 21 days after submission, the District Office to which it was submitted should be contacted.

There is no registration fee.

Requests for Information from FDA

Requests for additional information about the temporary alternative federal wholesale distributor registration procedure or other provisions of the Amendments or the PDMA should be directed to the local FDA District Office (see 21 *CFR* 5.115).

Significant loss or theft of drug samples must be reported in writing to:

Office of Compliance (HFD-300)
Center for Drug Evaluation and Research
Food and Drug Administration
5600 Fishers Lane
Rockville, MD 20857

Questions about the law can be directed to the:

Division of Regulatory Affairs (HFD-360)
Center for Drug Evaluation and Research
Food and Drug Administration
5600 Fishers Lane
Rockville, MD 20857
(301) 295-8038

DOCTOR AND PHARMACIST SENTENCED IN ILLEGAL DRUG SALES*

John Henkel

An anonymous letter first tipped off authorities two years ago that a Tennessee pharmacist and doctor were selling physician samples of various prescription drugs at a Memphis pharmacy. A subsequent seizure and search confirmed the trafficking and provided evidence to charge both men with felony violations of the Prescription Drug Marketing Act.

Last Dec. 3, Edward J. Lazarus, owner of the Georgian Hills Pharmacy, received a sentence of one year's probation, 100 hours of community service, and a $2,500 fine after pleading guilty to a single count of trading a physician drug sample.

Earlier, on July 26, 1993, James M. Anthony, M.D., was sentenced to two year's probation, six months of home detention, and a $2,000 fine. Like Lazarus, Anthony pleaded guilty to one count of trading a physician sample. The Tennessee Health Related Boards, acting on evidence of misconduct, had suspended Anthony's license on July 10, 1992. Further charges against both men were pending at press time.

Lazarus and Anthony's wrongdoing first surfaced in March 1992, when the Tennessee Board of Phar-

macy received an unsigned letter alleging that Anthony was providing physician samples to Georgian Hills Pharmacy. An investigator for the board visited the pharmacy March 30 and seized 44 containers of prescription drug products suspected of being physician samples. (Tennessee law allows such seizures without a court order if inspectors suspect violations.)

The board immediately notified FDA's Nashville district office, which teamed with the state, the Drug Enforcement Administration, the U.S. Attorney, and the U.S. Magistrate Judge to investigate Anthony and Lazarus. FDA examined the seized products and found evidence such as tablets marked "sample" mixed into an unlabeled vial with non-sample tablets.

From March 31 through May 18, 1992, the investigative team interviewed Anthony's relatives and former and current employees, patients and friends, as well as former and current employees of the pharmacy.

What emerged was the story of how Lazarus, whose business was a few doors down from the doctor's in the same strip mall, actively recruited Anthony to set up practice in the mall. To help Anthony get established, Lazarus let Anthony charge office supplies, drugs,

and other materials at the pharmacy. Anthony, in turn, sent the pharmacist customers, says Earl E. Davis, investigator in FDA's Nashville district. Such an arrangement in itself is not illegal. But Anthony broke the law when he repaid Lazarus' favors by giving him significant quantities of prescription drug samples. Lazarus then resold the drugs to his customers, some of whom were Anthony's patients.

"Anthony probably supplied Lazarus with 75 percent of his pharmacy business," says Davis. "It's very profitable for a pharmacy to have this kind of arrangement with a doctor."

With affidavits from customers, patients and others, the investigative team obtained a warrant to search the doctor's office and the pharmacy, which they served on May 21, 1992. The searches continued for a week, yielding more evidence of physician sample misuse. FDA also seized backup tapes from the pharmacy computer system, which indicated discrepancies between the amounts of suspect physician sample drugs dispensed and non-samples received at the pharmacy.

Anthony and Lazarus entered guilty pleas on Feb. 23 and Sept. 21, 1993, respectively, in the U.S. District Court for the Western District of Tennessee.

---

*Reprinted from *FDA Consumer* (June 1994).

SALES REP CONVICTED FOR SELLING PRESCRIPTION DRUG SAMPLES*

Dori Stehlin

A sales representative for a Missouri drug company who tried to sell prescription drug samples became the first person to be prosecuted and convicted under the Prescription Drug Marketing Act (PDMA) of 1988. His case led to charges being brought against eight others for similar PDMA violations.

David B. Snyder of Elizabethtown, Pa., pleaded guilty on June 26, 1990, to one count of violating the PDMA. On Dec. 7, 1990, he was sentenced to two years' probation and fined $5,050. Charges and sentencing of the others followed.

The PDMA prohibits selling, buying, trading, or offering to sell, buy or trade prescription drug samples. Pharmaceutical manufacturers and distributors routinely provide samples of their prescription drugs free to physicians who, in turn, give them to their patients either in place of a prescription, or to get the patient started on medication until the prescription can be filled. Diversion of samples from their intended use creates a risk that counterfeit, adulterated, misbranded, subpotent, or expired drugs will be sold to American consumers.

One thing that concerns FDA about these cases, says Eugene Schultz, a compliance officer in FDA's Philadelphia district office, is that "some sales reps gather the [stolen drug samples], throw them in the trunk [of their cars], and keep them there for possibly six months." That may affect the quality of the drugs, he explains, since the storage conditions are not properly controlled.

He adds that the agency is also concerned about the integrity of the drugs if the samples are re-

moved from their original packaging.

Pharmacist Helps

A pharmacist in Harrisburg brought Snyder's illegal activities to the attention of federal authorities. According to the pharmacist, Snyder had overheard him complain about how discount store prescription drug prices were hurting his business. Snyder offered to sell to the pharmacist samples of prescription drugs that were intended to be distributed free to physicians. Snyder indicated that the pharmacist would have to pay much less for the samples than he would normally pay for the same drugs purchased through a legitimate wholesaler.

The pharmacist reported Snyder's offer to the Drug Enforcement Administration's Harrisburg office in the middle of April 1989. Because the drugs Snyder was offering were not controlled substances, DEA contacted Charles Thorne, FDA's director of compliance in the agency's Philadelphia district office, on April 26, 1989, and Thorne called the pharmacist the next day.

Thorne said the pharmacist thought Snyder would be back within the week, expecting to make a sale, and asked the agency's advice on how to proceed.

After consulting with several FDA offices, Thorne and Dave Chesney, director of investigations, decided to set up undercover surveillance at the pharmacy in anticipation of Snyder's next visit. They enlisted the help of the Federal Bureau of Investigation.

FBI agents James Barnacle and John Hartmann set up electronic surveillance equipment on the morning of May 5 and, with FDA investigators William Griffin and

Marsha Major and supervisory investigator James Warn, watched the pharmacy from a van parked across the street.

Their wait was short. Snyder arrived at the pharmacy that afternoon and sold the pharmacist 18 different prescription drug products from 16 different manufacturers, including the antidepressant Prozac; ulcer treatments Tagamet, Carafate and Zantac; the anti-inflammatory Feldene; and the asthma drug Alupent.

Snyder had used acetone to remove the "sample" logo from about half of the 351 capsules of Feldene he sold to the pharmacist. Altering the capsules in that way is considered adulteration under the Federal Food, Drug, and Cosmetic Act, but the risk from any acetone residue would be minimal, according to Malcolm Williams, a toxicologist with the national Centers for Disease Control. "If he used any significant amount of acetone, it would dissolve the whole capsule," says Williams.

The pharmacist paid Snyder $1,600, which FDA had supplied to him. However, the agency estimates that the equivalent amount of bulk drugs would have had a wholesale price of approximately $3,200. After the drugs and the money changed hands, the FBI agents detained Snyder.

Others Violate PDMA

Following the detention, the U.S. attorney for the Middle District off Pennsylvania, with assistance from the FBI and FDA's general counsel, reached a plea agreement with Snyder and his attorney on May 24, 1989.

Under the plea agreement. Snyder was to help the FBI and the Department of Health and Human Services' inspector general identify

---

*Reprinted from *FDA Consumer* (October 1991).

other sales representatives and pharmacists who might be illegally buying and selling prescription drug samples. On Aug. 17, 1989, Snyder met with Saliba Shunnara, one of the pharmacists Snyder identified, in Mechanicsburg, PA, and completed a sale of drug samples. Shunnara was summoned to court and eventually charged with PDMA violations.

Information obtained from Shunnara and Snyder led to charges against three other sales representatives and four other pharmacists for PDMA violations. FDA assisted in these cases by providing technical information on the drugs involved.

Snyder and the other eight were charged in June 1990 with the sale, purchase, or offer to sell or purchase prescription drug samples.

Shunnara was sentenced on March 5, 1991, to one year's probation and fined $3,000. Michael Stephan, a sales representative for a Pennsylvania drug company, was sentenced on Jan. 25, 1991, to one year of probation and fined $250.

The charges may be dismissed for four of the pharmacists, Philip Winand of New Oxford, PA, William Welfley of Newport, PA, Herbert Gilbert of Harrisburg, PA and Gerald Wynn of Camp Hill, PA, and two of the sales representatives, Paul Carls and William

Hoover, both of Harrisburg, after a period of time set by the court if they meet the requirements of a pre-trial diversion program. The program requirements include regularly working in a lawful occupation, reporting to a government supervisor as directed, and performing 50 hours of community service. The court set the diversion program time at 12 months for all but Welfley, for whom it was set at six months.

Under the provisions of the PDMA, the pharmacist who helped the government apprehend Snyder is entitled to half of Snyder's $5,050 fine.

QUESTIONS: CHAPTER 14

1. Which president of the United States signed the Dingell Bill into law?

    a. George Bush
    b. Ronald Reagan
    c. Jimmy Carter
    d. Richard Nixon
    e. Abraham Lincoln

2. The Prescription Drug Marketing Act of 1987 prohibits:

    a. Distribution of drug samples by pharmaceutical manufacturers' sales representatives
    b. Written requests for drug samples by prescribers
    c. Written receipt for drug samples upon delivery
    d. Oral requests for drug samples by prescribers

3. The Prescription Drug Marketing Act of 1987 allows:

    a. Trading of drug samples
    b. Oral requests for drug samples by prescribers
    c. Written requests for drug samples by pharmacists
    d. Distribution of drug samples by pharmaceutical manufacturers' sales representatives upon written request by prescribers

4. The Prescription Drug Marketing Act of 1987 may also be referred to as the:

    a. Dingbat Bill
    b. Dingell Bill
    c. Diversion Bill
    d. Dingdong Bill
    e. b. and c.

5. Which of the following are allowed or required under the federal Prescription Drug Marketing Act of 1987? Indicate your answers by circling the letter to the left of each correct statement.

    a. Trading of drug samples
    b. Distribution of drug samples by manufacturer's sales representatives upon written request by prescribers
    c. Oral requests for samples by licensed practitioners
    d. Sale of drugs among hospitals under common control
    e. Written requests for drug samples by licensed practitioners
    f. Purchase of "coupons"
    g. Written receipt for drug samples upon delivery
    h. Written requests for drug samples by pharmacists
    i. Manufacturers/distributors must maintain records of all drug samples distributed for at least two years
    j. Drug samples may be distributed to a hospital pharmacy upon written request of a physician

CHAPTER 15

Narcotic Treatment Programs (Methadone Clinics)

Introduction

The Food and Drug Administration (FDA) and the National Institute on Drug Abuse (NIDA) regulation of the medical use of methadone began with Congress' passage of the Comprehensive Drug Abuse Prevention and Control Act of 1970 (P.L. 91-513). Section 4 of this Act instructed the Secretary of Health, Education, and Welfare to determine "appropriate methods of professional practice in the medical treatment of . . . narcotic addiction."

The legislative history of the act recognized that, historically, practitioners ran a significant risk of criminal prosecution under the Harrison Narcotic Act of 1914 if they used a narcotic drug in the treatment of drug addiction. Congress referred to the Supreme Court's holding in *Linder v. United States*, 268 U.S. 5, 45 S.Ct. 446, 69 L.Ed. 819 (1925) that prescribing "in the ordinary course and in good faith [a quantity of a narcotic drug], for relief of conditions incident to addition" was not violative of Federal law. Congress also pointed out that the Bureau of Narcotics' [a predecessor of the Drug Enforcement Administration (DEA)] regulations were, apparently, not in accord with the Court's language. In 1970, the Bureau's regulations stated:

> An order purporting to be a prescription issued to an addict or habitual user of narcotics, not in the course of professional treatment but for the purpose of providing the user with narcotics sufficient to keep him comfortable by maintaining his customary use, is not a prescription within the meaning and intent of the (Harrison) Act; and the person filling such an order, as well as the person issuing it, may be charged with violation of the law.   26 CFR 151.392 (1970)

Congress passed the Act of 1970 to clarify this confusing situation. Congressional intent was clear that practitioners who complied with the standards set forth in Section 4 would be assured that their action would not lead to prosecution under the Act (21 *U.S.C.* 801 et seq.).

In the early 1970s, diversion of methadone (Dolophine®, Lilly) from legitimate commerce into the illegal marketplace was becoming a serious problem. Congress wished neither to ignore this diversion nor to eliminate methadone as a treatment for narcotic drug addition. Therefore, Congress passed the Narcotic Addict Treatment Act of 1974 (P.L. 93-281, 88 Stat. 124), which allowed methadone to be dispensed for detoxification and maintenance only by practitioners who held a registration with DEA. In order for a practitioner to obtain the registration, FDA had to determine that the practitioner was complying with the standards that were established under Section 4 of the Comprehensive Drug Abuse Prevention and Control Act of 1970. During the invervening years, FDA and NIDA have issued regulations setting forth the conditions under which narcotic drugs could be dispensed for the treatment of drug addition, and establishing methadone as the only narcotic drug approved for such use.

Over the years, the regulation accumulated language that recommended certain practices in addition to requiring other practices. In order to clarify matters, the agencies have issued a guidance document. Most of the provisions are "recommended practices" originally contained in the former regulation, while other provisions were formerly mandatory provisions that are being reissued as recommendations.

This guidance document is intended to provide recommendations for providing medical and other services in addition to the regulation under 21 *CFR* 291.505. Following these recommendations should facilitate treatment for narcotic addicts. The guidance document does not represent the formal legal opinion of either FDA or NIDA.

The guidance document and the regulations contained in 21 *CFR* 291.505 are not meant to preclude States from regulating the practice of medicine in the treatment of narcotic drug addicts. States are free to provide additional requirements for practitioners dispensing methadone for treatment of narcotic addicts. The recommendations of the agencies follow.

Services

Required medical services and counseling, rehabilitative, and other social services (e.g., vocational and educational guidance, employment placement) should normally be made available directly by the sponsor at the primary outpatient facility, but the program sponsor may enter into a formal agreement, which must be documented [21 *CFR* 291.505(b)(2)(iii)], with private or public agencies, organizations, or institutions for these services to be provided on site or elsewhere. Such facilities should be easily accessible to the patient. The patient's progress at the referral agency should be periodically updated.

Hospital Affiliation

If a program is not physically located within a hospital that has agreed to provide any needed medical care for drug-related problems for the program's patients, there should be a formal, documented agreement between the program sponsor and a responsible official of a licensed and accredited hospital demonstrating that hospital care, including emergency, inpatient, and ambulatory care, is fully available to any patient who may need it for such problems. It is suggested that the program sponsor enter into an agreement with the hospital official to provide general medical care for patients. Neither the program sponsor nor the hospital is required to assume financial responsibility for the patient's medical care.

Medication Units

Medication units should normally be located at some distance from the program's primary facility and other medication units so as to serve a separate and distinct geographic area. The enrollment in a medication unit should be of reasonable size in relation to the space available for treatment.

Current Physiological Dependence

In determining current physiologic dependence, the physician should consider signs and symptoms of intoxication, a positive urine specimen for a narcotic drug, and old or fresh needle marks. Other evidence of current physiologic dependence may be obtained by noting early signs of withdrawal (lacrimation, rhinorrhea, pupilary dilation and piloerection) during the initial period of abstinence. Withdrawal signs may be observed during the initial period of hospitalization or while the person is an outpatient undergoing diagnostic evaluation (e.g., medical and personal history, physical examination, and laboratory studies). Increased body temperature, pulse rate, blood pressure, and respiratory rate are also signs of withdrawal, but their detection may require inpatient observation. It is unlikely but possible that a person could be currently dependent on narcotic drugs without having a positive urine test for narcotics. Conversely, it is possible that a person could have a positive urine test for narcotics and not be currently physiologically dependent. Thus, a urine sample that is positive for narcotics is not a requirement for admission to detoxification or maintenance treatment.

Drug Screening Urinalysis

The person(s) responsible for the program who uses the results of presumptive urinalysis for patient management should show evidence of reasonable access to confirmatory laboratory analysis for use on occasions when this is necessary, e.g., for intake urine testing on all prospective methadone patients, for any loss of patient privileges based on urinalysis, and for indicating frequency of use of other drugs not detectable by a screening method.

After the initial drug screening urinalysis, urine specimens for each patient should be collected and analyzed on a randomly scheduled basis at least monthly. More frequent testing for a specific drug(s) and for a specific person should occur when clinically indicated as determined by the reasonable clinical judgment of the medical director. Results of urine testing should be used as one clinical tool for the purposes of diagnosis, and in the determination of treatment plans, as well as used as one technique for overall program evaluation by monitoring patient drug-using patterns before and during treatment.

Contents of Medical Evaluation

The following laboratory examinations should be conducted for each patient on admission to a program in addition to the required examinations stated in 21 *CFR* 291.505(d)(3)(i):

1. complete blood count and differential
2. routine and microscopic urinalysis
3. liver functions profile, e.g., SGOT and SGPT
4. when the tuberculin skin test is positive, a chest X-ray or other appropriate tests
5. Hepatitis B surface antigen (HBsAg) testing
6. when clinically indicate, an EKG
7. when appropriate, pregnancy test and a Pap test
8. other tests when clinically indicated

When a person is readmitted to a program, it is recommended that the decision determining the appropriate laboratory tests to be conducted be based on the intervening medical history and a physical examination.

Admission Evaluation

A patient's history should include information relating to his or her psychosocial, economic, and family background, and any other information deemed necessary by the program that is relevant to the application or economic, educational, and vocational strengths and weaknesses, that a patient brings to the treatment setting. Each program should establish its own methods for measuring those strengths and weaknesses to assess the severity of the patient's problem, establish realistic treatment goals, and develop an appropriate treatment plan to achieve these goals. Such assessments should be made on admission or as soon as the patient is stable enough for appropriate interviewing. Treatment plans should reflect individualization geared to the patient's needs.

Initial Treatment Plan

The short-term goals contained in the initial treatment plan should be designed to expect completion within a finite time period, e.g., up to 180 days.

The information contained in the initial treatment plan should be in sufficient detail to demonstrate that each patient has been assessed and that the services provided are based on the patient assessment findings and the available program and community services.

Patients need varying degrees of treatment and rehabilitative services which are often dependent on or limited by a number of variables, e.g., patient resources, available program, and community services. It is not the intent of 21 *CFR* 291.505 or the guidance document to prescribe a particular treatment and rehabilitative service or the frequency at which a service should be offered.

The program physician or the primary counselor shall review, re-evaluate, and alter where necessary each patient's treatment plan at least once each 90 days during the first year of treatment, and then at least twice a year after the first year of continuous treatment.

The program physician shall ensure that the periodic treatment plan becomes part of each patient's record and that it is signed and dated in the patient's record by the primary counselor and is countersigned and dated by the supervisory counselor.

At least once a year, the program physician shall date, review, and countersign the treatment plan recorded in each patient's record and ensure that each patient's progress or lack of progress in achieving the treatment goals is entered in the patient's record by the primary counselor. When appropriate, the treatment plan and progress notes should deal with the patient's mental and physical problems, apart from drug abuse. The treatment plan is required to include the name of and the reasons for prescribing any medication for emotional or physical problems.

Pregnant Patients

If a pregnant patient refuses direct prenatal services or appropriate referral for prenatal services, the treating program physician should consider using informed consent procedures, i.e., to have the patient acknowledge in writing that she had the opportunity for this treatment but refused it.

Caution should be taken in the maintenance treatment of pregnant patients. Dosage levels should be maintained at the lowest effective dose if continued methadone treatment is deemed necessary. Detoxification treatment is not recommended for a pregnant patient.

Minimum Standards for Short-Term Detoxification Treatment

For short-term detoxification from narcotic drugs, the narcotic drug is required to be administered by the program physician or by an authorized agent of the physician, supervised by and under the order of the physician. The narcotic drug is required to be administered daily under close observation, in reducing dosages over a period not to exceed 30 days. All requirements for maintenance treatment apply to short-term detoxification treatment with the following exceptions:

Take-home medication is not allowed during short-term detoxification.

A history of 1 year physiologic dependence is not required for admission to short-term detoxification.

Patients who have been determined by the program physican to be currently physiologically narcotic dependent may be placed in short-term detoxification treatment, regardless of age.

A patient is required to wait at least 7 days between concluding a short-term detoxification treatment episode and beginning another.

Initial Dose

The initial dose of methadone should be given in an amount considered sufficient to control or mitigate abstinence symptoms concomitant to withdrawal of narcotic drugs. Currently, there is no absolutely reliable method available to determine narcotic tolerance levels. Thus, determination of the optimum initial dose is made on a case-by-case basis. Methadone dosages that are lower than the patient's current level of narcotic tolerance may result in the patient's experiencing withdrawal symptoms. Dosages sufficiently greater than the current level of narcotic tolerance can result in central nervous system depression, coma, and death. Therefore, it is important that the initial dose be adjusted individually to the narcotic tolerance of the patient. If the patient has been a heavy user of heroin up to the day of admission, he or she may require an initial dose of 30 to 40 milligrams with additional smaller increments 4 to 8 hours later. It is recommended practice that if the patient enters treatment with little or no narcotic tolerance (e.g., recently released from jail or using poor quality heroin), the initial dose be one-half these quantities. If there is any doubt, the smaller dose should be used initially and the patient kept under observation; if the symptoms of abstinence are distressing, an additional 5- to 10-milligram dose should be administered as needed. Subsequently, the dosage should be adjusted individually as tolerated and required. The stabilization dose frequently, but not necessarily, is higher than the dose needed to reduce withdrawal severity. The usual range of methadone maintenance dosages in the United States is between 30 and 100 milligrams daily.

Maintenance Dosage

The program physician should regularly review each patient's dosage level, carefully considering either increasing or decreasing the dosage as indicated. It should be noted that, according to the official approved labeling, therapeutic doses of meperidine have precipitated severe reactions in patients currently receiving monoamine oxidase inhibitors or those who have received such agents within 14 days. Similar reactions have not yet been reported with methadone, but if the use of methadone is necessary in such patients, it is recommended that a sensitivity test be performed in which repeated small incremental doses are administered over the course of several hours while the patient's condition and vital signs are under careful observation. Likewise, physicians should also be aware that according to the official approved labeling, concurrent administration of rifampin may possibly reduce the blood concentration of methadone to a degree sufficient to produce withdrawal symptoms. The mechanism by which rifampin may decrease blood concentrations of methadone is not fully understood, although enhanced microsomal drug-metabolized enzymes may influence drug disposition.

Minimum Standards for Long-Term Detoxification Treatment

For long-term detoxification from narcotic drugs, the narcotic drug is required to be administered by the program physician or by an authorized agent of the physician, supervised by and under the order of the physician. The narcotic drug is required to be administered on a regimen designed to reach a drug-free state and to make progress in rehabilitation in 180

days or less. All requirements for maintenance treatment apply to long-term detoxification treatment with the following exceptions.

In long-term detoxification treatment it is required that the patient be under observation while ingesting the drug daily or at least 6 days a week, for the duration of the long-term detoxification treatment.

A history of 1 year physiologic dependence is not required for admission to long-term detoxification.

The program physician shall document in the patient's record that short-term detoxification is not a sufficiently long enough treatment course to provide the patient with the additional program services he or she deems necessary for the patient's rehabilitation. The program physician shall document this information in the patient's record before long-term detoxification may begin.

A patient is required to wait at least 7 days between concluding a long-term treatment episode and beginning another. Before a long-term detoxification attempt is repeated, the program physician shall document in the patient's record that the patient continues to be or is again physiologically dependent on narcotic drugs. The provisions of these requirements apply to both inpatient and ambulatory long-term detoxification treatment.

Methadone Formulation

Hospitalized patients under care for a medical or surgical condition are permitted to receive methadone in parenteral form when the attending physician judges it advisable. Although tablet, syrup concentrate or other formulations may be distributed to the program, all oral medication is required to be administered or dispensed in a liquid formulation. The oral dosage form is required to be formulated in such a way as to reduce its potential for parenteral abuse. Take-home medication is required to be labeled with the treatment center's name, address, and telephone number and must be packaged in special packaging as required by 16 CFR 1700.14 in accordance with the Poison Prevention Packaging Act (P.L. 91-601, 15 U.S.C. 1471 et seq.) to reduce the chances of accidental ingestion. Exceptions may be granted when these provisions conflict with State law with regard to the administering or dispensing of drugs.

Take-Home Requirements

The requirement of time in treatment is a minimum reference point after which a patient may be eligible for take-home privileges. The time reference is not intended to mean that a patient in treatment for a particular time has a specific right to take-home medication. Thus, regardless of time in treatment, a program physician may, in his or her reasonable judgment, deny or rescind the take-home medication privileges of a patient.

In maintenance treatment it is required that a patient come to the clinic for observation daily or at least 6 days a week. If, in the reasonable clinical judgment of the program physician, a patient demonstrates that he or she has satisfactorily adhered to program rules *for at least 3 months,* has made substantial progress in rehabilitation and responsibility in handling narcotic drugs and would improve his or her rehabilitative progress by decreasing the frequency of attendance at the clinic for observation, the patient may be permitted to reduce his or her attendance at the clinic for observation to three times weekly. *The patient may receive no more than a 2-day take-home supply of medication.*

If a patient demonstrates that he or she has satisfactorily adhered to program rules *for at least 2 years* from his or her entrance into the program, the patient may be permitted to reduce his or her clinic attendance at the clinic for observation *to twice weekly. Such a patient may receive no more than a 3-day take-home supply of medication.*

If a patient demonstrates that he or she has satisfactorily adhered to program rules *for at least 3 consecutive years* from his or her entrance into the maintenance treatment program, has made substantial progress in rehabilitation, has no major behavioral problems, is responsible in handling narcotic drugs, and would improve his or her rehabilitative progress by decreasing the frequency of his or her clinic attendance for observation, the patient may be permitted to reduce clinic attendance for observation to once weekly, provided that the following additional criteria are met: The program physician has written into the patient's record an evaluation that the patient is responsible in handling narcotic drugs; the patient is employed (or actively seeking employment), attends school, is a homemaker, or is considered unemployable for mental or physical reasons by a program physician; the patient is not known to have abused drugs including alcohol in the last year; and the patient is not known to have engaged in criminal activity; e.g., drug dealing, in the last year. *A patient permitted to reduce clinic attendance for observation to once weekly may receive no more than a 6-day take-home supply of medication.*

Compounder

An entity engaging in maintenance treatment or detoxification treatment which also changes the dosage form of a narcotic drug for use in maintenance treatment or detoxification treatment at other locations.

There are six (6) registration categories (business activities) of Narcotic Treatment Programs:

1. Maintenance Program Only
2. Detoxification Program Only
3. Maintenance and Detoxification Program
4. Compounder with a Maintenance Program
5. Compounder with a Detoxification Program
6. Compounder with both a Maintenance and Detoxification Program

Every program must register under the category which applies to its business activity.

A program may register for detoxification and/or maintenance or compounder with detoxification and/or maintenance. The program must register as a compounder if they compound narcotics on the premises for use at a program on-site and off-site. If compounding or distribution for other programs occurs at a location where no program exists, then the compounding location must register with DEA as a manufacturer and/or distributor.

Problems have arisen regarding narcotic prescription orders (primarily in methadone). According to DEA regulations, a physician may prescribe methadone or any other narcotic for a patient in severe pain only. A patient who is to be or is being maintained or detoxified cannot receive a narcotic prescription order for this purpose. The patient must receive the necessary narcotics at a registered narcotic treatment program. In this case, the narcotic can be dispensed or administered to the patient, but not prescribed.

Furthermore, the regulations state that only four specific individuals employed by the narcotic treatment program can dispense or administer narcotics to the patients: (1) the licensed physician, (2) a registered nurse under the direction of the licensed physician, (3) a licensed practical nurse under the direction of the licensed physician, or (4) a pharmacist under the direction of the licensed physician. This regulation prohibits the receptionist or counselor or another untrained individual (in some cases even a patient) from administering narcotics to the patient.

21 *CFR* Sections 1306.07(b) and (c) have also raised several questions regarding narcotic treatment programs:

A physician who is not a part of a narcotic treatment program may administer narcotic drugs to an addicted individual on a daily basis for not more than a three (3) day period to relieve that individual's acute withdrawal symptoms while the physician makes arrangements to enroll the individual in a narcotic treatment program. This treatment cannot last more than three (3) days and may not be renewed or extended.

A hospital that has no program on the premises or a physician who is not part of a treatment program may administer narcotics to a drug dependent individual for either detoxification or maintenance purposes if the individual is being treated for a condition other than the addiction. It is assumed that the physician or hospital staff will not take advantage of this situation and detoxify or maintain a drug dependent person who has sustained a very minor injury or illness which will not prevent the person from going to a registered program. Also, a physician is allowed to exercise sound medical judgment and to dispense or administer narcotics to an individual for extended periods for the purpose of relieving intractable pain for which no other relief or cure is known. An example of this would be terminal cancer patients or patients with painful chronic disorders.

Definitions

Detoxification Treatment means the dispensing of a narcotic drug in decreasing doses to an individual to alleviate adverse physiological or psychological effects incident to withdrawal from the continuous or sustained use of a narcotic drug and as a method of bringing the individual to a narcotic drug-free state within such period. There are two types of detoxification treatment: short-term detoxification treatment and long-term detoxification treatment.

21 CFR 291.505(a)(1)

Short-Term Detoxification Treatment is for a period not in excess of 30 days.

21 CFR 291.505(a)(1)(i)

Long-Term Detoxification Treatment is for a period more than 30 days but not in excess of 180 days.

21 CFR 291.505(a)(1)(ii)

Maintenance Treatment means the dispensing of a narcotic drug in the treatment of an individual for dependence on heroin or other morphine-like drug.

21 CFR 291.505(a)(2)

Narcotic Dependent means an individual who physiologically needs heroin or a morphine-like drug to prevent the onset of signs of withdrawal.

21 CFR 291.505(a)(5)

Narcotic Treatment Program is an organization (or a person, including a private physician) that administers or dispenses a narcotic drug to a narcotic addict for maintenance or detoxification treatment, provides, when appropriate or necessary, a comprehensive range of medical and rehabilitative services, is approved by the State authority and the Food and Drug Administration, and that is registered with the Drug Enforcement Administration to use a narcotic drug for the treatment of narcotic addiction.

21 CFR 291.505(a)(6)

Program Sponsor is a person (or representative of an organization) who is responsible for the operation of a narcotic treatment program and who assumes responsibility for all its employees including any practitioners, agents, or other persons providing services at the program (including its medication units).

21 CFR 291.505(a)(7)

Methadone may be used as an analgesic in severe pain, for the detoxification of narcotic addicts, and as an oral substitute for heroin or other morphine-like drugs, in the maintenance treatment of narcotic addicts, pursuant to the conditions established in 21 CFR 291.505. Further data and information are required to establish the safety and effectiveness of methadone under a variety of conditions during widespread and long-term use. In view of the tremendous public health and social problems associated with the use of heroin, the demonstrated usefulness of methadone in treatment, the lack of a safe and effective

alternative drug or treatment modality, the need for additional safety and effectiveness data on methadone for narcotic addict treatment and the danger to health that could be created by uncontrolled distribution and use of methadone for narcotic addict treatment, the Commissioner of Food and Drugs finds that it is not in the public interest either to withhold the drug from the market until it has been proved safe and effective under all conditions of use for narcotic addict treatment or to grant full approval for unrestricted distribution, prescription, dispensing, or administration of methadone for this use. The Commissioner therefore concludes that it is essential to the public interest to prescribe detailed conditions for safe and effective use of methadone for narcotic addict treatment, utilizing the IND and NDA control mechanisms and the authority granted under the Comprehensive Drug Abuse Prevention and Control Act of 1970, to assure that the required additional information for assessing the safety and effectiveness of methadone is obtained, to maintain close control over the safe distribution, administration, and dispensing of the drug, and to detail responsibilities for such control. The conditions established in 21 CFR 291.505 constitute a determination of the appropriate methods of professional practice in the medical treatment of the narcotic addiction of various classes of narcotic addicts with respect to the use of methadone, pursuant to Section 4 of the Comprehensive Drug Abuse Prevention and Control Act of 1970.

21 CFR 310.304(b)

Initial Detoxification Dose

The recommended initial dose in detoxification treatment is 30 to 40 milligrams total dose for the first day.

Discontinuation of Methadone Use

Involuntary termination from treatment. The person(s) responsible for a program should develop and post prominently about the program premises at least one copy of a written policy establishing criteria for involuntary termination from treatment. This policy should describe patients' rights as well as the responsibilities and rights of the program staff. At the time a patient enters treatment, an appropriate program staff member designated by the person(s) responsible for the program should inform the patient where the copy of the policy is posted and should inform him or her of the reasons for which he or she might be terminated from treatment, his or her right under the involuntary termination procedure, and the fact that information about him or her shall be kept confidential in accordance with 42 CFR Part 2.

Voluntary withdrawal from methadone use. As with most types of medical treatment that require prolonged daily administration of medication, patients in a methadone treatment program should be evaluated periodically regarding the risks and benefits of continuing the medication. For some, the eventual withdrawal from methadone is a realistic goal. However, years of experience demonstrate that for others this goal is not yet realistic, even though these patients show vocational, educational, and psychosocial improvement, and are productive members of society. Research and clinical experience have not yet identified all the critical variables that determine when a patient can be successfully withdrawn from methadone and remain drug free. Thus, the determination to withdraw voluntarily from methadone maintenance is empirical and is left to the patient and the reasonable clinical judgment of the physician. Upon reaching a drug-free state, the patient should be encouraged to remain in the program for as long as the program considers it necessary to ensure stability in the drug-free state. The frequency of required program visits for patients for drug-free state may be adjusted at the discretion of the medical director.

Source: Guidance on the Use of Methadone in Maintenance and Detoxification Treatment of Narcotic Addicts. Center for Drug Evaluation and Research, FDA, DHHS and 21 *CFR* 291.505.

Alternative to Methadone

A longer acting alternative to methadone is available, which, like methadone, blocks cravings for heroin and is currently used to treat heroin addicts in most states. The drug, levomethadyl acetate hydrochloride, commonly known as LAAM is marketed in the United States by Roxane Laboratories by the brand name Orlaam.

QUESTIONS: CHAPTER 15

1. In which dosage form must methadone be dispensed to a narcotic addict enrolled in a narcotic treatment program?
   a. Tablet or capsule
   b. Tablet or oral liquid
   c. Oral liquid or parenteral
   d. Oral liquid
   e. Parenteral

2. Which one of the following statutes allowed methadone to be dispensed for the detoxification and maintenance to narcotic addicts?
   a. Comprehensive Drug Abuse Prevention and Control Act of 1970
   b. Narcotic Addict Treatment Act of 1974
   c. Harrison Narcotic Act of 1914
   d. Federal Food, Drug, and Cosmetic Act

3. In which controlled substance schedule does methadone belong?
   a. I
   b. II
   c. III
   d. IV
   e. V

4. The liquid vehicle for the oral dosage form of methadone may be:
   a. Bittersweet
   b. Non-sweetened
   c. Sweetened with Sweet-'N-Low®
   d. A syrup base

5. Which one of the following is the trade name for methadone?
   a. Lomotil
   b. Percodan
   c. Dolophine
   d. Methophine
   e. Napadone

6. The long-term detoxification period of an addict using methadone is:

    a. 7–10 days

    b. 10–21 days

    c. 30–60 days

    d. 60–180 days

    e. 30–180 days

7. The maintenance treatment period of an addict using methadone is in excess of:

    a. 21 days

    b. 30 days

    c. 60 days

    d. 90 days

    e. 180 days

8. Which of the following is the generic name for Dolophine?

    a. Meprobamate

    b. Meperidine

    c. Methophine

    d. Methadone

    e. Napadone

9. An addict enrolled in a treatment program for at least three months may be provided with a ____ days supply of take-home medication:

    a. 2

    b. 3

    c. 6

    d. 10

    e. 21

10. How many days supply of take-home methadone is allowed if the addict has been enrolled in a treatment program for two years?

    a. 2

    b. 3

    c. 6

    d. 10

    e. 180

11. How many days supply of take-home methadone is permitted to be dispensed to an addict if he/she has been enrolled in a treatment program for at least three years?

    a. 2

    b. 3

    c. 6

    d. 21

    e. 180

12. The short-term detoxification treatment period of an addict using methadone is limited to:

    a. 7 days

    b. 10 days

    c. 21 days

    d. 30 days

    e. 60 days

13. Which of the following is not an FDA approved use for methadone?

    a. Detoxification treatment

    b. Maintenance treatment

    c. Analgesic

    d. Analgesic against severe pain

    e. Temporary maintenance treatment of patient hospitalized for a medical condition other than addiction

14. In which dosage form are hospitalized patients under care for a medical or surgical condition permitted to receive methadone if deemed advisable by the attending physician?

    a. Tablet or capsule

    b. Tablet or oral liquid

    c. Oral liquid or parenteral

    d. Oral liquid

    e. Parenteral

15. To reduce the chances of accident ingestion of a liquid formulation of take-home methadone, it must be packaged pursuant to the:

    a. Comprehensive Drug Abuse Prevention and Control Act of 1970

    b. Harrison-Ford Narcotic Act of 1914

    c. Federal Food, Drug, and Cosmetic Act of 1938

    d. Poison Prevention Packaging Act of 1970

    e. Drug Addict Treatment Act of 1981

16. Which of the following statements is **correct** in regard to treatment of an addict with methadone?

    1) Take home medication is not allowed during short-term detoxification

    2) Oral medication is required to be dispensed in a liquid formulation

    3) Take home medication must be packaged pursuant to the provisions of the Federal Food, Drug, and Cosmetic Act of 1938

    4) Short-term detoxification treatment is for a period not in excess of 60 days

    5) Long-term detoxification treatment is for a period more than 30 days but not in excess of 100 days

        a. 1) and 2) are correct

        b. 1), 2), and 3) are correct

        c. 3), 4), and 5) are correct

        d. 2) and 4) are correct

        e. 1), 2), 3), and 5) are correct

17. Which of the following statements is **incorrect** in regard to treatment of an addict with methadone?

    1) Take home medication is not allowed during short-term detoxification

    2) Oral medication is required to be dispensed in a liquid formulation

    3) Take home medication must be packaged pursuant to the provisions of the Federal Food, Drug, and Cosmetic Act of 1938

    4) Short-term detoxification treatment is for a period not in excess of 60 days

    5) Long-term detoxification treatment is for a period more than 30 days but not in excess of 100 days

        a. 1) and 2) are correct

        b. 1), 2), and 3) are correct

        c. 3), 4), and 5) are correct

        d. 2) and 4) are correct

        e. 1), 2), 3), and 5) are correct

CHAPTER 16

The Orange Book

THE FOOD AND DRUG ADMINISTRATION'S ADVICE ON THERAPEUTIC EQUIVALENCE*

Don Hare and Thomas Foster, Pharm. D.

Following the repeal of the brandname antisubstitution laws by the states, the Food and Drug Administration (FDA) received numerous requests for assistance in developing drug formularies.

The FDA Commissioner, in response to these requests, notified appropriate state health officials of FDA's intention to compile a list of all marketed prescription drug products that have been approved for safety and effectiveness. This list would include therapeutic equivalence recommendations for all multisource drug products identified. The list would be useful to the states in implementing their drug product selection laws.

This list, entitled the *Approved Drug Products with Therapeutic Equivalence Evaluations*, more commonly known as the "Orange Book," was first published in October 1980. The Orange Book is now also printed as Volume III of the *USP DI*.

In the list, FDA provides guidance to the state authorities rather than to community pharmacies. More than 50% of the states provide a formulary based on this list for use by pharmacists. However, in states that do not have a formulary, the Orange Book can guide the community pharmacist in drug product selection.

PHARMACEUTICAL EQUIVALENTS

The Orange Book lists all multisource drug products grouped as "pharmaceutical equivalents." Pharmaceutical equivalents are drug products that contain the same active ingredient in the same concentration, dosage form, and route of administration. For example, under "oral dicyclomine hydrochloride capsules," the 1989 Orange Book lists Bentyl (dicyclomine hydrochloride, Merrell Dow), the innovator, and three generic products.

All drug products listed within a pharmaceutically equivalent category are assigned a two-letter code in which the first letter refers to therapeutic equivalence or inequivalence with other products in the category. Drug products with the first letter code of "A" are considered therapeutically equivalent. For example, Atarax (hydroxyzine hydrochloride, Roerig) and the 16 generic oral hydroxyzine hydrochloride tablets all have an A code and, therefore, are rated therapeutically equivalent.

Drug products with a "B" code—for example, Decadron (dexamethasone) and the eight generic oral dexamethasone tablets—are not considered therapeutically equivalent. The B code indicates that the products have a documented therapeutic inequivalence or have potential equivalency problems that have not been resolved and are not recommended for substitution by FDA.

The second letter of the code used in the Orange Book provides additional information about therapeutic equivalence or inequivalence.

A more complete definition of the codes can be found in the preface to the Orange Book. It should be noted that the percentage of B-rated drugs to the total number of multisource drugs listed in the Orange Book is now less than 10%.

OTHER INFORMATION

Single-source drug products are listed in the Orange Book as are nonprescription preparations that require FDA approval, such as insulin injections and 200-mg ibuprofen tablets, but without a therapeutic equivalence code. The Orange Book also contains other lists, such as available biopharmaceutic guidances. The Orange Book does not contain "pre-38" or "grandfathered" drugs—drugs marketed before pas-

---

*Reprinted from *American Pharmacy*, NS30:35–41 (July 1990).

sage of the Federal Food, Drug, and Cosmetic Act of 1938. Excluded are such legally marketed drugs as thyroid tablets or Lanoxin (digoxin) tablets. They are not included because the FDA has not reviewed these drugs for safety and efficacy and does not have the information necessary to make a recommendation for therapeutic equivalence. Some related pre-38 products such as Synthroid (levothyroxine sodium) tablets that are marketed without approved New Drug Applications (NDAs) or Abbreviated New Drug Applications (ANDAs) are also not listed.

Three other classes of drugs, although small, are not listed in the Orange Book because they have not been approved as safe and effective by FDA:

• Drug Efficacy Study Implementation (DESI) drug products (approved for safety only between 1938 and 1962) for which efficacy has not been demonstrated by the applicant and for which FDA has issued a notice of opportunity for hearing (NOOH) to withdraw approval of the application, e.g., Librax capsules and Donnatal tablets.

DESI drug products for which clinical efficacy studies are being conducted but are not yet completed, such as nitroglycerin patches.

Drug products that have never been approved but are similar and related to a DESI drug product that was raised to the effective status, such as Fiorinal with Codeine capsules, Naldecon, and Azo Gantrisin tablets.

For products not listed in the Orange Book, FDA makes no recommendation regarding drug product selection.

PROFESSIONAL JUDGMENT NEEDED

The introduction to the Orange Book cautions that it *is a source of information and advice* on drug

---

Questions Frequently Asked about the Orange Book

Reprinted with Permission from the Preface of Volume III of *USP DI*

The following questions and answers were abstracted and compiled from a survey of questions asked by State Boards of Pharmacy and responded to by FDA representatives at the annual meeting of the National Association of Boards of Pharmacy in 1988.

Question: Does the FDA ever plan to cover all legend drugs authorized for manufacturing in the U.S.A.? If not, why not?

Answer: There are two classes of unapproved prescription* drug products that are presently permitted by the FDA to remain on the market:

1. copies of drugs first marketed before 1938; and

2. certain DESI ineffective products awaiting completion of the FDA's administrative procedures. FDA is planning to initiate a program to declare all versions of pre-1938 drugs to be new drugs and require an approved application for a drug product to either stay or come on the market. Products deemed ineffective after the administrative and legal procedures of the DESI process are

---

*****Editor's Note:** Relatively few nonprescription medications enter the market through the New Drug Application procedures.

completed will come off the market. There are currently only a few drugs remaining in this category.

Question: How does the FDA revise its evaluation of a product based on adverse reports?

Answer: Adverse events, including therapeutic failures, may be reported for any drug. Therapeutic failures occur even when the drug product is not changed, as is evident from the reports we receive. Blood pressures can rise on previously effective therapy; heart failure can worsen on a stable digoxin/diuretic regimen; seizures can break through, etc. We would not consider changing our therapeutic equivalence evaluations unless evidence exists that the adverse reports (e.g., therapeutic failures) were due to the specific drug product rather than to a patient or drug substance problem. If such data were presented to us, we would change the code to therapeutically inequivalent or remove the product from the market.

Question: How long does it take for a drug to appear in the Orange Book?

Answer: The Orange Book is updated monthly. Each cumulative supplement indicates the time period covered by it.

Question: Is the Orange Book an official national compendium and authoritative source which can be used to provide protection in civil suits? Does it have force of law?

Answer: The Orange Book is not an official national compendium. The Orange Book displays the FDA's therapeutic equivalence recommendations on approved multiple source drug products. The FDA's evaluation of therapeutic equivalence is a scientific judgment based upon data submitted to the FDA. Generic substitution is a social and economic policy administered at the state level intended to minimize the cost of drugs to consumers. The programs are administered by the states, because the practices of pharmacy and medicine are state functions. The question of liability is not one in the FDA's area of expertise. We suggest that counsel in your state be consulted. The Orange Book does not have force of law. The preface of the Orange Book addresses this issue.

Question: [Can FDA] provide tips on how to explain to physicians that drugs that are bioequivalent are indeed therapeutically equivalent?

Many believe that drugs are not necessarily therapeutically equivalent, just because they are bioequivalent.

Answer: 1. The FDA is not aware of one clinical study that compared two drug products evaluated by the FDA as bioequivalent/therapeutic equivalent that demonstrate therapeutic inequivalence.

2. In the majority of cases the marketed innovator's product is not the formulation that was tested in clinical trials. The marketed innovator's drug product was shown to be therapeutically equivalent to the formulation that was used in the clinical trials by a bioavailability/bioequivalence study. Therefore, a generic drug product and the innovator's drug product stand in the same relationship to the formulation that was originally tested for safety and effectiveness.

Question: How does the Orange Book relate to and/or impact on state formularies?

Answer: It became apparent to the FDA soon after the repeal of the anti-substitution laws by the states that it could not serve the needs of each state on an individual basis in the preparation of their formularies. In 1978 the Commissioner of Food and Drugs notified appropriate officials of all states of the FDA's intention to provide a list of all prescription drug products that had been approved by the FDA for safety and effectiveness, with therapeutic equivalence recommendations being made on all multiple source drug products in the list. This list could be used by each state in implementing its own law and would relieve the FDA of expending an enormous amount of resources to provide individualized service to all states. Three copies of the Orange Book continue to be sent to state officials for their use in implementing their respective state laws. The states are under no mandate to accept the therapeutic equivalence recommendations in the Orange Book.

Question: What is the applicability of the Orange Book in a community pharmacy setting?

Answer: It was never the FDA's intention to have the Orange Book used in community pharmacies. However, a state could implement its law with this as a requirement.

Question: What is the legal status of pharmaceutical substitution of a different dosage form of a given drug entity? Can the FDA provide any assistance in identifying potential therapeutic problems (or therapeutic comparisons) between available dosage forms?

Answer: The Orange Book does not mandate which drug products may or may not be substituted. The therapeutic equivalence evaluations in the Orange Book are recommendations only. However, the FDA does not recommend substitution between different dosage forms. The Agency has very few bioequivalence studies in its files comparing different dosage forms of a given drug entity.

Question: Does the FDA have any way of identifying which distributors are marketing a given manufacturer's product and providing that information in the Orange Book?

Answer: No. Since an approved supplement is not required for an applicant with an approved drug product to license a distributor, FDA has no good mechanism to monitor distributors and to know when they change manufacturers.

---

product selection, *not a substitute for the professional judgment* of pharmacists and physicians. Drugs that share A codes may still vary in ways that could affect patient acceptance (such as color, flavor, shape, and packaging) and selection (such as preservatives, expiration date, and sometimes labeling). Therapeutic alternatives—for example, different salts or esters of the same active drug—are not listed as equivalent even though some physicians may prescribe them interchangeably.

In conclusion it should be emphasized that FDA believes it is the pharmacists's prerogative to decide whether to practice drug product selection. However, FDA firmly believes that generic drug products reviewed by FDA and recommended as therapeutically equivalent—those with an A code—can be dispensed with the full expectation that the patient will receive the same clinical effect as that of the innovator product or other generic products listed within that pharmaceutically equivalent category.

Purchasing the Orange Book

A subscription to the Orange Book, which includes the 1990 Basic Manual and monthly supplements, is available for $91 from the Superintendent of Documents, U.S. Government Printing Office, Washington, DC 20402-9372.

A subscription to the *USP DI Approved Drug Products and Legal Requirements*, Volume III, includes one book and six bimonthly updates, which is available for $59 from the United States Pharmacopeial Convention, Inc., Order Processing Department, 12601 Twinbrook Parkway, Rockville, MD 20852.

GUIDELINES FOR PHARMACISTS PERFORMING PRODUCT SELECTION

Dispensing Decisions

APhA's Bioequivalency Working Group recommends that pharmacists consider the following factors when selecting drug products to be dispensed to their patients. Not all of these factors will apply to each situation nor are they of equal weight. We believe if pharmacists consider these points as part of the professional judgment process when making drug product selections, it is likely that the best interests of the patients will be served. It is the responsibility of the pharmacist to use professional judgment in selecting the product.

• *State Rules and Regulations.* All states have legal requirements that address the issue of drug product selection. Pharmacists should be cognizant of these requirements and how they may impact their role in drug product selection. State regulations also might provide information and guidance in drug product selection through positive or negative formularies.

• *Bioequivalency Information/ Orange Book Ratings.* Only products with proven bioequivalency should be selected to be dispensed in lieu of the innovator product. Products being dispensed in response to a prescription drug order that is written generically should be expected to produce a therapeutic benefit for the patient at a reasonable cost. Products that are listed in the FDA's *Approved Drug Products and Therapeutic Evaluation* [1] (the Orange Book) as ''A'' rated should be selected when such products are available. For pre-1938 drugs, the selection should be based on data obtained from the literature, because bioequivalency testing is not required by the FDA for these drug products. FDA's review of the applicant's bioequivalency study is available under Freedom of Information (FOI) [2].

• *Dosage Form.* The type of dosage form should be considered whenever one drug product is selected from among multisource drug products. This is especially true with extended or delayed release medications. The Orange Book does not rate any different dosage forms as therapeutically equivalent.

• *Previous Drug Use.* Two questions should be considered regarding previous drug product usage. First, is the prescribed drug a continuation of already successful therapy? If it is, only a bioequivalent product should be selected, and the impact of any change in source of the medication should be considered. The pharmacist should also know which product the patient was using previously, including any medications in the hospital if the patient was recently discharged. Second, was the original product dispensed a generic product? If so, preference should be given to continuing to dispense

the same generic product from the same source.

• *Patient Status.* The pharmacist should consider how well controlled the patient is and how susceptible that patient might be to small changes in drug absorption. If a patient has labile control or has experienced great difficulty in achieving control, the pharmacist should continue therapy with a product from a single source throughout therapy.

• *Diseases.* The seriousness of the disease and its potential impact on the patient may influence the pharmacist's willingness to change products.

• *Drug Class or Category.* Drugs with narrow therapeutic ranges and with known clinically significant bioavailability problems should be substituted with care and/or after discussion with the prescriber.

• *Cost.* The cost of the product, while an important consideration, should be a secondary consideration in selecting among products judged by the pharmacist to be bioequivalent.

• *Patient Opinion.* An informed patient, cooperating with a physician and pharmacist in his or her drug therapy, is an important element in ensuring the best possible therapeutic outcomes. The pharmacist should take into account the patient's needs when selecting from multisource drug products and inform the patient of any potential consequences associated with alternate product selections.

Purchase Decisions

APhA's Bioequivalency Working Group recommends that pharmacists consider the following factors when purchasing products from multisource vendors. Not all of these factors are of equal importance in each purchasing decision, but all are worthy of consideration.

• *Current State Laws and Regulations.* States have legal requirements that address the issue of drug product selection. Some

states have positive or negative formulary systems that place regulatory restrictions on the products considered therapeutically equivalent. The state formulary may not always be in agreement with classifications listed in the FDA's Orange Book. Therefore, pharmacists should be familiar with both. Some states also have regulations that define the role of the pharmacist, physician, and patient in the drug product selection process.

• *Bioequivalency Information/ Orange Book.* Products shown to be bioequivalent through reference to the Orange Book or other reliable source of bioequivalency information are preferred. Purchase decisions for drugs marketed prior to 1938 should be based on data obtained from the literature or the manufacturer, because bioequivalency testing may not be required by the FDA for these drug products.

• *Drug Category.* Greater attention should be given to purchasing strategies for drug products used for serious or life-threatening diseases and in situations where therapeutic activity of the product is confined to a narrow range of biologic fluid concentration.

• *Availability.* A continuous supply from the same manufacturer is essential even in the event that the distributor has changed to ensure that refills of prescriptions will contain the same product as originally dispensed. However, in those instances when the manufacturer of a generic drug product has to be changed, care should be exercised to ensure that the new drug product is equivalent to the formerly stocked drug product.

• *Supplier's Reputation.* The reputation of the manufacturer in terms of its ability to adhere to good manufacturing practices (GMP) that ensure that each dosage form is manufactured correctly and in a consistent manner is an important consideration. When purchasing a product from a distributor rather than directly from the manufacturer, the procedure used by that supplier in selecting manufacturers for multisource products is also an important consideration. Establishment Inspection Reports and recall reports [3] are available from FDA through a Freedom of Information (FOI) request. These are valuable tools in this decision.

• *Cost.* Cost of the product is an important consideration for both the patient and the pharmacy.

REFERENCES

1. A subscription to the Orange Book, which includes the 1990 *Basic Manual* and monthly supplements, is available for $91 from the Superintendent of Documents, U.S. Government Printing Office, Washington, DC 20402-9372. A subscription to the *USP-DI, Approved Drug Products and Legal Requirements*, Volume III, includes one book and monthly updates. It is available for $59 from the U.S. Pharmacopeial Convention, Inc., Order Processing Department, 12601 Twinbrook Parkway, Rockville, MD 20852.

2. Freedom of Information Staff, HFW-35, Food and Drug Administration, 5600 Fishers Lane, Rockville, MD 20857; (301) 433-6310.

3. Recall/Regulatory Analysis, P.O. Box 6353, Silver Spring, MD 20906; (301) 460-8821.

GENERIC SUBSTITUTION*

Paul L. Doering, MS, R.Ph.

Prior to the 1940s, few prescription products were prefabricated by pharmaceutical manufacturers to the extent that they are today. Rather, the pharmacist used his unique skills and training to prepare a precise and elegant product compounded to the needs of the individual patient. Physicians depended upon the knowledge and experience of the pharmacist to meticulously prepare lotions, ointments, capsules, tablets, powders, and other dosage forms containing the specific active ingredients in the precise amounts called for. Until very recently, the mortar and pestle were the very symbols of the practice of pharmacy.

By the mid 1940s, there was a shift away from prescribing products that required compounding and toward the use of products that were manufactured in bulk by large drug firms. Much of the technology for mass producing industrial products and materials was adapted to pharmaceutical manufacturing. Assembly line concepts were adapted to the large scale manufacture of finished dosage forms of drugs. Prefabricated products could now be produced with greater consistency and with longer shelf-life in a fraction of the time (and hence, cost) required to individually compound a product. Prescribing was made easier for the physician because he could count on the high quality of drugs manufactured to exacting standards. Like it or not, the role of the pharmacist as mixer and maker of the drug product was rapidly fading.

The system functioned well until scandal struck the drug industry. A few unscrupulous manufacturers and businessmen found that they could take advantage of the success of the large firms to earn quick profits. They began to counterfeit versions of popular brand name drugs in low budget operations, and these products began appearing on drugstore shelves. These operators learned that by taking shortcuts in the manufacturing process, they could stretch their profits. It was not uncommon for illegal manufacturers to scrimp on the active ingredients or, in some cases, to leave out the active ingredient altogether. Poor quality tablets and capsules were manufactured in identical shapes and sizes as the products they were mimicking and were passed off as the genuine article. Unsuspecting pharmacists (and some who were not entirely innocent victims) began to dispense these inferior products in the course of filling prescriptions.

When news of these abuses became public, citizens groups, governmental agencies, and professional organizations were outraged. They banded together to fight this threat to the integrity of the healthcare system and to restore confidence in the medications taken by Americans. Drug companies fought back by creating distinct capsule and tablet shapes and other unique features for their products. Eli Lilly's unique bullet-shaped Pulvule® capsule was developed, in large part, to give identity and distinction to Lilly products. Since this shape was hard for counterfeiters to duplicate, consumers found confidence in the quality of the product when

*Reprinted with permission from *Pharmacy PoweRx-Pack.*

they recognized the familiar shape of the capsule. SmithKline and French adopted the beveled ends of the Spansule® dosage form to set them apart from cheap imitations. Soon, other companies began to create distinctive shapes and other features for their products. But perhaps the most effective tool for combating "passing off" was the enactment of state laws that required pharmacists to dispense the exact brand of a drug specified by the prescriber. Thus, if Luminal® brand of phenobarbital was prescribed by a doctor, the pharmacist had no choice but to dispense Luminal® by Winthrop. This was true despite the fact that several other reliable manufacturers were making their own versions of phenobarbital, which probably were equal to Luminal® in quality and reliability. That the product specified might be much more expensive than a similar product by a different manufacturer was of little concern. People were willing to pay whatever price necessary to get a product upon which they could rely. Drug manufacturers, governmental agencies, citizens groups, and the various professions banded together in a rare partnership to protect the integrity of America's drugs.

Over the years, the threat to the drug supply from unscrupulous profiteers diminished. Replacing worry about drug quality was the newfound concern about the high cost of prescription drugs. Consumer groups began to ask questions: Why can't a less expensive product containing the same amounts of the same active ingredient(s) be substituted for the brand name product specified by the doctor? They argued that the "generic" drug must be just as effective as the brand name product called for in the prescription, since, after all, it contained the same amount of the same active ingredient(s). Governmental agencies involved in funding healthcare joined in the discussion, envisioning large savings in drug expenditures if pharmacists were permitted

to substitute a less expensive generic equivalent for the specified brand name product. Pharmacists, whose training by then included careful study of product formulation and bioavailability, saw a new opportunity to use their knowledge by selecting the individual product to be dispensed when a drug was available from multiple manufacturers. Thus, what started as a groundswell of support for repeal of the antisubstitution laws soon became a mandate.

In 1970, the American Pharmaceutical Association adopted an official policy seeking the repeal of state antisubstitution laws. Pharmacists argued that physicians should choose the drug and the dosage form, but the brand of the drug should be chosen by the professional with the most training and education about drugs and drug products, the pharmacist. There was considerable debate over this issue, primarily between pharmacists and physicians. However, consumer groups, health insurers, and the federal and state governments spoke in an increasingly louder voice. One by one the states began to repeal these prohibitive laws. The first state to repeal its law was Kentucky in 1972. By 1978, about 40 states had enacted generic drug product selection laws and in 1984 Indiana removed its antisubstitution laws from the books, making it the 50th state to do so.

Extent of Generic Substitution

Generic drugs currently claim about a 25% share of the prescription drug market. This number is expected to increase an estimated 40% by 1995 [1]. New prescriptions for which a generic drug was dispensed totaled 127,926,000 in 1991, representing 13.9% of all new prescriptions, compared with 13.5% in 1990. Sales for generic drugs reached $5 billion in 1991 [2]. The rapid growth of the practice of generic substitution can be attributed to several factors, including the following:

• Patents for many popular, high

volume prescription drugs are expiring. Over the next 10 years, drugs with current sales of $21 billion will be coming off patent. From 1992 to 1995, drugs losing patent now have total sales of $8 billion. By 1995, approximately 40 of the 50 top selling drugs will be available for generic manufacturers to duplicate. In 1993, Naprosyn, a Syntex drug with an estimated $550 million market. Upjohn's Xanax®, and Ciba-Geigy's Voltaren® and Lopressor®, lead the top-selling branded drugs that will be available as generics. In 1994, SmithKline Beecham loses exclusivity on Tagamet® and Marion Merrell Dow loses its protection on Seldane®. In 1995, Glaxo's Zantac®, with worldwide sales approaching $3 billion and U.S. sales estimated at $1.5 billion, will go off patent [3].

• Both public and private third party payers have increased pressure on pharmacists to use generics as a means to control the cost of healthcare. Managed care environments often have restricted formularies which mandate that generics be dispensed.

• Under the provisions of the Title XIX Medicaid Program, the federal government has established limits for reimbursement of selected drugs by setting Maximum Allowable Costs (MAC). These regulations and specific state laws regulating Medicaid programs force the substitution of lower cost products.

• Many new incentive programs promote the selection and dispensing of generic products by pharmacists, physicians, and/or patients.

• Media attention has increased consumers' awareness of and desire for generic alternatives that could save them money.

• Recent federal legislation has made it easier for generic manufacturers to gain approval for generic versions of popular brand name drugs.

Mechanisms designed to allow substitution vary considerably from state to state. Some states are more aggressive in promoting drug substitution and their laws actually *require* substitution unless expressly forbidden by the prescriber or rejected by the patient. Other states have laws which are less proactive in encouraging substitution, permitting substitution only if certain steps are taken.

Some states allow substitution among products that are specified on a list (positive formulary approach), while others encourage (or require) substitution for all drugs *except* those specified on a separate list (negative formulary approach).

Assumptions

When the role of the pharmacist in product selection was being advanced, certain assumptions had to be made. The first of these was that the practicing pharmacist would look upon this new responsibility with enthusiasm and truly embrace the opportunities afforded by it. Second was the assumption that pharmacists had the proper training to evaluate products to determine equivalency and, hence, interchangeability. Pharmacists trained within the past 15–20 years were certain to have been exposed to the course content on which to base substituting decisions, but those trained earlier may not have the proper training to competently participate in product selection decision making. Another assumption was that practicing pharmacists would have ready access to necessary information about individual products, available at the time it was needed and in a format appropriate to their practice setting. Indeed, this last assumption proved to be erroneous, at least for the average practicing pharmacist.

About the same time as the repeal of antisubstitution laws was taking place, information was coming to light to challenge the notion that two products with the same amount of the same active ingredient could be expected to perform the same way in the body. The earliest examples of product inequivalence involved digoxin. A now-classic article published in the *New England Journal of Medicine* in 1971 revealed that vast differences in blood levels of digoxin could result when different brands of the drug were administered. The science of biopharmaceutics had indeed come out of the laboratory and into the clinic. Yet, as this information came to light, little of it found its way into the literature read by practicing pharmacists. Much of it was buried in the basic pharmaceutical science literature or the medical literature, neither of which were regularly read by those facing substitution decisions. While much was being written and said about product inequivalency, little definitive information to assist in product selection decisions filtered into the practice literature.

A Review of Biopharmaceutics and Product Evaluation

In order for a drug to work in the body it must be present at the site of action in sufficient concentration to evoke the desired response. The majority of drugs in the ambulatory setting are taken orally, and it is these products which can suffer most from problems of poor bioavailability and product inequivalence.

Systemic absorption of an orally administered drug consists of a series of steps (Figure 1). Before a drug can begin to work, it must be liberated from the dosage form in which it is administered. For tablets, the first step towards bioavailability is the disintegration of the tablet. Capsules release their contents in the presence of fluid in the stomach. Next, the drug is dissolved in the fluids of the gastrointestinal (GI) tract and is absorbed across the membrane barrier that lines the GI tract, resulting in the appearance of the drug in the blood.

Physical factors in tablet formulation and manufacture can affect each of these steps. For example, changing the disintegrating agent from potato starch to rice starch could conceivably alter the rate of

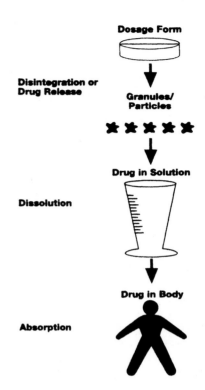

FIGURE 1.

disintegration. Similarly, the crystalline form of the active ingredient used in tablet manufacture can affect the rate of solubility of the drug in the gastric fluid. Even the hardness with which the tablet is compressed can affect the rate of absorption of certain drugs. Hence, it is possible that two products with the very same drug combined with the same inactive ingredients could vary in bioavailability simply by the manner in which the tablet is manufactured. Enteric coated tablets or specialized dosage forms (e.g., sustained- or delayed release products) are particularly prone to problems because of the variable materials and methods of their manufacture.

Since it is true that a solid form must disintegrate and dissolve in the GI fluids before absorption can occur, *in vitro* measurements of these parameters can be performed. Early product comparisons used *in vitro* methods almost exclusively, although problems exist with this type of testing. For example, results among different laboratories (and

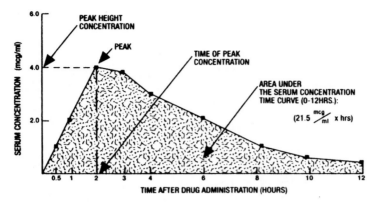

FIGURE 2.

even *within* the same laboratories) may vary. There is no established standard method of dissolution testing. The conditions of testing may not approximate the conditions encountered in the human GI tract. Factors such as gastric pH, gastric emptying, concurrent diseases of the patient, and additional drugs being taken by the patient may all influence *in vivo* bioavailability. It is difficult to draw firm conclusions about the *in vivo* comparison of two products based on *in vitro* data alone. Some examples demonstrate a good correlation between a dissolution test and *in vivo* bioavailability. In these instances, the Food and Drug Administration has recognized *in vitro* testing as adequate for comparing therapeutic equivalence of marketed products. Certainly, *in vitro* testing is easier, cheaper, and less invasive than *in vivo* methods, but for many products it is inadequate to uncover clinically significant bioequivalence problems.

The most commonly used method for determining bioavailability involves the administration of a single dose of the drug product to a group of subjects and the collection of blood samples over a period of time. Blood level determinations of the drug in question are plotted against time to give a picture of the amount of drug that reaches the circulation and the rate at which it does so. Figure 2 is a typical blood-level-versus-time curve. The three parameters of in-terest when comparing products for bioequivalence are: the area under the blood level-time curve (AUC), the maximum concentration of drug achieved in the blood after administration (C_{max}), and the time of maximum drug concentrations (T_{max}).

If the area under the curve is considerably less for one product, it is roughly equivalent to decreasing the dose of the drug. The rate of absorption (as reflected by T_{max} and C_{max}) can affect the effectiveness of the drug by not permitting the drug to reach therapeutic concentrations at the site of action or it could result in toxic side effects by achieving very high concentrations.

Regulators must determine if *rate* of absorption is the most important determinant of a drug's action, or if *extent* of absorption is more important. For many drugs, both parameters are important. Two drugs have identical bioavailability when their blood-level-versus-time curves match precisely; they are therefore said to be bioequivalent. Figure 3 shows a typical bioavailability comparison in which the drugs are considered bioequivalent. Under FDA guidelines, bioequivalent drugs are considered therapeutically equivalent when administered to patients under conditions specified in the product labeling and thus are expected to produce the same clinical response.

A single-dose bioequivalence study is usually performed in normal, healthy, male volunteers. Bioavailability studies are always done in a crossover fashion to control for variability among individuals. In this way, each subject serves as his own control. Every subject receives each drug product with an adequate washout period in between to allow for the body to eliminate any trace of the previous drug.

To achieve adequate information on which to make final conclusions, a sufficiently large number of subjects must be tested. A typical crossover bioequivalence study

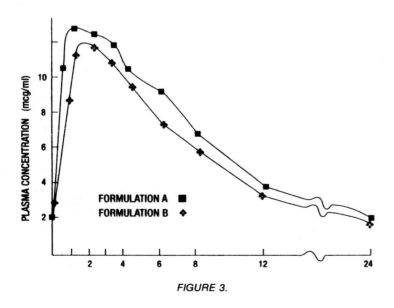

FIGURE 3.

may use 12 to 24 research subjects. This is usually satisfactory to learn how one or more products compares to the standard. The product which was on the market first is the one which has established itself as the "gold standard" against which other products will be compared. Sometimes this gold standard is not a perfect formulation of the drug, but it serves as the reference standard (sometimes called the "innovator" or "pioneer" product) by virtue of its proven clinical efficacy. Inequivalence can take the form of increased or decreased bioavailability compared with the innovator product.

The Need for Bioequivalence Data

As the frequency of generic substitution increased, the lack of bioequivalence data on which to base substitutions became a concern of government regulators. In 1974, the Drug Bioequivalence Study Panel of the Office of Technology Assessment (OTA) was founded. The panel's task was to study the issue of drug equivalence to determine what technology was necessary to ensure that drug products with the same physical and chemical composition would produce comparable therapeutic effects. The panel issued 11 conclusions and recommendations in its report. Acknowledging the importance of bioequivalence for many drugs, the panel also concluded that not all products pose bioequivalence problems. They rejected the notion that *in vivo* bioequivalence testing on *all* products should be required. The panel urged development of a system by which health professionals could be informed of the interchangeability of drug products. They suggested publication of an "official list" on which drugs would be listed in two categories: those for which evidence of bioequivalence is not considered essential and those for which evidence of bioequivalence is critical.

Proposed   bioavailability/bio-

equivalence regulations were published in the *Federal Register* on June 20, 1975. In those proposed regulations, the FDA listed 137 drugs which might pose real or potential bioequivalence problems. In January 1976, the FDA published a list of drugs entitled "Holders of Approved Drug Applications for Drugs Presenting Actual or Potential Bioequivalence Problems." This list included manufacturers' products that were subjects of concern but did not include companies which had conducted studies to prove the equivalence of their products to branded counterparts.

On February 7, 1977, the FDA issued final regulations defining certain terms relating to bioavailability and procedures for establishing a bioequivalence requirement. An update of the regulations became effective on July 14, 1981. The regulations provided a list of drugs with the greatest potential for bioequivalence problems.

Meanwhile, the states were struggling with the issue of product equivalence when trying to establish statewide formularies to assist with substitution. Several states turned to the FDA for help and guidance in establishing their respective formularies. In 1978, the FDA cooperated with the New York State Department of Health to provide a list of therapeutically equivalent drugs. In a letter to the Commissioner of the Department of Health of New York, FDA Commissioner Donald Kennedy stated:

We believe that all pharmaceutically equivalent drug products can be considered therapeutically equivalent providing they are marketed under approved new drug application, are manufactured under the same standards, meet identical or comparable specifications, and in those instances where positive evidence of bioequivalence is necessary, are shown to be bioequivalent. To the best of our knowledge the drug products on this list meet these criteria.

After publication of the New York list, the FDA received numer-

ous requests from other states for assistance in preparing similar lists. It became apparent that the FDA could not serve the needs of each individual state and that a single list based on common policies would be preferable to the evaluation of drug products based on differing criteria from each state law. Partly in response to the New York request, in mid-1978 the FDA revealed that it was preparing a list of all marketed prescription drug products that had been approved for safety and effectiveness by the FDA. In the case of multisource products, the list would identify products containing the same active ingredients and identical strength or concentration, dosage form, and route of administration that were considered therapeutically equivalent. The list was first published in October 1980 and was called *Approved Drug Products with Therapeutic Equivalence Evaluations* (more commonly known as the "Orange Book" for the distinctive color of its cover). Originally contemplated for use mostly by state governmental agencies and regulators, it is now viewed as an important tool for all pharmacists involved in the interchange of prescription drug products.

The Prescription Drug Products List and Other Lists in the Orange Book

Ideally, all pharmaceutical equivalents available in the United States should be approved by the FDA as bioequivalent. However, many drugs are currently marketed without the assurance of bioequivalence by the FDA. First, drugs marketed before 1938 were not subject to the Food, Drug, and Cosmetic Act, yet they can still be legally marketed without specific FDA approval. Examples of these "grandfathered" drugs include digoxin, morphine, codeine, phenobarbital, and certain thyroid medications (see Table 1).

When these pre-1938 drugs are formulated into new dosage forms,

---

Table 1
Common Examples of Drug Products Available before 1938
and Currently Marketed without an Approved NDA or ANDA
"Grandfathered Drugs"

Amobarbital
Aspirin with codeine
Atropine sulfate (oral and ophthalmic)
Chloral hydrate
Codeine
Colchicine
Digoxin
Digitoxin
Ephedrine preparations
Epinephrine preparations
Ergonovine maleate
Hydromorphone
Levothyroxine sodium
Magnesium sulfate
Methylene blue
Morphine sulfate
Nitroglycerin (sublingual and transdermal)
Phenazopyrine
Phenobarbital
Potassium chloride oral preparations
Pseudoephedrine
Thyroid
Quinine

This is only a small representation of products in this category that are still in common use. For a more extensive list, see Lewis, B.P., Jr., Castle, R. V., Jr. "Grandfathered Drugs of 1938." *Am. Pharmacy*, 1978; 18:36–9.

---

they are considered New Drugs under the Food, Drug, and Cosmetic Act. Hence, Burroughs-Wellcome was required to file a New Drug Application (NDA) for its capsule dosage form of digoxin (Lanoxicap®) and to include adequate studies of the capsule's bioavailability. The tablet dosage form does not appear in the Orange Book, although digoxin tablets are often cited among examples of drugs with notorious bioavailability problems. The FDA does not have regulatory authority to require comparative bioavailability evaluation for these older drugs. In some instances, the FDA has proposed that these drugs be reclassified as New Drugs under the Food, Drug, and Cosmetic Act and thus would require proof of efficacy as well as bioequivalency testing.

Certain drug products marketed between 1938 and 1962 were approved for safety but not for effectiveness (administratively termed "deemed approved") and are still

under the scientific and legal administrative review procedures of the Drug Efficacy Study Implementation (DESI) process. Before the enactment of a new law in 1984, only generic versions of drugs approved and marketed after 1938 but before 1962 could be processed by an Abbreviated New Drug Application (ANDA), and duplicates of products that were approved for marketing on or after October 10, 1962, could be handled by an administrative process known as the "Paper NDA" (a literature supported New Drug Application). In September 1984, the Drug Price Competition and Patent Term Restoration Act (also known as the Waxman-Hatch Act) became effective. These 1984 Amendments extended the eligibility for ANDA processing to drugs marketed after 1962 and also codified the "Paper NDA" process. The ANDA process does not require the sponsor of a product to repeat clinical research on active ingredients already found

to be safe and effective, making marketing of generic versions of products approved after 1962 economically feasible. Since the 1984 amendments went into effect, generic versions have been introduced for several hundred drugs previously available only as brand name (innovator or pioneer) products.

With the passage of the Waxman-Hatch Bill came the requirement that the FDA publish an up-to-date list of all marketed drug products, nonprescription as well as prescription, that have been approved for safety and efficacy and for which NDAs are required. The FDA considers the Orange Book and its monthly Cumulative Supplements to fulfill this requirement. As a result of the 1984 amendments, additional information was required in the Orange Book beginning with the sixth (1985) edition: nonprescription drug product marketed by the NDA route (e.g., ibuprofen 200 mg and all drug products administered by the Division of Blood and Blood Products.

A provision of the Waxman-Hatch amendments allows for patent term extensions to give back to the applicant the time spent while the NDA was being reviewed. Manufacturers are granted exclusive marketing rights for a specified period. If ANDAs are allowed to be submitted during this exclusive period, approval is granted with a delayed effective (marketing) date. The sixth and succeeding editions of the Orange Book also provide patent information concerning the listed drugs. Drug products that have been discontinued from marketing or that have had their approvals withdrawn for reasons other than safety or efficacy concerns are also listed. Other lists provided in the Orange Book are the Orphan Drug Product List, Drug Products Which Must Demonstrate *in vivo* Bioavailability Only if Products Fail to Achieve Adequate Dissolution, Biopharmaceutic Guidance Available, and ANDA Suitability Petitions. These lists may or may not be immediately useful to the practicing pharmacist in making substitution decisions.

Basis of Therapeutic Equivalence Determinations

The issue of therapeutic equivalence is addressed only in the Prescription Drug Products List of the Orange Book. In order for two drugs to be designated as therapeutic equivalents, they must first be pharmaceutical equivalents and then must be expected to have the same clinical effect when administered to patients under the conditions specified in the labeling. Although some confusion exists when the term "therapeutic equivalents" is used in pharmacy and medicine, when used by the FDA, the concept of therapeutic equivalence applies only to products containing the same active ingredients. Some have used this same terminology to denote chemically distinct drugs in the same therapeutic category that are, for practical purposes, equivalent in therapeutic effect. Table 2 lists important definitions applicable to bioequivalence/bioavailability issues. The Food and Drug Administration classifies as therapeutically equivalent those products that meet the following criteria:

1. They are approved as both safe and effective;

2. They are pharmaceutical equivalents, in that they (a) contain the identical amount of the same active ingredients in the same dosage form and route of administration, and (b) meet compendia or other applicable standards of strength, quality, purity, and identity;

3. They are bioequivalent, in that (a) they do not present a known or potential bioequivalence problem and they meet an acceptable *in vitro* standard, or (b) if they do present such a known or potential problem, they are shown to meet appropriate bioequivalence standards;

4. They are adequately labeled; and

5. They are manufactured in compliance with FDA Good Manufacturing Practice regulations.

Bioequivalent drug products are those pharmaceutically equivalent products that, for example, display comparable bioavailability (i.e., the rate and extent to which the active or therapeutic ingredient is absorbed from a drug product and becomes available at the site of drug action) when studied under similar experimental conditions. Bioequivalence alone does not guarantee the clinical effectiveness

of a particular marketed drug product. Conversely, just because a product is not bioequivalent does not mean that it is clinically ineffective. This is true when bioavailability differences are not important in the treatment of patients. Drugs with reported bioinequivalence that have no documented clinical significance include ampicillin, acetazolamide, propoxyphene, and nitrofurantoin.

In the preface to the Orange Book, the FDA is careful to point out that considerations other than

---

Table 2
Bioavailability/Bioequivalence Terms

Bioavailability. A measure of the rate and extent (amount) of the active ingredient which reaches the general circulatory system.

Bioequivalents. Pharmaceutical equivalents which, when administered under similar conditions, will produce comparable bioavailabilities. In a bioequivalent drug product, the rate and extent of absorption of the active ingredients do not show a significant difference from the rate and extent of drug absorbed from the reference product. In some cases the rate may differ if it is the intention, as reflected in the labeling and is not essential to the attainment of effective drug concentrations on multiple dosing and is considered clinically insignificant for the drug.

Generic substitution. The act of dispensing a different branded or unbranded drug product for the drug product prescribed (i.e., a pharmaceutical equivalent distributed by a different company). Examples are:
 a. Rufen® brand of ibuprofen for Motrin® brand of ibuprofen.
 b. unbranded generic ampicillin for Polycillin®.

Pharmaceutical alternates. Drug products which are administered by the same route and contain the same therapeutic moiety and strength but differ in the salt, ester, or dosage form.

Pharmaceutical equivalents. Multiple source drug products which contain the same active ingredients(s), in identical amounts, in identical dosage forms administered by the same route of administration and which meet existing standards in the *USP*. The products may differ in characteristics such as color, flavor, shape, packaging, inert ingredients, and expiration time.

Pharmaceutical substitution. The act of dispensing a pharmaceutical alternate for the drug product prescribed.
Examples are:
 a. *Salt.* Codeine sulfate for codeine phosphate or tetracycline hydrochloride for tetracycline phosphate complex.
 b. *Ester.* Propoxyphene hydrochloride for propoxyphene napsylate or erythromycinethyl succinate for erythromycin base.
 c. *Dosage form.* Ampicillin suspension for ampicillin capsule.

Therapeutic alternates. Drug products containing different therapeutic moieties which are of the same pharmacologic and/or therapeutic class that can be expected to have similar therapeutic effects when administered to patients in therapeutically equivalent doses.

Therapeutic equivalent. Pharmaceutical equivalents which will provide the same therapeutic effect, as measured by control of a disease or a disease symptom.

Therapeutic substitution. The act of dispensing a therapeutic alternate for the drug product prescribed. Examples are:
 a. chlorothiazide for hydrochlorothiazide
 b. cephradine for cephalexin

bioequivalence may be important when selecting a product to dispense. Products determined to be bioequivalent may differ in certain characteristics, such as shape, scoring configuration, packaging, excipients (including colors, flavors, presentations), expiration time, and minor aspects of labeling. The FDA cautions that "when such differences are important in the care of a particular patient, it may be appropriate for the prescribing physician to require that a particular brand be dispensed as a medical necessity." Suppose, for example, that two marketed products are pharmaceutically equivalent, yet one contains sodium metabisulfate as an antioxidant and the other does not. If the patient has a known hypersensitivity to sulfites, then obviously it would be a medical necessity for the patient to obtain the specific designated brand which does not contain this particular preservative.

Designation of Equivalence

As described above, the Prescription Drug Products List in the Orange Book contains drug products that are both single source (i.e., there is only one approved product available for that active ingredient and dosage form) and multisource (pharmaceutical equivalents available from more than one manufacturer). Currently, of just over 10,000 drugs on the Prescription Drug Product List, 20% are single source and 80% are multisource. Naturally, there is no product with which to compare single source products; bioequivalence evaluations are available only for multisource products. Of the approximately 8,000 multisource products listed, about 7,200, or 90%, are considered therapeutically equivalent.

A two-letter coding system is used to help pharmacists quickly determine the status of a drug product found in the Orange Book. The first letter signifies whether the product is therapeutically equivalent to other drugs for which

bioavailability data are required. The second letter provides additional information to help the reader understand the basis for the classification by the first letter.

Products are classified into one of two groups, signified by the appropriate first letter.

A. *Drug products* that are considered to be therapeutically equivalent to other pharmaceutically equivalent products; and

B. *Drug products* that are not at this time considered to be therapeutically equivalent to other pharmaceutically equivalent products.

Products for which there are no known or suspected bioequivalence problems are broken down into several categories (the second letter) according to dosage form (see Table 3). Products for which there are known or suspected bioequivalence problems, but where the problem has been resolved with adequate *in vitro* or *in vivo* testing, receive the AB rating. This signifies that the product meets necessary bioequivalence requirements. Thus, pharmacists can be reasonably confident that "A" rated products they dispense can be expected to produce the same clinical effect as other sources of the product which also carry the "A" rating.

Significance of B-Rated Drugs

Numerous B-rated drugs are listed in the Orange Book, including some brands of prednisone, extended release quinidine gluconate, warfarin, sulfasalazine, and most brands of extended-release theophylline. While all B-rated products lack proof of bioequivalence, this classification does not mean that the products are without effect. In some instances, a product was approved on the basis of clinical efficacy and safety studies. For

Table 3 Summary of FDA Codes for Therapeutic Equivalence Evaluations	
A—A generic drug product that is bioequivalent and, therefore, "therapeutically equivalent" to the brand name or reference product.	B—A generic drug product that is not considered to be bioequivalent and, thus, "not therapeutically equivalent" to the brand name or reference product.
AA—Products not presenting bioequivalence problems AB—Products meeting necessary bioequivalence requirements AN—Solutions and powders for aerosolization AO—Injectable oil solutions AP—Injectable aqueous solutions AT—Topical products	BC—Controlled-release tablets, capsules, injections BD—Active ingredients and dosage forms with documented bioequivalence problems BE—Enteric coated dosage forms BN—Products in aerosol drug delivery systems BP—Active ingredients and dosage forms with potential bioequivalence problems BR—Suppositories or enemas for systemic use BS—Products having drug standard deficiencies BT—Topical products with bioequivalence issues BX—Insufficient data to prove bioequivalence B*—Previously A or B drug requiring further FDA investigation in light of new information questioning therapeutic equivalence.

The first letter designates whether two drugs are therapeutically equivalent. A-rated drugs are considered equivalent, whereas B-rated drugs are not considered therapeutically equivalent. The second letter in the above table explains the basis for the equivalency/inequivalency determination.

example, DiaBeta® (Hoechst-Roussel) and Micronase® (Upjohn), two brand name pharmaceutical equivalents of glyburide, were compared with placebo in separate controlled trials but were not compared with each other in a bioequivalence study. Thus, while each is effective, it cannot be assumed that they produce the same clinical effect. In this instance, the pharmacist should not dispense one for another without the physician's knowledge. This way the physician can monitor the patient and adjust the dosage, if indicated.

It is possible for some pharmaceutical equivalents to be B-rated while others are A-rated. This is because some particular manufacturers have chosen to perform required bioequivalence testing while others have chosen not to. B-rated products should be assumed to be therapeutically inequivalent unless the manufacturer can provide data to the contrary. Clinical differences or serious bioequivalence problems with B-rated products have been reported for nortriptyline, extended-release quinidine, phenytoin, prednisone, levodopa, and thioridazine, etc. (see Table 4).

Limitations of the Orange Book

Because ratings for drugs in the Orange Book change as the FDA reviews and approves data, pharmacists should verify a drug's current status if a question of equivalence arises. Monthly supplements to the FDA's listing of equivalent drug products document additions, deletions, and changes in any particular drug's status. However, there is a two month lag time in publication.

Some products, sustained- or controlled-release dosage forms in particular, are not equivalent by the very nature of methods used to control the rate of release of medication from the dosage form. Thus, these products are rated B unless equivalence has been shown by *in vivo* testing using

Table 4
Multisource Drug Products Not Considered to Be Therapeutically Equivalent "B-Rated Drugs"

Rating	Drug
BN	Albuterol (metered-dose inhaler)
BD	Aminophylline (tablets)
BP	Amitriptyline (tablets)*
BP	Amitriptyline with perphenazine (tablets)*
BN	Beclomethasone dipropionate (metered-dose inhaler)
BN	Beclomethasone dipropionate monohydrate (intranasal)
BP	Benzthiazide (tablet)
BR	Caffeine with ergotamine (rectal suppositories)
BP	Chlorothiazide with reserpine (tablet)
BC	Chlorpheniramine with phenylpropanolamine (extended release)*
BP	Chlorpromazine (tablets)
BT	Clotrimazole (topical and vaginal cream)
BP	Colchicine with probencid (tablets)
BC	Corticotropin (injectable)
BP	Cortisone acetate (tablets and injectable)
BX	Desmopressin acetate (nasal solution)
BP	Dexamethasone (tablets and injectable suspension)
BC	Diethylpropion (extended release tablet)
BP	Diethylstilbestrol (tablets)
BE	Diethylstilbestrol (extended release tablets)
BC	Diltiazem (extended release capsule)
BX	Disulfiram (tablets)
BP	Dyphylline (tablets)
BS	Estrogens, esterified (tablets)
BP	Estrone (injectable)
BP	Fluoxymesterone (tablets)
BP	Fluphenazine (tablets)*
BX	Glyburide (tablets)
BP	Hydralazine with hydrochlorothiazide and reserpine
BP	Hydrochlorothiazide with reserpine (tablets)
BP	Hydrocortisone (tablets and injectable)
BX	Hydrocortisone with pramoxine (rectal foam)
BP	Hydroflumethiazide with reserpine (tablets)
BX	Ibuprofen (oral suspension)
BN	Isoetharine mesylate (metered-dose inhaler)
BN	Isoproterenol (metered-dose inhaler)
BC	Isosorbide dinitrate (extended release capsules)
BX	Leucovorin (tablets)*
BD	Levodopa (tablets)
BP	Mazindol (tablets)
BP	Medroxyprogesterone acetate (tablets)*
BP	Methylprednisolone (injectable suspension)
BP	Methyltestosterone (capsules and buccal tablets)
BC	Morphine sulfate (extended release tablets)
BC	Nicotine (Transdermal patches)
BD	Nortriptyline*
BC	Penicillin G benzathine
BC	Phendimetrazine (extended release capsules)
BX	Phenytoin sodium prompt (capsules)
BP	Phytonadione (injectable)
BC	Potassium chloride (extended release)*
BX	Prednisolone (tablets)
BP	Prednisolone (injectable)
BP	Prednisolone tebutate (injectable)
BX	Prednisone (tablets)*
BC	Procainamide (extended release)*
BP	Promethazine (tablet)
BR	Promethazine (rectal suppository)
BD	Propylthiouracil (tablets)

(continued next page)

Table 4 (continued)	
Rating	**Drug**
BC	Quinidine gluconate (extended release)*
BP	Rauwolfia serpentina (tablets)
BP	Reserpine (tablets)
BP	Reserpine with trichlormethiazide (tablets)
BP	Terbutaline (tablets)
BP,BX	Theophylline (capsules)
BC	Theophylline (extended release capsules and tablets)*
BP	Thyroglobulin (tablets)
BP	Triamcinolone (tablets and injectable)
BP	Trichlormethiazide (tablets)
BX	Warfarin (tablets)

*Some products in this category carry AB (equivalent) ratings or other ratings.
Source: *Approved Drug Products with Therapeutic Equivalence Evaluations, 12th Edition, 1992.*

repeated doses; because medication is not released and absorbed immediately, single-dose studies are not adequate to ensure bioequivalence. Once data from appropriate bioequivalence studies have been submitted, the FDA may rate the products AB. Thus, some sustained-release theophylline or potassium chloride tablets, for instance, are rated AB, whreas others continue to be rated B. Because of the diversity of pharmaceutical technology used to formulate controlled release dosage forms and the unique nature of some of these, pharmacists should be extra cautious when contemplating substitution of such products. Of course, B-rated controlled release medications should not be interchanged.

The FDA has not required comparative bioequivalence testing for transdermal nitroglycerin patches (TNPs). TNPs have been "conditionally" approved based on evidence of efficacy and safety. However, the FDA has been trying to change the status of TNPs to require further evidence of efficacy. In the absence of data documenting equivalence, it must be assumed that the products are inequivalent. In essence, these products take on a *de facto* "B" rating and therefore should not be substituted one for the other. This is especially true considering the complex nature of the controlled release mechanisms of transdermal products and the varying technology used by the different companies. Furthermore, there are important differences in the inert ingredients, for example the adhesive systems, that make designation of one brand over the other particularly important. Add to this the critical nature of the disease being treated, namely ischemic heart disease, and it becomes clear why substitution of nitroglycerin patches is unwise. Although transdermal nitroglycerin products do not appear in the Orange Book, they should be considered B-rated drugs.

In some instances the holder of the NDA is not the same as the manufacturer or distributor. Many smaller companies purchase products from dozens of manufacturers to complete their product lines. Similarly, a consistent source of supply may not be available to a particular distributor and, hence, the actual manufacturer of the products distributed may change periodically. This makes evaluation of the equivalency status difficult at times. Pharmacists should ask for bioequivalence information from the distributors from whom they purchase products.

The Orange Book and the Hospital Formulary

The Orange Book should be used by hospitals when purchasing drugs for their formulary. It should be used similarly as community pharmacists use it when deciding drugs for generic interchange. That is, drugs with "A" ratings can be purchased with the confidence that interchanging the formulary product for the product taken before hospitalization will not affect therapeutic outcome Drugs with a "B" rating cannot be assured to be therapeutically equivalent to the product used outside the hospital. For drugs not included in the Orange Book, the same steps should be taken in order to obtain necessary bioequivalence data from the manufacturer.

Many hospitals participate in buying groups to take advantage of the purchasing power that accompanies volume buying. Most buying groups, however, have stringent requirements when it comes to selecting the products it will accept for bid. The Orange Book is used extensively in the bidding process. In order to even be considered, drugs appearing in the Orange Book must have an "A" rating. For drugs not appearing in the book, special efforts are made to insure bioequivalence data are considered. Furthermore, most buying groups will set other criteria in order for a vendor to be considered "qualified" to submit bids. Vendors must have a good recall history, must be in compliance with Current Good Manufacturing Practices of the FDA, and vendors must have a reliable history of supplying their buyers with the products ordered. A highly qualified product manager and a quality assurance supervisor are also needed. The foundation of the process, however, is the Orange Book status of the product.

QUESTIONS: CHAPTER 16

1. The "Orange Book" is formally known as FDA's:

    a. Approved Drug Products and Legal Requirements
    b. Safe and Effective Drugs with Therapeutic Equivalence
    c. Approved Drug Products with Therapeutic Equivalence Evaluations
    d. Therapeutically Equivalent Drug Products

2. The established name of a drug is its:

    a. Brand name
    b. Generic name
    c. Chemical name
    d. Trademark name
    e. Proprietary name

3. Which one of the following alphabet letters used in the "Orange Book" indicates that drug products have a therapeutic equivalence problem?

    a. A
    b. B
    c. C
    d. D

4. How often is the "Orange Book" published?

    a. Every year
    b. Biennially
    c. Every three years
    d. Quintennially

5. Which drug products are not included in the "Orange Book"?
1) DESI
2) "Pre-1938"
3) Those not subject to FDA enforcement action as unapproved drugs

    a. 1) and 2) are correct.
    b. 1) and 3) are correct.
    c. 2) and 3) are correct.
    d. 1), 2), and 3) are correct.

6. What is a purpose of the "Orange Book"?

    a. Provides FDA's therapeutic equivalence evaluations for multi-source prescription drug products approved by the FDA
    b. Acts as a standard and supplement to the USP/NF
    c. Identifies competitive drug products to reduce prescription costs.
    d. Identifies manufacturers, distributors and repackagers of equivalent drug products

7. Which federal government agency compiles the list of drugs published in the "Orange Book"?

    a. USP/NF
    b. FBI
    c. FDA
    d. FTC
    e. CPSC

8. How often is the "Orange Book" revised (updated)?

    a. Monthly

    b. Semi-annually

    c. Biannually

    d. Annually

    e. Every five years

9. Which United States statute requires that the FDA publish an up-to-date list of all marketed drug products?

    a. Fair Packaging and Labeling Act

    b. Prescription Drug Marketing Act

    c. Omnibus Budget Reconciliation Act

    d. Drug Price Competition and Patent Restoration Act

10. Drug products which contain the same therapeutic moiety, but are different dosage forms and strengths, and differ as to ester, salt are:

    a. Therapeutic alternates

    b. Pharmaceutical alternates

    c. Therapeutic equivalents

    d. Generic substitutes

11. Which one of the following alphabet characters used in the "Orange Book" indicates that drug products are therapeutically equivalent?

    a. A

    b. B

    c. C

    d. D

12. The Drug Price Competition and Patent Restoration Act is also known as the _____ amendment to the FDC Act:

    a. Waxman-Hatch

    b. Durham-Humphrey

    c. Kefauver-Harris

    d. Reagan-Bush

    e. Harrison-Ford

13. A "grandfathered" drug product:

    a. Has been marketed in the U.S. over 65 years

    b. Is included in the "Orange Book"

    c. Was marketed prior to the 1938 FDC Act

    d. Is equivalent to a generic drug product

14. An example of a "grandfathered" drug product is:

    a. Tetracycline

    b. Penicillin G

    c. Acetaminophen

    d. Digoxin

15. Which one of the following is not common with the others?

    a. Aspirin w/codeine

    b. Thyroid

    c. Penicillin

    d. Digoxin

    e. Phenobarbital

16. A formulary of drug products deemed to be chemically and therapeutically equivalent to and interchangeable is referred to as a(n):

    a. Negative formulary

    b. Positive formulary

    c. Interchangeable open formulary

    d. Closed formulary

17. A _____ requires that substitution be permitted for all drugs except those prohibited by a particular list:

    a. Negative formulary

    b. Closed formulary

    c. Open formulary

    d. Positive formulary

18. The "Orange Book" was first published in October:

    a. 1905

    b. 1970

    c. 1975

    d. 1980

    e. 1985

19. How many categories of drug products exist in the "Orange Book"?

    a. One

    b. Two

    c. Three

    d. Four

20. FDA's Approved Drug Products with Therapeutic Equivalence Evaluations is a(n):

    a. Statute

    b. Regulation

    c. Law

    d. Guideline

CHAPTER 17

Prescription Drug User Fee Act of 1992

User Fees

The road to gaining FDA approval to market a new prescription drug or biologic can be a lengthy one. By law, FDA must review clinical test results for any new drug to ensure the product is safe and effective. Owing to staff shortages, limited resources, and incomplete submitted applications, it takes an average of 22 months for approval from the time companies apply to market products. But that is about to change.

Armed with resources provided by the Prescription Drug User Fee Act of 1992, FDA plans to shorten review time significantly over the next five years. To accomplish this, the agency has started collecting "user fees"—charges levied on pharmaceutical companies for certain new drug and biologic applications, drug products, and manufacturing establishments covered under the act. FDA will use these funds for hiring more reviewers to assess applications. The agency also plans to streamline drug and biologic review processes and use information technology to help speed reviews. At the same time, pharmaceutical companies will ensure that applications are complete and contain data needed for product approval.

Ultimately, FDA's goal is to employ about 700 new drug reviewers and support staff by the end of fiscal year 1997. To do this, the agency expects to collect more than $325 million in user fees over the five years covered by the 1992 act. [See chart.] Unless Congress renews the act, the user fee law will expire at the end of FY 1997.

FDA is now recruiting for the new positions and is working to hire up to 200 persons by this Sept. 30. Most new employees will work in either FDA's Center for Drug Evaluation and Research or Center for Biologics Evaluation and Research. They include medical officers, chemists, microbiologists, and pharmacologists, along with other professionals and support staff. FDA plans to acquire new space for the expanded staff, most of whom will be situated in or around FDA headquarters in Rockville, Md.

The new employees also will help FDA with its backlog of overdue applications, which the agency plans to eliminate within two years.

As for new applications, FDA aims to reduce review times to 12 months for "standard" applications and to six months for "priority" applications. Applications for drugs similar to those already marketed are designated standard, while priority applications represent drugs offering significant advances over existing treatments. (Drugs for AIDS and cancer typically fall in the priority category.) Goals for shortening review times and for hiring more staff will be phased in gradually over the five-year statutory period.

Although FDA is accelerating its review time, the agency is committed to high review standards. Newly initiated programs are helping to ensure the quality and integrity of the review process.

The prescription drug and biotechnology industries, particularly the Pharmaceutical Manufacturers Association and several biologic product trade associations, support user fees that bolster FDA's review process. About 175 drug and biologic companies are affected by the user fee law.

The pharmaceutical industry also will play a major part in helping the agency achieve user fee performance goals. For example, FDA will depend on companies to improve the overall quality of submissions and to provide timely responses to questions about applications. The agency plans to work closely with industry on programs to improve the quality of the drug and biologics submissions. FDA also will enlist information technology to help speed review of the massive amounts of data submitted

User Fee Estimates FY 93–97					
	FY 93	FY 94	FY 95	FY 96	FY 97
Applications	$100,000	$150,000	$208,000	$217,000	$233,000
Supplements & applications without clinical data	$50,000	$75,000	$104,000	$108,000	$116,000
Fee revenue	$12 million	$18 million	$25 million	$26 million	$28 million
Establishment fee	$60,000	$88,000	$126,000	$131,000	$138,000
Fee revenue	$12 million	$18 million	$25 million	$26 million	$28 million
Product fee	$6,000	$9,000	$12,500	$13,000	$14,000
Fee revenue	$12 million	$18 million	$25 million	$26 million	$28 million
Total fees	$36 million	$54 million	$75 million	$78 million	$84 million

in drug and biologics applications.

FDA has begun billing companies for FY 1993 fees. An FDA senior-level steering committee is guiding the transition to the fee system, while working groups handle specifics such as fee management, tracking progress toward meeting user fee performance goals, and the new staff's needs for training and computers.

A Long History

User fees are not a new concept. FDA has charged fees for color certification and insulin certification for over 40 years. FDA first considered the idea of drug review fees more than 20 years ago when the General Accounting Office recommended to Congress that FDA charge such fees. GAO's 1971 report cited the authority federal agencies were given to levy user fees under the Independent Offices Appropriation Act of 1952. But after weighing pros and cons—such as whether fees would burden small businesses or be passed on by firms that pay them in the form of higher prices—FDA's parent agency, the former Department of Health, Education, and Welfare, rejected the idea.

FDA user fees resurfaced in 1982 when President Reagan's Private Sector Survey on Cost Control recommended that FDA begin charging for many of its services, including new drug applications. That proposal failed to gain significant support. In 1985, however, FDA, in the midst of an eroding employment base and increased responsibilities, published a proposed rule in the *Federal Register* for collecting user fees. The administration followed suit by proposing $5 million in FDA user fees for the FY 1985 budget and again in FY 1986, but Congress refused to act either year. Both proposals specified that user fees would substitute for appropriate funds, meaning there would be no net boost in FDA resources.

In 1986, the Pharmaceutical Manufacturers Association strongly opposed the administration's user fee proposal, fearing funds would be diverted to the Treasury for federal deficit reduction. The association said the proposal amounted to a tax on drug applications. However, the trade group stated it would support user fees if funds were targeted to improving FDA review procedures. No action was taken that year. In subsequent years, the administration continued to propose a system of collecting user fees to replace appropriations, but Congress repeatedly dismissed it. In 1992, things changed.

As budget proceedings for FY 1993 began, FDA Commissioner David A. Kessler, M.D., testified before Congress that the user fee issue was one of critical importance to FDA's future and that it should be considered very seriously. FDA worked with the pharmaceutical industry to create performance goals and determine what fees would be needed to reach those goals. Though earlier fee suggestions encompassed numerous FDA-regulated products, the final proposal included only prescription drugs and certain biologics. (Biologics exempted were whole blood products or blood components for transfusion, some human drugs made from bovine blood products, allergenic extract products, and *in vitro* diagnostics. Large-volume parenterals, and generic drugs also were excluded.)

FDA and Congress then drafted legislation that said user fees would be used strictly to augment regular funds, which could not fall below the previous year's level. The drafts did not incorporate goals for improved performance, such as reducing drug application review times, an issue important to industry.

The Pharmaceutical Manufacturers Association said it would support legislation only if fees:

- supplemented existing FDA appropriations
- were fully dedicated to reviewing new drugs and biologics
- were reasonable
- were based on a long-term government commitment to improving the drug review process.

By Aug. 10, 1992, FDA and industry had reached a consensus. A bill emerged from committee on Sept. 15 that included the PMA provisions. The House passed an early version of the User Fee Act on Sept. 22. On Oct. 5, the House passed H.R. 6181, which became the Prescription Drug User Fee Act of 1992. The Senate passed the bill Oct. 7, and President George Bush signed it into law Oct. 29.

Fee Structure

The law provides for three categories of user fees:

- fees for drug and biologics applications and supplements
- annual establishment fees
- annual product fees

Each category accounts for one-third of the total revenue to be collected. For example, in FY 1993, FDA plans to take in $12 million for each user fee category for a total of $36 million [see chart]. But before FDA can collect any fees, Congress must appropriate the anticipated user fee revenue annually. For FY 1993, Congress enacted the necessary user fee appropriation on July 1, and President Clinton signed it on July 2. FDA now plans to collect FY 1993 user fees.

Based on estimates from the drug industry, FDA believes that by the end of FY 1993, it will receive 90 applications containing clinical data, 20 without clinical data, and 40 supplements to earlier applications. All application/supplemental fees are paid 50 percent at the time of submission and 50 percent upon receipt of an FDA "action letter." (Action letters indicate either approval or deficiencies that must be corrected for approval.) Not all applications for drug approval are equal. Some require more resources than others to review. The fee structure only takes into account the application's complexity based on whether or not clinical data are included. It makes no distinction based on application size. In FY 1993, for example, applications with clinical data will be charged $100,000, while those without will be charged $50,000, as will supplements (usually efficacy supplements) with clinical data. FY 1993 application fees are retroactive to Sept. 1, 1992.

The other two components of the fee structure—the annual establishment and product user fees—are set fees charged to the 200 drug establishments that manufacture drugs covered by the user fee law and on some 2,000 drug products in commercial distribution. The Prescription Drug User Fee Act defines an establishment as a business that makes at least one prescription drug product at one physical location, consisting of buildings within five miles of each other. A prescription drug product is defined as a specific strength or potency of a prescription drug, in

final dosage form, that has an approved human drug application.

Under the law, fees will increase each year. By FY 1997, FDA should collect $28 million per category, making total revenue for that year $84 million.

Waivers and Fee Reductions

The law provides for waivers and fee reductions if:

- the waiver is necessary to protect the public health
- the fee presents a "significant barrier" to innovation
- the fee exceeds FDA's cost of the review process
- the fee would be inequitable because the product is similar to certain generic drugs that are not part of the user fees program.

Businesses with fewer than 500 employees and without another prescription product on the market will be charged half the application fee, which will be due one year after submission.

FDA officials say if the current user fee program goes well, the agency might seek congressional authorization to expand it to medical devices and other areas.

Benefits of User Fees

- Reduction of Approval Times
  —12 months average product
  —6 months for prior product
  —FDA to hire additional staff

PRESCRIPTION DRUG USER FEE ACT OF 1992[*]

Donald O. Beers, Esq.

Introduction

On October 29, 1992, President Bush signed into law the Prescription Drug User Fee Act of 1992 [1]. This bill, which may ultimately be a model of similar legislation affecting other Food and Drug Administration (FDA)-regulated products, combined a new set of fees applicable to prescription drug manufacturers with a commitment that those fees will be used to speed the drug approval process. The bill provides for fees for five years (fiscal year 1993 through fiscal year 1997) [2], after which it expires if not extended by Congress [3]. Fees will not actually be assessed until a new appropriation bill is passed by the new Congress in early 1993.

Congressman Waxman estimates that the fees required to be paid by drug manufacturers under this bill will raise $327 million for the Food and Drug Administration over five years [4]. Dr. David Kessler, FDA Commissioner, represented to Congress that the fees would enable the FDA to cut approval times for new drug applications about in half within that five year period. The FDA's goal, as asserted by Dr. Kessler, would be to reach a decision on most approval applications for "breakthrough" drugs within six months and to reach such a decision with respect to most other applications within twelve months [5].

This article will summarize the law's requirements with respect to fees and describe the commitments the FDA has made on use of the funds those fees will generate [6].

New Fees

There are three types of fees established by this law: A fee for the submission of a human drug approval application or supplement [7], an annual fee for each prescription drug establishment [8], and an annual fee applicable to each holder of an approved human drug approval application [9].

Drug Application Fees

This fee does not apply to abbreviated new drug applications (ANDAs). It does apply to full new drug applications (NDAs) [10]. It also applies to "paper NDAs" (more specifically, NDAs described in § 505(b)(2) of the Federal Food, Drug, and Cosmetic Act), but only if those applications are for a previously unapproved molecular entity or indication for use of a drug [11]. Fees apply to the initial certification or initial approval of an antibiotic drug [12], and to the licensing of a biological product [13]. Fees also apply to supplements to any of those types of applications if those supplements require clinical trials for approval [14].

Fees for drug applications and supplements are applicable to over-the-counter drugs as well as prescription drugs.

There are two levels of fees for applications. A higher fee is payable for drug approval applications for which clinical data, other than bioavailability or bioequivalence studies, are necessary to show safety and effectiveness [15]. The lower fee is required for drug approval applications that do not require such clinical data [16]. That lower fee is also applicable to supplements that do require clinical data for approval [17]. No fee applies to supplements for which clinical data with respect to safety and effectiveness are not required for approval.

The fees increase by increments each year from fiscal year 1993 through fiscal year 1997. The higher drug application fees stated in the statute start at $100,000 during the first year, increasing in subsequent years to $150,000 (1994), $208,000 (1995, $217,000 (1996), and $233,000 (1997) [18]. The lower level fee, for new drug applications not requiring clinical data for approval and for supplements that do require such data, start at $50,000 (1993) with projected increases to $75,000 (1994), $104,000 (1995), $108,000 (1996), and $116,000 (1997) [19].

For years after the 1993 fiscal year, however, there is a strong likelihood that the fees will differ somewhat from those cited in the statute. This is because the fees stated here, and the other fees discussed below, may be adjusted each year so as to produce the projected fee revenues for each category of fee in the statute [20]. Those projections in turn may be adjusted upward to reflect the greater of the total percentage increase in the consumer price index for urban consumers or the total percentage increase in basic pay for federal employees [21].

The first payment for each of these fees is due upon submission of the application or the supplement [22]. Payment of the remaining 50% of the fee is due 30 days after the FDA sends the applicant an "action letter" on the application or after the application of supplement is withdrawn (unless the FDA waives the fee or a portion of the fee because no substantial work was performed on the application or supplement after it was filed) [23]. If the application is not accepted for filing, 50% of the fee that was paid is refunded [24].

An "action letter" for purposes of the fee provision is defined as one that approves the application or "which set[s] forth in detail the specific deficiencies in such ap-

*Reprinted with permission from *Regulatory Affairs*, 4:461–484 (1992).

plication[ ] and, where appropriate, the actions necessary to place such application[ ] in condition for approval" [25]. Once an application or supplement has been accepted for filing, if it is not approved or is withdrawn (and the fee is not waived), no fee is required for the resubmission of that application [26].

There is a reduced drug application fee for small businesses, which are defined as businesses with fewer than 500 employees, including employees of affiliates, which do not have a prescription drug product on the market. Such small businesses pay one-half of the amount of the fee for the basic human drug application, but pay the full fee for supplements [27].

Prescription Drug Establishment Fee

The prescription drug establishment fee applies to establishments that manufacture at least one prescription drug product that is not approved under an ANDA or a "paper NDA" (§ 505(b)(2) NDA), and which is "not the same as" a product approved under such an application [28]. Thus, this provision does not apply to generic drug manufacturers and to manufacturers of drugs all of which face generic competition. The fee only applies to establishments that had pending at the FDA a human drug application or supplement after September 1, 1992 [29].

The owner of a prescription drug establishment to which the fee applies is required to pay, on or before January 31 of each year, a prescription drug establishment fee [30]. That fee rises each year, starting at $60,000 in 1993, and with projected raises to $88,000 (1994), $126,000 (1995), $131,000 (1996), and $138,000 (1997) [31]. This provision does not apply to establishments that only manufacture over-the-counter drugs. It does apply to manufacturers of prescription antibiotics and biologics as well as non-antibiotic and non-biologic drugs [32].

The fee is applicable to prescription drug establishments either in the United States or abroad. "Prescription drug establishment" is further defined as being one general physical location consisting of one or more buildings, all of which are within five miles of each other, at which one or more prescription drug products are manufactured in final dosage form and which are under the management of a company that is listed as applicant in a human drug application for at least one prescription drug product [33]. For purposes of that definition, manufacturing does not include packaging [34].

Prescription Drug Product Fee

Each application holding a human drug application for a prescription drug product listed with the FDA who had a drug approval application pending with the FDA after September 1, 1992, is required to pay an annual fee for each such prescription drug product [35]. The fee is to be paid at the time of the first such listing of that product in each calendar year [36]. This provision does not apply, however, to prescription drugs covered by ANDAs or paper NDAs (§ 505(b)(2) applications) or to products that are the same as products approved under such applications (*i.e.,* products facing direct generic competition) [37]. The fee for each product starts at $6,000 in 1993 and is projected to increase to $9,000 (1994), $12,500 (1995), $13,000 (1996), and $14,000 (1997) [38].

Waivers

The FDA is to waive or reduce the fees described if it finds (1) that the waiver or reduction "is necessary to protect the public health," (2) that the fee "would present a significant barrier to innovation because of limited resources available to such person or other circumstances," (3) that the fees will exceed the anticipated present and future costs incurred by the FDA in

reviewing the application, or (4) that the fee for a full new drug application or supplement would be inequitable because a paper NDA (§ 505(b)(2) NDA) filed by another applicant for the same drug would not be assessed fees because it is not for a new molecular entity or new indication [39].

Failure to Pay Fees

If a company owes fees to the FDA, any human drug application or supplement it submits will be considered incomplete and will not be accepted for filing [40]. In addition, the government can collect fees due to the FDA in the same way that it collects other monies owed to the government [41].

Condition for Continuation of Fees

Congress and the Administration, and the pharmaceutical manufacturers who supported this legislation, expressed a common and strong commitment that the user fees would not simply go to pay for general expenses of the FDA or go to reduce the deficit. To assure that that does not happen, the law provides that no fees can be assessed in a fiscal year after 1993 unless appropriations for salaries and expenses of the FDA for that fiscal year (excluding the amounts obtained through fees) are equal to or greater than the amount of appropriations for the FDA for fiscal year 1992 multiplied by an adjustment factor. That factor will require at least an increase in appropriations at the lower of the percentage of the consumer price index increases for urban consumers or the percentage of increase in the total discretionary domestic budget [42]. Thus, should a future Congress or Administration seek effectively to decrease (by not keeping up with inflation) the budget of the FDA that comes from general revenues, or the proportion of the discretionary domestic budget that is allocated to the FDA, the fees could not be assessed.

If the total fees for a fiscal year exceed the costs for resources allocated for review of human drug applications, the fees will have to be adjusted downward [43]. The cost associated with the review that may be counted are expenses associated with officers, employees of the FDA and employees under contract to the FDA who work in FDA facilities, and advisory committees [44]. Notably, the statue does not include in this calculation costs of contractors conducting outside review of product approval applications. Management and overhead costs and any costs of collecting fees and accounting for them are included [45]. The statute states that the activities that may be considered for this purpose include not only direct application review, but inspections of prescription drug establishments and facilities related to that review, activities necessary for review of establishment license applications submitted by manufacturers of biologics or for the release of biologics, and monitoring of research conducted in connection with the review of human drug applications [46].

Increase in Speed of Review Process

The user fee bill was passed in exchange for a commitment from the FDA to use the revenues to achieve quite specific goals in speeding the approval of drug product approval applications. Those goals were outlined in a letter to Congress from Commissioner David Kessler [47]. Five year goals were stated as follows:

1. Action on "priority" drug product approval applications within six months after submission (with major amendments received in the last three months extending the review time frame by three months).

2. Action on standard applications within twelve months after submission (with the same extension for major amendments).

3. Action on "priority" supplements (supplements include "amendments" to product license applications and establishment license applications for biologics) within six months after submission.

4. Action on supplements that do not require review of clinical data (e.g., manufacturing supplements) within six months after submission.

5. Action on standard amendments requiring review of clinical data within twelve months after submission.

6. Action on applications resubmitted following a non-approval letter within six months after resubmission.

The action in each case would be an approval, an approvable letter, or a letter setting forth in detail specified deficiencies and, where appropriate, the actions necessary to put the application in condition for approval.

In the interim, the FDA commits to eliminate its overdue backlog of NDA, PLAs, ELAs, and amendments to PLAs within 24 months of initiation of user fee payments and to eliminate overdue backlogs of efficacy and manufacturing supplements within 18 months. In addition, the FDA commits to review 55% of new drug application, product license application, and establishment license application submissions received during fiscal year 1994 (starting October 1, 1993) within 12 months. A similar deadline is to apply to efficacy supplements. 55% of manufacturing supplements received during fiscal year 1994 are to be reviewed within 6 months, as are 55% of the resubmitted applications received during that time. The next year, the 55% goal is to be increased to 70%, with an increase to 80% in fiscal year 1996 and to 90% in fiscal year 1997.

The FDA has established a goal of having 50% of the incremental review staff related to these fees on board by the first quarter of fiscal year 1995 (the last quarter of calendar year 1994) with all staff on board by the end of fiscal year 1997. The FDA also states that it will take other management initiatives designed to manage and speed the drug approval process.

The FDA noted in a follow-up letter that most of these goals apply to over-the-counter as well as prescription drugs, but that the interim goals on reducing the backlog do not apply to those products [48].

Conclusion

The prescription drug user fee legislation represents an expensive experiment that will demonstrate whether providing more money to the FDA actually produces dividends in speeding the approval process. If it does, everyone seems to agree that the investment will be worthwhile and one could anticipate that manufacturers of other FDA-regulated products would become convinced that user fees may be appropriate for their products as well.

There will undoubtedly, however, be a period of frustration as the FDA struggles to use effectively the additional revenue that it expects to obtain from the statute. The agency has always had difficulty in bringing in and training reviewers. Nothing in the statute will increase the salaries that can be paid to such reviewers or otherwise enhance the incentives to come to the FDA and take on the task of reviewing drug applications.

The FDA believes, however, that it can accomplish this task and that its experience with drugs such as AIDS, in which assigning a proportionally larger number of staff persons to a drug has speeded approval, shows that progress can be made. We will all be watching with great interest.

References

1. Pub. L. No. 102-571 (1992).
2. *Id.*, § 103, adding § 736(b)(1) to the Federal Food, Drug, and Cosmetic Act. In subsequent footnotes, provisions added to that Act by § 103 will be cited only by reference to the section number of the added provision.
3. *Id.*, § 105.
4. 138 Cong. Rec. E2655 (Daily Ed., Sept. 16, 1992).
5. 138 Cong. Rec. E2657 (Daily Ed., Sept. 16, 1992).
6. The statute as passed includes a provision requring the FDA to study the possible usefulness of user fees for animal drugs, § 108, and provisions dealing with Dietary Supplements inserted at the insistence of Senator Hatch, §§ 201-06. This article does not address those provisions.
7. § 736(a)(1).
8. § 736(a)(2).
9. § 736(a)(3).
10. § 735(1)(A).
11. § 735(1)(B).
12. § 735(1)(C).
13. § 735(1)(D). There are specific exclusions for applications with respect to whole blood or a blood component for transfusion, bovine blood products for topical application licensed before September 1, 1992, allergenic extract products, *in vitro* diagnostic biologic products, and large volume parenteral drug products approved before September 1, 1992. § 7335(1).
14. § 736(a)(1)(A)(ii).
15. § 736(a)(1)(A)(i).
16. § 736(a)(1)(A)(ii).
17. § 736(a)(1)(A)(iii).
18. § 736(b)(1).
19. *Id.*
20. § 736(c)(2). In 1993 each category of fee is to yield a total revenue of $15 million, escalating to $18 million (1994), $25 million (1995), $26 million (1996), and $28 million (1997), § 736(b)(1).
21. § 736(c)(1).
22. § 736(a)(1)(B)(i).
23. § 736(a)(1)(B)(ii).
24. § 736(a)(1)(D).
25. § 735(6)(B).
26. § 736(a)(1)(C).
27. § 736(b)(2).
28. § 736(a)(2)(A).
29. § 736(a)(2)(B).
30. § 736(a)(2).
31. § 736(b)(1)) Note that the projected increases may be modified to produce revenues resulting in the statutory goals for each year.
32. § 735(3)(B). The exclusions recited in note 13 above apply here as well. § 735(3).
33. § 735(5).
34. *Id.*
35. § 736(a)(3)(A). Again, the exclusions in note 13 above apply. § 735(3).
36. § 736(a)(3)(A).
37. § 736(a)(3)(B).
38. § 736(b)(1).
39. § 736(d).
40. § 736(e).
41. § 736(h).
42. § 736(f)(1).
43. § 736(d)(3).
44. § 735(7)(A).
45. § 735(7)(B).
46. § 735(7)(C), (D).
47. 138 Cong. Rec. H9099 (Daily Ed. Sept. 22, 1992) (Commissioner Kessler's letter, Sept. 14, 1992).
48. 138 Cong. Rec. H9100 (Daily Ed. Sept. 23, 1992) (Commissioner Kessler's letter, Sept. 21, 1992).

User Fees

- Human drugs—prescription drugs, OTC drugs, and antibiotic drugs
- Biologic, by definition, is a drug, so it is encompassed by the drug definition

Exceptions

- Small emerging company given 50% decrease in application fee
- Due one year after submission
- Small emerging company—less than 500 employees and does not have product on the market
- Fees waived for orphan drugs, drug to protect public where fees significant barrier, and medical devices

User Fees

Excluded from User Fees:
- Generic antibiotics
- Allergenic extracts
- Whole blood or blood components for transfusion
- IVDs
- Medical devices

CHAPTER 18

Rx to OTC Switch

HOW DRUGS ARE MOVED FROM Rx TO OTC STATUS*

Max Sherman, R.Ph. and Steven Strauss, Ph.D., R.Ph.

During the course of the FDA/OTC drug review, now scheduled to be completed in 1993, 27 drugs for 31 indications have been switched from prescription to OTC status.

Most prescription drugs are regulated by the Food and Drug Administration as "new drugs" and are marketed subject to New Drug Applications (NDAs) approved by the FDA. Some OTC medicines are also regulated as "new drugs," and those products are subject to the same procedures and criteria for proof of safety and effectiveness as prescription drugs that are marketed under an NDA. The great majority of OTC medicines are, however, not subject to NDAs. For those medicines, FDA established a comprehensive procedure—the OTC drug review, which began in 1972, to ensure that all such products meet the regulatory requirements for general recognition of safety and effectiveness and are fully and informatively labeled [1]. The difference between OTC and Rx drugs is based upon "qualified experts" determination relative to safety and effectiveness and that prescription drugs are not safe enough for a layman to use as self medication. (This will be discussed later.)

The OTC Drug Review required the Commissioner of the Food and Drug Administration to appoint advisory review panels of qualified experts to evaluate the safety and effectiveness of OTC drugs, to review OTC drug labeling and to advise him on the promulgation of monographs establishing conditions under which OTC drugs are generally recognized as safe and effective and are not misbranded. This was not a trivial undertaking since more than 70 separate products categories had to be reviewed [2]. Initially there were more than 300,000 products to consider.

Included in the advisory review panel report to the Commissioner is a recommended monograph covering the category of OTC drugs and establishing conditions under which the drugs involved can be used safely and effectively. The monograph may include any conditions relating to active ingredients, labeling indications, warnings and adequate directions for use, prescription or OTC status, or any other conditions necessary and appropriate for the drug's use covered in the monograph [3].

After reviewing the conclusions and recommendations of the advisory review panel, the Commissioner publishes in the *Federal Register* a proposed order containing: (1) a monograph or monographs establishing conditions under which the category of OTC drugs is generally recognized as safe and effective and not misbranded—this would be Category I, or (2) a statement of the conditions excluded from the monograph on the basis of the Commissioner's determination that they would result in the drugs not being generally recognized as safe and effective and would result in misbranding—Category II. The third option would be a statement of the conditions excluded from the monograph on the basis of the Commissioner's determination that the available data are insufficient to classify either of the above conditions—Category III.

Once a product has been generally recognized as safe and effective in a final over-the-counter drug monograph, the product is no longer considered a "new drug." Products, of course, that are not considered "new drugs" do not require an approved NDA for marketing. The FDA provides an opportunity for the manufacturer of an affected product to comment on withdrawing approval of its NDA. A manufacturer of a drug product that complies with a final OTC drug monograph is not required to submit either supplemental, ab-

*Reprinted with permission from *U.S. Pharmacist* (June 1988).

Overview

- In 1972, the FDA concluded that it was appropriate to conduct a review of OTC drugs for safety and efficacy. One of the consequences of this move was a decision by the OTC advisory review panel to recommend that certain drugs be switched from Rx-only to OTC status.
- The FDA has initiated several changes in Rx status on its own outside of the OTC review process.
- The first drug to be switched under this policy was metaproterenol in a pressurized metered dose inhalation form. This marketing move was rescinded, but it did provide a legal framework for future decisions involving Rx-to-OTC switches.

breviated (ANDA) or a full NDA to cover such product [3].

History

There was no distinction under the 1906 Pure Food and Drugs Act [4] between OTC and Rx drugs. The purpose of the statute was to control drug labeling in a manner that assured it to be neither false nor misleading. The Harrison Narcotic Act did, however, specifically designate certain habit-forming drugs as available only by prescription from a licensed physician. When the Federal Food, Drug, and Cosmetic Act (the Act) [5] became law in 1938, it was silent with respect to the dispensing status of drugs by pharmacists. Soon after the passage of the Act, the FDA in its first public notice announced that sulfanilamide-containing drugs were dangerous unless their dosage was properly adjusted and used intelligently and expertly directed. The FDA stated that the "indiscriminate use" of such drugs would violate a provision of the law and deem the drug "misbranded" [6]. In this instance, the

drug would be dangerous to health when used in a dosage or manner, or with the frequency or duration prescribed, recommended or suggested in its labelling. To avoid "misbranding," the FDA indicated that drugs containing sulfanilamide should be labeled with a warning against unsupervised use by the public. No doubt this was a reaction to the sulfanilamide elixir disaster just one year earlier when 107 individuals died from ingesting the poisonous solvent diethylene glycol used in the elixir's formulation [7].

In December 1938 (the Act became law in June), the FDA issued a regulation which exempted drugs from the statutory requirement that labeling bear adequate instructions for use [8]. It advised that the statement "CAUTION: To be used only by or on the prescription of a physician," on the label constituted an exemption from the requirement for adequate labeling. This regulation clarified OTC from Rx drugs. In 1941 and again in 1944, in two *Federal Register* notices [9,10], the FDA prohibited any labeling representation concerning conditions of use for a drug that carried the "Caution" statement and sought to preclude the same statement for drugs that a layman could use safely.

Despite the early FDA activity in clarification of Rx and OTC drugs, the Durham-Humphrey Amendment [11] to the Act was the initial statute which distinguished between Rx and OTC drugs. The fundamental purpose of the amendment was to provide the pharmacist with clear guidance as to which drugs may not be sold without a prescription and may not be refilled without the prescriber's authorization as distinguished from those sold to the layman for self medication.

Before the amendment, many drugs were, as now, restricted to sale only upon prescription. Drugs that could be legally sold over-the-counter to laymen, however, were often also labeled by some manufacturers for prescription sale only.

Thus, the validity of the prescription legend was severely compromised. The formal statutory guidelines specified three types of drugs to be available by prescription only: (1) drugs that are habit-forming; (2) new drugs, under their approved NDAs; and (3) drugs that are toxic, or have the potential for harmful effect, or require collateral measures for safe use. The Durham-Humphrey amendment further authorized FDA "by regulation" to remove the prescription-dispensing requirement for habit-forming drugs and for drugs subject to NDAs when such requirements are not necessary for the protection of the public health.

As a result of this statutory authority, FDA defined the procedure for switching a drug from prescription to OTC status [12]. This so-called "switch" regulation enabled any interested person to petition for an exemption from the prescription-dispensing requirements. That petition could be a supplement to an approved NDA. Even with this guidance, there is some thought that the provisions of the amendment did not provide a clear policy or resulting consistent decisions on the prescription/non-prescription status of drugs in the United States [13].

Until 1962 a "new drug" was defined as one that was not generally recognized by experts as "safe" for its intended use. The 1962 Kefauver-Harris Drug Amendment to the Act [14] changed the definition of a "new drug" to provide that a drug was a "new drug" unless it was generally recognized by experts, on the basis of substantial scientifically sound evidence, as effective, as well as safe. The new legislation had a massive impact on FDA's regulation of drugs. "New drugs" previously covered by NDAs that considered safety only now had to be supported by substantial evidence of efficacy. Similarly, for drugs claimed to be not new, general recognition now extended to efficacy, as well as safety. In short, FDA was faced with the immense task of reevaluating almost all drugs marketed in the United States, both those sold by prescription and those marketed OTC.

The 1962 Amendment thus required FDA to review the efficacy claims of those drugs introduced into the market between 1938 and 1962. Because prescription drugs posed the greater potential for harm, the FDA opted to review NDA drugs first. This review known as DESI, or Drug Efficacy Study Implementation, was done under contract with the National Academy of Science—National Research Council (NAS-NRC).

Some 3500 drugs in DESI required a prescription, while approximately 420 were OTC. Many of these OTC drugs were handled under DESI, and final orders were issued classifying the drugs as either lacking substantial evidence of safety or as not having been shown to be safe and ordering their removal from the market. For the remainder of the DESI/OTC drugs, FDA concluded that they be referred to an OTC review for a final determination. Then with the DESI review well under way, FDA in 1972 concluded that it was appropriate to conduct a similar review of OTC drugs, and they then proposed procedural regulations for that task [1].

OTC Drug Review

The FDA/OTC drug review in its assessment and categorization of ingredients and labeling condi-

tions generally recognized as safe and effective for lay use, will result in a determination that certain drug ingredients for certain uses have a definitive OTC status for FDA's regulatory purposes. During the course of the review, a number of the OTC advisory review panels recommended that 27 drugs for 31 indications be switched from prescription to OTC status [15]. The Food and Drug Administration has been willing to allow some of these changes to occur during the course of the review, the most notable perhaps being the switch of several strengths of topical hydrocortisone from prescription to OTC status [16].

FDA regulations allow these changes to occur in the marketplace at the time that the panel's report (advanced notice of proposed rulemaking) is published in the *Federal Register* unless the FDA disagrees with the panel at that time [17]. The FDA has dissented from 10 of these switch recommendations, and has subsequently rescinded one of these dissents. Petitions to rescind several more of these dissents have been submitted to FDA and are being evaluated. It is important to understand the sequence used by the FDA to establish conditions under which OTC drugs can be marketed. The first step is the *Federal Register* publication of an advanced notice of proposed rulemaking (ANPRM). Thirty days are allowed for general comments. This is followed by issuance of a notice of proposed

rulemaking (NPRM), or a tentative final monograph (Figure 1).

At the tentative monograph state, Category I is termed a monograph condition and Categories II and III, nonmonograph. Final FDA action occurs with publication of a final rule. Manufacturers then have 12 months to comply. Products which do not meet monograph conditions are declared "new drugs," and the manufacturer would be faced with filing an NDA to continue marketing the drug. The FDA has projected that the final monograph will be completed in 1993.

Metaproterenol and FDA Policy

The FDA has initiated several prescription to OTC switches on its own initiative, i.e., the drug was not reviewed by an OTC advisory review panel, but was considered by FDA for OTC status after the relevant panel has completed its work. The first was the bronchodilator drug metaproterenol in a pressurized metered dose inhalation form [18].

When the proposal was made, it was based on FDA's enforcement policy under which a prescription drug may be marketed OTC if the agency reaches a tentative conclusion in the relevant OTC drug review proceeding, that such marketing is safe and the drug otherwise qualifies for inclusion in Category I. Moreover, the agency believed that metaproterenol provided a useful alternative drug therapy for asthma sufferers who at that time

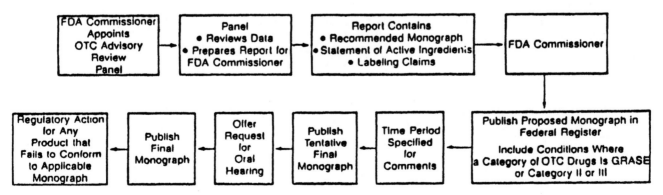

FIGURE 1. Procedure for classifying an over-the-counter drug as generally recognized as safe and effective (GRASE).

Glossary

"New Drugs" are defined by Section 201(p) of the Food, Drug, and Cosmetic Act to include drugs that are not generally recognized by experts as safe and effective for the use as recommended in their labeling.

An NDA or New Drug Application is an application requesting FDA approval to market a new drug in interstate commerce. The application must contain data from clinical studies and other information needed for FDA review including chemistry, pharmacology, toxicology, biopharmaceutics and statistics.

A nonprescription over-the-counter drug can be defined as a drug generally recognized among qualified experts as safe and effective, manufactured in accordance with good manufacturing practices, and labeled with directions under which the layman can use the drug safely and for the purpose for which it is intended.

Safety means a low incidence of adverse reactions or significant side effects under adequate instructions for use and warnings against unsafe use, as well as low potential for harm which may result from abuse under conditions of widespread availability.

Effectiveness means a reasonable expectation that, in a significant proportion of the target population, the pharmacological effect of the drug, when used under adequate directions for use and warnings against unsafe use, will provide clinically significant relief of the type claimed.

---

were limited to preparations containing epinephrine if they chose to treat asthma symptoms with an OTC-inhaled drug. The FDA also concluded that it would be in the interest of public health to allow marketing, rather than awaiting publication of a final monograph for OTC bronchodilator drugs, an event that might not occur for several years.

In terms of labeling, there was some controversy about whether patients can be depended upon to follow directions. The FDA believed that persons who suffer from severe asthma are capable of understanding and heeding instructions for safety using a product. Patients also have ready access to professional advice on the appropriate use of any drugs that may be taken. In reply to concerns that the product may be misused by children, the agency responded by stating that the key to such prevention is not the marketing status, but the degree of informed and effective control exercised by parents. Marketing of metaproterenol was rescinded because of criticism from physicians and an opinion from FDA's Pulmonary-Allergy Drugs Advisory Committee. However, the *Federal Register* announcement contained an important policy decision noting that

FDA had been given the statutory responsibility to make a broad range of decisions involving the suitability of drugs for and by the American public [19]. These decisions involve the safety and effectiveness of drugs, their status as a prescription or OTC drug, the indications for use, and other vital labeling information. While advisory committees are an important adjunct, the FDA stated that it does not believe that they should be viewed as an indispensable part of all FDA procedures for regulating drugs.

The initial action by the agency for metaproterenol is important because it illustrated FDA's early philosophy in changing drugs from prescription to OTC status. The FDA thus appeared to be more willing to recognize that even through a particular disease condition may have to be diagnosed by a physician, once such a diagnosis has been made, it is no longer essential that drugs used for the alleviation or treatment of that condition be limited to prescription status [20].

References

1. 37 FR 85, January 5, 1972.
2. 52 FR 40309, October 26, 1987.
3. 21 CFR 333.10.
4. Public Law 59-384, 34 Stat 768 (1906).
5. Public Law 75-717, 52 Stat 1040 (1938).
6. Food and Drug Administration, Trade Correspondence-1, August 26, 1938.
7. Sherman M: Infamous Drugs—a quick history, Drug & Cosmetic Industry 142(2):37, 1988.
8. 3 FR 3167, December 28, 1938.
9. 6 FR 1920, April 15, 1941.
10. 9 FR 12255, October 10, 1944.
11. Public Law 82-215, 65 Stat 648 (1951).
12. 21 CFR 310.200(e).
13. Hull PB: A legal framework for future decisions on transferring drugs from prescription to nonprescription status. Food Drug Cosmetic Laws 37:427, 1982.
14. Public Law J87-181, 76 Stat 780 (1962).
15. Rachanow GM: The switch of drugs from prescription to over the counter status. Food Drug Cosmetic Law J 39:201, 1984.
16. 44 FR 69768, December 4, 1979.
17. 21 CFR 330.13.
18. 47 FR 47520. October 26, 1982.
19. 43 FR 24925, June 3, 1983.
20. Kaplan AH: Over-the-counter and prescription drugs: The legal distinction under federal law. Food Drug Cosmetic Law, J37:441, 1982.
21. Prop. Assoc. Exec. Ltr. No. 48-86, December 12, 1986.

Regulatory Requirements for Rx and OTC Drugs

Regulatory Requirement	Marketing Status			
	Rx Drugs		OTC Drugs	
	NDA	No NDA	NDA	Monograph
FDA approval of safety	Yes	No	Yes	Yes
FDA approval of effectiveness	Yes	No	Yes	Yes
FDA approval of labeling	Yes	No	Yes	Yes
Applicability of adulteration requirements (Section 501)	Yes	Yes	Yes	Yes
Applicability of misbranding requirements (Section 502)	Yes	Yes	Yes	Yes
Applicability of Drug Listing Act (Section 510)	Yes	Yes	Yes	Yes
Establishment Inspection Authority (Section 704)	Yes	Yes	Yes	Yes
Submission of marketing experience prior to approval	Yes	No	Yes	Yes
Periodic submission of current marketing experience	Yes	Yes	Yes	No

Criteria for Rx to OTC Switch

- The drug must be safe. This is the primary criterion. Safety is defined as:
  —not habit forming
  —inherently non-toxic, i.e., a wide margin of safety to cover possible overdosing or abuse/misuse
  —acceptable side effect profile
  —no serious adverse experiences
  —unlikely to mask a more serious underlying disorder
- The product must be easily administered, i.e., no injectiables, dose titrating, etc.
- The product should be for therapy and not prophylaxis.
- The condition being treated must be of a non-serious nature and probably self-limiting (e.g., diarrhea).
- The condition should have recognizable symptoms, be self-diagnosable by the lay public, and generally require no medical intervention.

WHAT MAKES IT PRESCRIPTION*

Some physicians and consumers worry that there is danger in making a prescription drug freely available, the commonly held belief being that OTC drugs are "weaker" or "safer" than prescription-only drug products. This is not necessarily true. Aspirin can cause stomach bleeding in some people and antihistamines can cause drowsiness. Basically, what determines whether a particular drug will be marketed as a prescription or OTC product is spelled out in the Food, Drug, and Cosmetic Act. The definition of a prescription drug, incidentally, did not go on the books until 1951.

The FDC Act provides that all drugs are to be marketed OTC with certain exceptions. Slated for prescription use are drugs that are habit forming (17 habit-forming drugs and their derivatives are identified in FDA's regulations): drugs that are toxic, have a potential for harmful effects, or whose method of use or collateral measures for use make them unsafe for self-medication; and, finally, drugs that are limited by an approved New Drug Application for use only under supervision of a practitioner licensed by law to administer such drugs. In general, FDA decides which drugs meet these criteria.

The prescription status of a drug is not set in concrete, however. *A drug can be switched to OTC status by FDA initiative or on petition of another party if it is determined that the prescription-dispensing requirements are not necessary for the protection of the public health.* Factors that must be considered are

*Reprinted from *FDA Consumer* (July/August 1983).

whether the drug is safe to use without a doctor's supervision, whether follow-up care is needed (the "collateral measures" for use), and whether adequate directions for self-use can be written. Twenty-five new drugs have been switched from prescription to OTC status via this route, including sodium monofluorophosphate (a dentifrice) and dextromethorphan (a popular cough suppressant).

Manufacturers also can switch a drug from prescription to OTC status by filing a supplement to a New Drug Application. Several prescription drugs were switched via this mechanism during the OTC drug review. Examples include the popular cough-cold products Actifed, Benylin and Drixoral.

The OTC review process is the third way in which the Rx-to-OTC switch can be made. FDA's review of OTC drugs grew out of the mandate of the 1962 amendments to the Food, Drug, and Cosmetic Act that all drugs be both safe and effective for their intended use. (When the FDA Act became law in 1938, it required only that drugs be proved safe.) A mid-1960s review of drugs marketed between 1938 and 1962 revealed that only 25 percent of 512 OTC drug products were effective. The agency then decided it was time to take a good look at all the drugs on the OTC market. Many of these products had been "grandfathered"—that is, allowed to be sold because they had been on the market before the safety and effectiveness laws went into effect.

The OTC drug review got under way early in 1972. From the start it was evident that a product-by-product review was impossible. There were some 300,000 products containing over 700 ingredients.

FDA's approach was to evaluate the active ingredients by therapeutic category. The 74 product categories were assigned to 17 panels of nongovernment experts.

The first phase of the review, during which the panels made their evaluations and presented recommendations to FDA, is over. As of this writing, only one panel report is yet to be published for public comment.

During the second stage of the review, FDA evaluates the panel recommendations, public comments and new data. Out of this evaluation come "tentative final monographs," or proposed standards for the various classes of drugs. To date, FDA has published 19 tentative final monographs.

The final stage of the review involves publication of the final monographs, which represent the regulatory standards for the marketing of nonprescription drugs. Eight final monographs have been published.

From the beginning, FDA intended that the advisory review panels would consider the possibility of switching prescription drugs to OTC status. The authority to do so was included in the regulations establishing the procedures for the OTC drug review. It is FDA's policy to allow such drugs to be sold without a prescription once the panel's report has been published, if the agency has no objections and if the drug can be appropriately labeled for self-medication. However, manufacturers who take advantage of this opportunity do so at the risk that FDA might not approve a switch when it comes time to issue the final monograph.

Rx TO OTC—THE SWITCH IS ON*

Marian Segal

What do Dimetapp, Sominex, Bactine, Cortaid, Coricidin Nasal Mist, OcuClear, E-Z Scrub 241, Trosyd, and Actifed have in common? They, along with dozens of other drug products, have made the "switch" from prescription to over-the-counter (OTC) status.

The Nonprescription Drug Manufacturers Association estimates that more than 200 OTC drug products on the market today were available by prescription only a decade ago. Among them are antihistamines and nasal decongestants for colds and allergies, sleep aids, pain relievers, cough medicines, antifungals, antimicrobials, and anti-itch medicines. These products contain ingredients in dose strengths that the Food and Drug Administration has deemed safe enough to use without a doctor's prescription.

When this issue of *FDA Consumer* went to press, the most recent ingredient that FDA had approved for the switch from prescription to OTC sale was clotrimazole in cream and suppository dosage forms. Used to treat vaginal yeast infections, clotrimazole has been available by prescription for more than 10 years. It will be marketed OTC under the trade name Gyne-Lotrimin. In announcing the switch, Carl Peck, M.D., director of FDA's Center for Drug Evaluation and Research, said, "Clotrimazole is highly effective and carries a minimal risk. If initially diagnosed by a doctor, recurring symptoms of vaginal yeast in fection, or candidiasis, can be recognized by the patient, who can treat herself with the over-the-counter drug without the inconvenience and expense of going back to the doctor."

Some other prescription prod-

ucts the drug industry is interested in switching, according to the July 9, 1990, *Advertising Age*, are the antacids Zantac, Carafate, Tagamet, and Pepcid; the cold/allergy medications Claritin, Hismanal and Seldane; and the nonsteroidal anti-inflammatory drugs Naprosyn, Clinoril, Feldene, and Anaprox. The publication also reported a projection that the OTC drug market would reach $19 billion in manufacturer sales by the year 2000, up 72% from $11 billion in 1990.

OTC Drug Review

A major impetus for switching drugs from prescription to OTC status is FDA's comprehensive review, begun in 1972, of the active ingredients in OTC drug products. The review grew out of amendments to the drug law enacted in 1962, which require drugs to be proven effective before they can be marketed. (Before Congress passed this legislation, drugs had to be proven safe, but proof of their effectiveness was not required by law.)

Thus, FDA was obliged to reexamine all drugs—both prescription and OTC—that had been approved solely on the basis of safety. For OTC drugs, the endeavor involved about 730 active ingredients that were used in more than 300,000 drug products sold in the United States. The review separated the active ingredients in the products into therapeutic classes—for example, anti-itch medicines, antihistamines and antifungals. Seventeen panels of nongovernment experts were established to make recommendations about the safety and effectiveness of ingredients for their intended uses. As a result of the review, some ingredients were taken off the market because they were found ineffective; others were banned for safety reasons.

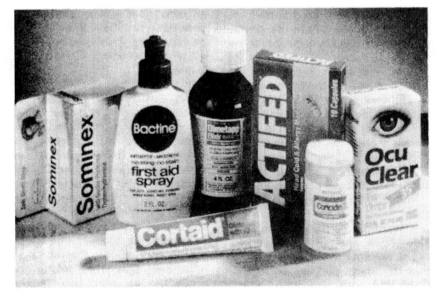

The ingredients or dosage strengths in these products were previously unavailable over the counter. The ingredients are: diphenhydramine (Sominex), hydrocortisone (Bactine and Cortaid), brompheniramine (Dimetapp), triprolidine (Actifed), and oxymetazoline (Coricidin Nasal Mist and OcuClear). Other brand-name products containing these ingredients, as well as generics, are also available.

*Reprinted from *FDA Consumer* (March 1991).

In addition to evaluating safety and efficacy of OTC drugs, the panels reviewed currently marketed prescription ingredients to determine whether some might be appropriate for OTC marketing. Some panels determined that dosages of certain OTC ingredients, such as antihistamines, needed to be raised to levels that were previously allowed by prescription only. So far, nearly 40 formerly prescription-only drug ingredients in at least 16 classes have been switched to OTC status.

What Determines Rx vs. OTC?

The distinction between prescription and nonprescription drugs is spelled out in the Durham-Humphrey Amendment to the Federal Food, Drug, and Cosmetic Act. Before this amendment was passed in 1951, there was no specific statutory requirement that any drug be labeled for sale by prescription only. With the amendment, prescription drugs were defined primarily as those unsafe for use except under professional supervision. They include certain habit-forming drugs and any drug that is unsafe "because of its toxicity or other potentiality for harmful effect, or the method of its use, or the collateral measures necessary to its use. . . ."

Nonprescription drugs are regarded as safe for consumers to use by following the directions and warnings required on the label.

To protect consumers, FDA regulations require that labeling of OTC drugs state:

• the intended uses and results of the product

• adequate directions for proper use

• warnings against unsafe use, side effects, and adverse reactions.

The labeling must be written so that ordinary people, including those with somewhat low reading comprehension skills, would be likely to understand it.

Toxicity is the major issue in deciding whether to switch a drug from prescription to OTC status.

Because almost any drug, if misused, can have some adverse side effect, one way to evaluate possible harm in switching is to consider the drug's overall margin of safety.

Gerald Rachanow, J.D., deputy director of FDA's division of OTC drug evaluation, explains that, "Drugs that have a high risk of causing toxicity and a low margin of safety, and that must be carefully used to achieve the appropriate level of effectiveness without endangering the consumer's safety, are appropriately classified as prescription drugs."

On the other hand, Rachanow says, "the mere possibility that a drug can be misused, with toxic results, is not a sufficient basis alone to classify it for prescription status."

OTC Labels

The process of switching some antihistamines to OTC status can serve as an example of the procedure. Antihistamines are used to relieve symptoms of hay fever and other upper respiratory allergies. They may cause drowsiness, however, presenting a hazard if taken in circumstances where alertness is important. Antihistamines also can be dangerous to patients with glaucoma, an enlarged prostate, or asthma.

In reviewing antihistamines, FDA's Cough/Cold Advisory Review Panel did not find these potential dangers sufficient cause to limit these ingredients to prescription use. It recommended instead that the labeling for OTC antihistamine drug products bear a warning that the product "may cause drowsiness" and caution consumers to "avoid driving a motor vehicle or operating heavy machinery" and to "avoid alcoholic beverages while taking this product." The panel also recommended that the label warn patients not to take these products except with the advice and supervision of a physician if they have glaucoma, asthma, or difficulty

urinating because of an enlarged prostate.

Self-Diagnosis

Another consideration in deciding whether or not a drug should be available without prescription is whether the condition being treated can be self-diagnosed. Inability to self-diagnose a condition, however, does not automatically preclude OTC status for products intended to treat its symptoms. Several drugs, such as bronchodilators, are marketed over the counter even though the conditions they are used to treat—asthma, in this case—cannot be self-diagnosed. FDA's Cough/Cold Advisory Review Panel recommended that bronchodilators could be marketed over the counter provided they were labeled with the warning: "Caution: Do not take this product unless a diagnosis of asthma has been made by a physician."

Most OTC drugs are labeled for the treatment of symptoms, such as sinus congestion, headache, pain, upset stomach, and itching. Consumers can readily recognize these symptoms and select an appropriate product to gain relief, but they may not know what underlying condition is causing the pain, cough or itch they are self-medicating. To help consumers judge when a physician should be consulted if a medical problem is not resolving itself through self-medication, products will carry warnings to consult a physician under appropriate conditions. An OTC hydrocortisone preparation to relieve itching from eczema, poison ivy, insect bites, and other causes, for example, carries the warning, "If condition worsens, or if symptoms persist for more than 7 days, discontinue use of this product and consult a doctor."

Timing of the Switch

The switch process has not been trouble-free. When the OTC drug review began, FDA did not have a

OTC Glossary

Drug: In common usage a term synonymous with the word medicine. By legal definition any substance which is intended for use in the diagnosis, cure, mitigation, treatment or prevention of disease. Any substance intended in any way to alter body functions also is a drug. Thus, a deodorant which claims only to mask body odor is by law a cosmetic while an antiperspirant which claims to reduce perspiration (a body function) is by law a drug.

Drug Misuse: Use of a drug in other than the recommended amount, frequency, strength or manner. Misuse may or may not result in damage to the person's health or ability to function.

Drug Abuse: A form of misuse in which a person deliberately uses a drug to achieve an effect which is not intended or recommended.

Effectiveness: The ability of an over-the-counter medicine to do what it claims to do. For example, relieve the symptoms of ailments such as headache, acid indigestion, constipation, coughs, nasal congestion, etc. Proof of effectiveness is required by federal law in order to market a drug for the first time.

Exclusivity: An FDA policy which seeks to limit the label descriptions (medical claims) of OTC medicines to those words specifically approved by the government. The policy—being reconsidered by FDA—would exclude all words not approved by the agency. Thus, "antiflatulent" would be allowed as a claim for an antacid but "anti-gas" would not be.

FD&C Act: The Federal Food, Drug, and Cosmetic Act, the basic law governing drugs sold in the U.S. Among other things, the Act prohibits the sale in interstate commerce of drugs that are adulterated, misbranded or dangerous to health; establishes minimum standards of strength, quality and purity for many drugs; and sets up specifications for drug labeling.

FDA: Food and Drug Administration. The federal agency responsible for approving all over-the-counter medicines on the basis of safety, effectiveness and proper labeling.

FTC: Federal Trade Commission. The federal agency responsible for preventing unfair and deceptive advertising of over-the-counter medicines.

Flag: A symbol, phrase or notation which OTC manufacturers voluntarily add to product labels to alert consumers to significant product changes, including new ingredients, dosage instructions or warnings.

Good Manufacturing Practice (GMP) Regulations: A set of federal (FDA) regulations that governs the processes and procedures followed by the makers of all medicines in order to assure safety and uniform quality of drugs.

Label: Any written, printed or graphic matter on the immediate container of an OTC medicine.

Labeling: All labels and other written, printed or graphic matter 1) on any OTC medicine or any of its containers or wrappers, or 2) accompanying an OTC medicine.

Monograph: A drug standard written by FDA to describe safe and effective ingredients, acceptable formulations and appropriate labeling for a specific category of over-the-counter medicines (laxatives, analgesics, antacids, etc.). A Monograph provides a regulatory "recipe book" and any product in conformance with all provisions of the Monograph may be marketed without specific FDA approval. Any product having ingredients, formulations or labeling outside an established Monograph must obtain separate approval by FDA prior to marketing.

Nonprescription Medicine: Any medicine which can be bought without a doctor's prescription. Distribution of nonprescription medicines is unrestricted and the medicines may be sold, for example, in grocery stores as well as pharmacies.

Over-The-Counter (OTC) Medicine: The same as "nonprescription medicine."

OTC Review: Shorthand name for FDA's process of evaluating the safety and effectiveness of ingredients used in nonprescription medicines. Monographs setting standards for acceptable ingredients, dosages, formulations and labeling in OTC medicines are the end product of the Review.

Patent Medicines: Now archaic. Originally used to describe English medicines for which letters of patent had been granted to manufacturers by the Crown.

Prescription Drugs: Medicines prescribed by a duly authorized practitioner and dispensed only by them or by a registered pharmacist. Also known as Rx, "legend," "caution," or prescription drugs. All drugs marketed in the U.S. are determined to be either prescription or nonprescription medicines by the FDA. All drugs by law must be nonprescription medicines if in FDA's judgment a label can be written to ensure safe and proper use by the consumer. When FDA judges that adequate consumer labeling cannot be written, the agency must restrict the medicine to prescription status.

Proprietary Medicines: Over-the-counter (nonprescription) medicines sold under a trademark and advertised to the general public.

"Rx-to-OTC": Popular term describing that part of the U.S. regulatory system under which appropriately safe and long-established prescription medicines are shifted by the Food and Drug Administration from prescription to over-the-counter availability.

Self-Medication: The use of nonprescription medicines as directed in the labeling.

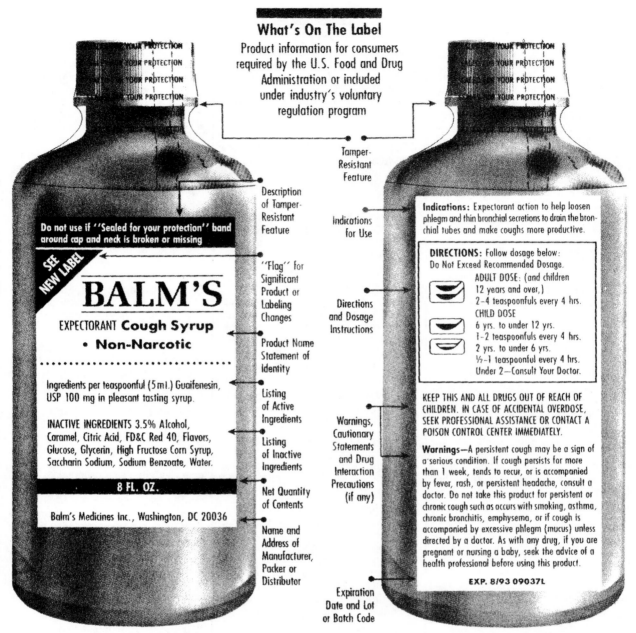

What's On The Label

Product information for consumers required by the U.S. Food and Drug Administration or included under industry's voluntary regulation program

Description of Tamper-Resistant Feature

Tamper-Resistant Feature

"Flag" for Significant Product or Labeling Changes

Indications for Use

Product Name Statement of Identity

Directions and Dosage Instructions

Listing of Active Ingredients

Listing of Inactive Ingredients

Warnings, Cautionary Statements and Drug Interaction Precautions (if any)

Net Quantity of Contents

Name and Address of Manufacturer, Packer or Distributor

Expiration Date and Lot or Batch Code

Do not use if "Sealed for your protection" band around cap and neck is broken or missing

SEE NEW LABEL

BALM'S
EXPECTORANT Cough Syrup
• Non-Narcotic

Ingredients per teaspoonful (5 ml.) Guaifenesin, USP 100 mg in pleasant tasting syrup.

INACTIVE INGREDIENTS 3.5% Alcohol, Caramel, Citric Acid, FD&C Red 40, Flavors, Glucose, Glycerin, High Fructose Corn Syrup, Saccharin Sodium, Sodium Benzoate, Water.

8 FL. OZ.

Balm's Medicines Inc., Washington, DC 20036

Indications: Expectorant action to help loosen phlegm and thin bronchial secretions to drain the bronchial tubes and make coughs more productive.

DIRECTIONS: Follow dosage below:
Do Not Exceed Recommended Dosage.
ADULT DOSE: (and children 12 years and over,)
2–4 teaspoonfuls every 4 hrs.
CHILD DOSE
6 yrs. to under 12 yrs.
1–2 teaspoonfuls every 4 hrs.
2 yrs. to under 6 yrs.
½–1 teaspoonful every 4 hrs.
Under 2—Consult Your Doctor.

KEEP THIS AND ALL DRUGS OUT OF REACH OF CHILDREN. IN CASE OF ACCIDENTAL OVERDOSE, SEEK PROFESSIONAL ASSISTANCE OR CONTACT A POISON CONTROL CENTER IMMEDIATELY.

Warnings—A persistent cough may be a sign of a serious condition. If cough persists for more than 1 week, tends to recur, or is accompanied by fever, rash, or persistent headache, consult a doctor. Do not take this product for persistent or chronic cough such as occurs with smoking, asthma, chronic bronchitis, emphysema, or if cough is accompanied by excessive phlegm (mucus) unless directed by a doctor. As with any drug, if you are pregnant or nursing a baby, seek the advice of a health professional before using this product.

EXP. 8/93 09037L

Whereas prescription drug labels for the patient carry minimal information, FDA requires that OTC labels be much more detailed so that consumers can properly use the products without the advice of a health professional.

FIGURE 1. Non-prescription, over-the-counter (OTC) drugs label.

clear policy that told industry at what point in the process it could market a product being considered for a switch. As a result, some manufacturers began marketing prescription products without waiting for publication of the panel's recommendation or issuance of FDA's final regulation.

In 1976, FDA published a statement of policy explaining that, unless the agency disagrees with the panel, products under review for the switch could be sold over the counter at the time that the advisory panel's report (called a "proposed monograph") is published in the *Federal Register*. The

drugs must be labeled as the panel recommends in its report or as the agency requires in a tentative final monograph. If at a later time FDA disagrees with the panel because of new or other evidence, the agency can then disallow the switch.

A company can also petition

Table 1
Top Selling RX-to-OTC Switches

Brand	Manufacturer	Therapeutic Category	Date Introduced
Advil	American Home Products	General pain reliever	1984
Monistat 7	Johnson & Johnson	Vaginal yeast infection	1991
Sudafed	Burroughs Wellcome	Cold medication	1978
Dimetapp	American Home Products	Cold medication	1985
Nuprin	Bristol-Myers Squibb	General pain reliever	1984
Benadryl	Warner-Lambert	Allergy medication	1985
Actifed	Burroughs Wellcome	Cold medication	1982
Afrin	Schering-Plough	Nasal decongestant	1976
Imodium A-D	McNeil Consumer	Antidiarrheal	1988
Drixoral	Schering-Plough	Cold medication	1982
Oxy-Line	SmithKline Beecham	Anti-acne	1975
Chlor-Trimeton	Schering-Plough	Allergy medication	1975
Micatin	Johnson & Johnson	Fungicidal preparation	1983
Cortaid	Upjohn	Topical hydrocortisone	1980
Lotrimin AF	Schering-Plough	Fungicidal preparation	1990
Benylin	Warner-Lambert	Cough syrup	1981
Nix	Burroughs Wellcome	Pediculicide	1990
Duration	Schering-Plough	Nasal decongestant	1976
Dimetane	American Home Products	Allergy medication	1976
Femstat 3	Procter & Gamble	Vaginal yeast infection	1995
Tagamet HB	SmithKline Beecham	Antacid	1995
Zantac 75	Glaxo Wellcome	Antacid	1996
Pepcid AC	Johnson & Johnson·Merck	Antacid	1995
Children's Motrin	McNeil	General pain reliever	1995
Actron Orudis KT	Bayer Whitehall Robins	General pain reliever	1995
Tavist-1	Sandoz	Allergy medication	1993
Rogaine	Pharmacia & Upjohn	Hair-growth stimulant	1996
Nicorette	SmithKline Beecham	Smoking cessation	1996
Axid AR	Whitehall-Robins Healthcare	Antacid	1996
Monistat 3	Ortho	Vaginal yeast infection	1996
Nicotrol	McNeil Consumer	Smoking cessation	1996
OcuHist	Pfizer	Eye care	1996
Gyne-Lotrimin	Schering-Plough	Vaginal yeast infection	1996
Nicoderm CQ	SmithKline Beecham	Smoking cessation	1996
Nasalcrom	McNeil Consumer	Allergy medication	1997
Vagistat-1	Bristol-Myers Squibb	Vaginal yeast infection	1997
Nizoral	Johnson & Johnson Consumer Products	Dandruff shampoo	1997
Zantac 75 Efferdose	Glaxo Wellcome	Antacid	1998

FDA to switch an ingredient from prescription to OTC status or, if the company itself manufactures the drug, it can submit a new drug application (NDA) or supplemental NDA for OTC status for the drug.

On occasion, the agency has rescinded an original decision to approve or disapprove a switch. For example, FDA initially disagreed with a panel recommendation to switch the drug diphenhydramine hydrochloride to OTC status for use as a nighttime sleep aid and antihistamine because more controlled studies were needed to satisfy the agency's concerns about the drug's safety and effectiveness in doses appropriate for OTC use. Twelve studies were submitted that compared diphenhydramine with a placebo. After reviewing the data, FDA concluded that the drug, at specified dosage levels, was safe and effective as an OTC nighttime sleep aid. In a later decision, diphenhydramine was also approved for OTC use as an antihistamine.

The converse has happened as well. In October 1982, FDA proposed OTC availability of the bronchodilator metaproterenol sulfate in a metered-dose inhalation aerosol. The proposal met with criticism from the medical community, particularly because of concerns that young children could be harmed by misusing the inhalers.

The agency agreed that there were some risks associated with self-diagnosis and treatment of asthma and that there was a potential for misuse of the product. It believed, however, that the risks did not outweigh the benefits of easy availability. The agency's required labeling for the inhalers warned that the product should be used only after asthma was diagnosed by a physician.

In May 1983, FDA's Pulmonary-Allergy Drugs Advisory Committee met in a public forum to hear reports, and discuss the issue. The committee concluded that the risks of OTC availability outweighed the benefits and recommended that FDA rescind its proposal to make metaproterenol an OTC drug. The agency did so the following month.

More recently, when the drug ibuprofen (Advil, Nuprin and Motrin IB) was approved for OTC sale, some experts wanted the label to carry a warning that it might cause kidney damage in people with preexisting kidney disease. FDA determined at that time that the warning was not needed, but is now reconsidering the need because of recent studies indicating an association.

A similar concern has been raised about the antihistamine Seldane, now being reviewed for OTC status. Unlike other antihistamines, Seldane has the advantage of not causing drowsiness. The drug can, however, cause abnormal heart rhythms in patients who have liver problems or take certain other drugs.

For Sale by Pharmacist Only

Some health professional organizations have petitioned FDA to establish a third class of drugs that would be available without prescription, but only through a pharmacist. Pharmacists would advise consumers about proper use of the drug and serve to identify problems that might arise. In 1974, in connection with an FDA monograph on OTC antacids, some pharmacy organizations commented that such a third class of drugs should be created. Others, including the Department of Justice, objected to a third class of drugs, stating that it would restrain competition, inconvenience the consumer, depart from U.S. economic policy, and cause price increases for the consumer with no attending benefit.

FDA concluded that "no controlled studies or other adequate research data have been supplied to support the position that any class of OTC drugs must be dispensed only by pharmacists in order to ensure their safe use. . . . There is at this time no public health concern that would justify the creation of a third class of drugs to be dispensed only by a pharmacist or in a pharmacy."

Whatever the mechanism, it's clear that we can expect many more drugs to be considered for the switch from prescription to over-the-counter sales. In recent years, Americans have become increasingly health conscious and have assumed more responsibility

Fact Sheet on Rx-to-OTC Switch

- Nonprescription medicines available under law to the general public without a prescription must be effective for their intended uses and must provide an appropriate margin of safety when used as directed. Label directions must be written in understandable language and must provide all information necessary for safe and effective use by the consumer.

- FDA has the authority to initiate an Rx-to-OTC transfer on its own. Any company, or interested party, may also petition FDA to switch an ingredient from prescription to OTC status.

- There have been 49 ingredients/dosages transferred from prescription to OTC status as a consequence of FDA's OTC Review.

- Trends identified as promoting Rx-to-OTC conversions include: the aging U.S. population; a population more informed and interested in self-medication; continuing popularity of OTC drugs; and cost savings that can be derived from OTC drugs.

- There are an estimated 125,000–300,000 OTC products (in a variety of sizes, dosages, strengths) marketed in the U.S.

Q: **How are OTCs regulated?**
A: The U.S. Food and Drug Administration regulates what ingredients and how much of each can be put into OTC medicines. FDA also decides what must be said in the labeling and how the medicines are to be packaged. The Federal Trade Commission regulates the way OTC medicines are advertised. All federal regulations are based on a congressional mandate that OTC medicines must be safe, effective and properly labeled to permit use without medical supervision. Congress also decreed that OTC medicines must be advertised to the public in a fair and nondeceptive way.

Q: **Do state and local governments have a say in the regulation of OTC medicines?**

A: Yes. Despite uniform national regulation by the federal government, individual states and localities continue to propose differing requirements for the distribution, packaging and labeling of OTC medicines. Such efforts nearly always conflict with or duplicate federal rules, other state or local rules, or both.

Q: **Who decides which medicines shall be OTC and which Rx (prescription)? And how is the decision made?**
A: The FDA decides and it does so under specific instructions from the Congress. Each decision is based on a safety judgment. If the use of a medicine involves serious risk, or if it requires professional guidance for proper use, it is allowed only by medical prescription. If the risk is not serious and if clear labeling can instruct the consumer in safe use of the product then it *must* be allowed for over-the-counter sale.

Q: **What about medicines formerly available only by prescription that are now sold over the counter?**
A: FDA will permit the over-the-counter marketing of carefully selected, safe and effective prescription medicines after long experience and the consensus of scientific opinion have shown them suitable for direct sale to the consumer. Rx-to-OTC "switch," as the process is called, is making ever better, more comprehensive self-medication a reality. Beyond symptomatic relief, recently switched drugs offer definitive treatment including, in some cases, prevention or cure for specified conditions.

---

for their health, evidenced by such trends as emphasis on diet and excercise and smoking cessation. This take-charge posture is also becoming apparent in self-treatment.

As John Naisbitt writes in his book *Megatrends: Ten New Directions Transforming Our Lives*, "Along with new habits, the medical self-help movement has brought an upsurge in self-care. No longer do Americans feel they must run to a doctor for every minor ailment: 75 percent of the people can successfully deal with medical problems without ever walking into a clinic or doctor's office."

James D. Cope, president of the Nonprescription Drug Manufacturers Association, says that self-care with self-medication is the largest component of our health-care system and the least costly.

"Six out of 10 medicines bought by consumers are nonprescription," says Cope, "yet total spending for [these medicines] is less than 2 cents of the U.S. health-care dollar." Cope maintains that in a single recent year, OTC medicines saved the nation $10.5 billion that otherwise would have been spent for prescription drugs, doctor visits, and lost time from work.

The trend toward more switches is generally greeted with enthusiasm by consumers, the drug industry, and many health professionals. Caution remains FDA's watchword, however. The continued success of these switches will depend on consumers' good judgment in using these products correctly and in following label directions and warnings.

CHAPTER 19

Federal Anti-Tampering Act

The Federal Anti-Tampering Act (P.L. 98-127), passed by Congress in 1983 and signed into law by President Ronald Reagan, as a result of a deliberate contamination of Tylenol capsules in 1982, makes it a federal offense to tamper with consumer products and gives regulatory authority to the FBI, USDA, and FDA.

The Food and Drug Administration has the authority under the *Federal Food, Drug, and Cosmetic Act* (the *Act*) to establish a uniform national requirement for tamper-resistant packaging of OTC drug products that will improve the security of OTC drug packaging and help assure the safety and effectiveness of OTC drug products. An OTC drug product (except a dermatological, dentrifice, insulin, or throat lozenge product) for retail sale that is not packaged in a tamper-resistant package or that is not properly labeled is adulterated under section 501 of the *Act* or misbranded under section 502 of the *Act*, or both.

The term *tamper*, when used in a criminal statute, has the limited meaning of improper interference "as for the purpose of alteration and to make objectionable or unauthorized changes." Tampering involves changing a product from what it was intended to be by the manufacturer. There are five sections of the *Federal Anti-Tampering Act:* (1) tampering with a consumer product that affects interstate or foreign commerce, with reckless disregard for the risk of death or bodily injury to another person; (2) tainting a consumer product with the intent of injuring a business; (3) communicating false information that a consumer product has been tainted; (4) threatening to tamper with a consumer product; and (5) conspiring to tamper.

A tamper-resistant package is defined as "one having an indicator or barrier to entry which if breached or missing, can reasonably be expected to provide visible evidence to consumers that tampering has occurred." The regulations do not require the use of specific packaging technologies; any technology that achieves the required effect is acceptable.

Although current packaging technologies have made products less vulnerable to tampering, tamper-*proof* packaging does not exist. Improvements in packaging technologies and heightened consumer awareness are needed for further protection against tampering.

Each manufacturer and packer who packages an OTC drug product (except a dermatological, dentifrice, insulin, or throat lozenge product) for retail sale shall package the product in a tamper-resistant package if this product is accessible to the public while held for sale. To reduce the likelihood of successful tampering and to increase the likelihood that consumers will discover if a product has been tampered with, the package is required to be distinctive by design (e.g., an aerosol product container) or by the use of one or more indicators or barriers to entry that employ an identifying characteristic (e.g., a pattern, name, registered trademark, logo, or picture).

The term "distinctive by design" means the packaging cannot be duplicated with commonly available materials or through commonly available processes, e.g., blister packs, aerosol containers, and individual foil pouches.

The term *aerosol product* means a product that depends upon the power of a liquified or compressed gas to expel the contents from the container.

A tamper-resistant package may involve an immediate-container and closure system or secondary-container or systems intended to provide a visual indication of package integrity. The tamper-resistant feature shall be designed to and shall remain intact when handled in a reasonable manner during manufacture, distribution, and retail display.

For two-piece, hard gelatin capsule products a minimum of two tamper-resistant packaging features is re-

Suggested Tamper-Resistant Packaging

• **Film wrappers.** A transparent film with distinctive design is wrapped securely around a product or product container. The film must be cut or torn to open the container and remove the product.

• **Blister or strip packs.** Dosage units (for example, capsules or tablets) are individually sealed in clear plastic or foil. The individual compartment must be torn or broken to obtain the product.

• **Bubble packs.** The product and container are sealed in plastic and mounted in or on a display card. The plastic must be torn or broken to remove the product.

• **Shrink seals and bands.** Bands or wrappers with a distinctive design are shrunk by heat or drying to seal the union of the cap and container. The seal must be cut or torn to open the container and remove the product.

• **Foil, paper or plastic pouches.** The product is enclosed in an individual pouch that must be torn or broken to obtain the product.

• **Bottle seals.** Paper or foil with a distinctive design is sealed to the mouth of a container under the cap. The seal must be torn or broken to open the container and remove the product.

• **Tape seals.** Paper or foil with a distinctive design is sealed over all carton flaps or a bottle cap. The seal must be torn or broken to open the container and remove the product.

• **Breakable caps.** The container is sealed by a plastic or metal cap that either breaks away completely when removed from the container or leaves part of the cap attached to the container. The cap must be broken to open the container and remove the product.

• **Sealed tubes.** The mouth of a tube is sealed and the seal must be punctured to obtain the product.

• **Sealed carton.** All flaps of a carton are securely sealed and the carton must be visibly damaged when opened to remove the product.

• **Aerosol containers.** Aerosol containers are inherently tamper resistant.

---

quired, unless the capsules are sealed by a tamper-resistant technology. For all other products, including two-piece, hard gelatin capsules that are sealed by a tamper-resistant technology, a minimum of one tamper-resistant feature is required.

Each retail package of an OTC drug product, except ammonia inhalant in crushable glass ampules, aerosol products, or containers of compressed medical oxygen, is required to bear a statement that is prominently placed so that consumers are alerted to the specific tamper-resistant feature of the package. The labeling statement is also required to be so placed that it will be unaffected if the tamper-resistant feature of the package is breached or missing. If the tamper-resistant feature is one that uses an identifying characteristic, that characteristic is required to be referred to in the labeling statement. For example, the labeling statement on a bottle with a shrink band could indicate "For your protection this bottle has an imprinted seal around the neck."

A manufacturer or packer may request an exemption from the packaging and labeling requirements.

Holders of approved new drug applications (NDAs) for OTC products are required to submit supplemental NDAs to provide for the changes in packaging and in the labeling to comply with the requirements of Tampering-Resistant Packaging (TRP).

Holders of approved premarket approval applications for products subject to TRP have to submit supplements to provide for changes in packaging to comply with the requirements of such packaging. If, however, these changes do not affect the container or the product then supplements to the PMA are not required. Any supplement PMA that is submitted should show that the changes made do not adversely affect the products.

If for any device or drug product the container closure is changed to comply with TRP requirements, the development of new stability data may be required. Stability data from accelerated studies are still appropriate to project a tentative expiration date as long as concurrent ambient temperature studies are conducted to verify the expiration date. Products in which major changes are made without appropriate stability testing would be in violation of the GMP regulations (21 *CFR* 211.137 and 211.166).

For tamper-resistant packaging to be fully effective, consumers need to examine the packaging carefully before consuming the contents, and they must be aware of specific tamper-resistant features that have been used. FDA regulations require that the labeling of products with tamper-resistant packaging bear a statement alerting the consumer to the tamper-resistant feature. This labeling statement must be placed so that it remains intact even if the tamper-resistant feature is breached or missing. If tampering is suspected, the closest FDA district office should be immediately notified.

The tamper-resistant packaging regulations for OTC drug products (21 *CFR* 211.132) are part of the CGMPs for finished drug product. For devices, the tamper-resistant packaging regulations are in 21 *CFR* 800.12, and those for cosmetics are in 21 *CFR* 700.25.

A *Compliance Policy Guide (7132a.17)* that describes specific tamper-resistant packaging technologies is available from the National Technical Information Service, 5285 Port Royal Road, Springfield, VA 22161.

QUESTIONS: CHAPTER 19

1. Tamper-resistant packaging regulations are implemented and enforced by:

    a. BNDD
    b. FDA
    c. FTC
    d. DEA
    e. CPSC

2. Which one of the following is exempt from tamper-resistant packaging pursuant to federal law?

    a. Oral prescription products dispensed by the pharmacist
    b. Controlled substances
    c. Aerosol products
    d. Vaginal cosmetic products
    e. OTC drugs intended for human use

3. Which one of the following is exempt from tamper-resistant packaging pursuant to federal law?

    a. Cosmetics
    b. Capsules
    c. Insulin
    d. Vaginal products
    e. Schedule V OTC drugs

4. Child-resistant packaging is synonymous with tamper-resistant packaging:

    a. True
    b. False

5. Tamper-resistant packaging may be "child-resistant":

    a. True
    b. False

6. Which one of the following presidents of the United States signed the Federal Anti-Tampering Act into law?

    a. John F. Kennedy
    b. James Earl Carter
    c. Ronald Reagan
    d. George H. W. Bush
    e. William Jefferson Clinton

> The FDA will require all OTC drug products sold in two-piece hard gelatin capsules to be sealed using tamper-evident technology. The requirement will take effect November 4, 1999.

CHAPTER 20

Homeopathic Drugs

HOMEOPATHIC DRUGS—REGULATORY CONCERNS*

Steven Strauss, Ph.D., R.Ph. and Max Sherman, R.Ph.

The eighth edition of the *Homeopathic Pharmacopeia of the United States* [1] is the sole authority in the United States for all homeopathic remedies which must be "proved" before they can be included. Homeopathic provings provide the experimental basis for learning what symptoms a substance causes and thus, according to the law of similars, what it uses. Provings are biological experiments on normal persons, simple and plain in execution. The substance to be investigated is given in a suitable preparation, dose and frequency, to a group of people, male and female, of varying ages and constitutions. These persons, "provers" as they are called, do not know what they are taking. Provings allow the practitioner to individualize a choice of medicine according to the totality of the patient's symptoms [2]. A homeopathic physician must be cognizant of the total or holistic nature of the patient's physiological disorder or disease. In addition to proving, there must be sufficient demand for the drug to justify its inclusion in the Pharmacopeia.

Now there is evidence of new interest in the subject by the Food

and Drug Administration (FDA). Until recently, homeopathic drugs were marketed on a limited scale by a few manufacturers who have predominantly served the needs of licensed practitioners. This has now changed, and this article will review regulatory issues, including the need for, and difficulties involved to prove that homeopathic drugs are safe and effective. According to the adherents of homeopathy, there is an obvious difference between allopathic or standard medicine and their beliefs. Allopathic medical treatment requires that a drug be administered in a sufficient quantity to realize specific blood levels. The drug is then incorporated into the cellular substance which may affect its metabolism. Hemeopathic therapeutics attempts, instead, to employ the remedial capacity (vital force) of the organism [3]. Homeopathic drugs cause no physiological action and take no part in the reaction which occurs in the disordered (sensitized) body. The correct homeopathic medicine, therefore, effectively stimulates the person's natural defense system, helps heal the illness, and raises the general level of health. It the toxic effect of the drug closely mimics a patient's symptoms, then the physiological reaction provoked by that substance in sub-

toxic amounts can aid the patient's recovery.

Regulatory Issues

The very nature of homeopathic drugs, and the fact that the *Federal Food, Drug, and Cosmetic Act* (the *Act*) recognizes the drugs and standards in the *Homeopathic Pharmacopeia*, presents a dichotomy in new drug development processes. (Inclusion of the reference to homeopathic drugs in the 1938 Act was largely due to the effort of Senator Royal Copeland (D,NY), the foremost homeopathic physician of his time.) That is, there are significant differences between the methods needed to introduce new allopathic (conventional) and new homeopathic drugs into the marketplace in the United States. When the manufacturer (sponsor) of a conventional drug wants to test its potential effect in treating disease, a sponsor is required to file an application for an investigational new drug exemption (an IND) with the Food and Drug Administration before testing the drugs in humans. This application must include a general investigational plan, protocols for each planned study, a description of drug chemistry and manufacturing process, copies of labeling provided to the investigators, detailed

---

*From a presentation at the *Annual Meeting of the American Society for Pharmacy Law*, April 8, 1989, Anaheim, CA.

pharmacology and toxicology information, and a summary of previous drug experience. This information is required to assure that potential risks are balanced by benefits, and that the proposed clinical trials could be expected to provide reliable and substantial evidence of safety and effectiveness data.

When the sponsor completes clinical trials and feels that they provide evidence of effectiveness in conjunction with acceptable risk, the sponsor must submit a new drug application (NDA) for FDA approval before marketing the compound. An NDA is approved if the FDA, often in consultation with an advisory committee, determines that the drug meets the statutory standards for safety and effectiveness, manufacturing and controls, and labeling. The clinical investigation underlying claims of effectiveness must be "adequate and well-controlled studies."

An NDA includes sections on chemistry, manufacturing and controls, drug substance, drug product, environmental impact, nonclinical pharmacology and toxicology, human pharmacokinetic and bioavailability, microbiology, clinical data (evidence for both safety and efficacy), statistical analyses, samples, case report forms, and the proposed text of labeling for the drug.

Homeopathic drugs are not subjected to the same rigorous standards for inclusion in the *Homeopathic Pharmacopeia of the United States*. There is, however, a research procedure that requires careful principles of double blind testing (although the patients are healthy individuals). A method to record and describe all symptoms accurately to a research director, a period of observation up to 60 days, frequent interrogation and patient examination, and finally, segregation of reports from the participants receiving placebos as opposed to participants receiving the drug that is being studied. In the latter, all the symptoms are evaluated as to frequency of appear-

ance, severity, location, and time of occurrence. This compilation of symptoms represents the pathogenesis or symptom picture of the drug. The research director then submits this information to a committee on standards of the American Institute of Homeopathy who then determines whether the drug shall or shall not be included in the pharmacopeia based on sufficient proof of safety and probable efficacy.

Thus, the public protection regarding "new drugs" which is based on a framework of federal laws and regulations is not applied to homeopathic remedies. The 1938 *Act* exempted homeopathic products from safety review. The 1962 Kefauver-Harris drug amendments to the *Act* [4] left the homeopathic exemption intact so that while allopathic drugs are scientifically tested and reviewed for safety and effectiveness, homeopathic products are checked for neither [5]. In essence, homeopathic drugs are presumed to be safe, but they have not been proven effective against disease by scientific means, such as randomized controlled double blind trials.

Labeling

Homeopathic products that are offered for testing serious disease conditions must be dispensed by the pharmacist pursuant to a prescription from a homeopathic practitioner. Because of this, homeopathic products have historically borne little or no labeling for the customer. Only products offered for use in self-limiting conditions recognized by consumers may be marketed without a prescription [6]. Because of increasing sales and some evidence of false claims, the Compliance Division, Food and Drug Administration, has been alerted and asked whether a homeopathic drug is being offered for use or promoted significantly beyond recognized or customary practices of homeopathy. Regulatory interest is evident from regulatory letters issued by the FDA and

recent issuance of a *Compliance Policy Guide* [6]. Action has been taken against firms which manufacture homeopathic products labeled as immune system alterers to treat AIDS, anticancer stimulant tablets which were offered for stimulating the body's own natural defense system against degenerative cells, and for remedies labeled for treatment of serious diseases such as hypoglycemia, gout, disturbances in cerebral function, and lung abscesses. It was the FDA position that all these homeopathic products are drugs as defined in Section 201(g) of the *Act*. Furthermore, the FDA was unaware of any substantial scientific evidence which demonstrates that any of the homeopathic drugs are generally recognized as safe and effective for their advertised use. A product's compliance with requirements of the *Homeopathic Pharmacopeia*, therefore, does not establish that it has been shown by appropriate means to be safe, effective, and not misbranded for its intended use.

As mentioned, while the law gives FDA no premarket review of true homeopathic drugs, FDA and traditional homeopaths have been concerned about other instances of untrained, unlicensed practitioners treating people for serious ailments and about recent attempts by companies to produce nonprescription products under the homeopathic umbrella in order to avoid FDA regulations. For example, some producers of nonprescription diet dermal patches claimed the products to be homeopathic, but FDA rules that their drug delivery systems required premarket approval.

Homeopathic drug product labeling must comply with the labeling provisions of Sections 502 and 503 of the *Act* and Title 21, Part 201, of the *Code of Federal Regulations*. Homeopathic drugs must list on the label the name and place of business of the manufacturer and provide adequate directions for use in conformance with Section 502(f) of the *Act* and 21 *CFR* 201.5.

The ingredient information must appear on homeopathic drug labels in accordance with 502(e) of the *Act* and 21 *CFR* 201.10. Labeling must bear a statement of the quantity and amount of ingredient(s) in the product in conformance with Section 502(b) of the *Act* as well as 21 *CFR* 201.10, expressed in homeopathic terms, e.g., 1X, 2X. Documentation must be provided to support those products or ingredients which are not recognized in the *Homeopathic Pharmacopeia* or its supplements.

The product must be in conformance with Section 502(e)(1) of the *Act* and must bear an established name in accord with Section 502(e) of the *Act* and 21 *CFR* 201.10. Many homeopathic products bear Latin names which correspond to listings in the *Homeopathic Pharmacopeia*. Since Section 502(c) of the *Act* and 21 *CFR* 201.15(c)(1) require that all labeling be in English, the industry is required to translate these names from Latin to their common English names as current labeling stocks are depleted or by June 11, 1990, whichever occurs first. It is permissible for industry to include in the labeling both English and Latin names.

Homeopathic prescription drugs must comply with the general labeling listed previously which also includes the statement "Caution: Federal law prohibits dispensing without prescription," a statement of identity, declaration of net quantity of contents and statement of dosage, and a package insert bearing information for the homeopathic practitioner.

Homeopathic non-prescription drugs, in addition to the general labeling provisions, must contain a principal display panel as provided under 21 *CFR* 201.62, a statement of identity, a declaration of net quantity of contents, indications for use in terms likely to be understood by lay persons, and warning statements in conformance with 21 *CFR* 201.63.

Good Manufacturing Practices

Homeopathic drug products must be packaged in accordance with Section 502(g) of the *Act* and be manufactured in conformance with Good Manufacturing Practices, Section 501(a)2(b) of the *Act* and 21 *CFR* 211. However, due to the unique nature of these drug products, some requirements of 21 *CFR* 211 are not applicable as follows:

1. Section 211.137 specifically exempts homeopathic drug products from expiration dating requirements [7].

2. Section 211.165: Several years ago, the FDA proposed to amend 21 *CFR* 211.165 to exempt homeopathic drug products from the requirement for laboratory determination of identity and strength of each active ingredient prior to distribution [8]. Pending a final rule of this exemption, this testing requirement is not being enforced for homeopathic drug products.

Homeopathic drugs, however, will be subject to the over-the-counter drug review [9]. They will be examined separately after all of the reviews have been completed.

Conclusion

Homeopathy has not been readily accepted by the current scientific and medical establishment [10]. Despite this, the FDA is faced with a renewed challenge and must now grapple with means to regulate this centuries old treatment method. Certainly if these drugs are ineffective, they are dangerous when used to treat serious or life-threatening disease. On the other hand, it could be that homeopathy's popularity and long survival are evidence that it works [11]. It will be interesting to see if increased demand and sales cause the FDA to take further action or to ask Congress to change the *Act* to seek parity between conventional and homeopathic drugs.

References

1. *The Homeopathic Pharmacopeia of the United States, Eighth Edition.* Washington, DC: American Institute of Homeopathy, 1974.

2. *Compendium of Homeopathic Therapeutics, The Homeopathic Pharmacopeia of the United States, Eighth Edition Addendum.* Washington, DC: American Institute of Homeopathy, 1974.

3. 21 U.S.C. 301-392.

4. P.I.. 87-181; 76 Stat. 780 et. seq.

5. FDA Talk Paper T-88-68, September 15, 1988.

6. Food and Drug Administration Compliance Policy Guide 7132.15 May 31, 1988.

7. Strauss, S. and M. Sherman. "Regulations Pertaining to Expiration Dating of Drug Products in the United States," *Food Drug Cosm. Law. J.*, 41(2):160, 1986.

8. Rados, B. "Riding the Coattails of Homeopathic Revival," *FDA Consumer*, 19(2):30, 1985.

9. Wertheimer, A. I. "The Status of Homeopathy Today," *NJ J. Pharm.*, 7:20, 1983.

10. Scofield, A. M. "Experimental Research in Homeopathy—Critical Revision," *Br. Homeopathy J.*, 73(4):211, 1984.

11. Barrett, S. 1987. "Homeopathy, Is It Medicine?" *Nutritional Forum*, 4(1):1, 1987.

CONDITIONS UNDER WHICH HOMEOPATHIC DRUGS MAY BE MARKETED*

Background

The term "homeopathy" is derived from the Greek words *homeo* (similar) and *pathos* (suffering or disease). The first basic principles of homeopathy were formulated by Samuel Hahnemann in the late 1700's. The practice of homeopathy is based on the belief that disease symptoms can be cured by small doses of substances which produce similar symptoms in healthy people.

The *Federal Food, Drug, and Cosmetic Act* (the *Act*) recognizes as official the drugs and standards in the *Homeopathic Pharmacopeia of the United States* and its supplements [Sections 201(g)(1) and 501(b), respectively]. Until recently, homeopathic drugs have been marketed on a limited scale by few manufacturers who have been in business for many years and have predominantly served the needs of a limited number of licensed practitioners. In conjunction with this, homeopathic drug products historically have borne little or no labeling for the consumer.

Today the homeopathic drug market has grown to become a multimillion dollar industry in the United States, with a significant increase shown in the importation and domestic marketing of homeopathic drug products. Those products that are offered for treatment of serious disease conditions, must be dispensed under the care of a licensed practitioner. Other products, offered for use in self-limiting conditions recognizable by consumers, may be marketed OTC.

This document provides guidance on the regulation of OTC and

prescription homeopathic drugs and delineates those conditions under which homeopathic drugs may ordinarily be marketed in the U.S.

Discussion

Section 201(g)(1) of the *Act* defines the term "drug" to mean articles recognized in the official *United States Pharmacopeia* (USP), the official *Homeopathic Pharmacopeia of the United States* (HPUS), or official *National Formulary* (NF) or any supplement to them; and articles intended for use in the diagnosis, cure, mitigation, treatment, or the prevention of disease in man or other animals; articles (other than food) intended to affect the structure or any function of the body of man or other animals; and articles intended for use as a component of any articles specified in the above. Whether or not they are official homeopathic remedies, those products offered for the cure, mitigation, prevention, or treatment of disease conditions are regarded as drugs within the meaning of Section 201(g)(1) of the *Act*.

Homeopathic drugs generally must meet the standards for strength, quality, and purity set forth in the *Homeopathic Pharmacopeia*. Section 501(b) of the *Act* (21 U.S.C. 351) provides in relevant part:

Whenever a drug is recognized in both the United States Pharmacopeia *and the* Homeopathic Pharmacopeia of the United States *it shall be subject to the requirements of the* United States Pharmacopeia *unless it is labeled and offered for sale as a homeopathic drug, in which case it shall be subject to the provisions of the* Homeopathic Pharmacopeia of the United States *and not to those of the* United States Pharmacopeia.

A product's compliance with requirements of the *HPUS, USP,* or *NF* does not establish that it has been shown by appropriate means to be safe, effective, and not misbranded for its intended use.

Labeling

Homeopathic drug product labeling must comply with the labeling provisions of Sections 502 and 503 of the *Act* and Part 201 Title 21 of the *Code of Federal Regulations (CFR)*, as discussed below, with certain provisions applicable to extemporaneously compounded OTC products. Those drugs in bulk packages intended for manufacture or preparation of products, including those subsequently diluted to various potencies, must also comply with the provisions of Section 502 of the *Act* and Part 201 (21 *CFR* 201).

General Labeling Provisions

Name and Place of Business: Each product must bear the name and place of business of the manufacturer, packer, or distributor in conformance with Section 502(b) of the *Act* and 21 *CFR* 201.1.

Directions for Use: Each drug product offered for retail sale must bear adequate directions for use in conformance with Section 502(f) of the *Act* and 21 *CFR* 201.5. An exemption from adequate directions for use under Section 503 is applicable only to prescription drugs.

Statement of Ingredients: Ingredient information shall appear in accord with Section 502(e) of the *Act* and 21 *CFR* 201.10. Labeling must bear a statement of the quantity and amount of ingredient(s) in the product in conformance with Section 502(b) of the *Act,* as well as 21 *CFR* 201.10, expressed in homeopathic terms, e.g., 1x, 2x.

Documentation must be provided to support that those prod-

*Reprinted from *Food and Drug Administration, Compliance Policy Guide,* 7132.15 (May 31, 1988).

ucts or ingredients which are not recognized officially in the *HPUS*, an addendum to it, or its supplements are generally recognized as homeopathic products or ingredients.

Established Name: The product must be in conformance with Section 502(e)(1) of the *Act* and must bear an established name in accord with Section 502(e)(3) of the *Act* and 21 *CFR* 201.10. Many homeopathic products bear Latin names which correspond to listings in the *HPUS*. Since Section 502(c) of the *Act* and 21 *CFR* 201.15(c)(1) require that all labeling be in English, the industry is required to translate these names from Latin to their common English names as current labeling stocks are depleted, or by June 11, 1990, whichever occurs first. It is permissible for industry to include in the labeling both English and Latin names.

Container Size—Labeling Exemption: For those products packaged in containers too small to accommodate a label bearing the required information, the label-

ing requirements provided under Section 502 of the *Act* and 21 *CFR* 201 may be met by placing information on the carbon or outer container, or in a leaflet with the package, as designated in 21 *CFR* 201.10(i) for OTC drugs and in 21 *CFR* 201.100(b)(7) for prescription drugs. However, as a minimum, each product must also bear a label containing a statement of identity and potency, and the name and place of business of the manufacturer, packer, or distributor.

Language: The label and labeling must be in the English language as described and provided for under 21 *CFR* 201.15(c)(1), although it is permissible for industry to include foreign language in the labeling, as well.

Prescription Drugs

The products must comply with the general labeling provisions above, as well as the provisions for prescription drugs below.

Prescription Drug Legend: All prescription homeopathic drug

products must bear the prescription legend, "Caution: Federal Law prohibits dispensing without prescription," in conformance with Section 503(b)(1) of the *Act*.

Statement of Identity: The label shall bear a statement of identity as provided for under 21 *CFR* 201.50.

Declaration of Net Quantity of Contents and Statement of Dosage: The label shall bear a declaration of net quantity of contents as provided in 21 *CFR* 201.51 and a statement of the recommended or usual dosage as described under 21 *CFR* 201.55.

General Labeling Requirements: The labeling shall contain the information described under 21 *CFR* 201.56 and 21 *CFR* 201.57. For all prescription homeopathic products, a package insert bearing complete labeling information for the homeopathic practitioner must accompany the product.

OTC Drugs

Product labeling must comply with the general labeling provisions above and the provisions for

---

Definitions

Homeopathy: The practice of treating the syndromes and conditions which constitute disease with remedies that have produced similar syndromes and conditions in healthy subjects.

Homeopathic Drug: Any drug labeled as being homeopathic which is listed in the *Homeopathic Pharmacopeia of the United States* (HPUS), an addendum to it, or its supplements. The potencies of homeopathic drugs are specified in terms of dilution, i.e., 1x (1/10 dilution), 2x (1/100 dilution), etc. Homeopathic drug products must contain diluents commonly used in homeopathic pharmaceutics. Drug products containing homeopathic ingredients in combination with non-homeopathic active ingredients are *not* homeopathic drug products.

Homeotherapeutics: Involves therapy which utilizes drugs that are selected and administered in accordance with the tenets of homeopathy.

Homeopathic Pharmacopeia of the United States (HPUS): A compilation of standards for source, composition, and prepration of homeopathic drugs. HPUS contains monographs of drug ingredients used in homeopathic treatment. It is recognized as an official compendium under Section 201(j) of the Act.

Compendium of Homeotherapeutics: An addendum to the HPUS which contains basic premises and concepts of homeopathy and homeotherapeutics; specifications and standards of prepration, content, and dosage of homeopathic drugs; a description of the proving process used to determine the eligibility of drugs for inclusion in HPUS; the technique of prescribing the therapeutic application of homeopathic drugs; and a partial list of drugs which meet the criteria of the proving process and are eligible for inclusion in HPUS and other homeopathic texts. [A proving is synonymous with the homeopathic procedure (identified in HPUS as a "Research Procedure") which is employed in healthy individuals to determine the dose of a drug sufficient to produce symptoms.]

Extemporaneously Compounded OTC Products: Those homeopathic drug products which are often prepared by dilution to many variations of potency from stock preparations, and which: (1) have at least one OTC indication; (2) are prepared pursuant to consumers' oral or written requests; and (3) are not generally sold from retail shelves. Those products which are prescription drugs only cannot be provided to consumers as extemporaneously compounded OTC products but, may only be prepared pursuant to a prescription order.

OTC drugs below, as current labeling stocks are depleted or by June 11, 1990, whichever occurs first.

Principal display Panel: The labeling must comply with the principal display panel provision under 21 *CFR* 201.62.

Statement of Identity: The label shall contain a statement of identity as described in 21 *CFR* 201.61.

Declaration of Net Quantity of Contents: The label shall conform to the provisions for declaring net quantity of contents under 21 *CFR* 201.62.

Indications for Use: The labeling for those products offered for OTC retail sale must bear at least one major OTC indication for use, stated in terms likely to be understood by lay persons. For extemporaneously compounded OTC products, the *labeling* must bear at least one major OTC indication for use, stated in terms likely to be understood by lay persons. For combination products, the labeling must bear appropriate indication(s) common to the respective ingredients. Industry must comply with the provisions concerning indications for use as current labeling stocks are depleted, or by June 11, 1990, whichever occurs first.

Directions for Use: See the general labeling provisions above.

Warnings: OTC homeopathic drugs intended for systemic absorption, unless specifically exempted, must bear a warning statement in conformance with 21 *CFR* 201.63(a). Other warnings, such as those for indications conforming to those in OTC drug final regulations, are required as appropriate.

Prescription/OTC Status

The criteria specified in Section 503(b) of the *Act* apply to the determination of prescription status for all drug products, including homeopathic drug products. If the *HPUS* specifies a distinction between nonprescription [over-the-counter (OTC)] and prescription status of products which is based on strength (e.g., 30x)—and which is more restrictive than Section 503(b) of the *Act*—the more stringent criteria will apply. Homeopathic products intended solely for self-limiting disease conditions amenable to self-diagnosis (of symptoms) and treatment may be marketed OTC. Homeopathic products offered for conditions not amenable to OTC use must be marketed as prescription products.

Home Remedy Kits

Homeopathic home remedy kits may contain several products used for a wide range of conditions amenable to OTC use. When limited space does not allow for a list of those conditions on the labels of the products, the required labeling must appear in a pamphlet or similar informational piece which is enclosed in the kits. However, as a minimum, each product must also bear a label containing a statement of identity and potency.

Other Requirements

All firms which manufacture, prepare, propagate, compound, or otherwise process homeopathic drugs must register as drug establishments in conformance with Section 510 of the *Act* and 21 *CFR* 207. Further, homeopathic drug products must be listed in conformance with the sections above. (*Note:* For a given product, variations in package size and potency are not required to be listed on separate forms 2657 but instead, may be listed on the same form). Homeopathic drug products must be packaged in accordance with Section 502(g) of the *Act*. Homeopathic drug products must be manufactured in conformance with current good manufacturing practice, Section 501(a)(2)(B) of the *Act* and 21 *CFR* 211. However, due to the unique nature of these drug products, some requirements of 21 *CFR* 211 are not applicable, as follows:

1. Section 211.137 (Expiration dating) specifically exempts homeopathic drug products from expiration dating requirements.

2. Section 211.165 (Testing and release for distribution): In the *Federal Register* of April 1, 1983 (48 FR 14003), the Agency proposed to amend 21 *CFR* 211.165 to exempt homeopathic drug products from the requirement for laboratory determination of identity and strength of each active ingredient prior to release for distribution.

Pending a final rule on this exemption, this testing requirement will not be enforced for homeopathic drug products.

Regulatory Action Guidance

Firms marketing homeopathic drugs which are not in compliance with the preceding conditions will be considered for regulatory follow-up. In general, minor misbranding violations should be considered as a basis for issuance of a Notice of Adverse Findings Letter (NAF Letter) or if imports, Release with Comment. The Office of Compliance, HFD-304, Center for Drug Evaluation and Research, should be consulted before such letters are issued.

Those homeopathic drug products which are not in compliance and do not meet the criteria for issuance of an NAF Letter are candidates for the issuance of Regulatory Letters, and should be referred to the Office of Compliance, HFD-304, for review.

Recommendations for the issuance of regulatory letters or other regulatory sanctions must be submitted in conformity with the *Regulatory Procedures Manual* and other Agency guidance concerning the review of regulatory actions.

The Legal Status of Homeopathic Drug Products Since 1897

The initials "HPUS" on the label of a drug product assure that legal standards of strength, quality, purity, and packaging exist for the drug product within the package. The active ingredients are official Homeopathic Drug Products and are found in the current *Homeopathic Pharmacopoeia of the United States*. The standards that must be met in order to append *HPUS* to a substance or a product are established by the Homeopathic Pharmacopoeia Convention of the United States, a non-governmental, non-profit scientific organization composed of experts in the fields of medicine, arts, biology, botany, chemistry, and pharmacy who have had appropriate training and experience and have demonstrated additional knowledge and interest in the principles of homeopathy. The Convention is an autonomous body that works closely with the Food and Drug Administration and homeopathic organizations, notably the American Institute of Homeopathy and the American Association of Homeopathic Pharmacists. Guidelines are published for the prescription or over-the-counter status of homeopathic drug products.

The *HPUS* is declared a legal source of information on drug products (along with the USP/NF) in the Federal Food Drug and Cosmetic Act. 21 U.S.C. § 301. Section 201(g)(1) of the Act. 21 U.S.C. § 321 defines the term *drug* as "articles recognized in the official *United States Pharmacopeia*, official *Homeopathic Pharmacopoeia of the United States*, or official *National Formulary* or any supplement to any of them."

§ Section 201(j) of the Act (221 U.S.C. § 321) defines the term *official compendium* as the "official *United States Pharmacopeia*, official *Homeopathic Pharmacopeia of the United States*, official *National Formulary* or any supplement to them."

The *Homeopathic Pharmacopoeia of the United States* is included in 42 U.S.C. § 801 of the Medicaire-Medicaid statute and 21 U.S.C. § 801 of the Controlled Substances Act. The FDA Compliance Policy Guide 7132.15 treats the subject of "Conditions Under Which Homeopathic Drugs May Be Marketed."

The Convention is responsible for the production and constant updating of the *HPUS*. The board appoints a Monograph Review Committee, a Pharmacopoeia Revision Committee, and a Council on Pharmacy to assist in the discharge of its ongoing responsibility. The Convention has a panel of experts that assists the Convention as required.

The *HPUS* is published as "Homeopathic Pharmacopoeia of the United States Revision Service"; thus, it can be kept current without delays implicit in a permanently bound form.

The *HPUS* has been in continuous publication since 1897 but was preceded by unofficial homeopathic pharmacopoeiae since 1841, a total period of 150 years.

CHAPTER 21

Color Additives

COLOR ADDITIVES*
David C. Oppenheimer, R.Ph.

History

Until the mid-nineteenth century, color additives used in foods, drugs, and cosmetics were generally derived from natural sources, e.g., vegetables or minerals. This all changed in 1856 with William Henry Perkin's unintentional discovery of the first commercial practical synthetic organic dye, aniline purple. Many aniline dyes were subsequently developed; they are still sometimes referred to as "coal tar colors," although this is incorrect, as synthetic colorants can be produced from other starting materials.

The presence of colors in foods, drugs, and cosmetics, and especially the proliferation of colored foods and drugs during the 19th century, caused the federal government to regulate color additives. The first U.S. government regulation of color additives occurred in 1886 when Congress passed the Oleomargarine Act [1].

By 1900 many foods contained color additives, and there was increasing use of colorants in drugs and cosmetics. Congress recognized the potential health problems resulting from the unregulated use of color additives and,

as a result of investigations by the U.S. Department of Agriculture (USDA), colorant guidelines were included in the Pure Food and Drugs Act of 1906, the first federal food and drug legislation [2]. The color additives guidelines addressed only their use in foods, even though the 1906 law itself included "drug" in its title. It seemed safe, however, to presume that only colors deemed appropriate for foods would be used to color drug products.

During the years following 1906, provision was made for the review of new colorants after the USDA had determined that appropriate pharmacological and toxicological tests had proven them harmless [3]. Some of these colors are still used today, e.g., FD&C Yellow No. 5 (tartrazine) and FD&C Red No. 4.

Color Additives for Drug Products

The inadequacies of the 1906 food and drug statutes and subsequent regulations led to the enactment by Congress in 1938 of the Federal Food, Drug, and Cosmetic Act. This Act superseded the 1906 law and, with its many amendments, remains the federal law governing foods, drugs, medical devices, and cosmetics [4]. The Act expanded on the adulteration provisions of the 1906 stat-

ute by stating that a drug or device shall be deemed to be adulterated if it contains an unsafe color additive. "Unsafe" means a colorant that is not appropriately listed by the FDA for its intended use [5].

The Act instituted several new and significant practices concerning color additives. It stated that only certified coal-tar colorants could be used in foods, drugs, and cosmetics. (Thus drugs and cosmetics were drawn into the regulatory fold.[1]) Any regulated product containing an uncertified coal-tar dye would be deemed to be adulterated and, hence, illegal. Certification, formerly voluntary, became mandatory. Also, the Act created three categories of certified colors:

1. FD&C colors: colorants certifiable for use in Foods, Drugs, and Cosmetics
2. D&C colors: colorants certifiable for use in ingested and externally applied Drugs and Cosmetics (but not for use in foods)
3. External D&C colors: colorants certifiable for use in externally applied Drugs and Cosmetics (but not for use in ingested products; not permitted for use on any mucous membrane)

There is no significance to the

---

*Reprinted with permission from U.S. Pharmacist (March 1982).

[1]Color additives are not permitted in injectable drug products; certain dyes are designated for coloring surgical sutures.

numbers used after the letters identifying each dye, e.g., FD&C Yellow No. 5.

The certification procedure established by the Act requires that each lot of each color be individually sampled for submission to the Food and Drug Administration (FDA) with a request for certification accompanied by the prescribed fee for certification services. The procedure is detailed in the regulations promulgated by the FDA to ensure compliance with the Act [6]. The specific lot represented by the certification request must be labeled, sealed, and held in quarantine by the manufacturer until the FDA has certified that the given lot has met all the specifications for that color. The FDA's laboratories perform a quality control function which is, in effect, the purpose of the certification requirement in the Act.

The 1938 Act continued to describe the regulated color additives as "coal-tar" colors. Even though the early synthetic dyes were derived from coal-tar, based upon Perkin's work with aniline, (a constituent of coal-tar), color additives were subsequently developed using other synthetic organic chemical processes. By 1938, therefore, the term "coal-tar" in connection with dyes had become archaic and inaccurate. The all-inclusive term "color additive" was not used in the statute and regulations until enactment of the Color Additive Amendments of 1960 [7] (discussed below).

The Act contained an exemption which is still current: coal-tar hair dyes, which were specifically exempt from the provisions of the law regarding certification of colors, were permitted with certain restrictions; these restrictions differed little from the language of the current law, which follows:

. . . the label of which (coal-tar hair dye) bears the following legend conspicuously displayed thereon: "Caution—this product contains ingredients which may cause skin irritation on certain individuals and a preliminary test according to ac-

companying directions should first be made. This product must not be used for dyeing the eyelashes or eyebrows; to do so may cause blindness", and the labeling of which bears adequate directions for such preliminary testing. For the purposes of this . . . the term "hair dye" shall not include eyelash dyes or eyebrow dyes [8].

A more significant problem for the manufacturers of color additives arose from the statement in the 1938 Act requiring that the colors must be "harmless and suitable for use"—hardly an unreasonable statement. However, "harmless" came to be defined as "harmless when fed to animals in any amount" [9]. This position was supported by a United States Supreme Court decision in 1958 which held that "harmless" in the law meant harmless regardless of the quantity of color used [10]. Thus the FDA had to remove several FD&C colorants from its approved list and it began to proceed against many more. It became apparent that virtually every new toxicological study of a color would result in its demise, as far as foods, drugs, and cosmetics were concerned. Both the FDA and the industry sought relief from Congress.

The Color Additive Amendment of 1960

Relief for the manufacturers and users of color additives was provided by Congress in the form of comprehensive amendments to the Act [11]. This new law established the "safety of use" principle, which ended the problems created by the 1958 Supreme Court's "harmless per se" pronouncement. Thus the FDA could specify safe conditions of use, the latter to include levels of use and certain restrictions where appropriate. These color additive amendments replaced the phrase "coal-tar" dyes with the all-inclusive term "color additives". (The only exception is in the previously described coal-tar hair dye exemption, which remains.) Thus the new law estab-

lished uniform criteria of acceptability for all colorants. In addition, the law determined that there be two groups of colors: those that required certification of individual batches, and those that the FDA could grant exemption from the certification requirement on the basis that it was not necessary for protecting the public health. Examples of the latter are limited to GRAS substances, i.e., those Generally Recognized As Safe by qualified experts. Practically all synthetic organic colorants require certification [12].

The 1960 amendments also mandated that the FDA create a permanent list of acceptable color additives and a provisional list. (Within both lists there could be colors requiring certification and those exempt from certification.) The permanent list consists of colorants for which sufficient scientific data exists to establish safety under conditions of use. The law placed upon the manufacturers the burden of proving safety.

The provisional list contains colorants which were commercially available when the 1960 amendments were enacted. A two-and-a-half year grace period was provided so that testing could be completed to meet the new requirements of proof of safety. The amendments also allowed this "closing date," i.e., the end of the grace period, to be postponed "for such period or periods as (the FDA) finds necessary to carry out the purposes" of the law [13]. This grace period has, in fact, been extended for more than 20 years, since safety data are still being accepted by the FDA. Thus the provisional colors can be used on an interim basis pending completion of scientific studies to determine whether they should be permanently approved or prohibited. (This will be mentioned later in the article.)

The amendments legally defined a color additive as a substance which:

(A) is a dye, pigment, or other

substance made by a process of synthesis or similar artifice, or extracted, isolated or otherwise derived, with or without intermediate or final change of identity from a vegetable, animal, mineral, or other source, and

(B) when added or applied to a food, drug, or cosmetic, or to the human body or any part thereof, is capable (alone or through reaction with other substance) of imparting color thereto; . . .

2. The term "color" includes black, white, and intermediate grays [14].

An additional statement is included in the regulatory definition of a color additive:

An ingested drug the intended function of which is to impart color to the human body is a "color additive" [15].

The inclusion of black, white, and grays to the definition means that substances not usually thought of as colorants are now regulated by the FDA as such, e.g., calcium carbonate, titanium dioxide, talc, zinc oxide. Generally, however, such substances are exempt from batch certification [16].

The "Delaney Clause," named for its Congressman (NY) author was first enacted as a part of the Food Additive Amendments to the Act in 1958. It was also included in the Color Additive Amendments. Also known as the "anti-cancer clause," it prohibits the use of any color additive known to produce cancer in man or animals or that has been found, by appropriate tests, to induce cancer in man or animals [17]. The FDA decided in 1971 to require studies of teratological and reproductive effects of all certifiable synthetic organic color additives designated for ingested drug products [18].

Color Additives—Present Status and Their Future

In 1976, the FDA terminated the provisional listing for FD&C Red No. 2, banning it for all use because of the uncertainties about its safety. FD&C Red No. 4 fol-

lowed a similar route of unresolved safety concerns and, in 1976, was also banned by the FDA for use in *ingested* drugs. In this case, however, FDA permanently listed FD&C Red No. 4 for use in *external* drugs and cosmetics. ("External" means applied only to external parts of the body and not to the lips or any body surface covered by mucous membrane.) Interestingly, Canada's Health Protection Branch (equivalent to the U.S. FDA) permits full use of both red colorants because it believes that the concerns are not substantiated by the available scientific evidence [19]. FD&C Red No. 40, on the other hand, is allowed for use in ingested and external drugs and cosmetics in the U.S., but cannot be used for these purposes in Canada. The opposing viewpoints of the U.S. and Canada regarding these dyes create obvious difficulties for multinational companies who manufacture only in the U.S.

FD&C Yellow No. 5 (tartrazine) is permanently listed for use in ingested drugs, but is provisionally listed for use in external drugs and cosmetics. However, since tartrazine has been shown to cause allergic reactions in some sensitive people when ingested, the FDA mandated that ingested drugs containing this dye must have "FD&C Yellow No. 5 (tartrazine)" stated on their labels. Ingested, in this case, means human drugs administered orally, nasally, rectally, or vaginally. The labeling for prescription drugs must have the additional statement in the package inserts: "This product contains FD&C Yellow No. 5 (tartrazine) which may cause allergic-type reactions (including bronchial asthma) in certain susceptible persons. Although the overall incidence of . . . sensitivity in the general population is low, it is frequently seen in patients who also have aspirin hypersensitivity" [20]. Anaphylactic shock is the acute manifestation of allergic reaction to tartrazine [21]. Topically-applied drugs require no precautionary statement concerning tartrazine because the FDA is not

aware of any published report of allergic-type responses in persons sensitive to the dye [22].

In addition to the aforementioned FD&C Red No. 2, certain other dyes are prohibited in drugs because they either are carcinogenic, could be carcinogenic, or have not been proven safe e.g., FD&C Violet No. 1, D&C Blue No. 6, D&C Reds Nos. 10, 11, 12, and 13, and the external D&C colors Green No. 1 and Yellows Nos. 1, 9, and 10 [23]. FD&C Red No. 40, on the other hand, has survived years of intensive investigation which include lifetime studies in mice and rats [24].

The status of the still provisionally listed dyes is detailed in the FDA's "Rules and Regulations" of March 27, 1981 [25], in which the FDA has mandated staggered dates for submission of supporting safety data and for the "closing" of each color additive's provisional listing. The latter range from May, 1982, through September, 1984. Theoretically, then, by late-1984 all color additives used in foods, drugs, medical devices, and cosmetics will be permanently listed. (A color additive used on or in a medical device is subject to the Act only if the colorant comes in direct contact with the body for a significant period of time [26]. Any new colorants which the industry wishes to introduce henceforth must be supported by a complete range of acute and chronic long-term safety data in accordance with current scientific capabilities. This applies to natural as well as to synthetic colorants.

Toxicity problems associated with color additives are generally related to their absorption. One California company hypothesized that these risks could be reduced if the color additives were not absorbed in the gastrointestinal tract. The company developed high-molecular weight (40,000–45,000) non-absorbable dyes, as opposed to the current FD&C dyes with an average molecular weight of about 500. These new colorants, known as polymeric dyes, have demonstrated clinically significant non-absorption. Their physical characteristics of flowability, solubility, and their thermal and photochemical properties are equal to or better than the FD&C dyes. Insoluble pigments (lakes) of polymeric dye can be prepared by adsorbing the dye onto an alumina hydrate substrate as is now done to manufacture FD&C lakes. Safety studies of these polymeric dyes have been completed and the Color Additive Petitions are being prepared for the FDA [27].

Two regulatory situations involving color additives developed during 1981. Oral tanning products containing beta-carotene and canthaxanthine were marked as cosmetics, but the FDA objected because these ingredients were not approved for this use. A major U.S. supplier has ceased distribution of its product until the legal aspects are clarified [28]. The other color additive confrontation involves a natural iron oxide used *in toto* as a cosmetic and, as such, was not considered by the manufacturer to be an "additive." The FDA disagreed, and the firm plans to submit a color additive petition to remove doubt about the legal status of the product [29].

The importance of color additives lies primarily in their value for product identification—to the manufacturer, to the dispensing pharmacist, and to the patient. Although not an excuse to avoid Good Manufacturing Practices (GMPs), use of color is certainly an adjunct to GMP and to effective dispensing control. Just imagine if all solid oral dosage forms were round and white! Product colors

assist health professionals and poison control center personnel in identifying unlabeled tablets and capsules, and other products. They provide reassurance to patients that they are taking the correct medicine, especially in chronic situations. Other uses include product appeal, standardization of finished product appearance, and cosmetic value in topical drugs.

Permanently listed colors will continue to be reviewed by the FDA under its cyclic program. Although the FDA well recognized that the objective of *absolute* safety is beyond current scientific capability, the agency must ensure that the element of risk is reduced to the minimum that can be achieved by informed scientists. As chemical and toxicological sciences advance, both existing colors and proposed new colors will be evaluated by appropriately advanced techniques [30]. Thus the public—all of us—will continue to be assured that color additives are as safe as science can demonstrate them to be.

References

1. Schaffner RM: Current regulations and future activities of the Food and Drug Administration for regulating colors. Presentation to the Food Colorants Symposium, ACS Meeting, New Orleans LA, 1977.
2. Bulhack P: Food and Drug Administration certified colors: History and procedures. Presentation to the annual meeting, Society of Cosmetic Chemists, New York, NY, 1980.
3. USDA FDA service and regulatory announcement, Food and Drugs No. 3, 1931.
4. Public Law No. 75-717, 1938.
5. Federal Food, Drug, and Cosmetic Act, As Amended, Section 501 (a)(4), 1980.
6. 21 CFR 80(Color Additive Certification), 1981.
7. Public Law No. 86-618, 1960.
8. Op.cit. Note 5, Section 601(a).
9. Op.cit. Note 1, p. 7.
10. U.S. Supreme Court, 358 U.S. 153, Dec. 15, 1958.
11. Op.cit. Note 7.
12. Berdick M: Safety studies on cosmetic colors. Presentation to the Symposium on Cosmetic Safety, CTFA, New York, NY, 1973.
13. Kirk-Othmer: "Colorants for foods, drugs, and cosmetics. Encyclopedia of chemical technology, New York, NY, John Wiley & Sons, Inc. 1979, Vol 6, p 563.
14. Op.cit. Note 5, Section 201 (t) (1).
15. 21 CFR 70.3 (f), 1981.
16. 21 CFR 73, 1981.
17. 21 CFR 70.50, 1981.
18. FR 36:18336, 1971.
19. Canadian government press release, 1976-12, Feb. 2, 1976.
20. 21 CFR 74.1705 and 201.20 1981.
21. No. 103 Tartrazine, Selections from Clin-Alert. US Pharm 6(9):61, 1981.
22. FR 44:37218, 1979.
23. Corwin E: Why FDA bans harmful substances. FDA Consumer 12(10):8, 1978.
24. FDC Reports. The Rose Sheet 2(42):4, 1981.
25. FR 46:18954, 1981.
26. Op.cit. Note 5, Section 706(a).
27. Meggos H: Non-absorbable dyes as the colors of the future. Pharm Tech, 5(10):41, 1981.
28. FDC Reports. The Rose Sheet 2(37):5, 1981.
29. FDC Reports. The Rose Sheet 2(40):4, 1981.
30. Op.cit. Note 1, p. 17.

REGULATORY ASPECTS OF COLOR ADDITIVES*

Martha M. Rumore, Steven Strauss, and Alka B. Kothari

According to the *Code of Federal Regulations*, color additives are: "Any substance, synthetic or otherwise, that when added or applied to a food, drug, or cosmetic, or to the human body or any part thereof, is capable . . . of imparting a color thereto" [1,2]. Coloring additives are used for aesthetics, as sensory adjuncts to flavors, and for product differentiation (see Glossary).

Before the development of synthetic color additives, food and cosmetic colorants were obtained from mineral, animal, and vegetable sources. Synthetic coloring agents, which were extracted from coal tar (pix carbonis), a byproduct of coal distillation, date back to the mid-19th century. By 1900, nearly 700 colors had been synthesized from aniline, a derivative of benzene produced from coal tar, and a major industry developed in the field of coal-tar dyes [3].

Approximately 90% of color additives in prescription and OTC drugs are synthesized from aniline that is currently obtained from petroleum or petroleum products [3]. Before the development of the oil industry, those chemicals could be derived only from coal tar—hence their unflattering but straightforward name. Most pharmaceutical colorants today are synthetic (Table 1), but they are still referred to as "coal-tar" dyes [4].

Early coal-tar dyes were used in foods and beverages without careful selection between those that were harmless and those that were toxic. By the 19th century, the use of mineral colors, such as red lead, copper sulfate, and lead chromate, as well as industrial dyes, had become a serious health problem. For example, in a 1910 court ruling, a macaroni product containing

"martius yellow," a poisonous dye, was deemed adulterated and subsequently prohibited [5]. Although many states passed laws prohibiting the use of harmful color additives, the laws were so limited and diverse that the U.S. public had minimal protection. Finally, Congress banned the use of harmful color additives.

The first federal statute dealing with coloring agents was the Oleomargarine Act of 1886, which permitted butter to be colored with beta carotene. In May 1900, Congress allocated funds to the Bureau of Chemistry (the original FDA) to investigate the character of proposed color additives, to determine their effect on digestion and health, and to establish guidelines for their use [5].

The 1906 Pure Food and Drug Act designated a few colors as certified or permitted colors [6]. This law established a voluntary certification system for synthetic food colors and required that any synthetic color be indicated on the label of foods (except butter, cheese, and ice cream). The law contained a list of seven permitted color additives for use in food. It provided for voluntary certification of individual batches of color additives.

Federal Food, Drug, and Cosmetic Act of 1938

The Federal Food, Drug, and Cosmetic Act of 1938 (the Act) marked the first time that the U.S. government controlled the use of color additivies in drug and cosmetic products. In addition, the Act required that a color be *harmless* at any level or *harmless per se* before it could be used. Harmless, according to the law, meant safe when fed to animals in any amount or regardless of the quantity of

color used [7]. The Act deemed products that contain unsafe color additives to be adulterated and consequently prohibited them from being introduced into interstate commerce. A color additive was deemed to be safe if it was listed in the regulation issued; its uses, intended or actual, complied with the conditions and limitations specified in the regulation; and it was batch certified in accordance with the regulation issued under section 706(c) of the Act or exempted by regulation from the requirement of certification [7]. Therefore, certification became mandatory, and manufacturers were charged a fee for the service.

Early in 1938, FDA began a series of conferences with manufacturers of food, drugs, cosmetics, and coal-tar colors for the purpose of creating a list of colors then in use. the food list contained only the colors certified under the voluntary system. The drug and cosmetic list, however, contained more than 1300 colors. These colors were rated according to known toxicity, extent of use, degree to which the color was essential to the industry, duplication of shade, stability (including fastness to light, acids, and alkalies), chemical purity, and identity.

Elimination of duplicates resulted in a list with fewer than 200 colors. These colors were grouped, according to the test results, in three categories:

- those suitable for food, drugs, and cosmetics
- those suitable for drugs and cosmetics, internally as well as externally
- those suitable only for external use in drugs and cosmetics

The resulting nomenclature established the prefixes FD&C, D&C, and External D&C (Table 2 [9,10]). This nomenclature for certifiable coal-tar colors was proposed in

*Reprinted with permission from *Pharmaceutical Technology,* 16(3):68–82 (1992).

Table 1: Natural Sources of Color Additives.

Mineral	Vegetable	Animal
Alumina (aluminum hydroxide)	Canthaxanthin	Guanine (fish scales)
Red ferric oxide (ferric oxide)	(natural beta carotene, carrots)	Tyrian purple (snails)
Yellow ferric oxide (ferric oxide)	Saffron (*Crocus sativis* plant)	Cochineal (insect)
Titanium dioxide	Indigo (indigo plant)	Carmine (lake of cochineal)
Azurite	Chlorophyll (green plants)	
Carbon black (carbon)	Beet juice (beets)	
Ultramarine blue (kaolin, sulfur, sodium	Xanthantine (microalgae)	
carbonate, carbon)	Tagetes	
Calcium carbonate	(Aztec marigold petals)	
Mica (muscovite mica)	Caramel (carbohydrates)	
Pyrophyllite	Grape color extract (Concord	
Chromium oxide greens	grapes)	
(chromic sequioxide)	Alizarin (madder plant)	
	Henna (henna plant)	
	Annatto extract (annatto seed)	
	Turmeric (*Curcuma longat*)	
	Logwood extract (leguminous	
	trees)	

February 1939 at an open hearing attended by representatives of both government and interested industries and was adopted unanimously [3,8]. Although the names are relatively clear, they are not consistent; i.e., they do not reliably correspond to the current usages of the colors. For example, Ext. D&C Violet No. 2 is permitted only in externally applied cosmetics even though a literal interpretation of the name would imply acceptability for use in drugs. There is no significance to the numbers used after the letters identifying each dye [11].

In the 1950s, several cases of illness from excessive use of color additives in candy and popcorn were reported [8,9]. Disagreements developed between industry and FDA over the definition of the term

harmless. The Act required that a color be harmless in any quantity or it could not be used at all. In 1958, in *Fleming v. Florida Citrus Exchange* [12], *absolute harmlessness* under the Act was interpreted to mean that the use of any coal-tar additive that was not harmless in any amount was prohibited. A change in the law was necessary to permit the continued use of most colors [5]. The court's rejection of the "safe-for-use" principle was largely responsible for the Color Additive Amendments of 1960. These amendments revised the statutory language and explicitly authorized the listing and certification of color additives, which, in the absence of tolerance limitations or other use limitations, could not be considered safe within the scope of the FDC Act.

The Color Additive Amendments of 1960

The Color Additive Amendments of 1960 amended the FD&C Act and established the basic statutory framework that still governs the regulation of color additives today (Table 3). It established, for the first time, a comprehensive system for premarket approval of all color additives [9–11]. Before the adoption of the amendments, the require-

ment for the listing and certification of colors extended only to coal-tar colors. Pursuant to this law, there is an FDA regulation for every color additive, specifying its physical, botanical, or chemical identity and the types of products in which it may be used. Limits have been established for impurities, and batch-by-batch certification is considered necessary because of the complex organic chemical reactions that take place during synthesis. The overriding concern is the presence of impurities beyond those that are permitted [9].

Colorants Exempt from Certification

Certain color additives are exempt from certification, including

No other country has so carefully monitored the coloring agents that can be used in food, drugs, and cosmetics as has the United States. To assist formulators in understanding these requirements, the present article reviews existing U.S. regulations for color additives, with particular attention to the Color Additive Amendments of 1960. The article also reviews safety issues and limitations on the uses of different coloring agents.

Table 2
COLOR ADDITIVE CLASSIFICATIONS

FD&C Dyes
May be legally used in foods, drugs, and cosmetics.

D&C Dyes
May be legally used in drugs and cosmetics.

External D&C Dyes
May be legally used to color topical drugs and cosmetics.

Glossary

COLOR ADDITIVE
A material that is a dye, pigment, or other substance made by a process or similar artifice, or extracted, isolated, or otherwise derived with or without intermediate or final change of identity, from a vegetable, animal, mineral, or other source, and when added or applied to a food, drug, or cosmetic, or to the human body or any part thereof, is capable (alone or through reaction with other substances) of imparting color. (*Color* includes black, white, and intermediate grays.)

CERTIFICATION
FDA has authority to require batch-by-batch testing to confirm that colors actually marketed meet the listing regulation specifications.

PIGMENT
An insoluble material that colors by dispersion.

LAKE PIGMENT
A pigment consisting of a sub-stratum of alumina hydrate on which dye is adsorbed.

PROVISIONAL LIST
Colors in use when the Color Additive Amendments were enacted and that have not yet qualified for "permanent" listing because all of the safety tests that FDA requires have not been completed.

DELANEY CLAUSE
An amendment to the FD&C Act which provides that no color additive is safe if it induces cancer when ingested by humans or animals or if it is found, after tests that are appropriate for the evaluation of the safety of food additives, to induce cancer in humans or animals.

BATCH
A homogeneous lot of color additive produced by an identified production operation, which is set apart and held as a unit for the purposes of obtaining certification of such quantity.

some that are referred to as *natural*. However, synthetic colors must be certified [9]. For foods, exempt color additives include beet powder, caramel, saffron, and cochineal extract. For drugs, exempt color additives are derived mostly from minerals and include chromium hydroxide green, copper powder, and aluminum powder. For cosmetics, exempt color additives include titanium dioxide, ultramarines, and henna. However, all color additives are subject to GMP regulations. Exemptions are allowed pursuant to law when certification is unnecessary to protect public health. However, exempt colorants are subject to surveillance by FDA to ensure that they meet government specifications and are used in accordance with the law.

Provisionally Listed Color Additives

All colorants in use at the time the amendments were enacted were provisionally listed pending completion of the studies needed to justify their permanent listing. This group consisted mostly of colors derived from mineral, animal, or vegetable products [4]. The provisional listing was established to permit continued use of pre-1960 colors while retesting was accomplished [12–14]. Although it was intended that this list would be eliminated after 2½ years, the grace period has been in existence more than 30 years because safety data are still being accepted by FDA. However, from 1960 to 1976, FDA either permanently approved or terminated the provisional listing of about 75 color additives.

The Color Additive Amendments of 1960 substitute *safety of use* for the *harmless per se* interpretation formerly used. Thus, marketing of noningested colors may be allowed if their risk is so minimal that it presents no public health or safety concern. With regard to ingested colors, however, FDA has officially proclaimed a zero-risk policy [12]. The agency's position, as reflected in the Constituents Policy, prohibits approval when the color "as a whole" is found to induce cancer [13]. As a result of increased sensitivity to the presence of carcinogens, it has been argued that maintaining the absolute Delaney Clause prohibition of carcinogenic additives is no longer practical [14].

The Color Additive Amendments of 1960 further provide that FDA, in determining whether a color additive may be listed for use in foods, drugs, and cosmetics, must consider the scientific data that establish its safety under conditions

Table 3: Provisions of the Color Additive Amendments of 1960.

Authorizes use of colors in safe amounts. Substitutes the "safety of use" principle for the "harmless per se" interpretation.

Separate listing and certification of batches of color additives.

Premarket safety testing.

Uniform criteria for admissibility or listing.

Determination that the use will not result in deception of consumers.

FDa authorization to restrict colors, including limitations on usage levels and product specifications.

Placed all exempt colorants into a provisional list, pending completion of scientific studies.

Shifted the burden of proof on the issue of safety from government to industry.

Included the Delaney Clause, which prohibits use of any color additive known to produce cancer in humans or animals.

of use. In determining safety, FDA must consider the probable consumption, the cumulative effect, safety factors, and the availability of analytical methods for determining identity and quantity of the pure dye, intermediates, and impurities, as well as the amount of additive in or on any article of food, drug, or cosmetic [9,15]. FDA must find with reasonable certainty that the color additive poses no risk to human health, that it accomplishes the intended effect, and that its use will not result in deception of consumers [10]. The use of colors to deceive the public is amply documented in the history of food and drug regulations, e.g., to conceal inferiority or damage that would result in charges of misbranding or adulteration of the product. In addition, color additives must be shown not to interfere with the therapeutic efficacy of the pharmaceutical product or with the product's assay procedure [3].

As mentioned, the burden of proving safety shifted from government to industry. Because of the great expense involved in performing the pharmacological and chemical experiments necessary for permanent listing, work was begun only with colors of economic importance to the food, drug, and cosmetic industry, and many of the previously certifiable colors were eliminated by default. Beyond the effective date of the Amendments, FDA would consider any food, drug, or cosmetic manufactured with a banned dye to be adulterated [2]. Often, however, even though a color has been banned, the product may not be recalled if there is no acute hazard to public health.

An effective date is usually provided for reformulation. The certification status of color additives is continually reviewed, and changes are made in the list of certified colors [1]. These changes include withdrawal of certification, transfer to another certification category, or addition of a new color to the list. The "permanent" listing of colors is not literally permanent [9]. Col-

ors can be banned under the same procedures applicable for initial listing [16] (Figure 1). The number of colors approved for use in cosmetics and drugs has been reduced since 1960 [5], and provisional color additives may be banned without recourse to the rule-making procedures [9]. Color additive regulations appear in Title 21 *Code of Federal Regulations (CFR)*, Parts 70 to 82, which is published on 1 April each year and contains all *Federal Register* contents from the previous calendar year.

FD&C aluminum lakes are dilute solutions of color additives that contain 10–40% pure color additive (see Glossary). With the exception of FD&C Red No. 40, all the current FD&C dyes are permanently listed, and their corresponding lakes are provisionally listed. This is an important difference because provisionally listed colorants can be removed by termination of the provisional listing. Permanently listed colorants can be removed only by a change in regulation, a lengthy process. This explains the recent action on FD&C

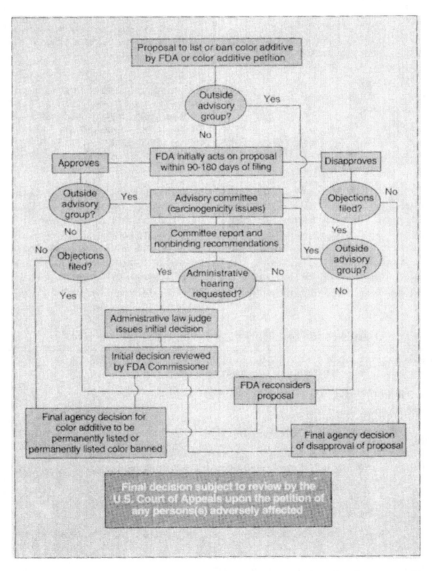

FIGURE 1. Procedures for permanently listing new colors or banning "permanently" listed colors.

Color	Reason
Violet 6B (FD&C Violet No. 1)	Safety cannot be shown
Guinea Green (D&C Green No. 1)	Inadequate analytical methods
Graphite	Contamination with polynuclear aromatic hydrocarbons
Napthol Yellow S (extract D&C Yellow No. 1)	Contamination with 4-amino-biphenyl
Amaranth (FD&C Red No. 2)	Cancer in rodents
Ponceau SX (FD&C Red No. 4)	Safety cannot be shown
Canary Yellow (extract D&C Yellow No. 10)	Contamination with β-naphthyl-amine
Carmoisin (D&C Red No. 19)	Contamination with β-naphthyl-amine
Geranine 2G (D&C Red No. 11)	Contamination with β-naphthyl-amine
Carbon Black	Safety cannot be shown
D&C Green No. 6	No petition-to-list filed
D&C Orange Nos. 10 and 11	No petition-to-list filed
D&C Red No. 36*	Cancer in rodents

*Can be used in ingested drugs.

Red No. 3. The lake form was removed quickly because of its provisional status, although the dye is still permitted for use until some future regulatory action.

Safety

Safety problems are not a new phenomenon. For example, Lash Lure, a coal-tar dye that was popular in the 1930s for eyebrows and eyelashes, in a few cases caused devastating effects such as blindness and death. In addition, paraphenylenediamine, a crucial ingredient in coal-tar dyes, has long been recognized as a strong sensitizer and as a carcinogen in rodents. In the 1970s, Russian reports indicated that FD&C Red No. 2 (amaranth) caused cancer in rats. Media attention then focused on the safety of several color additives and led FDA to ban several colors. In 1976, amaranth as well as FD&C Red No. 4 and carbon black were delisted because of unresolved safety questions [5]. Examples of color additives for which provisional listing was revoked for safety and other reasons are found in Table 4 [14,17,18].

FD&C Yellow No. 5 (tartrazine) was suspected of producing allergic-type reactions, including asthmatic symptoms, urticaria, angioedema, or nasal symptoms, especially in persons allergic to aspirin. Since 1980, this color additive must be listed on the labels of foods and OTC drugs to alert consumers who may be sensitive to it [17]. In addition, oral prescription drugs that contain tartrazine must have an additional warning statement in the package insert. Many companies have reformulated their products to remove this color. In 1990, two regulatory situations involved color additives: Oral tanning products containing beta carotene and canthaxanthin were marketed as cosmetics without FDA approval, and natural iron oxide used in toto as a cosmetic was not approved as a color additive [11]. In the same year, FD&C Red No. 3 (erythrosine sodium) was eliminated from use in coloring cosmetics and externally applied drugs. FDA acted in response to studies showing that laboratory rats developed benign thyroid tumors after consuming large amounts of this dye over their lifetime. FDA stated that there was no human health risk, but certain uses of the colorant were banned for legal reasons. Currently, FD&C Red No.

3 dye remains approved for use in both foods and ingested drugs.

Limitations

If necessary to ensure safe use of a color, FDA can impose tolerance limitations, labeling or packaging requirements, and other use-related conditions [9]. For example, coal-tar hair dyes currently include warnings to consumers to patch-test the dye for allergic reactions before using and to avoid contact with the eyes. Changes in use of colors reflect industry trends and practices. Manufacturers who want to use color additives in foods, drugs, cosmetics, or medical devices should review the regulations to ascertain which colors are listed for various uses. For example, some colors contain warnings, such as "Do not use in products applied in the area of the eye." Color additives formulated in injectable drugs and surgical sutures must have a specific provision allowing such use. Examples of color additives used for medical purposes are found in Table 5.

Liquid pharmaceutical preparations contain between 0.0005 and 0.001% colorant. In contrast, solid dosage forms such as tablets, capsules, sugar-coated tablets, film-coated tablets, and chewable tablets contain ~0.1% dye. Ointments, suppositories, ophthalmic, and parenteral products usually contain no color additives. If exact quantitative amounts are not used each time a formulation is prepared, the appearance of the product may change significantly from batch to batch. In order to achieve greater accuracy in measurement of these minute quantities, color additives often are formulated as dilute solutions or lake pigments rather than concentrated dry powders. FD&C aluminum lakes are subject to certification and must be made from certified color additives [3]. The official lot-test number must accompany the colors through all subsequent packagings.

Products must be reformulated if

Table 5: Pharmaceutical Colorants with Medical Indications.

Antifungal	Antiseptic	Anti-Infective	Diagnostic Dyes	Chemotherapeutic Agents	Laxatives
Gentian Violet	Phenazopyridine Iodine Potassium permanganate	Acriflavine Aminacrine Proflavine Mepacrine (quinacrine)	Congo Red Scarlet Red Phenolphthalein Methylene Blue Sulfobromophthalein sodium Indigotindisulfonate sodium (soluble Indigo Blue) Phenolsulfonphthalein (Phenol Red) Evans Blue Methyl Red Fluoroscein sodium (Uranine Yellow) Azuresin (Azure A carbacrylic resin)	Doxorubicin Daunorubicin	Phenolphthalein Danthron

*Not all listed items are FDA approved.

the certification of a color additive is revoked. However, manufacturers are not required by law to notify consumers of a change in the appearance of a dosage form. Since 1987, more than 500 USP Drug Product Problem Reports described problems attributed to a color change or lot-to-lot color variations [18]. Color additives need not be listed on drug labels; FD&C Yellow No. 5 is the only exception [4]. Under the Fair Packaging and Labeling Act (FPLA), cosmetic labels must identify by name all color additives used in a product [7]. The Medical Device Amendments of 1976 require that coloring substances used in or on devices must be regulated as color additives if they come in direct contact with the body for a significant period of time [9].

The Cosmetic, Toiletries, and Fragrance Association (CTFA) has various committees dealing exclusively with color additives. This organization, the Certified Color Manufacturers Association (CCMA), and the Pharmaceutical Manufacturers Association (PMA) have sponsored scientific research on provisionally listed colors [15] (see Glossary). The Interindustry Color Committee was organized by CTFA in 1971 in response to regulations requiring teratogenicity and reproduction testing of 25 colors used in cosmetics that may be subject to ingestion (such as lipsticks), foods, and drugs. The Color Petition Review Committee, organized by CTFA in 1968, has been meeting to resolve questions related to safety and technical data developed to support color additive petitions.

Current toxicity data requirements for color additives intended for use in foods primarily include oral toxicity data. Oral, parenteral, topical, eye, and inhalation toxicity data are necessary for medicinal use. For cosmetic use, oral, topical, mucous membrane, eye, and inhalation toxicity data are appropriate [16]. When a sponsor requests permission to use provisionally listed color additives in an ingestible product, FDA requires reports of teratogenicity studies and multigeneration animal reproduction studies showing that the color additive produces no adverse effects on reproduction [15].

No other government has so carefully guarded the colors that may be used as has the United States. Most countries that regulate the use of colors have used U.S. regulations as a model [19]. European Economic Community color regulations are contained in the 1976 Cosmetic Directive. The Japanese regulations are listed under the Pharmaceutical Affairs Law of 1960 and the Ministry of Health and Welfare Ordinance No. 30 [19]. Certification is not limited to colors made by U.S. manufacturers. Colors certified by foreign governments must be certified by FDA if they are used in the United States.

The Future

Many petitions for color additive approval have been submitted to FDA by various industry groups and independent companies. In addition, a great deal of scientific research is being conducted with new and innovative colors, such as nonabsorbable polymeric dyes, which will require regulatory attention. As science advances, both existing and proposed new colors will be evaluated by appropriately advanced techniques. Thus, the public will continue to be assured that color additives are as safe as science can demonstrate them to be.

References

1. Title 21, *Code of Federal Regulations,* Chapter I, Sec. 70.3 (1991).
2. 21 *USC* 321(t) (1976).
3. H.C. Ansel and N.G. Popovich, *Pharmaceutical Dosage Forms and Drug Delivery Systems,* 5th ed. (Lea & Febiger, Philadelphia, PA, 1990), pp. 113–116.
4. H. Hopkins. "The Color Additive Scorecard," *FDA Consumer,* March 1980, pp. 24–27.
5. G.E. Damon and W.F. Janssen, "Additives for Eye Appeal," *FDA Consumer,* July–August 1973, pp. 15–18.
6. Act of 30 June 1906, ch. 3915, 34 Stat. 768.
7. 21 *USC* 301 et seq.
8. P. Bulhack, "Food and Drug Administration Certified Colors: History and Procedures," Presentation at the annual meeting, Society of Cosmetic Chemists, New York, 1980.
9. M.R. Taylor, "Food and Drug Administration Regulation of Color Additives—Overview of Statutory Framework," *Food Drug Cosmetic Law J.* **39,** 273–280 (1984).
10. *Public Law* 86–618, 74 Stat. 397 (1960).
11. S. Strauss, *Strauss's Pharmacy Law Examination Review,* 2d ed. (Technomic Publishing Co., Lancaster, PA, 1990), pp. 150–154.
12. J.S. Kahan, "The Effect of Proposed Food Safety Legislation on Colors," *Food Drug Cosmetic Law J.* **39,** 281–91 (1984).
13. 47 *Federal Register* 14463 (1982).
14. D.M. Strauss, "Reaffirming the Delaney Anticancer Clause: The Legal and Policy Implications of an Administratively Created De Minimis Exception," *Food Drug Cosmetic Law J.* **42,** 393–428 (1987).
15. M. Lanzet, "What the Future Holds for Cosmetic Color Additives," *Food Drug Cosmetic Law J.* **37,** 187–194 (1982).
16. H. Blumenthal, "Current Requirements in Approving a Color Additive for Use in Cosmetics," *Food Drug Cosmetic Law J.* **37,** 183–186 (1982).
17. 44 *Federal Register* 37212–37220 (1979).
18. "Ban on Erythrosine Sodium (FD&C Red No. 3)," *Pharmacy Update,* April 1991, p. 16.
19. E.G. Murphy, "Regulation of Cosmetic Colors in Other Countries," *Food Drug Cosmetic Law J.* **37,** 163–171 (1982).

QUESTIONS: CHAPTER 21

1. The first federal statute which pertained to color additives was the:
   a. Import Drugs Act of 1848
   b. Oleomargarine Act of 1886
   c. Pure Food and Drugs Act of 1906
   d. Federal Food, Drug, and Cosmetic Act of 1938
   e. Color Additive Amendments to the FD&C Act in 1960

2. Which one of the following federal statutes marked the first controlled use of color additives in drug and cosmetic products?
   a. Import Drugs Act of 1848
   b. Oleomargarine Act of 1886
   c. Pure Food and Drugs Act of 1906
   d. Federal Food, Drug, and Cosmetic Act of 1938
   e. Color Additive Amendments to the FD&C Act in 1960

3. Which one of the following federal statutes marked the first controlled use of color additives in drug and cosmetic products?
   a. Pure Food and Drugs Act of 1906
   b. Delaney Amendment to the FD&C Act in 1958
   c. Color Additive Amendments to the FD&C in 1960
   d. Import Drugs Act of 1848
   e. Federal Food, Drug, and Cosmetic Act of 1938

4. The Federal Food, Drug, and Cosmetic Act of 1938, as amended, requires that a color additive be:

a. Safe

b. Effective

c. Safe *and* effective

d. Harmless when fed to animals in any amount

5. The amendment to the FD&C Act that specifies that no color additive is safe if it induces cancer in humans and animals is referred to as the:

a. Waxman-Hatch Act

b. Delaney Act

c. Durham-Humphrey Act

d. Dingell Act

e. Harrison-Ford Act

6. Which one of the following is an example of colorant obtained from vegetable sources:

a. Azurite

b. Cochineal

c. Chlorophyll

d. Yellow ferric oxide

e. Mica

7. Which one of the following is an example of colorant derived from animal sources:

a. Pyrophyllite

b. Red ferric oxide

c. Carmine

d. Indigo

e. Henna

8. Which one of the following is an example of colorant derived from mineral sources:

a. Chlorophyll

b. Canthaxanthin

c. Caramel

d. Cochineal

e. Carbon black

9. Color additives are certified (approved) by the:

a. DEA

b. BFD&C

c. BNDD

d. FDA

e. FBI

10. Before the development of synthetic color additives, colorants were obtained from:

1) Vegetables

2) Minerals

3) Animal

4) Coal tar

a. 1) and 2) are correct.

b. 2) and 3) are correct.

c. 1), 2), and 3) are correct.

d. 1), 2), 3), and 4) are correct.

CHAPTER 22

Food and Drug Administration

THE FOOD AND DRUG ADMINISTRATION: AN OVERVIEW

The Food and Drug Administration touches the lives of virtually every American every day; for it is FDA's job to see that the food we eat is safe and wholesome, the cosmetics we use won't hurt us, the medicines and medical devices we use are safe and effective, and that radiation-emitting products such as microwave ovens won't do us harm. Feed and drugs for pets and farm animals also come under FDA scrutiny. FDA also ensures that all of these products are labeled truthfully with the information that people need to use them properly.

FDA is one of our nation's oldest consumer protection agencies. Its approximately 9,000 employees monitor the manufacture, import, transport, storage and sale of $960 billion worth of products each year. It does that at a cost to the taxpayer of about $3 per person.

First and foremost, FDA is a regulatory agency, charged with enforcing the Federal Food, Drug, and Cosmetic Act and several related public health laws. To carry out this mandate of consumer protection, FDA has some 1,100 investigators and inspectors who cover the country's more than 90,000 FDA-regulated businesses. These employees are located in district and local offices in 157 cities across the country.

Inspections and Legal Sanctions

These investigators and inspectors visit more than 30,000 facilities a year, seeing that products are made right and labeled truthfully. As part of their inspections, they collect more than 70,000 domestic and imported product samples for examination by FDA scientists or for label checks.

If a company is found violating any of the laws that FDA enforces, FDA can encourage the firm to voluntarily correct the problem or to recall a faulty product from the market. A recall is generally the fastest and most effective way to protect the public from an unsafe product.

When a company can't or won't correct a public health problem with one of its products voluntarily, FDA has legal sanctions it can bring to bear. The agency can go to court to force a company to stop selling a product and to have items already produced seized and destroyed. When warranted, criminal penalties—including prison sentences—are sought against manufacturers and distributors.

About 3,000 products a year are found to be unfit for consumers and are withdrawn from the marketplace, either by voluntary recall or by court-ordered seizure. In addition, more than 20,000 import

shipments a year are detained at the port of entry because the goods appear to be unacceptable.

Scientific Expertise

The scientific evidence needed to back up FDA's legal cases is prepared by the agency's 2,100 scientists, including 900 chemists and 300 microbiologists, who work in 40 laboratories in the Washington, D.C., area and around the country. Some of these scientists analyze samples to see, for example, if products are contaminated with illegal substances. Other scientists review test results submitted by companies seeking agency approval for drugs, vaccines, food additives, coloring agents, and medical devices.

FDA also operates the National Center for Toxicological Research at Jefferson, Arkansas, which investigates the biological effects of widely used chemicals. The agency also runs the Engineering and Analytical Center at Winchester, Massachusetts, which tests medical devices, radiation-emitting products, and radioactive drugs.

Assessing risks—and, for drugs and medical devices, weighing risks against benefits—is at the core of FDA's public health protection duties. By ensuring that products

The United States Food and Drug Administration (FDA) is responsible for ensuring the safety and efficacy of all pharmaceuticals and medical devices introduced into interstate commerce.

To accomplish this goal, FDA reviews approval applications for new products, tracks product performance after approval, inspects manufacturing facilities, and provides guidance for manufacturers.

and producers meet certain standards, FDA protects consumers and enables them to know what they're buying. For example, the agency requires that drugs—both prescription and over-the-counter—be proven safe and effective.

In deciding whether to approve new drugs, FDA does not itself do research, but rather examines the results of studies done by the manufacturer. The agency must determine that the new drug produces the benefits it's supposed to without causing side effects that would outweigh those benefits.

The Orphan Drug Act was signed in January 1983, enabling the FDA to promote research, approval, and marketing of drugs needed for treating rare diseases, which otherwise would not be profitable. After ten years, 87 drug and biological products have been brought to market. These 87 products help more than 2 million Americans and millions more worldwide. Also, in the last 10 years, more than 190 grants have been awarded. Six products supported by the orphan products grants program have been brought to market. It is the intent of the Orphan Drug Act to stimulate the development and approval of products to treat rare diseases.

Product Safety

Another major FDA mission is to protect the safety and wholesomeness of food. The agency's scientists test samples to see if any substances, such as pesticide residues, are present in unacceptable amounts. If contaminants are iden-

tified, FDA takes corrective action. FDA also sets labeling standards to help consumers know what is in the foods they buy.

The nation's food supply is protected in yet another way as FDA sees that medicated feeds and other drugs given to animals raised for food are not threatening to the consumer's health.

The safety of the nation's blood supply is another FDA responsibility. The agency's investigators routinely examine blood bank operations, from record-keeping to testing for contaminants. FDA also ensures the purity and effectiveness of biologicals (medical preparations made from living organisms and their products), such as insulin and vaccines.

Medical devices are classified and regulated according to their degree of risk to the public. Devices that are life-supporting, life-sustaining or implanted, such as pacemakers, must receive agency approval before they can be marketed.

FDA's scrutiny does not end when a drug or device is approved

Food and Drug Administration Responsibilities

- Licenses manufacturers of biologics, drugs, and medical devices
- Inspects manufacturing facilities for compliance with FDA standards
- Test products submitted for certification
- Establishes written and physical standards for biological products
- Conducts research related to the development, manufacture, testing, and use of new and old biological products
- Evaluates the claims for new drugs that are biological products
- Develops policy regarding the safety, effectiveness, and labeling of all drugs for human use
- Evaluates new drug applications and requests to approve drugs for experimental use
- Develops standards for the safety and effectiveness of over-the-counter drugs
- Monitors the quality of marked drugs through product testing, surveillance, and compliance programs

- Develops guidelines on (current) good manufacturing practices (GMPs)
- Conducts research and develops scientific standards on the composition, quality, safety, and efficacy of human drugs
- Distributes information on toxicity of household products and medicines
- Conducts research and develops standards on the composition, quality, nutrition and safety of food, food additives, colors, and cosmetics
- Develops regulations for food standards to permit the safe use of color and food additives
- Develops programs to reduce human exposure to radiation
- Conducts research on the effects of radiation exposure
- Develops regulations on the safety, efficacy, and labeling of medical devices
- Conducts research on the biological effects of potentially toxic chemical substances found in the environment

Food and Drug Administration Enforcement Policy

The Food and Drug Administration (FDA), the nation's first line of consumer protection, is a scientifically based law enforcement agency. The enforcement function of the FDA is twofold: to safeguard the public health and to ensure honesty and fair-dealing between the regulated industry and consumers.

- The FDA encourages and expects compliance with the laws and regulations it enforces. To this end the agency informs industry, healthprofessionals, and the public of those legal requirements.
- The FDA constantly investigates and conducts surveillance over the industry it regulates, to continuously assess compliance and discover noncompliance. Depending upon the nature of noncompliance, the FDA may afford an opportunity for correction by industry. If adequate correction does not occur within a reasonable period of time, the FDA is committed to swiftly initiate action to obtain compliance.
- The FDA protects the public by relying on all of its varied enforcement tools—both administrative and judicial—according to the seriousness of the violation.
- The FDA does not tolerate fraud, intentional violations, or gross negligence, and promptly seeks prosecution to punish and deter whenever appropriate.
- The FDA uses fair and scientifically sound law enforcement and regulatory work to ensure efficiency in its enforcement activities and to maintain the public trust and confidence.
- The FDA cooperates with, and enlists the cooperation of, other federal, state, and local agencies; foreign governments; associations of health professionals; and international organizations to extend the scope and increase the effectiveness of its consumer protection programs.
- The FDA continuously evaluates its law enforcement programs and needs. It initiates administrative action and proposes legislative action—and it judiciously allocates resources—to enhance its ability to meet its law enforcement responsibilities within its budget and priorities.

for marketing; the agency collects and analyzes tens of thousands of reports each year on drugs and devices after they have been put on the market to monitor for any unexpected adverse reactions.

Cosmetic safety also comes under FDA's jurisdiction. The agency can have unsafe cosmetics removed from the market. The dyes and other additives used in drugs, foods and cosmetics also are subject to FDA scrutiny. The agency must review and approve these chemicals before they can be used.

The Food and Drug Administration Act of 1988, signed into law on November 4, 1988 by President Ronald Reagan calls for future FDA commissioners to be appointed by the president and confirmed by the Senate.

Legal Basis of FDA Authority

1. Food, Drug & Cosmetic Act
2. Public Health Service Act
3. Fair Packaging & Labeling Act

DEPARTMENT OF HEALTH AND HUMAN SERVICES
PUBLIC HEALTH SERVICE
FOOD AND DRUG ADMINISTRATION

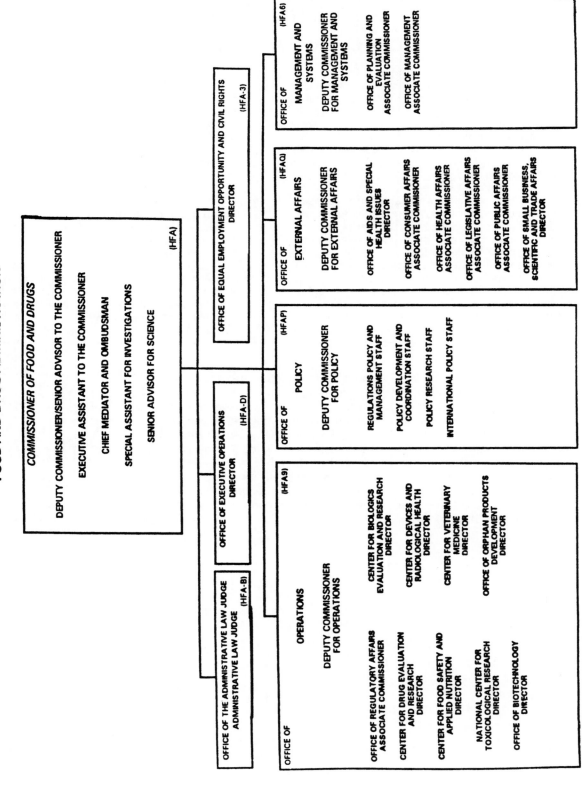

COMMISSIONER OF FOOD AND DRUGS

DEPUTY COMMISSIONER/SENIOR ADVISOR TO THE COMMISSIONER

EXECUTIVE ASSISTANT TO THE COMMISSIONER

CHIEF MEDIATOR AND OMBUDSMAN

SPECIAL ASSISTANT FOR INVESTIGATIONS

SENIOR ADVISOR FOR SCIENCE

(HFA)

OFFICE OF THE ADMINISTRATIVE LAW JUDGE
ADMINISTRATIVE LAW JUDGE
(HFA-B)

OFFICE OF EXECUTIVE OPERATIONS
DIRECTOR
(HFA-D)

OFFICE OF EQUAL EMPLOYMENT OPPORTUNITY AND CIVIL RIGHTS
DIRECTOR
(HFA-3)

OFFICE OF OPERATIONS
DEPUTY COMMISSIONER FOR OPERATIONS
(HFA9)

OFFICE OF REGULATORY AFFAIRS
ASSOCIATE COMMISSIONER

CENTER FOR DRUG EVALUATION AND RESEARCH
DIRECTOR

CENTER FOR FOOD SAFETY AND APPLIED NUTRITION
DIRECTOR

NATIONAL CENTER FOR TOXICOLOGICAL RESEARCH
DIRECTOR

OFFICE OF BIOTECHNOLOGY
DIRECTOR

CENTER FOR BIOLOGICS EVALUATION AND RESEARCH
DIRECTOR

CENTER FOR DEVICES AND RADIOLOGICAL HEALTH
DIRECTOR

CENTER FOR VETERINARY MEDICINE
DIRECTOR

OFFICE OF ORPHAN PRODUCTS DEVELOPMENT
DIRECTOR

OFFICE OF POLICY
DEPUTY COMMISSIONER FOR POLICY
(HFAP)

REGULATIONS POLICY AND MANAGEMENT STAFF

POLICY DEVELOPMENT AND COORDINATION STAFF

POLICY RESEARCH STAFF

INTERNATIONAL POLICY STAFF

OFFICE OF EXTERNAL AFFAIRS
DEPUTY COMMISSIONER FOR EXTERNAL AFFAIRS
(HFAQ)

OFFICE OF AIDS AND SPECIAL HEALTH ISSUES
DIRECTOR

OFFICE OF CONSUMER AFFAIRS
ASSOCIATE COMMISSIONER

OFFICE OF HEALTH AFFAIRS
ASSOCIATE COMMISSIONER

OFFICE OF LEGISLATIVE AFFAIRS
ASSOCIATE COMMISSIONER

OFFICE OF PUBLIC AFFAIRS
ASSOCIATE COMMISSIONER

OFFICE OF SMALL BUSINESS, SCIENTIFIC AND TRADE AFFAIRS
DIRECTOR

OFFICE OF MANAGEMENT AND SYSTEMS
DEPUTY COMMISSIONER FOR MANAGEMENT AND SYSTEMS
(HFA6)

OFFICE OF PLANNING AND EVALUATION
ASSOCIATE COMMISSIONER

OFFICE OF MANAGEMENT
ASSOCIATE COMMISSIONER

QUESTIONS: CHAPTER 22

1. The following question is applicable to answers 1 through 15. Which one of the following is *not* under the jurisdiction of the Food and Drug Administration?
   a. Spam
   b. Puppy food
   c. Chocolate-covered cherries
   d. Frozen spinach
   e. Imported caviar

2.
   a. Aspirin
   b. Anti-lice shampoo
   c. Insect repellent
   d. Eye shadow
   e. Lipstick

3.
   a. Pesticide residues in lettuce
   b. Canned tomatoes
   c. Oven cleaner
   d. Spaghetti
   e. Pet turtles

4.
   a. Airport security X-ray machines
   b. Laser products used in lumber mills
   c. Magnetic resonance imaging (MRI) diagnostic equipment
   d. Smoke detectors
   e. Microwave ovens

5.
   a. TV sets
   b. Over-the-counter antacid
   c. TV ads for aspirin
   d. Diptheria, pertussis, and tetanus vaccine
   e. Human plasma

6.
   a. Baby pacifiers
   b. Baby bottle nipples
   c. Ceramic ware for food use
   d. Coffee mugs
   e. Eye chart

7.
   a. Illegal heroin use
   b. Veterinary tetracycline
   c. Barbiturates
   d. Medicinal oxygen
   e. Methadone

8.
   a. Kidney dialysis machine
   b. Tongue depressor
   c. Toothpaste
   d. Fluoridated toothpaste
   e. Hair dryer

9.
   a. Label on beer
   b. Ground coffee
   c. Coffee beans
   d. Rabbit meat
   e. Canned tuna

10.
    a. Home canning equipment
    b. Food warehouse
    c. Drug warehouse
    d. Hearing aid dispenser (retailer)
    e. Exporting of drugs

11.
    a. Halloween make-up
    b. Theatrical make-up
    c. Soap
    d. Eye mascara
    e. Lipstick

12.
    a. Vaccine for horses
    b. Penicillin for horses
    c. Medicated feed for hogs
    d. Pet parrots
    e. Bird feed

13.
    a. Tap water
    b. Club soda
    c. Bottled mineral water
    d. Ginger ale
    e. Bottled water for water cooler

14.
    a. Tamper-resistant packaging for over-the-counter (OTC) drugs
    b. Child-resistant packaging for OTC drugs
    c. Plastic containers for soft drinks
    d. Valentine heart containing chocolates
    e. A tube containing medical ointment

15.
    a. Grooming cream for dogs
    b. Artificial limb for dogs
    c. Laser scanner at supermarket checkout
    d. Mercury vapor lamps
    e. Vitamin C tablets

CHAPTER 23

Ipecac Syrup

It is estimated that each year about 500,000 accidental poisonings occur in the United States and result in approximately 1,500 deaths, of which over 400 are children. In the emergency treatment of these poisonings, *ipecac syrup* is considered the emetic of choice. The immediate availability of this drug for use in such situations is critical, since rapid treatment may be the difference between life and death. The restriction of this drug to prescription sale limits its availability in emergencies. On the other hand, it is the consensus of informed medical opinion that ipecac syrup should be used only under medical supervision in the emergency treatment of poisonings. In view of these facts, the question of whether ipecac syrup labeled as an emergency treatment for use in poison-

Source: 21 CFR 201.308.

ings should be available over the counter has been controversial.

In connection with its study of this problem, the Food and Drug Administration has obtained the views of medical authorities. It is the unanimous recommendation of the American Academy of Pediatrics, the American Medical Association, and the Medical Advisory Board of the Food and Drug Administration that ipecac syrup in 1 fluid ounce containers be permitted to be sold without prescritpion so that it will be readily available in the household for emergency treatment of poisonings, under medical supervision, and that the drug be appropriately packaged and labeled for this purpose.

In view of the above recommendations, the Commissioner of Food and Drugs has determined that it is in the interest of the public health for ipecac syrup to be available for sale without prescription provided

that it is packaged in a quantity of 1 fluid ounce (30 milliliters), and its label bears, in addition to other required label information, the following, in a prominent and conspicuous manner:

(1) A statement conspicuously boxed and in red letters, to the effect: "For emergency use to cause vomiting in poisoning. Before using, call physician, the Poison Control Center, or hospital emergency room immediately for advice."

(2) A warning to the effect: "Warning—Keep out of reach of children. Do not use in unconscious persons. Ordinarily, this drug should not be used if strychnine, corrosives such as alkalies (lye) and strong acids, or petroleum distillates such as kerosene, gasoline, coal oil fuel oil, paint thinner, or cleaning fluid have been ingested."

(3) Usual dosage: 1 tablespoonful (15 milliliters) in persons over 1 year of age.

QUESTIONS: CHAPTER 23

1. What is the maximum quantity of Ipecac Syrup that may be sold at retail without a prescription?

    a. One ounce
    b. Two ounces
    c. Three ounces
    d. One pint
                                                               21 CFR 201.308

2. What is the intended use of Ipecac Syrup when sold over-the-counter as a drug?

    a. As an emetic
    b. As a flavoring
    c. For emergency use to induce vomiting
    d. For emergency use to induce vomiting in poisoning on advice
                                     21 CFR 201.308

3. What is the usual recommended dose of Ipecac Syrup in poisoning?

    a. One tablespoonful
    b. One teaspoonful
    c. One fluid ounce
    d. The contents of an entire container
                                     21 CFR 201.308

CHAPTER 24

Metric System

On February 14, 1992, President George Bush signed into law a requirement that the "statement of contents or quantity on food, cosmetic, and most nonprescription drug labels" be stated in metric units. The law became effective February 14, 1994. After this date, the system of pounds, gallons, inches, etc., may be used as an "optional, secondary statement of contents or quantity." These labeling changes result from amendments to the Fair Packaging and Labeling Act, P.L. 89-755, effective July 1, 1967, contained in Section 107 of the American Technology Preeminence Act of 1991.

The Fair Packaging and Labeling Act regulates various aspects of the packaging and labeling of consumer products. Regulation is for the purpose of (1) enabling consumers to obtain accurate information as to quantity of contents and (2) facilitating value comparisons by consumers (Sec. 2 at ¶502). Accordingly, while the law does regulate packaging and labeling practices that are or can be deceptive to consumers, the law also regulates practices that are not deceptive to consumers but can impair their ability to make the "best" choice or buy. Characteristic of the law, too, is its theme of control through industry-wide, rather than case-by-case, regulation.

Generally, the law is aimed at the packaging and labeling of the thousands of products appearing on supermarket and pharmacy shelves—those products taken into the household and consumed or expended. The actual scope of the law as to product coverage, however, is not clear from doubt.

Basically, the law applies to those who distribute consumer products in interstate commerce. It does not regulate the practices of retailers. But the law is not unmindful of the fact that many retailers also engage in packaging and labeling or control the packaging and labeling of the products they sell.

The Fair Packaging and Labeling Act is administered by two governmental agencies: the Secretary of Health and Human Services (HHS), through the Food and Drug Administration (FDA)—as to foods, drugs, devices, and cosmetics—and the Federal Trade Commission—as to other consumer products. Each has the authority to issue regulations as to the consumer products over which it has regulatory authority, and each has its own methods of enforcement.

CHAPTER 25

Foreign Prescriptions

FOREIGN PRESCRIPTIONS: LEGAL OR ILLEGAL?*

Richard A. Angorn, B.S. Pharm., J.D.

Pharmacists occasionally are faced with requests to fill prescriptions from foreign countries, especially pharmacists who practice in states that border Canada or Mexico or that have many foreign visitors.

The legal status of foreign drug prescriptions, with the exception of those for controlled substances, is dependent on state law and varies from state to state. Federal law restricts the prescribing of controlled substances to practitioners who are licensed to practice in the United States [1]. Most state laws do not address the issue of foreign prescriptions, and only vaguely specify that a prescription must be issued by a practitioner "licensed by law," [2] a "duly licensed medical practitioner," [3] a "licensed practitioner," [4] or a "prescriber" [5]. In some states, practitioners are specifically defined as being "licensed in this state" [6] or "other states" [7], "authorized by law" [8], or "licensed under specifically enumerated state licensing statutes" [9]. In other states, including Delaware, Kentucky, and Missouri, the statutes or rules do not define the term prescription except for controlled substances or narcotics.

Where state law is definite, restricting the issuance of prescriptions to practitioners licensed in the state or to specifically enumerated practitioners, no foreign prescriptions may be filled. Where state law is unclear, however, and the state attorney general has not ruled on the issue, the state pharmacy boards interpreted the validity of foreign prescriptions. Some boards (such as in Arizona) recognize foreign prescriptions (except those for controlled substances) on the basis of comity (courtesy) in cases where the legitimacy of the prescription and the validity of the physician-patient relationship can be verified. Other state boards (such as in New Mexico) do not permit the filling of foreign prescriptions.

The Federal Food, Drug, and Cosmetic Act restricts the prescribing of legend drugs to practitioners "licensed by law to administer such drugs" [10]. Some writers have interpreted the Act as prohibiting the filling of foreign prescriptions [11]. However, in a recent informal opinion, the Food and Drug Administration stated that Congress "did not alter state authority to determine who shall be authorized to prescribe drugs" and that "a state's recognition of a prescription from a foreign practitioner licensed by that foreign jurisdic-

tion to administer a prescription drug is not in conflict with either the language or legislative history of Section 503, but, indeed, supplements federal law" [12]. Therefore, state legislation that recognizes the validity of foreign prescriptions is not unconstitutional, since it does not conflict with federal law.

Some states have enacted legislation that specifically permits the filling of foreign prescriptions, although such laws impose restrictions and are of limited applicability. For example, Maine recognizes "nonresident prescriptions" provided by "a physician who has been licensed by the appropriate authorities to practice in the state of New Hampshire or the provinces of New Brunswick or Quebec and who is practicing in that state or province" [13]. Because of the many Canadian and South American visitors to Florida, state legislation recently was enacted there to permit the filling of prescriptions from a "jurisdiction other than Florida" under severely restricted conditions [14]. The term "jurisdiction" encompasses not only other states and federal territories but also foreign countries.

The Florida law includes several safeguards. The pharmacist must determine that, in his professional judgment: (1) the prescription

*Reprinted with permission from *Legal Aspects of Pharmacy Practice*, Vol. 5, No. 8.

order was issued pursuant to a valid physician-patient relationship, (2) the prescription order is authentic, and (3) the medication ordered is considered necessary for the continuation of treatment of a chronic or recurrent illness. If the prescribing physician is not known to the pharmacist, the pharmacist must obtain proof within reasonable limits that the prescription is valid. As a rule of thumb, prescriptions for maintenance medications would be considered valid because they are necessary for the continuation of treatment for a chronic or recurrent illness. Emergency prescriptions and prescriptions for new illnesses are not valid. Also in instances where the prescriber is not known by the pharmacist the Board requires the pharmacist to verify the physician-patient relationship and the validity of the prescription by telephoning the prescriber. This requirement would prevent filling of a foreign prescription if the prescriber cannot be contacted or communication is hampered by language difficulties.

Even if state law prohibits the filling of foreign prescriptions, however, legend drugs may be exported to most foreign countries. Except for controlled substances, for which a special exporter's license is required [15], federal law allows the export of a prescription drug provided that it: "(a) accords to the specifications of the foreign purchaser, (b) is not in conflict with the laws of the country to which it is intended for export, (c) is labeled on the outside of the shipping package that it is intended for export, and (d) is not sold or offered for sale in domestic commerce" [16]. An exported drug should be mailed directly by the pharmacist to the foreign patient or prescriber in the original manufacturer's container, with the labeling intact, and accompanied by the original written prescription order. It never should be given to the person presenting the prescription to prevent its possible diversion into domestic channels. A photocopy of the prescription order should be retained for the pharmacy records.

In summary, foreign prescriptions for drugs other than controlled substances are not illegal under federal law and are statutorily recognized in a few states. Even in states where they are not recognized, such drugs may be exported directly by the pharmacist, although they should not be given to the person presenting the prescription. In states in which the law is unclear or ambiguous, the attorney general's opinion should be solicited to clarify the legal status of foreign prescriptions.

References

1. Pub. L, No. 91-513 § 303 (f).
2. Code of AL 1975, § 34–23-1(16).
3. ARS § 36-1001(2); KSA 65-1626(h).
4. NM Stat. Ann. § 61-11-2.
5. CA Health & Safety Code (West) § 4036.
6. 1981 TX Gen. Laws, HB1628 § 5(30); IC § B54-1705(21); ORS 689.005.
7. CGSA § 20-184a.
8. ICA § 155.3(11).
9. IC25-26-10-12.
10. 21 USC § 353(b)(1).
11. Kaluzny, E. L.: *Pharmacy Law Digest* 1980, 441.
12. Dept. H& HS, informal legal opinion 5/24/82.
13. 32 MRSA § 2805.13A.
14. FL Stat. § 465.003(4).
15. Pub. L, No. 91-513 § 302(a), 21 CFR § 1312.21.
16. 21 USC § 381(d)(1).

CHAPTER 26

Pharmacy Compounding and Manufacturing

GOOD COMPOUNDING PRACTICES APPLICABLE TO STATE LICENSED PHARMACIES*

The question of what distinguishes compounding from manufacturing has been the subject of an on-going debate between the profession of pharmacy and enforcement agencies, such as the Food and Drug Administration (FDA) and the state boards of pharmacy.

During the past year [1992], the FDA issued a series of warning letters to retail establishments it believed were engaged in manufacturing, distributing, and promoting unapproved new drugs for human use in a manner clearly outside the bounds of traditional pharmacy practice. The Agency cited as one of the reasons for such action, the potential for causing harm to the public when drug products are manufactured and distributed in commercial amounts without prior approval from the FDA and without adequate record-keeping to facilitate the recall of harmful products.

What appeared to be a simple regulatory matter soon escalated into a full-blown crisis when various sectors within the profession denounced the FDA's actions as a further intrusion into the prac-

tice of pharmacy by the federal government and a blatant attempt to stop pharmaceutical compounding by pharmacists. In response to the criticism, FDA officials pointed to reports of serious injuries and data which indicated that some establishments were manufacturing over 300,000 dosage units of inhalation therapy per month for 6,000 patients, most of whom lived out of state.

Throughout the debate, the FDA maintained that it did not want to regulate or interfere with the activities of licensed pharmacists engaged in pharmaceutical compounding as part of the traditional practice of pharmacy. At several meetings with NABP and representatives of the profession, the FDA publicly expressed its willingness to defer matters of pharmaceutical compounding to the state boards of pharmacy. FDA emphasized that it was concerned about those large-scale operations that were using retail pharmacy licensure as a means to avoid registering as a manufacturer and adhering to Good Manufacturing Practice Standards (GMPs). During its meetings with NABP, the FDA asked that the Association develop guidelines for pharmacy compounding.

Following is the first of a two-part presentation of the resulting document. NABP intends to incorporate

these Good Compounding Practices into its *Model State Pharmacy Act (Model Act)*, a document used by state boards of pharmacy to develop laws/regulations in their states, to help distinguish pharmaceutical compounding from manufacturing, and to establish uniform standards for regulating pharmaceutical compounding. Part two will appear in the third quarter "National Pharmacy Compliance News" section of this *Newsletter*.

Good Compounding Practices

The following Good Compounding Practices (GCPs) are meant to apply only to the compounding of drugs by State-licensed pharmacies. Applicable portions of the *NABP Model State Pharmacy Act* formed the basis for the development of this document.

Subpart A—General Provisions

The recommendations contained herein are considered to be the minimum current good compounding practices for the preparation of drug products by State-licensed pharmacies for dispensing and/or administration to humans or animals.

Pharmacists engaged in the com-

*Reprinted from *National Pharmacy Compliance News*, National Association of Boards of Pharmacy, Park Ridge, IL, May 1993.

pounding of drugs shall operate in conformance with applicable State law regulating the practice of pharmacy.

The following definitions from the *NABP Model State Pharmacy Act* apply to these Good Compounding Practices. States may wish to insert their own definitions to comply with State Pharmacy Practice Acts.

"Compounding"—the preparation, mixing, assembling, packaging, or Labeling of a drug (including radiopharmaceuticals) or device (i) as the result of a Practitioner's Prescription Drug Order or initiative based on the Practitioner/patient/pharmacist relationship in the course of professional practice, or (ii) for the purpose of, or as an incident to, research, teaching, or chemical analysis and not for sale or Dispensing. Compounding also includes the preparation of Drugs or Devices in anticipation of Prescription Drug Orders based on routine, regularly observed prescribing patterns.

"Manufacturing"—the production, preparation, propagation, conversion, or processing of a Drug or Device, either directly or indirectly, by extraction from substances of natural origin or independently by means of chemical or biological synthesis, and includes any packaging or repackaging of the substance(s) or Labeling or relabeling of its container, and the promotion and marketing of such Drugs or Devices. Manufacturing also includes the preparation and promotion of commercially available products from bulk compounds for resale by pharmacies, Practitioners, or other Persons.

"Component"—any ingredient intended for use in the compounding of a drug product, including those that may not appear in such product.

Based on the existence of a pharmacist/patient/prescriber relationship and the presentation of a valid prescription, or in anticipation of Prescription Drug Orders based on routine, regularly observed prescribing patterns, pharmacists may compound, for an individual patient, drug products that are commercially available in the marketplace.

Pharmacists shall receive, store, or use drug substances for compounding that have been made in an FDA-approved facility. If unobtainable from an FDA-approved facility, pharmacists shall receive, store, or use drug components in compounding prescriptions that meet official compendia requirements. If neither of these requirements can be met, and pharmacists document such, pharmacists shall use their professional judgment in the procurement of acceptable alternatives.

Pharmacists may compound drugs in very limited quantities prior to receiving a valid prescription based on a history of receiving valid prescriptions that have been generated solely within an established parmacist/patient/prescriber relationship, and provided that they maintain the prescriptions on file for all such products compounded at the pharmacy (as required by State law). The compounding of inordinate amounts of drugs in anticipation of receiving prescriptions without any historical basis is considered manufacturing.

Pharmacists shall not offer compounded drug products to other State-licensed persons or commercial entities for subsequent resale, except in the course of professional practice for a prescriber to administer to an individual patient. Compounding pharmacies/pharmacists may advertise or otherwise promote the fact that they provide prescription compounding services; however, they shall not solicit business (e.g., promote, advertise, or use salespersons) to compound specific drug products.

The distribution of inordinate amounts of compounded products without a prescriber/patient/pharmacist relationship is considered manufacturing.

Subpart B—Organization and Personnel

As in the dispensing of all prescriptions, the pharmacist has the responsibility and authority to inspect and approve or reject all components, drug product containers, closures, in-process materials, and labeling; and the authority to prepare and review all compounding records to assure that no errors have occurred in the compounding process. The pharmacist is also responsible for the proper maintenance, cleanliness, and use of all equipment used in prescription compounding practice.

All pharmacists who engage in drug compounding, and State-authorized supportive personnel supervised by pharmacists who assist in drug compounding, shall be competent and proficient in compounding and shall maintain that proficiency through current awareness and training. Competency and proficiency in the art of compounding for all pharmacists and State-authorized supportive personnel shall be evaluated, documented, and maintained in the files of the pharmacy. Every pharmacist who engages in drug compounding and any supportive personnel who assist in compounding, must be aware of and familiar with all details of these Good Compounding Practices.

It is incumbent upon each State Board of Pharmacy to determine whether non-pharmacist personnel may assist in compounding prescriptions. If non-pharmacist personnel may assist in drug compounding, the State Board of Pharmacy shall determine the responsibilities of supportive personnel and the pharmacist.

Personnel engaged in the compounding of drugs shall wear clean clothing appropriate to the operation being performed. Protective apparel, such as coats/jackets, aprons, gowns, hand or arm coverings, or masks shall be worn as necessary to protect personnel from chemical exposure and drug products from contamination.

Only personnel authorized by the responsible pharmacist shall be in the immediate vicinity of the drug compounding operation. Any person shown at any time (either by medical examination or pharmacist determination) to have an apparent illness or open lesions that may adversely affect the safety or quality of a drug product being compounded shall be excluded from direct contact with components, drug product containers, closures, in-process materials, and drug products until the condition is corrected or determined by competent medical personnel not to jeopardize the safety or quality of the products(s) being compounded. All personnel who assist the pharmacist in compounding procedures shall be instructed to report to the pharmacist any health conditions that may have an adverse effect on drug products.

Subpart C—Drug Compounding Facilities

Pharmacies engaging in compounding shall have a specifically designated and adequate area (space) for the orderly compounding of prescriptions, including the placement of equipment and materials. The drug compounding area for sterile products shall be separate and distinct from the area used for the compounding of nonsterile drug products. The area(s) used for the compounding of drugs shall be maintained in a good state of repair.

Bulk drugs and other chemicals or materials used in the compounding of drugs must be stored in adequately labeled containers in a clean, dry area or, if required, under proper refrigeration.

Adequate lighting and ventilation shall be provided in all drug compounding areas. Potable water shall be supplied under continuous positive pressure in a plumbing system free of defects that could contribute contamination to any compounded drug product. Adequate washing facilities, easily accessible to the compounding area(s) of the pharmacy, shall be provided. These facilities shall include, but not be limited to, hot and cold water, soap or detergent, and air-driers or single-use towels.

The area(s) used for the compounding of drugs shall be maintained in a clean and sanitary condition. It shall be free of infestation by insects, rodents, and other ver-

min. Trash shall be held and disposed of in a timely and sanitary manner. Sewage and other refuse in and from the pharmacy and immediate drug compounding area(s) shall be disposed of in a safe and sanitary manner.

Sterile Products

If sterile (aseptic) products are being compounded, the following conditions shall be met: [*Reference the "NABP Model Regulations for Sterile Pharmaceuticals"*].

If radiopharmaceuticals are being compounded, the following conditions shall be met: [*Reference the "NABP Model Regulations for Nuclear Pharmacy"*].

Special Precaution Products

If drug products with special precautions for contamination, such as penicillin, are involved in a compounding operation, appropriate measures, including either the dedication of equipment for such operations or the meticulous cleaning of contaminated equipment prior to its use for the preparation of other drugs, must be utilized in order to prevent cross-contamination.

FOOD AND DRUG ADMINISTRATION COMPLIANCE POLICY GUIDES (MARCH 16, 1992; GUIDE 71.32.16)

CHAPTER 32—DRUGS GENERAL

Subject

Manufacture, distribution, and promotion of adulterated, misbranded, or unapproved new drugs for human use by state-licensed pharmacies.

Background

This compliance policy guide (CPG) reflects longstanding FDA policy that has been articulated in related CPGs, warning letters, and federal court decisions.

FDA recognizes that pharmacists traditionally have extemporaneously compounded and manipulated reasonable quantities of drugs upon receipt of a valid prescription for an individually identified patient from a licensed practitioner. This traditional activity is not the subject of this CPG.

With respect to such activities, it is important to note that 21 U.S.C. 360(g)(1) exempts retail pharmacies from the registration requirements that include, among other things, a mandatory biennial FDA inspection. The exemption applies to "pharmacies" that operate in accordance with state law and dispense drugs "upon prescriptions of practitioners licensed to administer such drugs to patients *under the care of such practitioners in the course of their professional practice, and which do not manufacture,* prepare, propagate, *compound,* or process drugs or devices for sale *other than in the regular course of their business of dispensing* or selling drugs or devices *at retail*" (emphasis added). See also 21 U.S.C. Sections 374(a)(2) (exempting pharmacies that meet the foregoing criteria from certain inspection provisions) and 353(b)(2) (exempting drugs dispensed by filling a valid prescription from certain misbranding provisions).

It should be noted, however, that, while retail pharmacies that meet the statutory criteria are exempted from certain requirements of the Federal Food, Drug, and Cosmetic Act (Act), they are not the subject of any general exemption from the new drug, adulteration, or misbranding provisions of the Act.

FDA believes that an increasing number of establishments with retail pharmacy licenses are engaged in manufacturing, distributing, and promoting unapproved new drugs for human use in a manner that is clearly outside the bounds of traditional pharmacy practice and that constitute violations of the Act. Some "pharmacies" that have sought to find shelter under and expand the scope of the exemptions identified above have claimed that their manufacturing, distribution, and marketing

practices are only retail dispensing; however, the practices of these entities are far more consistent with those of drug manufacturers and wholesalers than with retail pharmacies. The activities of the self-styled pharmacies are consistent with the activities of manufacturers in that they direct promotional activities at licensed practitioners and patients. The promotional activities include employing detail persons and hiring marketing consultants to promote the company's specialization of compounding specific products or therapeutic classes of drugs. The firms also receive and use in large quantity bulk drug substances to manufacture unapproved drug products and to manufacture drug products in large quantity, in advance of receiving a valid prescription for the products. Moreover, the firms serve physicians and patients with whom they have no established individual or professional relationship.

When less significant violations of the Act related to a pharmacy have occurred, FDA has worked cooperatively with state regulatory agencies; generally, FDA will continue to defer such actions to state authorities. However, FDA regards the more extreme examples of the foregoing conduct as significant violations that constitute deliberate efforts to circumvent the new drug, adulteration or misbranding provisions of the Act.

There is a very real potential for causing harm to the public health when drug products are manufactured and distributed in commercial amounts without FDA's prior approval and without adequate record keeping (to retrace and recall harmful products), without labeling, or without adequate manufacturing controls to assure the safety, purity, potency, quality, and identity of the drug product. In one recent instance, an outbreak of eye infections in regional hospitals and the loss of an eye by each of two patients were attributed to a drug product compounded by a pharmacy.

FDA has issued warning letters to several firms that were clearly manufacturing drugs for human use under the guise of traditional pharmacy practice. For example, one establishment manufactured over 300,000 dosage units of albuterol sulfate and other inhalation therapy drugs per month for 6,000 patients, most of whom live out of state. Another firm manufactured a large quantity of a drug product at dosage levels that have not been determined by adequate and well-controlled studies to be effective for the indicated use. A recent inspection of another company operating with a pharmacy license revealed that the firm had hundreds of bulk drug ingredients on hand to manufacture about 165 different products. A review of the manufacturing dates of the "compounded" drugs on hand during the inspection of this firm revealed that 37 products had been produced over a year prior to the inspection, six products had been made between six and eleven months prior to the inspection, and 111 products had no recorded manufacturing date.

The agency has initiated enforcement action when pharmacy practice extends beyond the reasonable and traditional practice of a retail pharmacy. The courts have upheld FDA's interpretation in those cases. See *United States v. Sene X Eleemosynary Corp.,* 479 F. Supp. 970 (S.D. Fla. 1979), aff'd, [1982–1983 Transfer Binder] Food Drug Cosm. L. Rep. (CCH) para. 38,207 at 39,117 (11th Cir. 1983); *Cedars N. Towers Pharmacy, Inc., v. United States* [1978–79] Transfer Binder] Food Drug Cosm. L. Rep. (CCH) para. 38,200 at 38,826 (S.D. Fla. Aug. 28, 1978). See also *United States v. Algon Chemical, Inc.,* 879 F.2d 1154 (3d Cir. 1989), *United States v. 9/1 Kg. Containers,* 854 F.2d 173 (7th Cir. 1988), cert. denied, 489 U.S. 1010 (1989), and *United States v. Rutherford,* 442 U.S. 544 (1979), regarding limitations on sale of unapproved and otherwise unlawful products to licensed practitioners.

Policy

FDA recognizes that a licensed pharmacist may compound drugs extemporaneously after receipt of a valid prescription for an individual patient (i.e., an oral or written order of a practitioner licensed by state law to administer or order the administration of the drug to an individual patient identified and treated by the practitioner in the course of his or her professional practice).

Pharmacies that do not otherwise engage in practices that extend beyond the limits set forth in this CPG may prepare drugs in very limited quantities before receiving a valid prescription, provided they can document a history of receiving valid prescriptions that have been generated solely within an established professional practitioner-patient-pharmacy relationship and provided further that they maintain the prescription on file for all such products dispensed at the pharmacy as required by state law.

If a pharmacy compounds finished drugs from bulk active ingredient materials considered to be unapproved new drug substances, as defined in 21 CFR 310.3(g), such activity must be covered by an FDA-sanctioned investigational new drug application (IND) that is, in effect, in accordance with 21 U.S.C. Section 355(i) and 21 CFR 312.

In certain circumstances, it may be appropriate for a pharmacist to compound a small quantity of a drug that is only slightly different than an FDA-approved drug that is commercially available. In these circumstances, patient-by-patient consultation between physician and pharmacist must result in documentation that substantiates the medical need for the particular variation of the compound.

Pharmacies may not, without losing their status as retail entities, compound, provide, and dispense drugs to third parties for resale to individual patients.

FDA will generally continue to defer to state and local officials regulation of the day-to-day practice of retail pharmacy and related activities. FDA anticipates that cooperative efforts between the states and the agency will result in coordinated investigations, referrals, and follow-up actions by the states.

Regulatory Action Guidance

Pharmacies engaged in promotion and other activities analogous to manufacturing and distributing drugs for human use are subject to the same provisions of the Act as manufacturers. District offices are encouraged to consult with state regulatory authorities to assure coherent application of this CPG to establishments that are operating outside of the traditional practice of pharmacy.

FDA-initiated regulatory action may include issuing a warning letter, seizure, injunction, and/or prosecution. Charges may include, but need not be limited to, violations of 21 U.S.C. Sections 351(a)(2)(B), 352(a), 352(f)(1), 352(o), and 355(a) of the Act.

FDA's Guidelines on Compounding vs. Manufacturing

Pursuant to FDA's "Compliance Policy Guide," any of the following practices would trigger FDA enforcement actions for violations of the federal Food, Drug, and Cosmetic Act. The list is "not intended to be exhaustive and other factors may be appropriate for consideration in a particular case," says FDA.

- Soliciting business (promoting, advertising, or using sales persons) to compound specific drug products, product classes, or therapeutic classes of drug products
- Compounding, regularly or in inordinate amounts, drug products that are commercially available in the marketplace and that are essentially generic copies of commercially available FDA-approved drug products
- Using commercial-scale manufacturing or testing equipment for compounding drug products
- Receiving, storing, or using drug substances without first obtaining written assurance from the supplier that each lot of the drug substance has been made in an FDA-approved facility
- Compounding inordinate amounts of drugs in anticipation of receiving prescriptions in relation to the amounts of drugs compounded after receiving valid prescriptions
- Offering compounded drug products at wholesale to other state licensed persons or commercial entities for resale
- Distributing inordinate amounts of compounded products out of state
- Failing to conform with applicable state law regulating the practice of pharmacy

Compounding: What's Allowed

The basic requirements for compounded products are that they be:

- Compounded for an identified individual patient
- Compounded pursuant to unsolicited receipt of a valid prescription order or of a notation, approved by the prescribing practitioner, that a compounded product is necessary for the identified patient, and
- Compounded by a licensed pharmacist in a state-licensed pharmacy or by a physician

Products may be compounded in limited quantities before receipt of a prescription if there is a history of receiving such orders and there is an established relationship between the compounder and the patient or the prescriber. The compounding, regularly or in inordinate amounts, of products that are essentially copies of commercial products is prohibited.

CHAPTER 27

Patient Package Inserts

The patient package insert (PPI) (and the manufacturer's package insert), which are provided by the manufacturer or distributor, are prime examples of labeling. Each relates to a drug product, category of drug, or medical device.

Each of the following categories requires a PPI each and every time the pharmacist dispenses such a product:

- Oral contraceptive

- Inhalant containing isoproterenol as an active ingredient
- Estrogen prescription product
- Diethylstilbestrol when used for post-coital contraception
- Progestational drug product marketed pursuant to an approved new drug application (NDA)
- Intrauterine contraceptive device (IUD)

When estrogens are prescribed for a hospitalized patient, the pharmacist is required to provide the patient package insert prior to the administration of the first dose and at least once every thirty (30) days, as long as therapy continues.

Patient package inserts do not have to be provided with prescriptions dispensed to patients when any of the above categories are compounded by the pharmacist pursuant to a bona fide prescription.

QUESTIONS: CHAPTER 27

1. Which drug product requires a patient package insert each time it is dispensed?

    a. Anadrol-50

    b. Winstrol

    c. Oxadrin

    d. Durabolin

    e. Ortho Novum 7/7/7

2. Which one of the following is correct in relation to PPIs?

    a. Isuprel and Proventil

    b. Medihaler-Iso and Isuprel

    c. Duo-Medihaler and Ventolin

    d. Isuprel and Medihaler-Iso

    e. Alupent and Metaprel

3. Which drug product requires a PPI when dispensed by the pharmacist?

    a. Ovulette

    b. Ovral

    c. Oretic-21

    d. Omicron 28

    e. Oxazepam

4. For which category of drug product is the pharmacist required to provide a patient package insert each time the product is dispensed?

    a. Anorectics

    b. Barbiturates

    c. Corticosteroids

    d. Diuretics

    e. Estrogens

5. How often and when is the pharmacist required to provide a PPI when an estrogen is prescribed to an in-patient?

    a. Prior to administration of first dose

    b. Upon discharge from the hospital

    c. At least every 30 days

    d. a. and b. are correct.

    e. a. and c. are correct.

Glossary of Legal Terms of Interest to Pharmacists

All professionals have a tendency to insulate themselves from the lay public by the development of a specialized language. The legal profession has achieved this insulation with spectacular success. Despite the increasing pervasiveness of the law in every facet of the pharmacy, the special language of the law has become a barrier to the pharmacist's basic understanding of the laws that govern the profession.

In order to help the pharmacist overcome the disadvantages inherent in reading or discussing the law, the author has prepared this glossary for pharmacists who wish a readily comprehensible explanation of unfamiliar yet common legal terms used in legal proceedings or in the literature. The glossary is not comprehensive; it is intended to be a convenient, quick reference in the absence of a law dictionary.

Abrogate to annul, revoke or cancel; to void a law by legislative repeal.

Accessory one who aids or contributed in a secondary way or assists in or contributed to a crime as a subordinate.

Act an enactment, as of a legislative body, such as the U.S. Congress or the state legislature.

Ad Hoc (Latin) for this. An *ad hoc* committee is one created for a special purpose, i.e., *for this* purpose.

Adjective Law rules of procedure or practice, as opposed to that body of law which the courts are established to administer (substantive law); it means the rules according to which the substantive law is administered; sometimes referred to as "remedial law."

Adjudication the determination of controversy and a pronouncement of a judgment based on evidence presented.

Administrative Agency board, commission; a subdivision of government created by the legislature to implement and administer the general policies specified by the legislature and statutes; a government agency having administrative, legislative or judicial powers.

Administrative Law the branch of law which pertains to the various branches of government, and mandates what, when, where, and how they are to govern.

Affiant the person making the oath.

Affidavit a written statement made under oath before an officer of the court, a notary public, or other person authorized to so act.

Agency relation in which one person acts (agent) on behalf of another (principal).

Agent a person who, by mutual consent, acts for the benefit of another. The acts of an agent are binding on his principal.

Allegation a statement by a party to a legal action of what he undertakes to prove.

Amendment a modification in an existing law, leaving some part(s) of the original as is.

Amicus Curiae (Latin) friend of the court; a person not party to the case, who files a written argument or provides information on a matter before the court. The intent is to call the court's attention to some matter which might otherwise escape its attention, and which it may need to make a proper decision, or to urge a particular decision on behalf of the public or private interest of third parties who will be indirectly affected by the resolution of the dispute.

Annul to make void, as to annul a (pharmacist's) license. Such a license is void *ab initio* (from the very beginning) as compared with a license which is revoked by decree. A revocation operates only to terminate the license from a certain date forward and does not affect the former validity of that license.

Answer the response by the defendant (respondent) to the charges made by the complainant (plaintiff).

Antedate to insert or place an earlier date on an instrument, such as a prescription, than the actual date on which it was executed.

A Posteriori (Latin) known only through experience of facts.

Appellant the person who appeals a decision of a lower court and brings the case to a reviewing court.

Appellate Court a court that has the jurisdiction to review, affirm, reverse, or modify the judgments of another court. It is a court which reviews a case, and which determines whether or not the ruling and judgment of a lower court were correct. It is not a trial court, and hence a new case cannot be made here.

Appellee the person who won in a lower court and who requests in a reviewing court that the judgment of the lower court be upheld in his favor.

Arraignment an initial step in a criminal proceeding where the defendant is read the charges against him and is asked to enter a plea (guilty, not guilty, nolo contendre). It is at this point in the procedure that the accused is given a copy of the complaint and informed of his constitutional rights, e.g., to plead not guilty, have a jury trial, have a right to a legal counsel.

Assault an attempt to inflict bodily injury upon someone else (see **Battery**).

Assign generally, an assignment is a transfer of one's interests to another. For example, an owner (assignor) selling his pharmacy may transfer (assign) the lease to the new owner (assignee).

Attest to affirm as true or genuine; to authenticate by signing as a witness; to put on oath that the statements are correct, as in an application of a license.

Bad Debt a debt (money, goods, services) owed by one (debtor) to another (creditor) which is not collectible and therefore worthless.

Bankruptcy popularly defined as the inability of a debtor to pay his debts as they become due. Technically, the term refers to the procedures under the federal Bankruptcy Act by which the assets of the debtor are liquidated to pay the creditors. In reorganization, liquidation may be avoided and the debtor may continue to function, carry on business, and pay the creditors under the supervision of the court.

Battery the unlawful beating or use of force on a person without his consent; the actual touching involved in an "assault and battery."

Bill a draft of a proposed law submitted to the legislature for enactment.

Bona Fide made in good faith without fraud or deceit; genuine, not counterfeit.

Breach of Duty an infraction or violation of a law, obligation, or standard. A breach of duty may be the failure of a pharmacist to dispense medication as prescribed by the physician; any violation to perform a duty owed to another (patient), whether willful or done through negligence.

Burglary the taking of property belonging to someone else by breaking into and entering certain premises with intent to steal.

Case Law the aggregate of reported cases; the law pertaining to a particular subject as formed by adjudged cases, in distinction to statutes and other sources of law.

Case Law the aggregate of reported cases; the law pertaining to a particular subject as formed by adjudged cases, in distinction to statutes and other sources of law.

Case System a method of teaching or studying the law based on cases.

Caveat (Latin) a warning; let him beware; in general, a warning or emphasis for caution.

Caveat Emptor (Latin) let the buyer beware; expresses a rule of commercial law that without a warranty the purchaser buys at his own risk, and thus takes the risk of quality upon himself.

Certification the process by which a nongovernmental agency or association grants recognition to an individual who has met certain predetermined qualifications specified by that agency or association.

Certiorari (Latin) a mandate of a superior (higher) court to an inferior (lower) court to provide it with the records of a case. The intent of the higher court is to review the proceedings in the lower court to determine whether or not any legal irregularities may have occurred, and this is a means of gaining appellate review.

Change of Venue the removal of a lawsuit from one place to trial (court) to another (see **Venue**).

Chattel any tangible, movable or immovable property, except real property; personal property.

Citation an official summons to appear, as before a court, on the date and time indicated, and do something mentioned therein; also, refers to a source of legal reference by page, volume, and date.

Class Action a legal action undertaken by one or more representatives on behalf of themselves and all other persons having an identical interest in the alleged wrong.

Code A systematic compilation of laws arranged into tables of content, chapters, and index, and promulgated by legislative authority.

Codicil a legal supplement or addition to a last will and testament.

Commercial Paper a negotiable instrument.

Common Law a system of law derived from principles based on justice, reason, and common sense (as decided in prior cases) rather than on absolute, fixed, and inflexible rules. The principles of common law are determined by the social needs of the community and are subject to adaptation by the courts to new conditions, interests, relations, and usages as the progress of society may require.

Comparative Negligence is the proportional sharing of compensation for injuries between plaintiff and defendant, or between defendants, based on the relative negligence of each.

Complainant the party who initiates the complaint in a legal action; synonymous with petitioner, plaintiff.

Complaint a formal accusation; the initial formal written allegations filed by the plaintiff in a legal proceeding.

Concurrent occurring at the same time or acting in conjunction. For example, two different authorities, such as the Drug Enforcement Administration (DEA) and a board of pharmacy, may have *concurrent* jurisdiction over the same matter (prescription for a controlled substance).

Consent; Consent Decree a voluntary agreement to comply with a proposal by another, e.g., board of pharmacy penalty in case of violation; does not constitute an admission of guilt nor that the law has been violated. A consent order is different than a plea bargain, in which guilt is admitted in exchange for a lesser penalty or criminal charge.

Contempt of Court may be classified as civil or criminal. The former refers to misconduct in the form of disobedience to an order of the court by one part to a judicial proceeding to the prejudice of the other litigant. Criminal contempt refers to an act which is disrespectful to the court, calculated to bring the court into disrepute, or is of such nature so as to obstruct the administration of justice.

Contiguous touching along a boundary or at a point. For example, the board of pharmacy of one state may legally recognize, and thus permit its licensed pharmacists to dispense, prescriptions authorized by physicians licensed and practicing in neighboring (*contiguous*) states.

Contingent Fee an attorney's compensation based on the successful result of a case and one which is agreed to be a percentage of the amount the client actually collects (recovers) as an outcome of a lawsuit.

Contract a legally enforceable agreement between two or more parties to do or not to do a particular thing; may be written or oral.

Contributory Negligence is conduct on the part of the plaintiff that falls below the standard to which he should conform for his own protection, and is a legally contributing cause in bringing about the plaintiff's harm.

Court of Claims a court which has jurisdiction over claims against a government. When a private citizen has a claim against the state, or certain government agencies, it must be brought in the court of claims.

Covenant an agreement or promise between two or more parties.

Damages monetary compensation which may be recovered in the courts by any person who has suffered loss, or injury to his person, property, or rights, through the unlawful act or negligence of another.

Debenture a written acknowledgment of a debt with a promise to pay.

Debt goods, services, or money that one person owes another.

Decree a decision or order of the court.

De Facto (Latin) in fact; in reality.

Defamation anything that may harm the reputation of another by libel or slander.

Default a failure to do something required by duty or law (e.g., failure to appear at the required time in a legal proceeding). A judgment entered in a civil case, where the defendant has failed to appear to contest the claim asserted against him, may result by *default*.

Defendant a person who is being sued in a civil action or is prosecuted in a criminal action.

Demurrer a defense to plaintiff's complaint wherein the defendant, for the sake of argument, admits plaintiff's alleged facts, but denies the plaintiff's conclusion (remedy for relief) is legally enforceable; in effect, defendant says "so what" to plaintiff's complaint.

Deponent a witness; one who gives evidence.

Deposition testimony under oath, in writing, outside the court.

Disclaimer a declaration of a refusal to accept responsibility or an obligation.

Discovery procedures for determining facts prior to the time of trial in order to eliminate the element of surprise in litigation.

Dissent a difference of opinion; to disagree. A dissenting opinion by a judge of an appellate court could indicate his reason for disagreeing with the results reached by the majority of judges.

District Court the trial court in the federal system which has jurisdiction over such matters as bankruptcy proceedings, cases arising under patent or copyright laws, cases involving a fine, penalty, or forfeiture under federal laws, civil rights cases, and disputes between citizens of different states.

Docket a court calendar.

Domicile a person's fixed, permanent, and principal home for legal purposes.

Due Process of Law the guarantee of procedural fairness; legal proceedings carried out in accordance with established rules and principles. The United States and the state constitutions refer to it, e.g., U.S. Bill of Rights, Articles V–VIII.

Duress forcing a person to commit an act he need not do.

Duty a moral or legal obligation. Under the law of negligence, a pharmacist owes a patient a duty of care in that he must conduct himself so as to avoid injury to the patient, e.g., dispense the prescribed medication according to the accepted standards of care.

Eminent Domain a right of government to take private property for public use.

Enacting Clause a preliminary section of a law which declares its enactment and serves to identify it as an act of legislation emanating from some legislative body. Various statements are used for this purpose, such as "Be it enacted by the People of the . . .," or "Be it enacted by the Senate and House of Representatives of the United States in Congress assembled," etc.

Enjoin to forbid; prohibit.

Escrow a deed, money, a bond, or property delivered to or held by a neutral third party (*escrow agent*) to an agreement. The escrow agent will hold the instrument until the terms of the contract are fulfilled.

Et al. (Latin) an abbreviation for et alia, "and others."

Et Seq. (Latin) an abbreviation for et sequentes, "and the following ones."

Ex Officio (Latin) by virtue of his office. The U.S. vice president serves *ex officio* as president of the Senate.

Expert Witness a person who has acquired special knowledge in a particular field of endeavor through practical experience and/or study, which gives him a superior knowledge so that his opinion is admissible at trial.

Express explicitly set forth in words; stated, not implied.

Express Warranty an affirmation of fact or promise made by the seller to the buyer in regard to goods purchased.

False Pretenses obtaining property, such as drugs from a pharmacist, by making false representation of a fact, e.g., posing as a licensed physician.

Federal Register sometimes referred to as "the daily newspaper of the federal government," which publishes regulations, orders, and other documents. It informs citizens of their rights, obligations, and benefits. Before FDA, DEA, or any other federal government agency can establish, amend, or repeal any of its rules and regulations, it is required by law to announce its intentions in the *Federal Register*.

Felony a generic term used to distinguish certain serious crimes, such as murder, arson, etc., from relatively minor offenses. The test of whether a crime is a felony generally is whether the act is declared by law to be such or when it is punishable by death or imprisonment in a state prison; for example, arson, murder, kidnapping.

Fiduciary a trustee; a person having a duty, created by his undertaking to act primarily for the benefit of another in matters pertaining to such endeavors. A pharmacist selecting and dispensing a generic drug product acts as a fiduciary.

Forgery falsely making or materially altering any writing, such as the signature of a physician on a prescription, which, if it were genuine, might have legal value.

Fraud intentional deceit or misrepresentation of truth in order to induce another to part with something of value or surrender a legal right, or misleading by nondisclosure or concealment. A person who obtains a pharmacist's license by concealing or misrepresenting certain facts required on the application for licensure can be accused of fraud.

Freedom of Contract the ability to enter into agreements with others without coercion or constraint. A pharmacist may or may not choose to participate in third-party payment programs; such action is voluntary under the concept of *freedom of contract*.

Garnishment a process whereby money (wages) or property (assets) belonging to a debtor are held by another.

Generic relating to or characteristic of a whole group; not protected by trademark or patent law, such as generic drugs.

Grandfather Clause provisions which create an exemption based on circumstances which existed prior to the enactment of a law. In some states druggists were licensed without meeting all the criteria that the new entrants into the profession (pharmacists) have to fulfill.

Grand Jury a jury generally consisting of no more than 25 persons, that considers evidence against persons charged with crime and if the evidence warrants makes formal charges on which the accused persons are later tried in court before a petit jury.

Home Rule limited autonomy granted by a state to a local government (county or municipal) in order for the latter to legislate without first obtaining permission from the state legislature.

Hung Jury a petit jury that is unable to agree upon a verdict.

Impeach process whereby charges of misconduct are brought against a public official.

Implied an intent not directly or explicitly stated; deduced from circumstances, conduct, or language; suggested or understood.

In Camera (Latin) in chambers. Discussion relating to a trial may be held *in camera*, e.g., in the judge's chambers.

In Personam (Latin) refers to a legal proceeding against a person for the purpose of imposing a liability or an obligation.

In Rem (Latin) in the case or matter of a *thing* rather than a person.

In Toto (Latin) totally; entirely.

Indictment a written accusation from a grand jury charging a person with a crime. It differs from a criminal complaint or information in that a grand jury, rather than a judge, determines if there is sufficient evidence to charge the person with the crime.

Informed Consent in tort law, a requirement that a person (patient) be given prior notice as to the risks, benefits, and nature of a medical procedure, e.g., surgery or use of drugs, by the physician.

Injunction a written order of a court whereby one is prevented from or required to do a specified act.

Injury/Damages any wrong done to another, either to his person, rights, representation, or property.

Interlocutory temporary, not final; a decision of a court which decides some matter prior to the final adjudication of the entire issue.

Interrogatories written questions of one adversary to another, and vice versa, in a lawsuit, who must provide written responses under oath outside the court. These questions and answers may be read at the trial and have the same force and effect as if the person were testifying personally.

Intestate a person who dies without leaving a will.

Ipso Facto (Latin) by the very nature of the facts.

Judiciary the branch of government in which judicial (the administration of justice) power is vested.

Judgment a formal decision by a court; the final sentence, order or decision at the conclusion of a legal case.

Jurisdiction the power, right, or authority (any one of which may be limited) to enact, interpret, or apply law.

Landmark Case a legal event or development that marks a turning point in a matter of great importance and establishes a precedent. The expression is usually used of a case presented to a supreme court, e.g., Whalen vs. Roe, Liggett vs. Baldridge.

Learned Intermediary Doctrine the principle that the drug manufacturer has responsibility to warn only physicians adequately about known or knowable risks and potential adverse effects of prescription drugs. The manufacturer has no duty to warn patients directly about prescription medications; this responsibility is left to the physician.

Lease a written agreement between the landlord (lessor) and the tenant (lessee) which contains the rights and duties of each.

Legal Duty that which the law requires to be done.

Lessee a tenant.

Lessor a landlord.

Libel any published matter that reflects upon and injures the reputation of a person.

License a privilege granted by some competent authority (licensor) to do something which otherwise could not be done legally. A board of pharmacy may grant a license to a qualified person to practice pharmacy (licensee, licentiate), and such license may be revoked, annulled, or suspended due to some infraction of the pharmacy statutes and/or regulations.

Licensure the process by which an agency of government grants permission to an individual to engage in a given occupation upon finding that the applicant has attained the minimal degree of competency necessary to ensure that the public health, safety, and welfare will be reasonably well protected.

Lien a hold or claim upon someone's real or personal property in order to satisfy some debt.

Litigate to be involved in a lawsuit.

Malefactor a person guilty of a crime.

Malfeasance a wrongful or illegal act; any act, say, of a board of pharmacy member, forbidden by the terms of his appointment.

Malice the intent to injure or cause harm.

Malpractice an intentional abandonment of professional duty or a failure to exercise an accepted degree of professional skill or knowledge by a person, such as a pharmacist, rendering professional services which results in harm, injury or damage.

Mandate an order or directive, usually issued by a court.

Miranda Rule statements issued by law enforcement officials to a person in custody, that said person has certain rights, such as to remain silent, to be represented by an attorney, and to be provided with an attorney. A warning must also be given to the effect that any statements of the accused may be used against him. Unless such rights are waived by the accused, evidence obtained during questioning may not be used at trial.

Misdemeanor a generic term used to distinguish certain relatively minor offenses, usually punishable by confinement in a county or city jail, or a fine, or both; for example, shoplifting, theft or larceny of small sums, and driving an automobile at excessive speed.

Misfeasance the improper performance of some legal act.

Mitigate to reduce or lessen. Circumstances which would tend to reduce damages caused by a tort or breach of contract, while not completely exonerating the person charged.

Moot unsettled; undecided. A moot point is one not settled by judicial decisions.

Negligence the omission to do something which, under ordinary circumstances, a reasonable person would do; the doing of something which a reasonable and prudent person would not do. If the negligence is the proximate cause of injury to another, it becomes an actionable tort.

Nolo Contendere (Latin) I will not contest it; a plea by which a defendant announces his intention not to defend the action. A plea that lets a suspect maintain his innocence while conceding there is sufficient evidence to convict him. The plea admits, for the purposes of the case, all the facts, but is not meant as a plea of "guilty." For all intents and purposes, it is practically equivalent to a "guilty" plea, and judgment can be entered against the defendant. Generally, the plea is made in hope of a reduced sentence.

Nonfeasance nonperformance of some acts which should be performed; the failure to perform a duty; neglect of duty.

Notary Public a public officer who has the legal authority to administer oaths and affirmations, certify documents, take depositions and affidavits.

Null and Void having no legal force or effect, as if something had not taken place at all.

Oath a pledge made in verification of statements made or to be made.

On Demand when asked for; when requested. For example, prescription records may be made available upon request by a board of pharmacy inspector during the course of a routine inspection.

Ordinance a statute enacted by the leglislative body of a municipality (see **Statute**).

Original Jurisdiction the authority possessed by a court to hear a case in the beginning, to try it, and pass judgment upon it.

Pecuniary relating to money or monetary affairs.

Per Curiam a legal opinion of the entire court rather than by one judge. Sometimes it may refer to an opinion of a presiding judge or chief justice.

Peremptory Challenge a number of questions or challenges allowed each litigant in the selection of a jury. A reason for the challenge need not be stated; however, the response may exclude a person from serving as a juror.

Perjury a false statement made under oath.

Petit Jury the trial jury, generally consisting of no more than 12 persons.

Plaintiff a person who initiates a lawsuit.

Plaintiff in Error a person who appeals a judgment against him in a lower court, regardless of whether he was the plaintiff or defendant in the case in the court; an appellant.

Plea Bargain is an agreement between the prosecution and the defendant in which the defendant agrees to plead guilty to a crime, in exchange either for the prosecution dropping a more serious charge or for a less than maximum sentence. A typical condition of a plea bargain is that the defendant will accept it only if the judge (court) agrees to impose the sentence recommended by the prosecution.

Police Power authority vested in state government by the United States Constitution to impose restrictions upon private rights which are related to promotion, protection, and maintenance of health, safety, morals, and general welfare of its citizens.

Postdate to insert or place a later date on an instrument, such as a prescription, than the actual date on which it was executed.

Power of Attorney a written statement authorizing another to act as one's agent or attorney regarding specified acts.

Preamble an introductory statement in a statute or some other legal document which explains the reasons for its enactment or objectives.

Precedent a prior decision or authority that serves as an example for an identical or similar question of law. A precedent may involve an interpretation of a statute/regulation, or it may relate to a unique situation in law.

Presumption of Innocence the presumption of fact that a person accused of a crime is innocent until it is proven that such person in fact is guilty of the offense charged.

Prima Facie (Latin) at first sight; on the face of it; not requiring further support of evidence and accepted as fact unless disproved by some evidence to the contrary. A written prescription of a licensed practitioner is sufficient proof of a particular fact, and may be admitted in a lawsuit as *prima facie* evidence.

Pro Bono Publico (Latin) for the public good.

Probate a determination by a court of competent jurisdiction, e.g., probate court or surrogate's court, establishing the validity of a last will and testament.

Promulgate to publish, to announce, to make known a law after its enactment.

Proprietary one who has exclusive title to a thing. The proprietary name is also the brand name of a drug product.

Proximate Cause that which produces an injury, and

without which the results would not have occurred; a negligent act contributory to an injury, without which such injury would not have resulted; the dominant or producing cause.

Punitive Damages   payment in excess of those required to compensate the plaintiff for the wrong or harm done, which are imposed by the court in order to punish the defendant because of the particularly cruel or willful character of the wrongdoing.

Purport   to imply, to have the appearance of being; meaning; differs from *tenor*, which means an exact copy.

Quasi   (Latin) as if it were, analogous to. This term is used to indicate that one subject resembles another with which it is compared. Certain actions of a board of pharmacy are *quasi-judicial* in character, in that they may be required to investigate facts, or ascertain the existence of facts, and draw conclusions from them as a basis for their official action, and to exercise discretion of a judicial nature.

Quid Pro Quo   (Latin) something given or received for something else.

Quorum   the minimum number of persons who must be present in order that business may be legally transacted.

Reasonable Care   the care that a prudent person would exercise under the same circumstances.

Reciprocity   the existence of a relationship between persons, businesses, or governments whereby privileges or favors granted by one are returned by the other. Thus, if state A licenses pharmacists already licensed by state Z, reciprocity or mutuality exists when Z similarly licenses pharmacists previously licensed by A.

Registrant   a person who is formally enrolled (registered), particularly for the purpose of securing a right or a privilege granted by law on condition of such registration. A licensed pharmacist may be a registered pharmacist by virtue of having his name enrolled/recorded with some authority, such as the board of pharmacy of a state, as required (annually, payment of a fee, etc.) and thereby being granted the privilege of practicing the profession in that state.

Regulation   a specific rule or order promulgated by an administrative agency of government which modifies, restates, or interprets the particular statute upon which it is based or from which it derives its authority.

Regulatory Process   the law-making process used by federal agencies (such as DEA or the FDA) and state agencies (such as the Board of Pharmacy or the state government body regulating Medicaid) to define, implement, and enforce specific statutes passed by the state legislative body or the U.S. Congress.

Reinstate   to place again in a former state from which a person has been removed. To reinstate a licensed pharmacist after having served a suspension of license does not mean granting a new license, but does mean that the pharmacist has been restored to all the benefits accruing to him under the laws of the licensing state.

Remand   to send back, as for further deliberation by the legal tribunal from which a case came.

Repeal   to abolish a law by the enactment of a subsequent statute which declares that the former law shall be revoked.

Reprimand   an expression of disapproval. A board of pharmacy may find fault with and subsequently formally and publicly criticize the professional conduct of a licensed pharmacist.

Respondeat Superior   (Latin) let the superior answer. This legal maxim is in effect when there is a master (employer, supervising pharmacist, pharmacist-preceptor)–servant (employee, pharmacy intern) relationship, in which the master is liable in certain instances for the wrongful acts of the servant, during the latter's course of employment and within the scope of his responsibilities. Hence, the doctrine is inapplicable where the wrongdoing occurred outside the legitimate scope of authority.

Restraining Order   a preliminary legal order sometimes issued by a court to keep a situation unchanged pending decision upon an application for injunction.

Revoke   to void or cancel by taking back, such as a license.

Rider   an addition to a document, such as an insurance policy or legislative bill, attached on a separate piece of paper for the purpose of changing it in some respect.

Robbery   the taking of someone else's property against that person's will and by force or by putting the person in fear.

Show Cause   an order of some judicial body to present to it facts and law for consideration to influence its decision of the case before it.

Show Cause Order   an "order" of the court requiring one party to a lawsuit to appear before the court and show cause (argue) why a certain thing should not be done or permitted.

Slander   defaming or injuring a person's character by spreading false and/or malicious oral statements about him.

Stare Decisis   (Latin) to stand by decided matters. It refers to the judicial policy of following legal principles established by previous court decisions.

Statute   written law enacted by a legislature other than that of a municipality (see **Ordinance**).

Statute of Limitations   any law which affixes a certain time after which rights cannot be enforced by legal action or offenses cannot be punished; a statutory time limit beyond which action cannot be taken.

Strict Products Liability   a theory in products liability law, which dictates that a manufacturer or other member in the chain of commerce is strictly liable (liable without a showing of fault) when a product that will be used without inspection for defects proves to have a defect that causes injury.

Subpoena ad Testificandum   (Latin) under penalty to give testimony. A written order of the court to compel the appearance of a witness to render testimony before it. Failure to appear on the date and time specified may result in a penalty.

Subpoena Duces Tecum   (Latin) under penalty you shall bring with you. A written order of the court to compel a person to produce in court designated documents or other evidence, e.g., prescriptions and prescription records.

Substantive Law   that part of law which creates, defines, and regulates rights and duties which are the sum and substance of the law.

Summons   an official notification to a person to appear, as before a court, on the date and time indicated, and do something mentioned therein.

Supra (Latin) above. In a written work it refers the reader to a preceding section.

Surrogate a local judicial officer who has jurisdiction over the probate of wills, the settlement of estates, and the appointment and supervision of guardians.

Suspension the temporary removal of a privilege, such as the privilege to practice pharmacy pursuant to license, which will be restored after a definite or indefinite period of time.

Testate having made a will.

Testator a person who leaves a will at the time of death.

Testimony oral statement by a witness under oath given in response to a question by a lawyer or authorized public official at the time of trial or a hearing.

Theft the wrongful taking of personal property belonging to someone else, with the intent to deprive the owner of possession.

Tort a private or civil wrong or injury upon the person or property, independent of a contract. It may be 1) a direct invasion of some legal right of the individual; 2) the infraction of some public duty by which special damage accrues to the individual; or 3) the violation of some private obligation by which like damage accrues to the individual. The three elements of every tort action are existence of a legal duty from defendant to plaintiff, breach of that duty, and damages as proximate result.

Tort-Feasor one who commits or is guilty of a tort.

Trademark a name, symbol, device, mark, that identifies or is capable of distinguishing goods or services, e.g., Valium, Pulvule, Abbo-Pac, Detecto-Seal.

Trade Secret may consist of any formula, pattern, device, or compilation of information used in one's business which gives the manufacturer an opportunity to obtain an advantage over competitors who do not know or use it.

Ultra Vires (Latin) beyond the powers; exceeding the powers granted a government agency.

Unprofessional Conduct that which violates an ethical code of a profession, or such conduct which is considered grossly unprofessional because it is immoral or dishonorable.

Venue a particular geographical location (county, city) in which a court with jurisdiction may hear and determine a case (see **Change of Venue**).

Verdict the decision of the petit jury on the matter submitted to them in trial.

Vicarious Liability a situation in a principle–agent, master–servant, or employer–employee relationship where the superior being may have to answer for the wrongdoing of the agent, servant, or employee pursuant to the *doctrine of respondeat superior.*

Void having no legal effect and not binding on anyone.

Waive(r) to completely give up a right, privilege, or claim.

Warranty an assurance by a seller that goods or products are as represented, or will be as promised. Warranties may be expressed (stated) or implied.

Warranty of Fitness assertion that a good or product is suitable for a particular purpose of a buyer (implied warranty).

Witness a person who has knowledge of a fact or an event and is called to testify.

Writ any written order of a court.

Glossary of Drug Regulatory Terms

Abbreviated New Drug Application, or ANDA a simplified submission permitted for a duplicate of an already approved drug. ANDAs are for products with the same or very closely related active ingredients, dosage form, strength, administrative route, use, and labeling as a product that has already been shown to be safe and effective. An ANDA includes all the information on chemistry and manufacturing controls found in a new drug application (NDA), but does not have to include data from studies in animals and humans. It must, however, contain evidence that the duplicate drug is bioequivalent (see "Bioequivalence") to the previously approved drug.

Action Letter an official communication from FDA to an NDA sponsor that informs of a decision by the agency, e.g., application approved, approvable, or not approvable.

Actual Yield is the quantity that is actually produced at any appropriate phase of manufacture, processing, or packing of a particular drug product.

21 CFR 210.3(a)(18)

Acceptance Criteria the product specifications and acceptance/rejection criteria, such as acceptable quality level and unacceptable quality level, with an associated sampling plan, that are necessary for making a decision to accept or reject a lot or batch (or any other convenient subgroups of manufactured units.)

21 CFR 210.3(a)(20)

Active Ingredient any component that is intended to furnish pharmacological activity or other direct effect in the diagnosis, cure, mitigation, treatment, or prevention of disease, or to affect the structure or any function of the body of man or other animals. The term includes those components that may undergo chemical change in the manufacture of the drug product and be present in the drug product in a modified form intended to furnish the specified activity or effect.

21 CFR 210.3(a)(7)

Adequate Directions for Use directions under which the layman can use a drug safely and for the purposes for which it is intended.

21 CFR 201.5

Administer means the direct application of a drug to the body of a patient or research subject by injection, inhalation, ingestion, or any other means.

Adverse Drug Reaction (Significant) means any drug-related incident that results in serious harm, injury, or death to the patient.

Advisory Committee a panel of outside experts convened periodically to advise FDA on safety and efficacy issues about drugs and other FDA-regulated products. FDA isn't bound to take committee recommendations, but usually does.

Approved Drug a drug product approved by the FDA for marketing in the United States.

Approvable Letter a written communication to an applicant from FDA stating that the agency will approve the application if specific additional information or material is submitted or conditions are met. An approvable letter does not constitute approval of any part of a new drug application (NDA) and does not permit marketing of the drug that is the subject of the application.

21 CFR 314.3(b)

Approval Letter a written communication to an applicant from FDA approving a new drug application (NDA). An approval letter permits marketing of the drug product that is the subject of the application.

21 CFR 314.3(b)

Batch a specific quantity of a drug or other material that is intended to have uniform character and quality, within specified limits, and is produced according to a single manufacturing order during the same cycle of manufacture.

21 CFR 210.3(b)(2)

Bioavailability the rate and extent to which the active drug ingredient or therapeutic moiety is absorbed from a drug product and becomes available at the site of drug action.

21 CFR 320.1(a)

Bioequivalence Requirement a requirement imposed by the FDA for in vitro and/or in vitro testing of specified drug products which must be satisfied as a condition of marketing.

21 CFR 320.1(f)

Bioequivalent Drug Products pharmaceutical equivalents or pharmaceutical alternatives whose rate and extent of absorption do not show a significant difference when administered at the same molar dose of the therapeutic moiety under simnilar experimental conditions, either single dose or multiple dose. Some pharmaceutical equivalents or pharmaceutical alternatives may be equivalent in the extent of their rate of absorption and yet may be considered bioequivalent because such differences in rate of absorption are intentional and are reflected in the labeling, are not essential to the attainment of effective body concentrations on chronic use, or are considered medically insignificant for the particular drug product studied.

21 CFR 320.1(e)

Biologics any virus, therapeutic serum, toxin, antitoxin, vaccine, blood, blood component or derivative, allergenic product, or analogous product . . . applicable to the prevention, treatment, or cure of diseases or injuries to man. [Human biological drug products are licensed by the FDA Center for Biologic Evaluation and Research (FDA-CBER)].

Bulk Drug Substance any substance that is represented for use in a drug and that, when used in the manufacturing, processing, or packaging of a drug, becomes an active ingredient or a finished dosage form of the drug, but the term does not include intermediates used in the synthesis of such substances.

21 CRF 207.3(a)(4)

Clinical Protocol is a critical document in the evaluation of a study, shaping both the conduct of the trial and the ultimate analyses. It sets out the objectives of the study in clinical terms and then relates these objectives to the statistical hypotheses that are tested. It describes critical features of the study's design and execution, such as the experimental design (single-investigator or multi-investigator; parallel or crossover), patient selection and exclusion criteria, the choice of control group(s), the method for treatment allocation, the level and method of blinding, the sample size, the efficacy and safety variables to be measured, and planned intermit analyses of the data, the procedures for early termination of study (if any), the roles and responsibilities of any data-monitoring board, and the proposed statistical methods. In defining, ahead of time, specific subgroups for separate analysis, and particular variables that are considered primary end-points, the protocol defines, and limits, the hypotheses the study is able to test.

Clinical Studies Clinical, or human, studies aim to distinguish a drug's effect from other influences—for example, a spontaneous change in disease progression or in the effect of a placebo (an inactive substance that looks like the test drug). Such studies conducted in the United States must be under an approved IND, under the guidance of an institutional review board, and in accord with FDA rules on human studies and informed consent of participants.

Cohort Study a study in which a defined group of patients (the cohort) is followed for a specific period of time.

Color Additive any material, not exempted under section 201(t) of the (Federal Food, Drug, and Cosmetic) Act that is a dye, pigment, or other substance made by a process of synthesis or similar article, or extracted, isolated, or otherwise derived, with or without intermediate or final change of identity, from a vegetable, animal, mineral, or other source and that, when added or applied to a food, drug, or cosmetic or to the human body or any part thereof, is capable (alone or through reaction with another substance) of imparting a color thereto. Substances capable of imparting a color to a container for foods, drugs, or cosmetics are not color additives unless the customary or reasonable foreseeable handling or use of the container may reasonably be expected to result in the transmittal of the color to the contents of the package or any part thereof. Food ingredients such as cherries, green or red peppers, chocolate, and orange juice which contribute their own natural color when mixed with other foods are not regarded as "color additives"; but where a food substance such as beet juice is deliberately used as a color, as in pink lemonade, it is a "color additive." Food ingredients as authorized by a definitions and standard of identity prescribed by regulations pursuant to section 401 of the Act are "color additives," where the ingredients are specifically designed in the definitions and standards of identity as permitted for use for coloring purposes. An ingredient of an animal feed whose intended function is to impart, through the biological processes of the animal, a color to the meat, milk, or eggs of the animal is a color additive and is not exempt from the requirements of the statute. This definition shall apply whether or not such ingredient has nutritive or other functions in addition to the property of imparting color. An ingested drug the intended function of which is to impart color to the human body is a "color additive."

21 CFR 70.3(f)

Commercial distribution any distribution of a human drug except for investigational use and any distribution of an animal drug or an animal feed bearing or containing an animal drug for non-investigational uses, but the term does not include internal or interplant transfer of a bulk drug substance between registered domestic establishments within the same parent, subsidiary, and/or affiliate company.

21 CFR 207.3(a)(5)

Compendium the official *United States Pharmacopeia,* official *Homeopathic Pharmacopeia of the United States,* official *National Formulary,* or any supplement to any of them.

21 U.S.C. 321(j)

Compounding means the preparation, mixing, assembling, packaging, or labeling of a drug or device (1) as the result of a practitioner's prescription drug order or initiative based on the pharmacist-patient-prescriber relationship or (2) for the purpose of or as an incident to research, teaching, or chemical analysis and not for sale or dispensing. Compounding also includes the preparation of drugs or devices in anticipation of prescription drug orders based on routine, regularly observed prescribing patterns.

Contract Research Organization a person that assumes, as independent contractor with the sponsor, one or more of the obligations, e.g., design of a protocol, selection or monitoring of investigations, evaluation or reports, and preparation of materials to be submitted to the Food and Drug Administration.

21 CFR 312.3(b)

Control number also lot number of batch number; any distinctive combination of alphabet characters, numerals or symbols which can provide a history of the manufacture, processing, packaging, distribution, or warehousing of a specific quantity (batch, lot) of a regulated product, e.g., drug, medical device.

Controls similar test specimens that are subjected to as nearly as possible the same conditions as the test object; provides critical scientific comparison against observations made on test object.

Correction repair, modification, adjustment, relabeling, destruction, or inspection (including patient monitoring) of a product under FDA's jurisdiction (drug, cosmetic, device, food) without its physical removal to some other location.

21 CFR 7.3(h)

Cosmeceutical Although the Food, Drug, and Cosmetic Act does not recognize the term "cosmeceutical," the cosmetic industry has begun to use this word to refer to cosmetic products that have drug-like benefits. The Food, Drug, and Cosmetic Act defines drugs as those products that cure, treat, mitigate or prevent disease or that affect the structure or function of the human body. While drugs are subject to an intensive review and approval process by FDA, cosmetics are not approved by FDA prior to sale. If a product has drug properties, it must be approved as a drug.

Cosmetic (1) articles intended to be rubbed, poured, sprinkled, or sprayed on, introduced into, or otherwise applied to the human body or any part thereof for cleansing, beautifying, promoting attractiveness, or altering the appearance, and (2) articles intended for use as a component of any such articles; except that such term shall not include soap.

21 U.S.C. 321(i)

Counterfeit Drug a drug which, or the container or labeling, of which, without authorization, bears the trademark, trade name, identifying mark, imprint, or device, or any likeness thereof, of a drug manufacturer, processor, packer, or distributor other than the person who in fact manufactured, processed, packed, or distributed such drug and which thereby falsely purports or is represented to be the product of, or to have been packed or distributed by, such other drug manufacturer, processor, packer, or distributor.

21 U.S.C. 321(g)(2)

Dating Period the period beyond which the product cannot be expected beyond reasonable doubt to yield its specific results.

21 CFR 600.3(1)

Debarment applies to a person who is prohibited from "providing services in any capacity to a person that has an approved or pending drug product application." Any firm with an approved or pending product application who uses the services of a debarred person is subject to civil money penalties. In addition, the FDA will not accept or review any approved or pending drug product application submitted by or with the help of a debarred individual.

FDCA 306(a)(2)

Designer Drug a substance other than a controlled dangerous substance that has a chemical structure substantially similar to that of a controlled dangerous substance or that was specifically designed to produce an effect substantially similar to that of a controlled dangerous substance.

Designer drugs are forms of synthetic or man-made narcotics that give the user the same "high" as the more traditional scheduled substances but which, until 1986, were not illegal because their structure had been chemically altered to avoid the proscription of the definition of controlled dangerous substances.

Detoxification Treatment the dispensing of a narcotic drug in decreasing doses to an individual to alleviate adverse physiological or psychological effects incident to withdrawal from the continuous or sustained use of a narcotic drug and as a method of bringing the individual to a narcotic drug-free state within such period. There are two types of detoxification treatment: short-term detoxification treatment and long-term detoxification treatment:
(1) *Short-term detoxification treatment* is for a period not in excess of 30 days.
(2) *Long-term detoxification treatment* is for a period more than 30 days but not in excess of 180 days.

21 CFR 291.505(a)(1)

Device generally, means an instrument, apparatus, implement, machine, contrivance, implant, in vitro reagent, or other similar or related article, including any component, part, or accessory, which is: (1) recognized in the official *National Formulary*, or the *United States Pharmacopeia*, or any supplement to them, (2) intended for use in the diagnosis of disease or other conditions, or in the cure, mitigation, treatment, or prevention of disease, in man or other animals, or (3) intended to affect the structure or any function of the body of man or other animals, and which does not achieve any of its principal intended purposes through chemical action within or on the body of man or other animals and which is not dependent upon being metabolized for the achievement of any of its principal intended purposes.

21. U.S.C. 321(h)

Dietary Supplement a product, other than tobacco, *intended to supplement the diet* that bears or contains one or more of the following dietary ingredients: (a) a vitamin, (b) a mineral, (c) an herb or other botanical, (d) an amino acid, (e) a dietary substance for use by man to supplement the diet by *increasing the total dietary intake*, or (f) a concentrate, metabolite, constituent, extract, or combination of the above. A dietary supplement may not be represented for use as a conventional food or as a sole item of meal or diet. Furthermore, a dietary supplement must be intended *to supplement the diet*. Consequently, topical products such as creams and ointments, as well as injectables, are unlikely to come within the definition of "dietary supplement." A dietary supplement may come in a variety of dosage forms. The law specifically authorizes galenical (dosage) forms such as tablets, capsules, powders, softgels, gelcaps and liquids. A dietary supplement may also be marketed in other forms as long as the supplement does not simulate and is not represented as a conventional food. For example, herbs and botanicals marketed in their natural form (seeds, flowers, etc.) are within the dietary supplement definition. The law also requires, for the first time, that a dietary supplement label must explicitly state that the product is a "dietary supplement." Characterization of a product as a dietary supplement does not immunize a product from FDA's drug regulations. *A single product is capable of being both a dietary supplement and a drug, largely depending upon the claims made for the product.* However, the law limits the ability to take an article that was approved by the FDA as a drug (including antibiotics and biologics) and thereafter market the article as a dietary supplement.

21 U.S.C. 321

District Director the director of the district of the Food and Drug Administration having jurisdiction over the port of entry through which an article is imported or offered for import, or such officer of the district as he may designate to act in his behalf in administering and enforcing the provisions of Section 801(a), (b), and (c).

21 CFR 1.83(b)

Drug (a) articles recognized in the official *United States Pharmacopeia,* official *Homeopathic Pharmacopeia of the United States,* or official *National Formulary,* or any supplement to any of them; and (b) articles intended for use in the diagnosis, cure, mitigation, treatment, or prevention of disease in man or other animals; and (c) articles (other than food) intended to affect the structure or any function of the body of man or other animals; and (d) articles intended for use as a component of any articles specified in clause (a), (b), or (c); but does not include devices or their components, parts, or accessories.

21 U.S.C. 321(g)(1)

Drug Product a finished form, for example, tablet, capsule solution, etc., that contains an active drug ingredient generally, but not necessarily, in association with inactive ingredients. The term also includes a finished dosage form that does not contain an active ingredient but is intended to be used as a placebo.

21 CFR 210.3(a)(4)

Drug Product Salvaging the act of segregating drug products that may have been subjected to improper storage conditions, such as extremes in temperature, humidity, smoke, fumes, pressure, age, or radiation, for the purpose of returning some or all of the products to the marketplace.

21 CFR 207.3(a)(6)

Drug Substance an active ingredient that is intended to furnish pharmacological activity or other direct effect in the diagnosis, cure, mitigation, treatment, or prevention of disease or to affect the structure of any function of the human body, but does not include intermediates used in the synthesis of such ingredient.

21 CFR 314.3(b)

Emergency Situation for the purpose of authorizing an oral prescription of a controlled substance listed in Schedule II of the Federal Controlled Substances Act, the term "emergency situation" means those situations in which the prescribing practitioner determines: (a) that immediate administration of the controlled substance is necessary, for proper treatment of the intended ultimate user; and (b) that no appropriate alternative treatment is available, including administration of a drug which is not a controlled substance under Schedule II of the Act, and (c) that it is not reasonably possible for the prescribing practitioner to provide a written prescription to be presented to the person dispensing the substance, prior to the dispensing.

21 CFR 290.10

Establishment a place of business under one management at one general physical location. The term includes, among others, independent laboratories that engage in control activities for a registered drug establishment (e.g., "consulting" laboratories), manufacturers of medicated feeds and of vitamin products that are drugs in accordance with section 201(g) of the act, human blood donor centers, and animal facilities used for the production or control testing of licensed biologicals, and establishments engaged in drug product salvaging.

21 CFR 207.3(a)(7)

Effectiveness Checks the purpose of effectiveness checks is to verify that all consignees at the recall depth specified by the strategy have received notification about the recall and have taken appropriate action. The method for contacting consignees may be accomplished by personal visits, telephone calls, letters, or a combination thereof. (A guide entitled "Methods for Conducting Recall Effectiveness Checks" that describes the use of these different methods is available upon request from the Dockets Management Branch (HFA-305), Food and Drug Administration, Room-4-62, 5600 Fishers Lane, Rockville, MD 20857.) The recalling firm will ordinarily be responsible for conducting effectiveness checks, but the Food and Drug Administration will assist in this task where necessary and appropriate. The recall strategy will specify the method(s) to be used for and the level of effectiveness checks that will be conducted.

21 CFR 7.42(b)(3)

Ex Parte Communication is an oral or written communication not on the public record for which reasonable prior notice to all parties is not given, but does not include requests for status reports on a matter.

21 CFR 10.3(a)

Expiration Date the date placed on the immediate container label of a drug product that designates the date through which the product is expected to remain within specifications. If the expiration date includes only a month and year, it is expected that the product will meet specifications through the last day of the month.

Expiration Dating Period the interval that a drug product is expected to remain within the approved specifications after manufacture. The expiration dating period is used to establish the expiration date of individual batches. It may be extended in an annual report only if the criteria set forth in the approved stability study protocol are met in obtaining the supporting data. Otherwise, a supplement requiring FDA approval will be necessary before the change is made.

21 CFR 314.70(b)(2)(ix)

Feminine Deodorant Spray any spray deodorant product whose labeling represents or suggests that the product is for use in the female genital area or for use all over the body.

21 CFR 740.12(a)

Fragrance any natural or synthetic substance or substances used solely to impart an odor to a cosmetic product.

21 CFR 700.3(d)

Generic Substitution the act of dispensing a different brand or non-brand drug product instead of the drug product prescribed, i.e., a pharmaceutical equivalent distributed by a different company. For example, Rufen brand of ibuprofen instead of Motrin brand of ibuprofen; generic ampicillin for Polycillin.

Guidelines establishes principles or practices of general applicability and do not include decisions or advice on particular situations. A guideline represents the formal position of FDA on a matter and obligates the agency to follow it until it is amended or revoked. Guidelines relate to performance characteristics, preclinical and clinical test procedures, manufacturing practices, product manufacturing practices, product standards, scientific protocols, compliance criteria, ingredient specifications, labeling, or other technical or policy criteria. Guidelines state procedures or standards of general applicability that are *not* legal requirements but are acceptable to FDA for a subject matter which falls within the laws administered by the Commissioner of FDA.

21 CFR 10.90

Human Subject an individual who is or becomes a participant in research, either as a recipient of the test article or as a control. A subject may be either a healthy human or a patient.

21 CFR 50.3(g)

Human Drug Product the active ingredient of a new drug, antibiotic drug, or human biologic product (as those terms are used in the FDC Act and the Public Health Service Act), including any salt or ester of the active ingredient, as a single entity or in combination with another active ingredient.

21 CFR 60.3(a)(10)

Immediate Container the bottle, vial, ampule, tube, unit or other receptacle which contains the product.

21 CFR 600.3(bb)

Imminent Hazard within the meaning of the Federal Food, Drug, and Cosmetic Act, an imminent hazard to the public health is considered to exist when the evidence is sufficient to show that a product or practice, posing a sig- nificant threat to health, creates a public health situation (1) that should be corrected immediately to prevent injury and (2) that should not be permitted to continue while a hearing or other formal proceeding is being held. The imminent hazard may be declared at any point in the chain of events which may ultimately result in harm to the public health. The occur-

rence of the final anticipated injury is not essential to establish that an "imminent hazard" of such occurrence exists.

21 CFR 2.5(a)

Inactive Ingredient any component other than an "active ingredient."

21 CFR 210.3(a)(8)

Informed Consent knowledgeable, written consent by a human being subject to medical experiments; written documentation that ensures that clinical investigations regulated under 21 *CFR* 50 by the Food and Drug Administration pursuant to the Food, Drug, and Cosmetic Act conform to ethical standards and the rights and safety of human participants in clinical research are protected in support of applications for permission to market regulated products in the United States.

In-Process Material any material fabricated, compounded, blended, or derived by chemical reaction that is produced for, and used in, the preparation of the drug product.

21 CFR 210.3(a)(9)

Institutional Review Board institutional review committee; means any board, committee, or other group formally designated by an institution to review biomedical research involving humans as subjects, to approve the initiation of and conduct periodic review of such research. The purpose of such review is to assure the protection of the rights and welfare of the human subjects.

21 CFR 56.102(g)

Investigational New Drug a new drug, or biological drug that is used in a clinical investigation. The term also includes a biological product that is used *in vitro* for diagnostic purposes. The terms "investigational drug" and "investigational new drug" are synonymous.

21 CFR 312.3(b)

Investigator an individual who actually conducts a clinical investigation, i.e., under whose immediate direction the drug is administered or dispensed to a subject. In the event an investigation is conducted by a team of individuals, the investigator is the responsible leader of the team. Subinvestigator includes any other individual member of that team.

21 CFR 312.3(b)

Label any display of written, printed, or graphic matter on the immediate container of any article, or any such matter

How Experimental Drugs Are Tested in Humans			
	Number of Patients	Length	Purpose	Percent of Drugs Successfully Completing*
Phase 1	20–100	Several months	Mainly safety	70 percent
Phase 2	100–200	Several months to 2 years	Some short-term safety, but mainly effectiveness	33 percent
Phase 3	Several hundred to several thousand	1–4	Safety, effectiveness, dosage	25–30 percent

*For example, of 100 drugs for which investigational new drug applications are submitted to FDA, about 70 will successfully complete phase 1 trials and go on to phase 2; about 33 will complete phase 2 and go to phase 3; 25 to 30 will clear phase 3 (and, on average, about 20 of the original 100 will ultimately be approved for marketing).

affixed to or appearing upon a package containing any consumer commodity.

21 CFR 1.3(b)

Labeling includes all written, printed, or graphic matter accompanying an article at any time while such article is in interstate commerce or held for sale after shipment or delivery in or interstate commerce, e.g., package insert.

21 CFR 1.3(a)

Lot a batch, or a specific identified portion of a batch having uniform character and quality within specified limits; or, in the case of a drug product produced by continuous process, it is a specific identified amount produced in a unit of time or quantity in a manner that assures its having uniform character and quality within specified limits.

21 CFR 210.3(a)(10)

Lot Number a distinctive combination of symbols, alphabet characters or numerals, or any combination of them which identifies a specific quantity of an item that is intended to have uniform character and quality, within specified limits, and is produced according to a single manufacturing order during the same cycle of manufacture. This identifying mark on the label should be able to yield the manufacturing history of the package/product. An incorrect lot number may be regarded as causing the product to be misbranded; sometimes referred to as "batch number" or "quality control number."

21 CFR 201.18
21 CFR 210.3(a)(10)

Maintenance Treatment the dispensing of a narcotic drug in the treatment of an individual for dependence on heroin or other morphine-like drug.

21 CFR 291.505(a)(2)

Manufacturing or *processing* means the "manufacture, preparation, propagation, compounding, or processing of a drug or drugs" as used in section 510 of the (FDC) Act and in the making by chemical, physical, biological, or other procedures of any articles that meet the definition of drugs in section 201(g) of the Act. The term includes manipulation, sampling, testing, or control procedures applied to the final product or to any part of the process. The term also includes repackaging or otherwise changing the container, wrapper, or labeling of any drug package to further the distribution of the drug from the original place of manufacture to the person who makes final delivery or sale to the ultimate consumer.

21 CFR 207.3(a)(8)

Marketing Application an application for a new drug submitted under section 505(b) of the FDC Act, a request to provide for certification of an antibiotic submitted under section 507 of the Act, or a product license application for biological product submitted under the Public Health Service Act.

21 CFR 312.3(b)

Market Withdrawal a firm's removal or correction of a distributed product which involves a minor violation that would not be subjected to legal action by the Food and Drug Administration or which involves no violation, e.g., normal stock rotation practices, routine equipment adjustments and repairs, etc.

21 CFR 7.3(i)

Multicenter Study a single study involving several centers (or clinical investigators) where the data collected from these centers are intended to be analyzed as a whole (as opposed to a post-hoc decision to combine data or results from separate studies).

National Formulary abbreviated as *NF* or *N.F.* The *National Formulary* was first published in 1888 by the American Pharmaceutical Association and was designated an official compendium by the Federal Pure Food and Drugs Act of 1906 and later by the 1938 FD&C Act.

The *NF* has been published with the *United States Pharmacopeia* in a single volume since 1980 as a consequence of the acquisition, by the United States Pharmaceutical Convention, Inc., of the *NF* in 1975. However, the *USP* and the *NF* have continued as two distinct official compendia, with the NF being limited to standards for pharmaceutical ingredients.

Narcotic Dependent an individual who physiologically needs heroin or a morphine-like drug to prevent the onset of signs of withdrawal.

21 CFR.505(a)(5)

Narcotic Treatment Program an organization (or a person, including a private physician) that administrators or dispenses a narcotic drug to a narcotic addict for maintenance or detoxification treatment, provides, when appropriate or necessary, a comprehensive range of medical and rehabilitative services, is approved by the State authority and the Food and Drug Administration, and that is registered with the Drug Enforcement Administration to use a narcotic drug for the treatment of narcotic addiction.

21 CFR 291.505(a)(6)

National Drug Code a ten numeral code. The first five numerals identify the manufacturer or distributor; the last five numerals identify the drug product, the trade package size and type. The segment that identifies the manufacturer or distributor is referred to as the "labeler code"; the segment that identifies the product is known as the "product code"; and the segment that identifies the trade package size and type is called the "package code."

21 CFR 208.35(b)(i)
and (ii)

New Drug (1) any drug (except a new animal drug or an animal feed bearing or containing a new animal drug) the composition of which is such that such drug is not generally recognized, among experts qualified by scientific training and experience to evaluate the safety and effectiveness of drugs, as safe and effective for use under the conditions prescribed, recommended, or suggested in the labeling thereof, except that such a drug not so recognized shall not be deemed to be a "new drug" if at any time prior to the enactment of this (FDC) Act it was subject to the Food and Drugs Act of June 30, 1906, as amended, and if at such time its labeling contained the same representations concerning the conditions of its use; or (2) any drug (except a new animal drug or animal feed bearing or containing a new animal drug) the composition of which is such that such drug, as a result of investigations to determine its safety and effectiveness for use under such conditions, has become so recognized, but which has not, otherwise than in such investigations, been used to a material extent or for a material time under such conditions.

21 U.S.C. 321(p)

Non-Prescription Drug means a drug that may be sold without a prescription, which is labeled for use by the consumer in accordance with the requirements of the statutes and rules of state and/or the federal government; commonly referred to as either OTC or over-the-counter drug.

Not Approvable Letter a written communication to an applicant from FDA stating that the agency does not consider the new drug application (NDA) approvable because one or more deficiencies in the application preclude the agency from approving it.

21 CFR 314.3(b)

Package any container or wrapping in which any food, drug, device or cosmetic is enclosed for use in the delivery or display of such commodities to retail purchasers.

21 CFR 1.20

Patient Counseling the effective oral communication by the pharmacist of information to the patient or care giver in order to improve therapy by ensuring proper use of drugs and devices.

Percentage of Theoretical Yield the ratio of the actual yield (at any appropriate phase of manufacture, processing, or packing of a particular drug product) to the theoretical yield (at the same phase), stated as a percentage.

21 CFR 210.3(a)(9)

Personal Identifiers individual names, identifying numbers, symbols, or other identifying designations assigned to individuals. Personal identifiers does not include names numbers, symbols, or other identifying designations that identify products, establishments, or actions.

21 CFR 21.3(d)

Pharmacopeial Forum the *USP* journal of drug standards development and official compendia revision. It is the working document of the USP Committee of Revision, the major portion of which presents proposals for revising standards of the *USP* and *NF.*

Pharmaceutical Alternates drug products which are administered by the same route and contain the identical therapeutic moiety and strength but differ in the salt, ester, or dosage form.

21 CFR 320.1(d)

Pharmaceutical Alternatives drug products that contain the identical therapeutic moiety, or its precursor, but not necessarily in the same amount or dosage form or as the same salt or ester. Each such drug product individually meets either the identical or its own respective compendial or other application standard of identity, strength, quality, and purity, including potency and, where applicable, content uniformity, disintegration times and/or dissolution rates.

21 CFR 320.1(c)

Pharmaceutical Equivalents drug products that contain identical amounts of the identical active drug ingredient, i.e., the same salt or ester of the same therapeutic moiety, in identical dosage forms, but not necessarily containing the same inactive ingredients, and that meet the identical compendial or other applicable standard of identity, strength, quality, and purity, including potency and, where applicable, content uniformity, disintegration times and/or dissolution rates.

21 CFR 320.1(c)

Pharmaceutical Substitution the act of dispensing a pharmaceutical alternate for the drug product prescribed. For example, codeine sulfate instead of codeine phosphate or tetracycline hydrochloride instead of tetracycline phosphate complex; propoxyphene hydrochloride instead of propoxyphene napsylate or erythromycin ethylsuccinate instead of erythromycin base; ampicillin suspension instead of ampicillin capsule.

Pharmacology is the science that pertains to the effect of drugs on living organisms.

Phase 1 includes the initial introduction of an investigational new drug into humans. Phase 1 studies are typically closely monitored and may be conducted in patients or healthy volunteer subjects. These studies are designed to determine the metabolism and pharmacological actions of the drug in humans, the side effects associated with increasing doses, and, if possible, to gain early evidence on effectiveness. During Phase 1, sufficient information about the drug's pharmacokinetics and pharmacological effects should be obtained to permit the design of well-controlled, scientifically valid, Phase 2 studies. The total number of subjects and patients included in Phase 1 studies varies with the drug, but is generally in the range of 20 to 100. Phase I studies also include studies of drug metabolism, structure-activity relationships, and mechanism of action in humans, as well as studies in which investigational drugs are used as research tools to explore biological phenomena or the disease process.

Phase 2 includes the controlled clinical studies conducted to evaluate the effectiveness of the drug for a particular indication or indications in patients with the disease or medical condition under study and to determine the common short-term adverse effects and risks associated with the drug. Phase 2 studies are typically well controlled, closely monitored, and conducted in a relatively small number of patients, usually involving no more than 100–200 subjects. Long-term tests for safety in animals usually continue during Phase 2.

Phase 3 studies are expanded controlled and uncontrolled trials. They are performed after preliminary evidence suggesting effectiveness of the drug has been obtained, and are intended to gather the additional information about effectiveness and safety that is needed to evaluate the overall benefit-risk relationship of the drug and to provide an adequate basis for physician labeling. Phase 3 studies usually include from several hundred to several thousand subjects.

Postmarketing Surveillance Postmarketing drug surveillance is the mechanism used to discover both the beneficial and the harmful effects of drugs used under conditions different from those of the premarket tests.

The most common form of postmarketing surveillance is the publication of observations or anecdotal reports by physicians, pharmacists, nurses or other health professionals. Alert clinicians are the most important and comprehensive source of new information about observed events in people for whom specific products are prescribed or made available.

Alert clinicians also play a central role in the most common of the government-sponsored methods of post-marketing surveillance—the voluntary adverse drug reaction (ADR) reporting system. To be effective this system requires that health professionals, pharmaceutical manufacturers and consumers of medicines report unexpected events associated with the use of the medicines to a national agency specifically established to receive, process, analyze and communicate such reports.

Potency interpreted to mean the specific ability or capacity of the product, as indicated by appropriate laboratory tests or by adequately controlled clinical dates obtained through the administration of the product in the manner intended, to effect a given result. (See *Strength*).

21 CFR 600.3(s)

Practice of Pharmacy means the interpretation, evaluation, and dispensing of prescription drug orders in the patient's best interest; participation in drug and medical device selection, drug administration, prospective drug reviews, and drug or drug-related research; patient counseling, acts or services necessary to provide pharmaceutical care, and the responsibility for compounding and labeling of drugs and medical devices (except labeling by a manufacturer, repackager, or distributor of non-prescription drugs and commercially packaged legend drugs and devices), proper and safe storage of drugs and devices and maintenance of proper records for them.

Privacy Act Record System consists of records about individuals under the control of the Food and Drug Administration from which information is retrieved by individual names or other personal identifiers. The term includes such a system of records whether subject to a notice published by the Food and Drug Administration, the Department (of Health and Human Services), or another agency. Where records are retrieved only by personal identifiers other than individual names, a system of records is not a Privacy Act Record System if the Food and Drug Administration cannot, by reference to information under its control, or by reference to records of contractors that are subject to this part under Section 21.30, ascertain the identity of individuals who are the subjects of the records.

21 CFR 21.3(c)

Processing or *manufacturing*, means the "manufacture, preparation, propagation, compounding, or processing of a drug or drugs" as used in section 510 of the (FDC) Act and is the making by chemical, physical, biological, or other procedures of any articles that meet the definition of drugs in section 201(g) of the act. The term includes manipulation, sampling, testing, or control procedures applied to the final product or to any part of the process. The term also includes repackaging or otherwise changing the container, wrapper, or labeling of any drug package to further the distribution of the drug from the original place of manufacture to the person who makes final delivery or sale to the ultimate consumer.

21 CFR 207.3(a)(8)

Proprietary Ingredient any product ingredient whose name, composition, or manufacturing process is protected from competition by secrecy, patent, or copyright.

21 CFR 700.3(f)

Public Advisory Committee or Advisory Committee any committee, board, commission, council, conference, panel, task force, or other similar group, or any subcommittee or other subgroup of an advisory committee that is not composed wholly of full-time employees of the Federal Government and is established or utilized by the Food and Drug Administration to obtain advice or recommendations.

21 CFR 10.3(a)

Public Warning the purpose of a public warning is to alert the public that a product being recalled presents a serious hazard to health. It is reserved for urgent situations where other means for preventing use of the recalled product ap- pear inadequate. The Food and Drug Administration in consultation with the recalling firm will ordinarily issue such publicity. The recalling firm that decides to issue its own public warning is requested to submit its proposed public warning and plan for distribution of the warning for review and comment by the Food and Drug Administration. The recall strategy will specify whether a public warning is needed and whether it will issue as: (i) General public warning through the general news media, either national or local as appropriate, or (ii) public warning through specialized news media, e.g., professional or trade press, or to specific segments of the population such as physicians, hospitals, etc.

CFR 7.42(b)(2)

Quality Assurance the continual verification of criteria used in the manufacturing process. It includes, but is not limited to, monitoring, reviewing, documenting, and validating of the process, from raw materials to finished dosage form.

Quality Control the continual process which measures (monitors) quality of a product and compares it with a standard.

Radioactive Drug any substance defined as a drug in section 201(g)(1) of the Federal Food, Drug and Cosmetic Act which exhibits spontaneous disintegration of unstable nuclei with the emission of nuclear particles or photons and includes any nonradioactive reagent kit or nuclide generator which is intended to be used in the preparation of any such substance but does not include drugs such as carbon-containing compounds or potassium-containing salts which contain trace quantities of naturally occurring radionuclides. The term "radioactive drug" includes a "radioactive biological product" as defined in 600.3(ee) of 21 CFR.

Raw Data a researcher's records of patients, such as patient charts, hospital records, X-rays, and attending physician's notes. They may or may not accompany an NDA, but must be retained in the researcher's file if FDA requests their submission.

"Real Life" Usage patterns of drug release use outside of controlled clinical studies, including the physician developed variations in dosage, delivery, and indications that do not conform to the package insert recommendations.

Recall a firm's removal or correction of a marketed product (drug, cosmetic, device, food) that the Food and Drug Administration considers to be in violation of the laws it administers and against which the agency would initiate legal action, e.g., seizure. "Recall" does not include a market withdrawal or a stock recovery.

21 CFR 7.3(g)

Recall Classification the numerical designation, i.e., I, II, or III, assigned by the Food and Drug Administration to a particular product recall to indicate the relative degree of health hazard presented by the product being recalled. *Class I* is a situation in which there is a reasonable probability that the use of, or exposure to, a violative product will cause serious adverse health consequences or death. *Class II* is a situation in which use of, or exposure to, a violative product may cause temporary or medically reversible adverse health consequences or where probability of serious health consequences is remote. *Class III* is a situation in which use of, or exposure to, a violative product is not likely to cause adverse health consequences.

21 CFR 7.3(m) and (n)

Recalling Firm the firm that initiates a recall or a requested recall by the Food and Drug Administration; the firm that has primary responsibility for the manufacture and marketing of the product to be recalled.

21 CFR 7.3(i)

Recall Strategy a planned specific course of action to be taken in conducting a specific recall of a drug, cosmetic, device or food product, which addresses the depth of recall, need for public warnings, and extent of effectiveness checks for the recall.

21 CFR 7.3(l)

Reminder Advertisement calls attention to the name of the drug product but does not include indications or dosage recommendations. These advertisements contain only the proprietary name of the drug product, if any; the established name of each active ingredient in the drug product; and, optionally, information relating to quantitative ingredient statements, dosage form, quantity of package contents, price, the name and address of the manufacturer, packer, or distributor or other written, printed, or graphic matter containing no representation or suggestion relating to the advertised drug product.

21 CFR 202.1(e)(2)(i)

Reportable Experience an experience involving any allergic reaction, or other bodily injury, alleged to be the result of the use of a cosmetic product under the conditions of use prescribed in the labeling of the product, under such conditions of use as are customary or reasonably foreseeable for the product or under conditions of misuse, that has been reported to the manufacturer, packer, or distributor of the product by the affected person or any other person having factual knowledge of the incident other than an alleged experience which has been determined to be unfounded or spurious when evaluated by a filed screening procedure.

21 CFR 700.3(q)

Representative Sample a sample that consists of a number of units that are drawn based on rational criteria such as random sampling and intended to assure that the sample accurately portrays the material being sampled.

21 CFR 210.3(a)(21)

Representative Sampling of Advertisements typical advertising material (excluding labeling) that gives a balanced picture of the promotional claims used for the drug, e.g., if more than one medical journal advertisement is used but the promotional content is essentially identical.

21 CFR 207.3(a)(a)

Respondent a person named in a notice who presents views concerning an alleged violation either in person, by designated representative, or in writing.

21 CFR 7.3(c)

Safe/Safety a reasonable certainty in the minds of competent scientists that the substance is not harmful under the intended conditions of use. Safety may be determined by scientific procedures or by general recognition of safety. It is impossible in the present state of scientific knowledge to establish with complete certainty the absolute harmlessness of the use of any substance. Also, the relative freedom from harmful effect to persons affected, directly or indirectly, by a product when prudently administered, taking into consideration the character of the product in relation to the condition of the recipient at the time.

21 CFR 170.3(i)

Safety Update Reports that an NDA sponsor must submit to FDA pertaining to any new safety information that may affect the draft labeling statements about contraindications, warnings, precautions, and adverse reactions. Safety update reports are required four months after the application is submitted, after the application receives an approvable letter, and other times when FDA requests.

Sample a unit of a prescription drug which is not intended to be sold and is intended to promote the sale of the drug (see **Starter Packs**).

Serious Adverse Experience any experience that suggests a significant hazard, contraindication, side effect, or precaution. With respect to human clinical experience, a serious adverse drug experience includes an experience that is fatal or life-threatening, is permanently disabling, requires inpatient hospitalization, or is a congenital anomaly, cancer, or overdose. With respect to results obtained from tests in laboratory animals, a serious adverse drug experience includes any experience suggesting a significant risk for human subjects, including any finding of mutagenicity, teratogenicity, or carcinogenicity.

21 CFR 312.32(a)

Sponsor a person who takes responsibility for and initiates a clinical investigation. The sponsor may be an individual or pharmaceutical company, governmental agency, academic institution, private organization, or other organization. The sponsor does not actually conduct the investigation unless the sponsor is a sponsor-investigator. A person other than an individual that uses one or more of its own employees to conduct an investigation that it has initiated is a sponsor, not a sponsor-investigator, and the employees are investigators.

21 CFR 312.3(b)
21 CFR 310.3(j)

Sponsor-Investigator an individual who both initiates and conducts an investigation, and under whose immediate direction the investigational drug is administered or dispensed. The team does not include any person other than an individual.

21 CFR 312.3(b)

Starter Packs also known as stock samples, trade packages, or starter stocks are prescription drug products distributed without charge by manufacturers or distributors to prescribers and pharmacists with the intent that the pharmacists place the prescription drugs in stock and sell them at retail. Under the PDMA, a sample is defined as a unit of drug ". . . not intended to be sold . . . and intended to promote the sale of the drug." Although starter packs are given without charge to a pharmacy, they are not intended to be free samples to the consumer nor are they packaged as such. Since starter packs do not meet both parts of the definition of a sample under the PDMA, they are *not* considered to be samples. However, starter packs are subject to regulation as prescription drugs under the FD&C Act the same as stock shipments of prescription drugs.

Stock Recovery a firm's removal or correction of a product that has not been marketed or that has not left the direct control of the firm, i.e., the product is located on premises owned by, or under the control of, the firm and no portion of the lot has been released for sale or use.

21 CFR 7.3(k)

Strength the a) concentration of the drug substance (for example, weight/weight, weight/volume, or unit dose/volume basis), and/or b) the potency, that is, the therapeutic activity of the drug product as indicated by appropriate laboratory tests or by adequately developed and controlled clinical data (expressed, for example, in terms of units by reference to a standard).

21 CFR 210.3(a)(16)

Subject a human who participates in an investigation, either as a recipient of the investigational new drug or as a control. A subject may be a healthy human or a patient with a disease.

21 CFR 312.3(b)

Supplemental NDA may be filed by one who has an approved original new drug application or an abbreviated new drug application; it is used to obtain FDA approval for changes in an existing product's formula, packaging, or labeling or for a new, related product.

Theoretical Yield the quantity that would be produced at any appropriate phase of manufacture, processing, or packing of a particular drug product, based upon the quantity of components to be used, in the absence of any loss or error in actual production.

21 CFR 210.3(a)(17)

Therapeutic Alternates drug products containing different therapeutic moieties which belong in the same pharmacologic and/or therapeutic category that can be expected to have similar therapeutic effects when administered to patients in therapeutically equivalent doses.

Therapeutic Equivalence refers to two drugs that, when administered to the same person in the same dosage regimen, provide the same therapeutic effect, even though they may not be chemically equivalent.

Therapeutic Equivalent Drug Product drugs of the same or similar therapeutic category which will accomplish the same results as the drug prescribed.

Therapeutic Substitution the act of dispensing a therapeutic alternate instead of the drug product prescribed. For example, chlorothiazide instead of hydrochlorothiazide (diuretic); cephradine instead of cephalexin (cephalosporin antibiotic).

Unit Dose one dose; a single dose of medication to be administered to the patient directly from the container.

Unit Dose Container a single-unit container for drugs intended for administration by other than injection as a single dose directly from the container to the patient.

Unit-of-Use-Container contains a sufficient quantity of medication for one normal course of therapy, e.g., therapy for seven days.

United States Pharmacopeia abbreviated as *USP* or *U.S.P*; the oldest (since 1820) continuously published pharmacopeia in the world recognized by the Federal (USA) Food, Drug, and Cosmetic Act as containing legally enforceable (by FDA) standards and specifications for strength, quality, and purity [Sec 501(b)], packaging and labeling [Sec 502(g)], and if applicable bioavailability for drugs. Also contains standards or medical devices, diagnostics, and nutritional supplements. Published and marketed every five years by the non-governmental, not-for-profit U.S. Pharmacopeial Convention, Inc.

Validation the defining and testing of processes, specifications and/or equipment used, and to prove the capability and suitability of achieving required results consistently; A requirement of the Current Good Manufacturing Practices Regulations for Finished Pharmaceuticals, 21 CFR Parts 210 and 211, and of the Good Manufacturing Practice Regulations for Medical Devices.

21 CFR Part 820

Validation Protocol a written plan stating how validation will be conducted, including test parameters, product characteristics, production equipment, and decision points on what constitutes acceptable test results.

Validation Prospective validation conducted prior to the distribution of either a new product, or product made under a revised manufacturing process, where the revisions may affect the product's characteristics.

Validation Retrospective validation of a process for a product already in distribution based upon accumulated production, testing and data.

Warning Letter a written communication from FDA notifying an individual or firm that the agency considers one or more products, practices, processes, or other activities to be in violation of the Federal Food, Drug, and Cosmetic Act, or other acts, to the extent that failure of the responsible party to take appropriate and prompt action to correct the violation may be expected to result in administrative and/or regulatory enforcement without further notice. The three most common deficiencies alleged in Warning Letters are deviations from current Good Manufacturing Practices (GMPs), deviations from FDA labeling requirements, and failure to obtain product approvals. Companies may receive Warning Letters from FDA district offices based on four criteria outlined in Chapters 8–10 of FDA'S Regulatory Procedures Manual (RPM). The four criteria that the FDA uses to determine whether or not to issue a Warning Letter after it becomes aware of an alleged violation are: (1) If FDA district officials think the agency's policy concerning the situation at issue is clear and unambiguous; (2) If district officials reasonably expect a company will correct the situation promptly after receiving the letter; (3) If the district officials think that failure to correct the alleged violation would necessitate further enforcement action; and (4) If the "circumstances surrounding the situation make the issuance of a letter appropriate"; a criterion designed to provide flexibility and promote delegation to FDA district offices.

Abbreviations and Their Meanings

ANDA Abbreviated New Drug Application, sometimes referred to as a supplemental NDA, is a report submitted to the FDA by the sponsor of a drug whenever the latter decides to make changes in the labeling, formulation, manufacturing process, etc., in its NDA-approved product.

CDC Centers for Disease Control; part of the Public Health Service which monitors epidemiological data and evaluates communicable disease in the United States.

CFR *Code of Federal Regulations;* an annually revised codification of the general and permanent rules published in the *Federal Register* by the executive departments and agencies of the federal government. The CFR is divided into fifty titles which represent broad areas subject to federal regulation.

CGMP Current Good Manufacturing Practices; regulations of the FDA which establish minimal standards for the manufacturing of pharmaceutical products.

CHAMPUS The civilian Health and Medical Program of the Uniformed Services; the health insurance program sponsored by the Department of Defense for military personnel and their dependents when medical treatment is required away from a military facility.

CPG Compliance Policy Guides; provides guidance to FDA field inspection and compliance staffs in a bound book (CPG Manual). The CPG Manual explains FDA's policy on regulatory issues related to FDA laws and regulations. The statements in the Manual are not intended to create or confer any rights, privileges, or benefits on or for any private person or to bind FDA, but are intended solely for internal FDA guidance. CPGs do not have the force of law.

CPSC Consumer Product Safety Commission; the federal regulatory agency which regulates, among other things, certain prescription and nonprescription substances and requires that such substances be packaged for consumer use in special packaging (*safety closures*) that will make it significantly difficult for children under five years of age to open, but not difficult for adults.

DEA Drug Enforcement Administration; a component of the U.S. Justice Department, is the primary federal drug law enforcement agency established to control the manufacture and distribution of *controlled substances,* such as narcotics, barbiturates, stimulants.

DESI Drug Efficacy Study Implementation; a regulation of the FDA which requires manufacturers of drugs marketed in the United States between 1938 and 1962 to prove claims of effectiveness for the indications specified in the labeling of such products.

DMF Drug Master File; a submission to the Food and Drug Administration (FDA) that may be used to provide confidential detailed information about facilities, processes, or articles used in the manufacturing, processing, packaging, and storing of one or more human drugs. The submission of a DMF is not required by statute or FDA regulation. A DMF is submitted solely at the discretion of the holder. The information contained in the DMF may be used to support an Investigational New Drug Application (IND), a New Drug Application (NDA), an Abbreviated New Drug Application (ANDA), another DMF, and Export Application, or amendments and supplements to any of these. A DMF is *not* a substitute for an IND, NDA, ANDA, or Export Application. It is not approved or disapproved by the FDA. Technical contents of a DMF are reviewed *only* in connection with the review of an IND, NDA, ANDA, or an Export Application. Drug Master Files are provided for in 21 CFR 314.420.

DSHEA Dietary Supplement Health and Education Act; establishes labeling requirements, provides a regulatory framework, and authorizes FDA to promulgate good manufacturing practice regulations for dietary supplements and dietary ingredients and classifies them as food. The Act also establishes a commission to recommend how to regulate label claims and an agency to promote scientific studies regarding dietary supplements.

DUR Drug Utilization Review, Drug Use Review; the use of information from the patient medication profile to conduct a review of drug therapy *before* a prescription is dispensed or delivered to an individual by the pharmacist. The drug review should include screening for potential drug therapy problems due to therapeutic duplication, drug-disease contraindications, food-drug and drug-drug interactions (including serious interactions with nonprescription or over-the-counter drugs), incorrect drug dosage or duration of drug treatment, drug-allergy interactions, and clinical abuse/misuse; a structured and continuing program that reviews, analyzes, and interprets patterns of drug usage in a given health care environment against predetermined standards. The objectives of DUR systems are: a) to improve quality of care; and b) to assist in containing health care costs.

FCI For Cause Inspections; study oriented or investigator oriented inspections conducted in the United States and in foreign countries by the Food and Drug Adminstration.

FDA Food and Drug Administration; the federal agency, part of the Department of Health and Human Services (HHS), which has jurisdiction over the interstate shipment of foods, drugs, medical devices, and cosmetics to insure that they are pure, safe, and effective for their intended uses.

FD&C Act or FDCA Food, Drug, and Cosmetic Act of 1938 regulates the interstate commerce of foods, drugs, cosmetics, and medical devices.

510(k) Device Notice; the section of the FDCA which requires manufacturers of medical devices who must register with FDA to notify the agency, at least ninety days in advance, of their intent to market a medical device in the United States.

FOI(A) Freedom of Information Act; governs the public's access to information held by federal agencies in the conduct of their business. The Act requires that agency documents be made available to the public for inspection and copying, with certain exceptions, and requires each federal agency to promulgate and publish regulations under which it will act on requests for such information. The Food and Drug Administration has established a system for handling FOI requests in its regulations and has analyzed its records in connection with the exceptions described below to determine what records are exempt from disclosure.

The FOI Act does not require an agency to disclose any of the following types of information: (1) material classified as secret pursuant to Executive Order in the interest of national defense; (2) material pertaining solely to international personnel rules and practices of an agency; (3) material specifically exempted from disclosure by another statue; (4) privileged or confidental trade secrets and commercial or financial information furnished by a person or corporation; (5) inter- and intra-agency memoranda that would not be available to a party to an action against the agency (ther than to the agency itself); (6) personnel, medical, and similar files, disclosure of which would constitute an invasion of privacy; (7) investigatory records of the agency compiled for enforcement proceedings, prevent a fair trial, constitute an invasion of privacy of an individual, or disclose confidental sources and confidental information furnished by such sources in criminal or national security investigations; (8) material prepared by or on behalf of agencies regulating or supervising financial institutions; and (9) geological and geographical data concerning wells (refer to Appendix K).

FR *Federal Register;* a serial publication which contains, as determined by the Federal Register Act, president documents, documents of general applicability and legal effect, and documents to be published by statute. There is an edition of the FR for each official federal working day. The FR is the printed source which keeps the CFR up-to-date.

FTC Federal Trade Commission; the agency that regulates advertising relating to nonprescription drugs and cosmetics, with the exception of labeling.

GAO General Accounting Office; the federal agency responsible for reviewing all federal government spending.

GMP Good Manufacturing Practices; (see CGMP).

GRAS Generally Recognized As Safe; a designation for regulated food products the FDA has determined are not harmful. If experts cannot agree whether or not a product is safe, it is up to the manufacturer to prove that it is safe.

HCFA Health Care Financing Administration; the federal agency which administers Medicare.

HHS Department of Health and Human Services (formerly HEW or DHEW, Department of Health, Education and Welfare); the federal agency, created in 1979, concerned generally with the health and welfare of the U.S. population.

HMO Health Maintenance Organization; provides basic and supplemental health services to its members, and, in connection with the prescription or provision of prescription drugs, maintains, reviews, and evaluates a drug-use profile of members, evaluates patterns of drug utilization to assure optimum drug therapy, and educates its members and health professionals in use of prescription and nonprescription drugs.

IDE Investigational Device Exemption; Section 502(g) of the FD&C Act authorizes FDA to exempt devices intended solely for investigational use from certain requirements of the FD&C Act in order to allow for their shipment and use on human subjects. This provision applies to investigational studies undertaken to develop safety and effectiveness data for a medical device when these studies use human subjects.

An applicant for IDE for a "significant risk" device must submit information to demonstrate that the testing will be supervised by an institutional review board, that appropriate informed consent will be provided, and that certain records and reports will be maintained.

IND Investigational New Drug Application; formally referred to as Notice of Claimed Investigational Exemption for a New Drug, one approved by the Food and Drug Adminstration only for human clinical trials after preclinical (laboratory) testing. It is not generally approved for medical use in the United States.

IRB Institutional Review Board; composed of at least five persons with varying backgrounds who are generally knowledgeable through training or experience in the research areas likely to be considered. Racial, ethnic and other interests must be represented, and at least one member must be from a non-scientific discipline, such as law or the clergy, and at least one must not be affiliated with the research institution. The purpose of the IRB review is to ensure, among other things, that risk to subjects is minimized, informed consent is obtained, selection of subjects is fair and equitable, risks to subjects are reasonable in relation to expected benefit, and there are safeguards to protect the privacy of subjects.

MAC Maximum Allowable Cost; part of the reimbursement plan to reduce costs for drugs under federally

(Medicare) and state (Medicaid) sponsored programs. MAC establishes a ceiling price for multiple source drug products. The disbursing authority (federal or state) will not reimburse for more than the established MAC or EAC limit, whichever may be less.

MedMARx This is USP's internet accessible medication-error database software program.

NDA New Drug Application; a report submitted by its sponsor to the FDA before a new drug (new chemical entity), a dosage form not previously marketed, and for an OTC timed-release version of an Rx combination is considered safe and effective for marketing; consists of, among other things, reports of scientific and clinical investigations, formulation of the drug product, description of manufacturing processes (GMP), samples of the drug, and examples of the label/labeling.

NDC National Drug Code; a ten numeral code. The first five numerals identify the manufacturer or distributor; the last five numerals identify the drug product, the trade package size and type. The segment that identifies the manufacturer or distributor is referred to as the "labeler code"; the segment that identifies the product is known as the "product code"; and, the segment that identifies the trade package size and type is called the "package code."

NIH National Institutes of Health; part of the Public Health Service of the HHS which has over twenty separate institutes having highly qualified researchers and clinicians seeking to understand and conquer *unsolvable* medical problems. Both basic research and patient services are offered on its Bethesda, Maryland, campus.

OBRA '90 Omnibus Budget Reconciliation Act of 1990 (P.L. 101-508); also known as the Pryor Bill (David Pryor D-Ark), Pharmaceutical Access and Prudent Purchasing Act, Medicaid Drug Rebate Law; signed into law by President George Bush and became effective January 1, 1993. The statute's intent is to reduce the costs of state Medicaid programs. Manufacturers must charge Medicaid no more than the lowest price charged to hospitals or other entities that serve indigent populations. For pharmacists, the law includes a four-year prohibition on reductions of Medicaid reimbursement, enhanced drug-use review programs, incentives to develop electronic claims processing systems, and demonstration projects for cognitive services and patient counseling.

PF *Pharmacopeial Forum;* the USP journal of drug standards development and official compendia revision. It is the working document of the USP Committee of Revision, the major portion of which presents proposals for revising standards of the *USP* and *NF.*

OTC Over-the-Counter drug product; one which does not require a prescription prior to its sale in the United States.

PDMA Prescription Drug Marketing Act of 1987; also known as the Drug Diversion Act or Dingell Bill; signed into law by President Ronald Reagan on April 22, 1988, and became effective on July 21, 1988. The statute amends several sections of the FD&C Act and is intended to reduce public health risks from adulterated, misbranded, and counterfeit drug products that enter the marketplace through drug diversion.

PDUFA Prescription Drug User Fee Act; authorizes the FDA to collect user fees for certain applications for approval of drug and biological products, on establishments where the products are made, and on such marketed products.

PHS Public Health Service; part of the HHS, was formed in the late 1700s to directly provide medical care for the merchant marine. Today, it coordinates many aspects of regulation, provision of services, research, and establishment of standards in health care in the United States.

PPI Patient Package Insert; contains information designed to inform the patient-consumer about prescribed medication he/she has been provided, and attempts to explain, among other things, the risks, benefits, and proper use that may be anticipated from the drug product.

PPPA Poison Prevention Packaging Act of 1970; provides for special packaging to protect children from serious injury or illness which could result from handling, using, or ingesting certain substances, such as poisons, drugs, or cosmetics.

ProDUR Prospective Drug Utilization Review requires a pharmacist to conduct a review of a patient's prescription and medication profile *before* each prescription is dispensed, to communicate information to the patient (or caregiver) about the drug therapy to improve therapeutic results, and to obtain, record, and maintain information about each patient, such as medication history, known allergies, gender, date of birth, drug reactions.

RDUR Retrospective Drug Utilization Review involves the study of and focus on patterns of drug therapy by patients to determine overuse, abuse, inappropriate use of medication, therapeutic duplication, duration of treatment, and unnecessary care of patients by health care professionals.

SMDA Safe Medical Devices Act of 1990; signed into law by President George Bush on November 28, 1990. Expands and strengthens regulation of medical devices. Requires postmarketing surveillance via user reports, new 510K requirements, and FDA recall authority with civil penalties. Permits the use of Premarket Approval (PMA) to approve subsequent (generic) devices and orphan device exemption. Requires manufacturer of Class III devices introduced into commerce before 1976 to submit safety and efficacy data by 1995.

USAN Council United States Adopted Names Council; a private not-for-profit organization sponsored since January 1964 by the American Pharmaceutical Association, the United States Pharmacopeia, and American Medical Association. Its secretariat is housed in the AMA headquarters building in Chicago.

USAN A program specially organized to produce simple and useful nonproprietary (generic) names for drugs while the drug is still in its investigational stage. The USAN Council chooses each U.S. Adopted Name with the expectation that it will be suitable for prescribing and dispensing purposes and for designation as the title of the monograph, should the article be recognized in the official *United States Pharmacopeia* or *National Formulary.* Section 508 of the Federal Food, Drug, and Cosmetic Act (added by the Kefauver-Harris Amendments of October 10, 1962) authorizes the Commissioner of Food and Drug Administration to designate an official name for any drug if he/she determines that such action is necessary or desirable in the interest of usefulness and simplicity. Although the FDA has legal authority to assign names, it has delegated this responsibility to the Council, which is sponsored by the AMA, APhA, and USP. Representatives from each organization, as well as a liaison from the FDA, comprise the Council.

USC United States Code; a compilation of federal statutes arranged by subject matter called "titles," such as food and drugs, education, labor, in one easily accessible set of books having a subject matter index.

USP/DPPR *United States Pharmacopeia*/Drug Product Problem Reporting Program. Serving the needs of health care professionals for more than 21 years, this program encourages pharmacists, nurses, and physicians to report any observations or complaints concerning the quality of drug products. All reports received become part of the *USP*/DPPR database and can directly influence the development or revision of *USP/NF* standards as well as information monographs in the *USP DI*. USP immediately screens each report for health hazards and forwards all information to the FDA and the drug manufacturer for review and evaluation. To report a problem to *USP*/DPPR, one can call 1-800-638-6725.

USPHS United States Public Health Service (see PHS).

USP/MDLP *United States Pharmacopeia*/Medical Device and Laboratory Product Problem Reporting Program. This voluntary program provides an effective way to report concerns about the quality, safety, performance, packaging, or design of medical devices. Each report is forwarded to the FDA and the product manufacturer for evaluation and any necessary action. Reports include products such as catheters, IV equipment, cardiac monitors, ventilators, X-ray equipment, contact lenses, and *in vitro* kits. To report a problem one can call 1-800-638-6725.

USP/MER *United States Pharmacopeia*/Medication Errors Reporting Program. Founded in 1975 by the Institute for Safe Medication Practices, Inc., this nationwide program enables health professionals to report confidentially to the USP any medication errors they observe. MER encompasses a wide variety of problems such as misadministration, unclear or confusing product names or packaging. To report a medication error, one can call 1-800-233-7767.

USP/NF *United States Pharmacopoeia*/*National Formulary*; designated as the official compendia pursuant to federal and some state statutes, and containing enforceable standards and specifications for strength, quality, purity, packaging, labeling, storage, and where applicable, bioavailability of drugs. Also contains standards for medical devices, diagnostics, and nutritional supplements.

USP/SNM *United States Pharmacopeia*/Society of Nuclear Medicine Drug Product Problem Reporting Program for radiopharmaceuticals. Since 1975 this program has enabled health professionals to report both adverse reactions and quality problems to a responsive nationwide network. Jointly sponsored by USP and the Society of Nuclear Medicine (SNM), the program shares reports with the FDA, SNM, and product manufacturers on radionuclide and radiochemical impurities, packaging and labeling problems, quality concerns, and patient reactions. To report a problem one can call 1-800-638-6725.

Glossary of Acronyms of Interest to Pharmacists and Regulatory Personnel

An acronym is a word formed from the initial letter or letters of each successive part or major parts of a compound term. It is not to be confused with a palindrome, anagram, lipogram, cryptogram, rhopalic or other word diversion.

The use of acronyms is proliferating in publications, regulations, correspondence and even in conversations. Some people contend that a regulation is hardly a regulation unless it has an acronym. Others claim that acronyms are used as a code to keep the uninitiated from learning too much. And still others say the use of linguistic shorthand is an absolute necessity to save time, paper and money. Further, we also get acronyms and abbreviations as new systems and new, easy to use communcations equipment come into being. Therefore, it's inevitable that the former increase simply because of the volumes of message traffic, thus creating a need for some form of shorthand.

AACP	American Association of Colleges of Pharmacy
AADA	Abbreviated Antibiotic Drug Application
AAPS	American Association of Pharmaceutical Scientists
ABPI	Association of the British Pharmaceutical Industry
ACA	American College of Apothecaries
ACCP	American College of Clinical Pharmacy
ACE	Adverse Clinical Event
ACPE	American Council on Pharmaceutical Education
ADA	Antiobiotic Drug Application
ADE	Adverse Drug Experience
ADME	Absorption, Distribution, Metabolism, Excretion
ADR	Adverse Drug Reaction
AE	Adverse Event
AHI	Animal Health Institute
AID	Agency for International Development
AIHP	American Institute of the History of Pharmacy
AMA	American Medical Association
ANDA	Abbreviated New Drug Application
ANMP	Association of Natural Medicine Pharmacists
AOAC	Association of Official Analytical Chemists
APhA	American Pharmaceutical Association
APT	Association of Pharmacy Technicians
ASCP	American Society of Consultant Pharmacists
ASHP	American Society of Health System Pharmacists
ASPEN	American Society for Parenteral and Enteral Nutrition
ASPL	American Society for Pharmacy Law
ATC	Anatomical-Therapuetic-Chemical
AUC	Area Under the Curve
AWP	Average Wholesale Price
BCE	Beneficial Clinical Event
BP	British Pharmacopeia
BPC	British Pharmaceutical Codex
BPS	Board of Pharmaceutical Specialties
CAMA	Computer Assisted Marketing Application
CANDA	Computer Assisted New Drug Application Review
CAPER	Computer Assisted Pharmacology Evaluation and Review
CAPLA	Computer Assisted Product License Application
CAS	Chemical Abstract Service
CBBB	Council of Better Business Bureaus
CBER	Center for Biologics Evaluation and Research

CDC	Centers for Disease Control
CDER	Center for Drug Evaluation and Research
CDRH	Center for Devices and Radiological Health
CE	Continuing Education
CEQ	Council on Environmental Quality
CFR	*Code of Federal Regulations*
CFSAN	Center for Food Safety and Applied Nutrition
CGMP	Current Good Manufacturing Practices
CHPA	Consumer Healthcare Products Association (formerly NDMA)
CIOMS	Council for International Organizations of Medical Sciences
CIRTS	Compliance Inspection Request Tracking System
CIS	Commonwealth of Independent States
CITS	Compliance Inspection Tracking System
CLIA	Clinical Laboratory Improvement Amendments (1988)
CME	Continuing Medical Education
CMMS	Centers for Medicare and Medicaid Services
COA	Certificate of Analysis
COBRA	Consolidated Omnibus Reconciliation Act (1985)
COMPASS	Computerized On-Line Medical Pharmaceutical Analysis and Surveillance System
COSTART	Coding Symbols for Thesaurus of Adverse Reaction Terms (FDA's)
CPG	Compliance Policy Guide
CPMP	Committee for Proprietary Medicinal Products
CPSC	Consumer Product Safety Commission
CRADA	Cooperative Research and Development Agreement
CRF	Case Report Form
CRL	Controlled Release Society
CRO	Contract Research Organization
CSA	Controlled Substances Act
CSR	Clinical Study Report
CTC	Clinical Trial Certificates (UK)
CTFA	Cosmetic, Toiletry and Fragrance Association
CTX	Clinical Trial Exemptions (UK)
CVM	Center for Veterinary Medicine
DCAT	Drug, Chemical and Allied Trades Association
DCI	Drug and Cosmetic Industry
DD	Department of Defense
DDD	Daily Defined Dose
DDS	Doctor of Dental Surgery
DEA	Drug Enforcement Administration
DESI	Drug Efficacy Study Implementation
DHHS	Department of Health and Human Services

DIA	Drug Information Association
DIC	Drug Information Center
DIS	Drug Information Service
DISNET	Drug Information Systems Network
DMB	Dockets Management Branch
DMD	Doctor of Dental Medicine
DMF	Drug Master File
DO	Doctor of Osteopathy
DOD	Department of Defense
DOH	Department of Health
DPM	Doctor of Podiatric Medicine
DQRS	Drug Quality Reporting System
DRA	Drug Regulatory Authority or Drug Regulatory Affairs
DRG	Diagnostic Related Groupings
DSHEA	Dietary Supplement and Health Education Act
DUR	Drug Utilization Review
DVM	Doctor of Veterinary Medicine
EA	Environmental Assessment
EC	European Community
ECDS	Eastern Caribbean Drug Service
ECJ	European Court of Justice
ECOSOC	Economic and Social Community of the EC
EEC	European Economic Community
EER	Establishment Evaluation Report
EFPIA	European Federation of Pharmaceutical Industries Association
EFTA	European Free Trade Association
EGA	European Generics Association
EIR	Establishment Inspection Reports
EIS	Environmental Impact Statement
ELA	Establishment License Application
EOQ	European Organization for Quality
EP	*European Pharmacopeia*
EPA	Environmental Protection Agency
ESRA	European Society of Regulatory Affairs
EUCOMED	European Confederation of Medical Device Association
FBI	Federal Bureau of Investigation
FDA	Food and Drug Administration
FDAMA	FDA Modernization Act
FDA-DQRS	FDA's Drug Quality Reporting System
FD&C Act	Food, Drug, and Cosmetic Act
FDCA	Food, Drug, and Cosmetic Act
FDLI	Food and Drug Law Institute
FFD&CA	Federal Food, Drug, and Cosmetic Act
FFDCA	Federal Food, Drug, and Cosmetic Act
FIC	For Cause Inspection
FIFRA	Federal Insecticide, Fungicide and Rodenticide Act
FOIA	Freedom of Information Act
FONSI	Finding of No Significant Impact

FPLA	Fair Packaging and Labeling Act		**MBR**	Master Batch Record
FR	*Federal Register*		**MD**	Doctor of Medicine
FTC	Federal Trade Commission		**MDR**	Medical Device Reporting
FTZB	Foreign Trade Zones Board		**MRC**	Medical Research Council (UK)
FY	Fiscal Year			

GAO	General Accounting Office
GATT	General Agreement on Tariffs and Trade
GCP	Good Clinical Practices
GDEA	Generic Drug Enforcement Act of 1992
GLP	Good Laboratory Practices
GMP	Good Manufacturing Practices
GNP	Gross National Product
GPIA	Generic Pharmaceutical Industry Association
GPO	Government Printing Office
GRAE	Generally Regarded As Effective
GRAS	Generally Recognized As Safe
GRASE	Generally Regarded As Safe and Effective
GSA	General Services Administration

HHS	Health and Human Services (Department of)
HMO	Health Maintenance Organization
HP	*Homeopathic Pharmacopeia of the United States*
HPB	Health Protection Branch (Canada)

ICC	Interstate Commerce Commission
IDE	Investigational Device Exemption
IFPMA	International Federation of Pharmaceutical Manufacturers Association
IG	Inspector General
INAD	Notice of Claimed Exemption for a New Animal Drug
IND	Investigational New Drug
INN	International Nonproprietary Name
IPA	International Pharmaceutical Abstracts
IRB	Institutional Review Board
IRS	Internal Revenue Service
ISO	International Organization for Standardization
IUB	International Union of Biochemistry
IUPAC	International Union of Pure and Applied Chemistry
IVD	In Vitro Diagnostic

JCAHO	Joint Commission on Accreditation of Health Care Organizations

LOC	Library of Congress
LVP	Large Volume Parenteral

MAC	Maximum Allowable Cost

NABP	National Association of Boards of Pharmacy
NACDS	National Association of Chain Drugstores
NADA	New Animal Drug Application
NAF	Notice of Adverse Findings (FDA)
NAI	No Action Indicated
NAPM	National Association of Pharmaceutical Manufacturers
NARD	National Association of Retail Druggists (see NCPA)
NBS	National Bureau of Standards
NCE	New Chemical Entity
NCPA	National Community Pharmacists Association (formerly NARD)
NCPIE	National Council on Patient Information and Education
NCTR	National Center for Toxicological Research
NDA	New Drug Application
NDC	National Drug Code
NDMA	Nonprescription Drug Manufacturers Association
NDS	New Drug Substance
NEPA	National Environmental Policy Act (1969)
NF	*National Formulary*
NICODARD	National Information Center for Orphan Drugs and Rare Diseases
NIH	National Institutes of Health
NIOSH	National Institute for Occupational Safety and Health
NIST	National Institute of Standards and Technology (formerly NBS)
NLRB	National Labor Relations Board
NLT	Not Less Than
NME	New Molecular Entity
NMT	Not More Than
NPA	National Pharmaceutical Association
NPC	National Pharmaceutical Council
NRC	Nuclear Regulatory Commission
NSF	National Science Foundation
NWDA	National Wholesale Druggists Association

OBRA	Omnibus Budget Reconciliation Act (1990)
OD	Doctor of Optometry
ODE	Office of Device Evaluation
OECD	Organization for Economic Cooperation and Development
OGD	Office of Generic Drugs
OJC	Official Journal of the EC-C series (information and notices)
OMB	Office of Management and Budget

OSHA	Occupational Safety and Health Administration		**SBA**	Small Business Administration
OTA	Office of Technology Assessment		**SMDA**	Safe Medical Devices Act (of 1990)
OTC	Over-The-Counter		**SNF**	Skilled Nursing Facility
OTT	Office of Technology Transfer		**SNOMED**	Systematized Nomenclature of Medicine
			SOP	Standard Operating Procedure
			SPC	Supplementary Protection Certificate
PA	Proprietary Association		**SSA**	Social Security Administration
PAC	Pharmaceutical Advertising Council			
PAHO	Pan American Health Organization		**TFM**	Tentative Final Monograph
PBR	Production Batch Record		**TRP**	Tamper Resistant Packaging
PCSO	Pharmaceutical Contract Support Organization		**TSCA**	Toxic Substances Control Act
PDA	Parenteral Drug Association		**USAN**	United States Adopted Names
PDMA	Prescription Drug Marketing Act (1987)		**USC**	United States Code
PDP	Product Development Protocol		**USDA**	United States Department of Agriculture
PF	Pharmaceutical Forum		**USGPO**	United States Government Printing Office
PhRMA	Pharmaceutical Research Manufacturers of America (previous name for Pharmaceutical Manufacturers Association)		**USIA**	United States Information Agency
			USITC	United States International Trade Commission
PHS	Public Health Service		*USP*	*United States Pharmacopeia*
PI	Package Insert		*USP-DDN*	*United States Pharmacopeia Dictionary of Drug Names*
PIC	Pharmaceutical Inspection Convention		**USP-DPPR**	United States Pharmacopeia Drug Product Problem Reporting Program
PLA	Product License Application			
PMA	Pharmaceutical Manufacturers Association (see PhRMA)		**USP-MERP**	United States Pharmacopeia Medication Errors Reporting Program
PMA	Premarket Approval Application		**USP-PRN**	United States Pharmacopeia Practitioners' Reporting Network
PMS	Post Marketing Surveillance			
PPG	Policy and Procedure Guide		**USP-SNM**	United States Pharmacopeia-Society of Nuclear Medicine Drug Product Problem Reporting Program for Radiopharmaceuticals
PPI	Patient Package Insert			
PPPA	Poison Prevention Packaging Act			
PPS	Prospective Payment System			
PQA	Preproduction Quality Assurance		**USPC**	United States Pharmacopeial Convention
PRO	Pharmaceutical Research Organization		**USPHS**	United States Public Health Service
PTO	Patent and Trademark Office		**USPS**	United States Postal Service
QA	Quality Assurance		**VA**	Veterans Affairs (Department of)
QC	Quality Control		**VAI**	Voluntary Action Indicated
			VAT	Value Added Tax
RAC	Regulatory Affairs Certificate (Certified)		**VP**	Vice President
RAPS	Regulatory Affairs Professionals Society			
R&D	Research and Development		**WHO**	World Health Organization
RINN	Recommended International Nonproprietary Name		**WHO-ART**	World Health Organization Adverse Reaction Terminology
RUG	Resource Utilization Groups			

Food and Drug Administration Forms and Applications

The Management Methods Branch (HFA-250) publishes an *FDA Forms Catalog* in order to provide interested parties the information for ordering forms and applications that are vital to doing business with the Food and Drug Administration.

Requests for the *catalog* and specific forms should be addressed to: Consolidated Forms and Publications Distribution Center, Washington Commerce Center, 3222 Hubbard Road, Landover, MD 20785.

Questions concerning the FDA Forms Management Program should be directed to: Mary J. Thomas, 301-443-1793; Dottie O'Neal, 301-443-4055.

FDA 356h	Application to Market a New Drug for Human Use/Antibiotic Drug for Human Use
FDA 457	Product/Establishment Surveillance Report
FDA 466	Section 305 Notice of Hearing
FDA 466a	Information Sheet for Section 305 Notice of Hearing
FDA 481	Establishment Inspection Report
FDA 482	Notice of Inspection
FDA 482a	Demand for Records
FDA 482b	Request for Information
FDA 483	Inspectional Observations
FDA 484	Receipt for Samples
FDA 486	Order of Condemnation & Forfeiture
FDA 487	Information Regarding Seized Material
FDA 718	Notice of Detention and Hearing
FDA 1571	Investigational New Drug Application (IND)
FDA 1572	Statement of Investigator (Clinical)
FDA 1639	Adverse Reaction Report (Drugs and Biologics)
FDA 1639b	Adverse Event Report
FDA 2252	Transmittal of Annual Reports for Drugs for Human Use
FDA 2253	Transmittal of Advertisements and Promotional Labeling for Drugs for Human Use
FDA 2334	Color Certification
FDA 2656	Registration of Drug Establishment
FDA 2656e	Annual Registration of Drug Establishment
FDA 2657	Drug Product Listing
FDA 2658	Registered Establishments' Report of Private Label Distributors
FDA 2714	Monthly Recall Status Report
FDA 2887a	Drug Product Complaint
FDA 3177	Recall Audit Check Report
FDA 3291	Request for Consultation
FDA 3318	Drug Quality Reporting Program
FDA 3351	Notice of Seizure

DEPARTMENT OF HEALTH AND HUMAN SERVICES
PUBLIC HEALTH SERVICE
FOOD AND DRUG ADMINISTRATION

APPLICATION TO MARKET A NEW DRUG FOR HUMAN USE
OR AN ANTIBIOTIC DRUG FOR HUMAN USE
(Title 21, Code of Federal Regulations, 314)

Form Approved: OMB No. 0910-0001
Expiration Date: June 30, 1992
See OMB Statement on Page 3.

FOR FDA USE ONLY	
DATE RECEIVED	DATE FILED
DIVISION ASSIGNED	NDA/ANDA NO. ASS.

NOTE: No application may be filed unless a completed application form has been received (21 CFR Part 314).

NAME OF APPLICANT	DATE OF SUBMISSION
	TELEPHONE NO. *(Include Area Code)*
ADDRESS *(Number, Street, City, State and Zip Code)*	NEW DRUG OR ANTIBIOTIC APPLICATION NUMBER (If previously issued)

DRUG PRODUCT

ESTABLISHED NAME *(e.g., USP/USAN)*	PROPRIETARY NAME *(If any)*	
CODE NAME *(If any)*	CHEMICAL NAME	
DOSAGE FORM	ROUTE OF ADMINISTRATION	STRENGTH(S)

PROPOSED INDICATIONS FOR USE

LIST NUMBERS OF ALL INVESTIGATIONAL NEW DRUG APPLICATIONS *(21 CFR Part 312)*, NEW DRUG OR ANTIBIOTIC APPLICATIONS *(21 CFR Part 314)*, AND DRUG MASTER FILES *(21 CFR 314 420)* REFERRED TO IN THIS APPLICATION:

INFORMATION ON APPLICATION

TYPE OF APPLICATION *(Check one)*

☐ THIS SUBMISSION IS A FULL APPLICATION *(21 CFR 314.50)*   ☐ THIS SUBMISSION IS AN ABBREVIATED APPLICATION (ANDA) *(21 CFR 314 55)*

IF AN ANDA, IDENTIFY THE APPROVED DRUG PRODUCT THAT IS THE BASIS FOR THE SUBMISSION

NAME OF DRUG	HOLDER OF APPROVED APPLICATION

STATUS OF APPLICATION *(Check one)*

☐ PRESUBMISSION
  ☐ ORIGINAL APPLICATION
☐ AN AMENDMENT TO A PENDING APPLICATION
  ☐ RESUBMISSION
☐ SUPPLEMENTAL APPLICATION

PROPOSED MARKETING STATUS *(Check one)*

☐ APPLICATION FOR A PRESCRIPTION DRUG PRODUCT *(Rx)*   ☐ APPLICATION FOR AN OVER - THE - COUNTER PRODUCT *(OTC)*

FORM FDA 356h (12/91)   PREVIOUS EDITION IS OBSOLETE   Page 1

FIGURE 1.

CONTENTS OF APPLICATION

This application contains the following items: (*Check all that apply*)

	1. Index
	2. Summary (21 CFR 314.50 (c))
	3. Chemistry, manufacturing, and control section (21 CFR 314.50 (d) (1))
	4. a. Samples (21 CFR 314.50 (e) (1)) (Submit only upon FDA's request)
	b. Methods Validation Package (21 CFR 314.50 (e) (2) (i))
▨	c. Labeling (21 CFR 314.50 (e) (2) (ii))
	i. draft labeling (*4 copies*)
	ii. final printed labeling (12 copies)
	5. Nonclinical pharmacology and toxicology section (21 CFR 314.50 (d) (2))
	6. Human pharmacokinetics and bioavailability section (21 CFR 314.50 (d) (3))
	7. Microbiology section (21 CFR 314.50 (d) (4))
	8. Clinical data section (21 CFR 314.50 (d) (5))
	9. Safety update report (21 CFR 314.50 (d) (5) (vi) (b))
	10. Statistical section (21 CFR 314.50 (d) (6))
	11. Case report tabulations (21 CFR 314.50 (f) (1))
	12. Case reports forms (21 CFR 314.50 (f) (1))
	13. Patent information on any patent which claims the drug (21 U.S.C. 355 (b) or (c))
	14. A patent certification with respect to any patent which claims the drug (21 U.S.C. 355 (b) (2) or (j) (2) (A))
	15. OTHER (*Specify*)

I agree to update this application with new safety information about the drug that may reasonably affect the statement of contraindications, warnings, precautions, or adverse reactions in the draft labeling. I agree to submit these safety update reports as follows: (1) 4 months after the initial submission, (2) following receipt of an approvable letter and (3) at other times as requested by FDA. If this application is approved, I agree to comply with all laws and regulations that apply to approved applications, including the following:

  1. Good manufacturing practice regulations in 21 CFR 210 and 211
  2. Labeling regulations in 21 CFR 201
  3. In the case of a prescription drug product, prescription drug advertising regulations in 21 CFR 202.
  4. Regulations on making changes in application in 21 CFR 314 70, 314 71, and 314.72.
  5. Regulations on reports in 21 CFR 314.80 and 314.81.
  6. Local, state and Federal environmental impact laws.

If this application applies to a drug product that FDA has proposed for scheduling under the controlled substances Act I agree not to market the product until the Drug Enforcement Administration makes a final scheduling decision.

NAME OF RESPONSIBLE OFFICIAL OR AGENT	SIGNATURE OF RESPONSIBLE OFFICIAL OR AGENT	DATE
ADDRESS (*Street, City, State, Zip Code*)	TELEPHONE NO. (*Include Area Code*)	

(**WARNING:** A willfully false statement is a criminal offense. U.S.C. Title 18, Sec. 1001.)

Public reporting burden for this collection of information is estimated to average 20 minutes per response, including the time for reviewing instructions, searching existing data sources, gathering and maintaining the data needed, and completing and reviewing the collection of information. Send comments regarding this burden estimate or any other aspect of this collection of information, including suggestions for reducing this burden to:

Reports Clearance Officer, PHS   and to: Office of Management and Budget
Hubert H. Humphrey Building, Room 721-B   Paperwork Reduction Project (0910-0001)
200 Independence Avenue, S.W.   Washington, DC 20503
Washington, DC 20201
Attn: PRA

Please DO NOT RETURN this application to either of these addresses.

FIGURE 1 (continued).

1. HOME DISTRICT	2. REPORTING UNIT SYMBOL	3. CENTRAL FILE NO	4. J D /T A	5. COUNTY	6. DATE
7. PRODUCT CODE	8. OPERATION	9. PROGRAM ASSIGNMENT CODE			10. HOURS

11. IDENTIFICATION *(Quote pertinent labeling including Establishment name and address)*

12. MANUFACTURER CONTROL CODES *(Labels, packaging and shipping containers)*	13. AMOUNT ON HAND	14. DATE LOT RECEIVED
	15. ESTIMATED VALUE	16. SAMPLE NO(s).

17. DEALER *(Name, street address, city, state, and ZIP code)*	18. ☐ DISTRIBUTOR ☐ SHIPPER ☐ MANUFACTURER ☐ OTHER *(Name, street address, city, state, Zip code, and telephone)*

19. ESTABLISHMENT TYPE(S)	INDUSTRY CODE						20. ESTABLISHMENT SIZE *(\$ VOLUME)*	21. INFORMATION OBTAINED BY *(Check one)*
	1	2	3	4	5	6		
a.								MAIL
b.								TELEPHONE
c.								VISIT

22. REMARKS

23. REPORT PREPARED BY *(Type or print name and title)*	24. EMPLOYEE NO.	25. PC	26. SIGNATURE

27. REPORTING UNIT ACTION
☐ REFERRED TO HOME DISTRICT   ☐ ADD TO ACTIVE OEI
  ☐ COLLECT OFFICIAL SAMPLES   ☐ ROUTINE FOLLOW-UP
☐ REFERRED TO STATE LOCAL OR   ☐ INSPECT
  OTHER FEDERAL AUTHORITIES
☐ REINSPECT   ☐ MAKE INVESTIGATION   ☐ NO ACTION
  ☐ REFERRED TO HDQTRS _____ *(Routing Symbol)*

28. NAME OF REVIEWING OFFICIAL *(Type or print)*	
29. TITLE	30. DATE REVIEWED

FORM FDA 457 (5/90)   PREVIOUS EDITION MAY BE USED   **PRODUCT/ESTABLISHMENT SURVEILLANCE REPORT**

FIGURE 2.

SUSPECTED VIOLATIONS *(Check appropriate box)*

HEALTH

DRUGS—DEVICES

Dangerous under any condition of use: 502(j).	Inadequate directions for use: 502(f)(1).
Dangerous when sold indiscriminately: 502(f).	Failure to bear list of active ingredients: 502(e).
Dangerous on account of excessive dosage: 502(j).	Possible variation from professed standard: 501(b), (c), (d).
Dangerous because of inadequate warnings: 502(f)(2).	Vitamin preparations—possible variation from professed standard: 501(b), (c), (d).
Drugs dangerous on account of impurities: 501(a)(2), (3), 502(j).	Extravagant therapeutic claims: 502(a).[1]

[1] If descriptive or promotional material employed in sale of product bears or contains extravagant therapeutic claims, indicate (in REMARKS on front or in separate memo) source, how received, and how employed in sale of product. See Section 201(m), Labeling; 301(b), 301(k), Prohibited Acts.

HYGIENIC

ECONOMIC

Deceptive packagaed: 502(i)	Suspect short weight or volume: 502(b)

NEW DRUG

HEALTH

FOODS

Presence of poisons: 402(a)(1), (2).	Therapeutic claims for food: Subject to 502.
Dangerous and non-nutritive substances (confectionery): 402(d).	Vitamin claims: 403(a), (j). May also be subject to 502.
Poisonous containers: 402(a)(6).	Special dietary foods: 403(j).

HYGIENIC

Stored under insanitary conditions: 402(a)(4).	Suspected filth or decomposition: 402(a)(3).

ECONOMIC

Deceptive packaging: 403(d).	Failure to declare mandatory statements: nonstandardized foods: 403(e), (f), (i), (k).
Short weight or volume: 403(e)(2).	Standardized foods, misbranding or nonconformity: 403(g), (h).
Misrepresentations in labeling: 403(a). See 201(m).	

COSMETICS

Dangerous cosmetics: 601(a)	Adulteration: 601.
Misbranding: 602.	

OTHER

EXPLAIN

FORM FDA 457 (5/90)   (BACK)

DH 79

FIGURE 2 (continued).

373

| SECTION 305 |
| NOTICE |

Investigation by this Administration indicates your responsibility for violation of the Federal Food, Drug, and Cosmetic Act, and other Federal Laws, as described in the attached Charge Sheet, with respect to the following:

An informal meeting has been scheduled for

to give you an opportunity to present your views on this matter. The enclosed INFORMATION SHEET and REGULATIONS explain the purpose and nature of the meeting, and how you may reply. Please note the regulations require that if you choose to be represented by a "designated representative," that individual must bring a written statement to the meeting authorizing him or her to speak on your behalf. (See regulation 7.84 (g).) If no response is received on or before the date set, our decision on whether to refer the matter to the Department of Justice for prosecution will be based on the evidence in hand.

By direction of the Secretary of the Department of Health and Human Services:

Compliance Officer

(IMPORTANT: NOTE ALL ENCLOSURES CAREFULLY)

Enclosures:
Legal Status Sheet
Charge Sheet
Information Sheet
Regulations

FORM FDA 466 (11/80)   PREVIOUS EDITION IS OBSOLETE

FIGURE 3.

DEPARTMENT OF HEALTH AND HUMAN SERVICES
PUBLIC HEALTH SERVICE
FOOD AND DRUG ADMINISTRATION

INFORMATION SHEET IN CONNECTION WITH ENCLOSED SECTION 305 NOTICE

OBJECT OF THE MEETING

This **meeting** is scheduled to give the person or persons who appear to be responsible for the violations of the **Federal Food, Drug, and Cosmetic Act,** and other Federal Laws, as specified in the attached Charge Sheet an opportunity to explain **voluntarily** any circumstances connected with the preparation, handling, shipment, or sale of the articles involved which would indicate that criminal action should not be taken. You are not compelled, however, to answer. Any civil action which may have been taken against the goods involved, such as seizure, does not preclude prosecution of those responsible for the violation; the meeting concerns the possible criminal action only. A copy of the Federal Food, Drug, and Cosmetic Act and regulations for its enforcement may be had upon request.

NATURE OF THE MEETING

This **meeting** is informal and confined to questions of fact. For your convenience in submitting required information concerning the status of your firm both on the date of response to this notice and on the date of alleged violation, the attached Legal Status forms may be filled out and returned with your answer, whether written or by personal appearance. Your answer may consist of the disclosure of any pertinent facts, letters, files, guaranties, shipping documents, analyses, arguments, etc., which you feel may present valid reasons why you should not be prosecuted.

GUARANTIES

In the case of articles that are adulterated or misbranded when introduced in interstate commerce the Federal Food, Drug, and Cosmetic Act places responsibility on the interstate shipper, even though he may be only the distributor and not the manufacturer. Distributors may relieve themselves of responsibility if they hold a legal guaranty under Section 303(c) of the act. If the articles were sold to you by a person residing in the United States and guaranteed by such person to comply with the provisions of the act, you should submit —

Evidence of that fact, and

A statement as to whether the product at the time of the apparent violation by you was in the identical condition and bore the same labels as when received by you from the guarantor, and

The full name of the person who, if called upon, can identify pertinent records and testify to the facts as you present them.

HOW TO ANSWER

You may appear in person or by attorney or other designated representative, or you may submit your response in the form of a letter in lieu of personal appearance. If written response is made, please submit your letter and all accompanying documents in **triplicate.** Documents submitted at personal appearance should be in **triplicate. All documents should be conspicuously identified by the reference number shown on the upper right corner of the Section 305 Notice.**

RESULT OF THE MEETING

After the meeting has been held and all the facts considered, if it is the conclusion of the Secretary of the Department of Health and Human Services that prosecution should be recommended, the facts in the matter will be transmitted to the Department of Justice for appropriate action.

FORM FDA 466a (7/80) PREVIOUS EDITION IS OBSOLETE.

FIGURE 4.

DEPARTMENT OF HEALTH AND HUMAN SERVICES
PUBLIC HEALTH SERVICE
FOOD AND DRUG ADMINISTRATION

1. DISTRICT ADDRESS & PHONE NO.

2. NAME AND TITLE OF INDIVIDUAL

3. DATE

TO

4. FIRM NAME

HOUR

a.m.

6. NUMBER AND STREET

p.m.

7. CITY AND STATE & ZIP CODE

8. PHONE # & AREA CODE

Notice of Inspection is hereby given pursuant to Section 704(a)(1) of the Federal Food, Drug, and Cosmetic Act [21 U.S.C. 374(a)]¹ and/or Part F or G, Title III of the Public Health Service Act [42 U.S.C. 262-264]²

9. SIGNATURE *(Food and Drug Administration Employee(s))*

10. TYPE OR PRINT NAME AND TITLE *(FDA Employee(s))*

Applicable portions of Section 704 and other Sections of the Federal Food, Drug, and Cosmetic Act [21 U.S.C. 374] are quoted below:

¹Sec. 704. (a)(1) For purposes of enforcement of this Chapter, officers or employees duly designated by the Secretary, upon presenting appropriate credentials and a written notice to the owner, operator, or agent in charge, are authorized (A) to enter, at reasonable times, any factory, warehouse, or establishment in which food, drugs, devices, or cosmetics are manufactured, processed, packed, or held, for introduction into interstate commerce or after such introduction, or to enter any vehicle being used to transport or hold such food, drugs, devices, or cosmetics in interstate commerce; and (B) to inspect, at reasonable times and within reasonable limits and in a reasonable manner, such factory, warehouse, establishment, or vehicle and all pertinent equipment, finished and unfinished materials, containers, and labeling therein. In the case of any factory, warehouse, establishment, or consulting laboratory in which prescription drugs or restricted devices are manufactured, processed, packed, or held, the inspection shall extend to all things therein (including records, files, papers, processes, controls, and facilities) bearing on whether prescription drugs or restricted devices which are adulterated or misbranded within the meaning of this Chapter, or which may not be manufactured, introduced into interstate commerce, or sold, or offered for sale by reason of any provision of this Chapter, have been or are being manufactured, processed, packed, transported, or held in any such place, or otherwise bearing on violation of this Chapter. No inspection authorized by the preceding sentence or by paragraph (3) shall extend to financial data, sales data other than shipment data, pricing data, personnel data (other than data as to qualifications of technical and professional personnel performing functions subject to this Act), and research data (other than data, relating to new drugs, antibiotic drugs and devices and, subject to reporting and inspection under regulations lawfully issued pursuant to section 505(i) or (k), section 507(d) or (g), section 519, or 520(g), and data relating to other drugs or devices which in the case of a new drug would be subject to reporting or inspection under lawful regulations issued pursuant to section 505(k) of the title. A separate notice shall be given for each such inspection, but a notice shall not be required for each entry made during the period covered by the inspection. Each such inspection shall be commenced and completed with reasonable promptness.

Sec. 704(e) Every person required under section 519 or 520(g) to maintain records and every person who is in charge or custody of such records shall, upon request of an officer or employee designated by the Secretary, permit such officer or employee at all reasonable times to have access to and to copy and verify, such records.

Section 512 (1)(1) In the case of any new animal drug for which an approval of an application filed pursuant to subsection (b) is in effect, the applicant shall establish and maintain such records, and make such reports to the Secretary, of data relating to experience and other data or information, received or otherwise obtained by such applicant with respect to such drug, or with respect to animal feeds bearing or containing such drug, as the Secretary may by general regulation, or by order with respect to such application, prescribe on the basis of a finding that such records and reports are necessary in order to enable the Secretary to determine, or facilitate a determination, whether there is or may be ground for invoking subsection (e) or subsection (m)(4) of this section. Such regulation or order shall provide, where the Secretary deems it to be appropriate, for the examination, upon request, by the persons to whom such regulation or order is applicable, of similar information received or otherwise obtained by the Secretary.
(2) Every person required under this subsection to maintain records, and every person in charge or custody thereof, shall, upon request of an officer or employee designated by the Secretary, permit such officer or employee at all reasonable times to have access to and copy and verify such records.

²Applicable sections of Parts F and G of Title III Public Health Service Act [42 U.S.C. 262-264] are quoted below:

Part F - Licensing — Biological Products and Clinical Laboratories and******

Sec. 351(c) "Any officer, agent, or employee of the Department of Health & Human Services, authorized by the Secretary for the purpose, may during all reasonable hours enter and inspect any establishment for the propagation or manufacture and preparation of any virus, serum, toxin, antitoxin, vaccine, blood, blood component or derivative, allergenic product or other product aforesaid for sale, barter, or exchange in the District of Columbia, or to be sent, carried, or brought from any State or possession into any other State or possession or into any foreign country, or from any foreign country into any State or possession."

Part F — ******Control of Radiation.

Sec. 360 A(a) "If the Secretary finds for good cause that the methods, tests, or programs related to electronic product radiation safety in a particular factory, warehouse, or establishment in which electronic products are manufactured or held, may not be adequate or reliable, officers or employees duly designated by the Secretary, upon presenting appropriate credentials and a written notice to the owner, operator, or agent in charge, are thereafter authorized (1) to enter, at reasonable times any area in such factory, warehouse, or establishment in which the manufacturer's tests (or testing programs) required by section 358 (h) are carried out, and (2) to inspect, at reasonable times and within reasonable limits and in a reasonable manner, the facilities and procedures within such area which are related to electronic product radiation safety. Each such inspection shall be commenced and completed with reasonable promptness. In addition to other grounds upon which good cause may be found for purposes of this subsection, good cause will be considered to exist in any case where the manufacturer has introduced into commerce any electronic product which does not comply with an applicable standard prescribed under this subpart and with respect to which no exemption from the notification requirements has been granted by the Secretary under section 359(a)(2) or 359(e)."

(b) "Every manufacturer of electronic products shall establish and maintain such records (including testing records), make such reports, and provide such information, as the Secretary may reasonably require to enable him to determine whether such manufacturer has acted or is acting in compliance with this subpart and standards prescribed pursuant to this subpart and shall, upon request of an officer or employee duly designated by the Secretary, permit such officer or employee to inspect appropriate books, papers, records, and documents relevant to determining whether such manufacturer has acted or is acting in compliance with standards prescribed pursuant to section 359(a)."

******

(f) "The Secretary may by regulation (1) require dealers and distributors of electronic products, to which there are applicable standards prescribed under this subpart and the retail prices of which is not less than $50, to furnish manufacturers of such products such information as may be necessary to identify and locate, for purposes of section 359, the first purchasers of such products for purposes other than resale, and (2) require manufacturers to preserve such information.

FORM FDA 482 (5/85)   PREVIOUS EDITION IS OBSOLETE

NOTICE OF INSPECTION

(Continued On Reverse)

Any regulation establishing a requirement pursuant to clause (1) of the preceding sentence shall (A) authorize such dealers and distributors to elect, in lieu of immediately furnishing such information to the manufacturer to hold and preserve such information until advised by the manufacturer or Secretary that such information is needed by the manufacturer for purposes of section 359, and (B) provide that the dealer or distributor shall, upon making such election, give prompt notice of such election (together with information identifying the notifier and the product) to the manufacturer and shall, when advised by the manufacturer or Secretary, of the need therefor for the purposes of Section 359, immediately furnish the manufacturer with the required information. If a dealer or distributor discontinues the dealing in or distribution of electronic products, he shall turn the information over to the manufacturer. Any manufacturer receiving information pursuant to this subsection concerning first purchasers of products for purposes other than resale shall treat it as confidential and may use it only if necessary for the purpose of notifying persons pursuant to section 359(a)."

Sec. 360 B.(a) It shall be unlawful—
(1) ***
(2) ***
(3) "For any person to fail or to refuse to establish or maintain

records required by this subpart or to permit access by the Secretary or any of his duly authorized representatives to, or the copying of, such records, or to permit entry or inspection, as required by or pursuant to section 360A."
***

Part G — Quarantine and Inspection

Sec. 361(a) "The Surgeon General, with the approval of the Secretary is authorized to make and enforce such regulations as in his judgement are necessary to prevent the introduction, transmission, or spread of communicable diseases from foreign countries into the States or possessions, or from one State or possession into any other State or possession. For purposes of carrying out and enforcing such regulations, the Surgeon General may provide for such inspection, fumigation, disinfection, sanitation, pest extermination, destruction of animals or articles found to be so infected or contaminated as to be sources of dangerous infection to human beings, and other measures, as in his judgement may be necessary."

FIGURE 5.

376

DEPARTMENT OF HEALTH AND HUMAN SERVICES
PUBLIC HEALTH SERVICE
FOOD AND DRUG ADMINISTRATION

1. DISTRICT ADDRESS AND PHONE NO.

TO

2. NAME AND TITLE OF INDIVIDUAL

3. DATE

4. FIRM NAME

5. HOUR   a.m.   p.m.

6. NUMBER AND STREET

7. CITY AND STATE

8. ZIP CODE

Written demand for examination and/or copying of the records required by 21 CFR 113, 21 CFR 114 and 21 CFR 507 is hereby given, pursuant to 21 CFR 108.25(g), 21 CFR 108.35(h) and 21 CFR 508.35(h) for the records described below in order to verify the pH, adequacy of processing, the integrity of container closures, and the coding of the products processed by your firm.

9. RECORDS NECESSARY

NAME FDA EMPLOYEE *(Print or type)*

SIGNATURE

TITLE FDA EMPLOYEE

FORM FDA 482a (6/82) PREVIOUS EDITION IS OBSOLETE.

DEMAND FOR RECORDS

FIGURE 6.

DEPARTMENT OF HEALTH AND HUMAN SERVICES PUBLIC HEALTH SERVICE FOOD AND DRUG ADMINISTRATION	1. DISTRICT ADDRESS AND PHONE NUMBER			

TO

2. NAME AND TITLE OF INDIVIDUAL	3. DATE	
4. FIRM NAME		a.m.
6. NUMBER AND STREET	5. HOUR	p.m.
7. CITY AND STATE	8. ZIP CODE	

Written request is hereby given pursuant to 21 CFR 108.25(c)(3)(ii), 21 CFR 108.35(c)(3)(ii) and 21 CFR 508.35(c)(3)(ii) for the information described below, concerning processes and procedures which is deemed necessary by the Food and Drug Administration to determine the adequacy of the processes for products processed by your firm.

9. INFORMATION NECESSARY

NAME FDA EMPLOYEE *(Print or type)*	SIGNATURE	TITLE FDA EMPLOYEE

FORM FDA 482b (8/82)   PREVIOUS EDITION MAY BE USED.   REQUEST FOR INFORMATION

FIGURE 7.

DEPARTMENT OF HEALTH AND HUMAN SERVICES PUBLIC HEALTH SERVICE FOOD AND DRUG ADMINISTRATION	DISTRICT ADDRESS AND PHONE NUMBER	
NAME OF INDIVIDUAL TO WHOM REPORT ISSUED TO:	PERIOD OF INSPECTION	C. F. NUMBER
TITLE OF INDIVIDUAL	TYPE ESTABLISHMENT INSPECTED	
FIRM NAME	NAME OF FIRM, BRANCH OR UNIT INSPECTED	
STREET ADDRESS	STREET ADDRESS OF PREMISES INSPECTED	
CITY AND STATE *(Zip Code)*	CITY AND STATE *(Zip Code)*	

DURING AN INSPECTION OF YOUR FIRM (I) (WE) OBSERVED:

SEE REVERSE OF THIS PAGE	EMPLOYEE(S) SIGNATURE	EMPLOYEE(S) NAME AND TITLE *(Print or Type)*	DATE ISSUED

FORM FDA 483 (5/85)   PREVIOUS EDITION MAY BE USED.   **INSPECTIONAL OBSERVATIONS** PAGE   OF   PAGES

The observations of objectionable conditions and practices listed on the front of this form are reported:

1. Pursuant to Section 704(b) of the Federal Food, Drug and Cosmetic Act, or

2. To assist firms inspected in complying with the Acts and regulations enforced by the Food and Drug Administration.

Section 704(b) of the Federal Food, Drug, and Cosmetic Act (21 USC 374(b)) provides:

"Upon completion of any such inspection of a factory, warehouse, consulting laboratory, or other establishment, and prior to leaving the premises, the officer or employee making the inspection shall give to the owner, operator, or agent in charge a report in writing setting forth any conditions or practices observed by him which, in his judgement, indicate that any food, drug, device, or cosmetic in such establishment (1) consists in whole or in part of any filthy, putrid, or decomposed substance, or (2) has been prepared, packed, or held under insanitary conditions whereby it may have become contaminated with filth, or whereby it may have been rendered injurious to health. A copy of such report shall be sent promptly to the Secretary."

FIGURE 8.

DEPARTMENT OF HEALTH AND HUMAN SERVICES

PUBLIC HEALTH SERVICE

FOOD AND DRUG ADMINISTRATION

1 DISTRICT ADDRESS & PHONE NUMBER

2 NAME AND TITLE OF INDIVIDUAL	3 DATE	4 SAMPLE NUMBER

5 FIRM NAME	6 FIRM'S DEA NUMBER	7 FDA'S DEA NUMBER

8 NUMBER AND STREET	9 CITY AND STATE (Include Zip Code)

10 SAMPLES COLLECTED (Describe fully. List lot, serial, model numbers and other positive identification)

The following samples were collected by the Food and Drug Administration and receipt is hereby acknowledged pursuant to Section 704(c) of the Federal Food, Drug, and Cosmetic Act [21 U.S.C. 374 (c)] and / or Part F, Sub Part 3, Section 356(b) of The Public Health Service Act [42 U.S.C. 263d] and/or 21 Code of Federal Regulations (CFR) 1307.02. Excerpts of these are quoted on the reverse of this form
(**NOTE**: If you bill FDA for the cost of the Sample(s) listed below, please attach a copy of this form to your bill.)

11 SAMPLES WERE	12 AMOUNT RECEIVED FOR SAMPLE	13 SIGNATURE (Person receiving payment for sample or person providing sample to FDA at no charge)
☐ PROVIDED AT NO CHARGE ☐ PURCHASED ☐ BORROWED (To be returned)	☐ CASH ☐ BILLED ☐ VOUCHER ☐ CREDIT CARD	

14 COLLECTOR'S NAME (Print or Type)	15 COLLECTOR'S TITLE (Print or Type)	16 COLLECTOR'S SIGNATURE

FORM FDA 484 (10/87) PREVIOUS EDITION MAY BE USED   **RECEIPT FOR SAMPLES**   PAGE   OF   PAGES

Section 704(c) of the Federal Food, Drug, and Cosmetic Act [21 U.S.C. 374(c)] is quoted below:

"If the officer or employee making any such inspection of a factory, warehouse, or other establishment has obtained any sample in the course of the inspection, upon completion of the inspection and prior to leaving the premises he shall give to the owner, operator, or agent in charge a receipt describing the samples obtained."

Part F, Sub Part 3, Section 356(b) of The Public Health Service Act [42 U.S.C. 263d] is quoted in part below:

"Section 356(b) In carrying out the purposes of subsection (a), the Secretary is authorized to -
(1) ****
(2) ****
(3) ****
(4) procure (by negotiation or otherwise) electronic products for research and testing purposes, and sell or otherwise dispose of such products "

21 Code of Federal Regulations 1307.02 is quoted below:

"1307.02 Application of State law and other Federal law.
Nothing in Parts 1301-1308, 1311, 1312, or 1316 of this chapter shall be construed as authorizing or permitting any person to do any act which such person is not authorized or permitted to do under other Federal laws or obligations under international treaties, conventions or protocols, or under the law of the State in which he desires to do such act nor shall compliance with such Parts be construed as compliance with other Federal or State laws unless expressly provided in such other laws."

An agreement between the Food and Drug Administration (FDA) and the Drug Enforcement Administration (DEA) provides that in the event any samples of controlled drugs are collected by FDA representatives in the enforcement of the Federal Food, Drug, and Cosmetic Act, the FDA representative shall issue a receipt for such samples on FDA form FDA 484, RECEIPT FOR SAMPLES, in lieu of DEA form 400, to the owner, operator, or agent in charge of the premises

Report of analysis will be furnished only where samples meet the requirements of Section 704(d) of the Federal Food, Drug, and Cosmetic Act [21 U.S.C. 374(d)] which is quoted below:

"Whenever in the course of any such inspection of a factory or other establishment where food is manufactured, processed, or packed, the officer or employee making the inspection obtains a sample of such food, and an analysis is made of such sample for the purpose of ascertaining whether such food consists in whole or in part of any filthy, putrid, or decomposed substance, or is otherwise unfit for food, a copy of the results of such analysis shall be furnished promptly to the owner, operator, or agent in charge."

FIGURE 9.

380

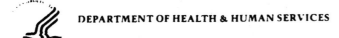

DEPARTMENT OF HEALTH & HUMAN SERVICES   Public Health Service

_____

Food and Drug Administration
Rockville MD 20857

TELEPHONE:

SEIZURE NO(S):

PRODUCT:

Dear Sir:

Order of condemnation and forfeiture, providing for disposition of the above product by you, was entered in this case on

When disposition is accomplished, please provide us with the following information, which may be furnished by filling in the captions on the extra copy of this letter enclosed and returning to this office.

Sincerely yours,

Enclosure:
cc this letter
Self-addressed franked envelope

_____

AMOUNT OF PRODUCT:

DATE OF DISPOSITION

METHOD OF DISPOSITION:

BY WHOM ACCOMPLISHED:

FORM FDA 486 (6/82)

FIGURE 10.

DEPARTMENT OF HEALTH & HUMAN SERVICES

Public Health Service

Food and Drug Administration
Rockville MD 20857

Reference:

SAMPLE NO.

FDC NO.

PRODUCT

Dear Sir:

Please refer to Complaint for Forfeiture which has been filed in the above referenced matter.

As soon as seizure has been effected, we will appreciate your providing us with the following information, which may be furnished by filling in the captions below, on the extra copy of this letter enclosed for that purpose.

Sincerely yours,

Enclosure
cc this letter
Self-addressed franked envelope

DATE SEIZED:

AMOUNT SEIZED:

RETURN DATE (date after which default will be entered):

SEIZED IN POSSESSION OF:

WHERE STORED AFTER SEIZURE:

SEIZED BY _____
U. S. Marshal or Deputy Marshal

FORM FDA 487 (6/82)

FIGURE 11.

NOTICE OF
DETENTION AND HEARING

NOTICE OF DETENTION AND HEARING

Examination of samples or their evidence indicates that the above described shipment as shown below appears to be in violation of the F D & C Act and other related Acts, and the Public Health Service Act. The merchandise should continue to be held intact pending final decision as to whether it shall be admitted or refused admission.

You have the opportunity to appear at the District office of the Food and Drug Administration at the above address to introduce testimony relative to the admissibility of the article or to file a statement in writing, within ten (10) days following the Date of Detention (Saturdays, Sundays, and holidays not included). The testimony which you may present may include evidence as to the manner in which the article can be brought into compliance with the Act or removed from its scope by rendering it not a food, drug, device, or cosmetic as defined by the Act.

DATE OF DETENTION	REASON FOR DETENTION

CONCLUSIONS

Distribution: Importer of Record (Orig)
HFC-131
U S. Customs
District File

FORM FDA 718 (10/88)

_____

Director of District

FIGURE 12.

383

DEPARTMENT OF HEALTH AND HUMAN SERVICES
PUBLIC HEALTH SERVICE
FOOD AND DRUG ADMINISTRATION
INVESTIGATIONAL NEW DRUG APPLICATION (IND)
(TITLE 21, CODE OF FEDERAL REGULATIONS (CFR) Part 312)

Form Approved OMB No 0910-0014.
Expiration Date December 31, 1992
See OMB Statement on Reverse.

NOTE. No drug may be shipped or clinical investigation begun until an IND for that investigation is in effect (21 CFR 312.40)

1. NAME OF SPONSOR	2. DATE OF SUBMISSION
3. ADDRESS *(Number, Street, City, State and Zip Code)*	4. TELEPHONE NUMBER *(Include Area Code)*
5. NAME(S) OF DRUG *(Include all available names Trade Generic, Chemical Code)*	6. IND NUMBER *(If previously assigned)*

7. INDICATION(S) *(Covered by this submission)*

8. PHASE (S) OF CLINICAL INVESTIGATION TO BE CONDUCTED ☐ PHASE 1 ☐ PHASE 2 ☐ PHASE 3 ☐ OTHER _____ *(Specify)*

9. LIST NUMBERS OF ALL INVESTIGATIONAL NEW DRUG APPLICATIONS *(21 CFR Part 312)* NEW DRUG OR ANTIBIOTIC APPLICATIONS *(21 CFR Part 314)* DRUG MASTER FILES *(21 CFR 314.420)*, AND PRODUCT LICENSE APPLICATIONS *(21 CFR Part 601)* REFERRED TO IN THIS APPLICATION

10. IND submissions should be consecutively numbered. The initial IND should be numbered "Serial Number: 000." The next submission (e.g., amendment, report, or correspondence) should be numbered "Serial Number: 001." Subsequent submissions should be numbered consecutively in the order in which they are submitted.

SERIAL NUMBER:
_ _ _

11. THIS SUBMISSION CONTAINS THE FOLLOWING *(Check all that apply)*

☐ INITIAL INVESTIGATIONAL NEW DRUG APPLICATION (IND) ☐ RESPONSE TO CLINICAL HOLD

PROTOCOL AMENDMENT(S).   INFORMATION AMENDMENT(S)   IND SAFETY REPORT(S).

☐ NEW PROTOCOL   ☐ CHEMISTRY/MICROBIOLOGY   ☐ INITIAL WRITTEN REPORT

☐ CHANGE IN PROTOCOL   ☐ PHARMACOLOGY/TOXICOLOGY   ☐ FOLLOW-UP TO A WRITTEN REPORT

☐ NEW INVESTIGATOR   ☐ CLINICAL

☐ RESPONSE TO FDA REQUEST FOR INFORMATION   ☐ ANNUAL REPORT   ☐ GENERAL CORRESPONDENCE

☐ REQUEST FOR REINSTATEMENT OF IND THAT IS WITHDRAWN,   ☐ OTHER _____
INACTIVATED, TERMINATED OR DISCONTINUED   *(Specify)*

CHECK ONLY IF APPLICABLE

JUSTIFICATION STATEMENT MUST BE SUBMITTED WITH APPLICATION FOR ANY CHECKED BELOW. REFER TO THE CITED CFR SECTION FOR FURTHER INFORMATION.

☐ TREATMENT IND 21 CFR 312.35(b) ☐ TREATMENT PROTOCOL 21 CFR 312.35(a) ☐ CHARGE REQUEST/NOTIFICATION 21 CFR 312.7(d)

FOR FDA USE ONLY

CDR/DBIND/OGD RECEIPT STAMP	DDR RECEIPT STAMP	IND NUMBER ASSIGNED:
		DIVISION ASSIGNMENT.

FORM FDA 1571 (6 92)   PREVIOUS EDITION IS OBSOLETE

FIGURE 13.

384

CONTENTS OF APPLICATION

This application contains the following items: (check all that apply)

☐ 1 Form FDA 1571 [21 CFR 312.23 (a) (1)]

☐ 2.Table of contents [21 CFR 312.23 (a) (2)]

☐ 3. Introductory statement [21 CFR 312.23 (a) (3)]

☐ 4. General investigational plan [21 CFR 312.23 (a) (3)]

☐ 5. Investigator's brochure [21 CFR 312.23 (a) (5)]

6. Protocol(s) [21 CFR 312.23 (a) (6)]

    ☐ a. Study protocol(s) [21 CFR 312.23 (a) (6)]

    ☐ b. Investigator data [21 CFR 312.23 (a) (6)(iii)(b)] or completed Form(s) FDA 1572

    ☐ c. Facilities data [21 CFR 312.23 (a) (6)(iii)(b)] or completed Form(s) FDA 1572

    ☐ d. Institutional Review Board data [21 CFR 312.23 (a) (6)(iii)(b)] or completed Form(s) FDA 1572

☐ 7. Chemistry, manufacturing, and control data [21 CFR 312.23 (a) (7)]

    ☐ Environmental assessment or claim for exclusion [21 CFR 312.23 (a) (7)(iv)(e)]

☐ 8. Pharmacology and toxicology data [21 CFR 312.23 (a) (8)]

☐ 9. Previous human experience [21 CFR 312.23 (a) (9)]

☐ 10. Additional information [21 CFR 312.23 (a) (10)]

---

13 IS ANY PART OF THE CLINICAL STUDY TO BE CONDUCTED BY A CONTRACT RESEARCH ORGANIZATION? ☐ YES   ☐ NO

IF YES, WILL ANY SPONSOR OBLIGATIONS BE TRANSFERRED TO THE CONTRACT RESEARCH ORGANIZATION? ☐ YES   ☐ NO

IF YES, ATTACH A STATEMENT CONTAINING THE NAME AND ADDRESS OF THE CONTRACT RESEARCH ORGANIZATION, IDENTIFICATION OF THE CLINICAL STUDY, AND A LISTING OF THE OBLIGATIONS TRANSFERRED

---

14 NAME AND TITLE OF THE PERSON RESPONSIBLE FOR MONITORING THE CONDUCT AND PROGRESS OF THE CLINICAL INVESTIGATIONS

---

15 NAME(S) AND TITLE(S) OF THE PERSON(S) RESPONSIBLE FOR REVIEW AND EVALUATION OF INFORMATION RELEVANT TO THE SAFETY OF THE DRUG

I agree not to begin clinical investigations until 30 days after FDA's receipt of the IND unless I receive earlier notification by FDA that the studies may begin. I also agree not to begin or continue clinical investigations covered by the IND if those studies are placed on clinical hold. I agree that an Institutional Review Board (IRB) that complies with the requirements set forth in 21 CFR Part 56 will be responsible for the initial and continuing review and approval of each of the studies in the proposed clinical investigation. I agree to conduct the investigation in accordance with all other applicable regulatory requirements.

---

16 NAME OF SPONSOR OR SPONSOR'S AUTHORIZED REPRESENTATIVE	17 SIGNATURE OF SPONSOR OR SPONSOR'S AUTHORIZED REPRESENTATIVE	
18 ADDRESS (Number, Street, City, State and Zip Code)	19 TELEPHONE NUMBER (Include Area Code)	20 DATE

(WARNING: A willfully false statement is a criminal offense U.S.C. Title 18, Sec 1001)

FIGURE 13 (continued).

DEPARTMENT OF HEALTH AND HUMAN SERVICES
PUBLIC HEALTH SERVICE
FOOD AND DRUG ADMINISTRATION
STATEMENT OF INVESTIGATOR
(TITLE 21, CODE OF FEDERAL REGULATIONS (CFR) Part 312)
(See instructions on reverse side.)

Form Approved: OMB No. 0910-0014
Expiration Date: November 30, 1990
See OMB Statement on Reverse.

NOTE: No investigator may participate in an investigation until he/she provides the sponsor with a completed, signed Statement of Investigator, Form FDA 1572 (21 CFR 312 53(c))

1. NAME AND ADDRESS OF INVESTIGATOR.

2. EDUCATION, TRAINING, AND EXPERIENCE THAT QUALIFIES THE INVESTIGATOR AS AN EXPERT IN THE CLINICAL INVESTIGATION OF THE DRUG FOR THE USE UNDER INVESTIGATION. ONE OF THE FOLLOWING IS ATTACHED:

☐ CURRICULUM VITAE   ☐ OTHER STATEMENT OF QUALIFICATIONS

3. NAME AND ADDRESS OF ANY MEDICAL SCHOOL, HOSPITAL, OR OTHER RESEARCH FACILITY WHERE THE CLINICAL INVESTIGATION(S) WILL BE CONDUCTED.

4. NAME AND ADDRESS OF ANY CLINICAL LABORATORY FACILITIES TO BE USED IN THE STUDY.

5. NAME AND ADDRESS OF THE INSTITUTIONAL REVIEW BOARD (IRB) THAT IS RESPONSIBLE FOR REVIEW AND APPROVAL OF THE STUDY(IES).

6. NAMES OF THE SUBINVESTIGATORS *(e.g., research fellows, residents, associates)* WHO WILL BE ASSISTING THE INVESTIGATOR IN THE CONDUCT OF THE INVESTIGATION(S).

7. NAME AND CODE NUMBER, IF ANY, OF THE PROTOCOL(S) IN THE IND FOR THE STUDY(IES) TO BE CONDUCTED BY THE INVESTIGATOR.

FORM FDA 1572 (7/90)   PREVIOUS EDITION IS OBSOLETE.

FIGURE 14.

8. ATTACH THE FOLLOWING CLINICAL PROTOCOL INFORMATION:

☐ FOR PHASE 1 INVESTIGATIONS, A GENERAL OUTLINE OF THE PLANNED INVESTIGATION INCLUDING THE ESTIMATED DURATION OF THE STUDY AND THE MAXIMUM NUMBER OF SUBJECTS THAT WILL BE INVOLVED.

☐ FOR PHASE 2 OR 3 INVESTIGATIONS, AN OUTLINE OF THE STUDY PROTOCOL INCLUDING AN APPROXIMATION OF THE NUMBER OF SUBJECTS TO BE TREATED WITH THE DRUG AND THE NUMBER TO BE EMPLOYED AS CONTROLS, IF ANY; THE CLINICAL USES TO BE INVESTIGATED; CHARACTERISTICS OF SUBJECTS BY AGE, SEX, AND CONDITION; THE KIND OF CLINICAL OBSERVATIONS AND LABORATORY TESTS TO BE CONDUCTED; THE ESTIMATED DURATION OF THE STUDY; AND COPIES OR A DESCRIPTION OF CASE REPORT FORMS TO BE USED.

9. COMMITMENTS:

I agree to conduct the study(ies) in accordance with the relevant, current protocol(s) and will only make changes in a protocol after notifying the sponsor, except when necessary to protect the safety, rights, or welfare of subjects.

I agree to personally conduct or supervise the described investigation(s).

I agree to inform any patients, or any persons used as controls, that the drugs are being used for investigational purposes and I will ensure that the requirements relating to obtaining informed consent in 21 CFR Part 50 and institutional review board (IRB) review and approval in 21 CFR Part 56 are met.

I agree to report to the sponsor adverse experiences that occur in the course of the investigation(s) in accordance with 21 CFR 312.64.

I have read and understand the information in the investigator's brochure, including the potential risks and side effects of the drug.

I agree to ensure that all associates, colleagues, and employees assisting in the conduct of the study(ies) are informed about their obligations in meeting the above commitments.

I agree to maintain adequate and accurate records in accordance with 21 CFR 312.62 and to make those records available for inspection in accordance with 21 CFR 312.68.

I will ensure that an IRB that complies with the requirements of 21 CFR Part 56 will be responsible for the initial and continuing review and approval of the clinical investigation. I also agree to promptly report to the IRB all changes in the research activity and all unanticipated problems involving risks to human subjects or others. Additionally, I will not make any changes in the research without IRB approval, except where necessary to eliminate apparent immediate hazards to human subjects.

I agree to comply with all other requirements regarding the obligations of clinical investigators and all other pertinent requirements in 21 CFR Part 312.

INSTRUCTIONS FOR COMPLETING FORM FDA 1572
STATEMENT OF INVESTIGATOR:

1. Complete all sections. Attach a separate page if additional space is needed.

2. Attach curriculum vitae or other statement of qualifications as described in Section 2.

3. Attach protocol outline as described in Section 8.

4. Sign and date below.

5. FORWARD THE COMPLETED FORM AND ATTACHMENTS TO THE SPONSOR. The sponsor will incorporate this information along with other technical data into an Investigational New Drug Application (IND). INVESTIGATORS SHOULD NOT SEND THIS FORM DIRECTLY TO THE FOOD AND DRUG ADMINISTRATION.

10. SIGNATURE OF INVESTIGATOR	11. DATE

Public reporting burden for this collection of information is estimated to average 1 hour per response, including the time for reviewing instructions, searching existing data sources, gathering and maintaining the data needed, and completing reviewing the collection of information. Send comments regarding this burden estimate or any other aspect of this collection of information, including suggestions for reducing this burden to:

Reports Clearance Officer, PHS
Hubert H. Humphrey Building, Room 721-B
200 Independence Avenue, S.W.
Washington, DC 20201
Attn: PRA

and to:

Office of Management and Budget
Paperwork Reduction Project (0910-0014)
Washington, DC 20503

⋆ U.S. Government Printing Office: 1990-261-200/13866

FIGURE 14 (continued).

DEPARTMENT OF HEALTH AND HUMAN SERVICES
PUBLIC HEALTH SERVICE
FOOD AND DRUG ADMINISTRATION (HFD-730)
ROCKVILLE, MD 20857

Form Approved OMB No. 0910-0230
See OMB Statement on the Reverse

FDA
CONTROL NO

ADVERSE REACTION REPORT
(Drugs and Biologics)

ACCESSION
NO

I. REACTION INFORMATION

1. PATIENT ID / INITIALS (In Confidence)	2. AGE YRS	3. SEX	4-6 REACTION ONSET			8-12 CHECK ALL APPROPRIATE
			MO	DA	YR	☐ PATIENT DIED

7. DESCRIBE REACTION(S)

☐ REACTION TREATED WITH R$_x$ DRUG
☐ RESULTED IN, OR PROLONGED, INPATIENT HOSPITALIZATION
☐ RESULTED IN PERMANENT DISABILITY

13. RELEVANT TESTS/LABORATORY DATA

☐ NONE OF THE ABOVE

II. SUSPECT DRUG(S) INFORMATION

14. SUSPECT DRUG(S) (Give manufacturer and lot no. for vaccines/biologics)

20. DID REACTION ABATE AFTER STOPPING DRUG?
☐ YES   ☐ NO   ☐ NA

15. DAILY DOSE	16. ROUTE OF ADMINISTRATION

17. INDICATION(S) FOR USE

21. DID REACTION REAPPEAR AFTER REINTRODUCTION?

18. DATES OF ADMINISTRATION (From/To)	19. DURATION OF ADMINISTRATION

☐ YES   ☐ NO   ☐ NA

III. CONCOMITANT DRUGS AND HISTORY

22. CONCOMITANT DRUGS AND DATES OF ADMINISTRATION (Exclude those used to treat reaction)

23. OTHER RELEVANT HISTORY (e.g. diagnoses, allergies, pregnancy with LMP, etc.)

IV. ONLY FOR REPORTS SUBMITTED BY MANUFACTURER	**V.** INITIAL REPORTER (In confidence)
24. NAME AND ADDRESS OF MANUFACTURER (Include Zip Code)	26.-26a. NAME AND ADDRESS OF REPORTER (Include Zip Code)

24a. IND/NDA NO. FOR SUSPECT DRUG	24b. MFR CONTROL NO.	26b. TELEPHONE NO. (Include area code)

24c. DATE RECEIVED BY MANUFACTURER	24d. REPORT SOURCE (Check all that apply) ☐ FOREIGN ☐ STUDY ☐ LITERATURE ☐ HEALTH PROFESSIONAL ☐ CONSUMER	26c. HAVE YOU ALSO REPORTED THIS REACTION TO THE MANUFACTURER? ☐ YES ☐ NO

25. 15 DAY REPORT? ☐ YES ☐ NO	25a. REPORT TYPE ☐ INITIAL ☐ FOLLOWUP	26d. ARE YOU A HEALTH PROFESSIONAL? ☐ YES ☐ NO	Submission of a report does not necessarily constitute an admission that the drug caused the adverse reaction.

NOTE: Required of manufacturers by 21 CFR 314.80

FORM FDA 1639 (12/91)   PREVIOUS EDITION MAY BE USED

FIGURE 15.

INSTRUCTIONS FOR COMPLETING FORM FDA - 1639

REPORTING ADVERSE REACTIONS TO FDA

All health care providers who observe *suspect* reactions to drugs or biologics are encouraged to report these to FDA. Serious reactions, observations of events not described in the package insert, and reactions to newly marketed products are of particular importance.

GENERAL

- Use a separate Form FDA-1639 for each patient.
- Additional pages may be attached if space provided on the Form FDA-1639 is inadequate.
- For questions call: 301-443-4580
- Patient and initial reporter identification is held in confidence by the FDA

SPECIFIC INSTRUCTIONS

I. Reaction Information
- Item 2. Age—For children under 5 years of age, also write date of birth (DOB) in Item 1. For congenital malformations, give the age and sex of the infant (even though the mother was exposed).
- Item 7. Describe Reaction(s)—Give signs and/or symptoms, diagnoses, course, etc.
- Item 13. Relevant Tests/Laboratory Data—Both pre- and post-drug values should be provided if known.

II. Suspect Drug Information
- Item 14. Suspect Drug—The trade name is preferred. If a generically produced product is involved, the manufacturer should be identified.
- Item 15. Dose—For pediatric patients, also give body weights.
- Item 20 and 21. NA—is defined as nonapplicable (*e.g. when only one dose given or outcome was irreversible*).

V. Initial Reporter
- Item 26c. Have you also reported this reaction to the manufacturer? Your answer facilitates identification of duplicates in the central adverse reaction file. FDA encourages direct reporting even if a report has been submitted to the manufacturer.

NOTE TO MANUFACTURERS *(Refer to 21 CFR 314.80 and 21 CFR 310.305).* Detailed instructions are contained in the "Guideline for Postmarketing Reporting of Adverse Drug Reactions."

Public reporting burden for this collection of information is estimated to average 5 hours per response, including the time for review instructions, searching existing data sources, gathering and maintaining the data needed, and completing and reviewing the collection of information. Send comments regarding this burden estimate or any other aspect of this collection of information, including suggestions for reducing this burden to:

Reports Clearance Officer, PHS
Hubert H. Humphrey Building, Room 721-B
200 Independence Avenue, S.W.
Washington, DC 20201
Attn: PRA

and to:

Office of Management and Budget
Paperwork Reduction Project (0910-0230)
Washington, DC 20503

Please DO NOT RETURN your questionnaire to either of these addresses.

After completing the form on the other side of this sheet, please triple fold, seal with tape, and mail to address shown below.
No postage is necessary.

**DEPARTMENT OF
HEALTH & HUMAN SERVICES**

Public Health Service
Food and Drug Administration
Rockville MD 20857

Official Business
Penalty for Private Use $300

NO POSTAGE
NECESSARY
IF MAILED
IN THE
UNITED STATES

BUSINESS REPLY MAIL

FIRST CLASS MAIL   PERMIT NO. 946   ROCKVILLE MD

POSTAGE WILL BE PAID BY ADDRESSEE

Food and Drug Administration
Division of Epidemiology and Surveillance (HFD-730)
Public Health Service
5600 Fishers Lane
Rockville MD 20852-9787

FIGURE 15 (continued).

TRANSMITTAL OF ANNUAL REPORTS FOR DRUGS FOR HUMAN USE (21 CFR 314.81)	DATE SUBMITTED	Form Approved: OMB No 0910-0001 Expiration Date: November 30, 1990 See Reverse for OMB Statement on Part 1

NOTE: This report is required by law (21 USC 355; 21 CFR 314.81). Failure to report can result in withdrawal of approval of the New Drug Application.

1 NDA OR ANDA NUMBER

N

INSTRUCTIONS

Complete a transmittal form for each application for which an annual report is being submitted. Retain the carbon copy labeled "applicant." Submit the remaining copies of the transmittal form along with two copies of the annual report to FDA.

If any part of the annual report applies to more than one application, list in item 7 all other applications to which such parts apply.

2. Report No. (FDA Complete)

Y-

APPLICANT NOTE
Reference NDA and Y numbers (entered on Acknowledgement Copy) in any subsequent correspondence regarding report.

4. APPLICANT

3. CFR SECTION NUMBER (Antibiotic only)

5. DRUG NAME

6. TYPE OF REPORT (Check one)
☐ ANNUAL   ☐ OTHER

7. OTHER NDA/ANTIBIOTIC APPLICATION NUMBERS (List all numbers if any part of report applies to more than one number.)

8. PERIOD COVERED BY REPORT

FROM		TO	
YEAR	MONTH	YEAR	MONTH

Fold Line

9. REPORT INFORMATION REQUIRED (See § 314.81 for description)
(Enter type of information attached under "Identification." If you have nothing to report, enter None.)
(INFORMATION IN "9b" and "9c" IS ALWAYS REQUIRED.)

TYPE OF INFORMATION	IDENTIFICATION (Volume No.(s)/Tab(s)/Page(s) of Report)
a. SUMMARY OF SIGNIFICANT NEW INFORMATION	
b. DISTRIBUTION DATA	
c. LABELING (Whether or not previously submitted)	
d. CHEMISTRY MANUFACTURING AND CONTROLS CHANGES	
e. NONCLINICAL LABORATORY STUDIES	
f. CLINICAL DATA	
g. STATUS REPORT POST-MARKETING STUDIES	
h. STATUS OF OPEN REGULATORY BUSINESS (Optional)	

Fold Line

TYPED NAME AND TITLE OF RESPONSIBLE OFFICIAL OR AGENT

FDA USE ONLY

10. REPORT FILED IN NDA NUMBER

N

SIGNATURE

11. DATE OF RECEIPT

APPLICANTS RETURN ADDRESS (Type within the window envelope tic marks)

FORM FDA 2252 (8/90)   PREVIOUS EDITION IS OBSOLETE.

FIGURE 16.

| TRANSMITTAL OF ADVERTISEMENTS AND PROMOTIONAL LABELING FOR DRUGS FOR HUMAN USE | 1. DATE SUBMITTED | Form Approved. OMB No. 0910-0001
Expiration Date: March 31, 1990.
See OMB Statement on Reverse of Part 1 |

	2. NDA NO	1	2	3	4	5	6
		N					

NOTE: This form is required by law (21 CFR 314.81). Failure to report can result in withdrawal of approval of NDA or Antibiotic Application.

INSTRUCTIONS

1. Submit a separate form (parts 1 through 3) for each NDA or Antibiotic Application for which advertisement or promotional labeling material is submitted.
2. Attach two copies of each piece of material to the form.
3. Enter in Column C the total number of types (not copies) of material submitted.
4. Forward form and attachments to Department of Health and Human Services, Food and Drug Administration (HFD-240), 5600 Fishers Lane, Rockville, Maryland 20857.

3. APPLICANT

4. DRUG NAME

5. ADVERTISEMENT/PROMOTIONAL LABELING MATERIAL

TYPE a.	DATE OF ISSUANCE b.	NUMBER c.	IDENTIFICATION (Use code or other designation. If necessary; continue on an 8 1/2 x 11" sheet.) d.
JOURNAL ADVERTISEMENT(S)			
PROMOTIONAL LABELING			
BROCHURE(S) LEAFLET(S)			
FILE CARD(S)			
HOUSE ORGAN(S)			
PRICE LIST(S)			
PHYSICIANS SAMPLE(S)			
PROMOTIONAL LETTER(S)			
LITERATURE REPRINT(S)			
OTHER (Audio-Visual material (films, tapes, etc.) or typed scripts of such material).			
LABELING ON WHICH THE ABOVE IS BASED (Include currently approved labeling with each submission)			
PACKAGE INSERT(S)			
OTHER LABELING (If no package insert(s) exists)			

6. TYPED NAME AND TITLE OF RESPONSIBLE OFFICIAL OR AGENT	7. SIGNATURE

8. APPLICANTS RETURN ADDRESS (Begin typing address directly below window dot)	9. FDA ACKNOWLEDGEMENT
•	

FORM FDA 2253 (10/89)

FIGURE 17.

391

Form Approved OMB No 0910-0045 Expiration Date September 30, 1992 See OMB Statement on Reverse.

DEPARTMENT OF HEALTH AND HUMAN SERVICES
PUBLIC HEALTH SERVICE
FOOD AND DRUG ADMINISTRATION
REGISTRATION OF DRUG ESTABLISHMENT
(In accordance with Public Law 92-387)

RECORD
PURPOSE OF FORM
☐ REGISTRANT
☐ DISTRIBUTOR ONLY
☐ FOREIGN COUNTRY

FOR FDA USE
CONTROL NO.
REPORT DATE MO. DA YR
FDA VALIDATION

REPORTING FIRM NAME
FULL NAME

ESTABLISHMENT REGISTRATION NO.
BUSINESS TYPE
C-HUMAN
V-VETERINARY
REASONS FOR SUBMISSION
NDC LABELER CODE

SHORT NAME

SITE ADDRESS
NUMBER AND STREET
CITY STATE ZIP CODE FOREIGN COUNTRY

MAILING ADDRESS (If different from site address)
NUMBER AND STREET
CITY STATE ZIP CODE FOREIGN COUNTRY

PARENT COMPANY (If any)
FULL NAME
SHORT NAME
PARENT ESTAB REG NO.

NAME OF PERSON SUBMITTING DATA
AREA CODE AND PHONE NO.

COMPLETE ITEMS WITHIN HEAVILY RULED BOX FOR REGISTRATION ONLY
NAME OF OWNER, OR NAMES AND TITLES OF PARTNERS CORPORATE OFFICERS; DIRECTORS OR BOARD OF MANAGEMENT MEMBERS
LAST NAME FI MI TITLE

OTHER FIRM NAMES USED BY REPORTING ESTABLISHMENT IN DRUG HANDLING ACTIVITIES AT SITE ADDRESS
FULL NAME
SHORT NAME

RECORD ID NO. HT OTHER LABELER CODE

SIGNATURE OF DISTRIBUTOR
SIGNATURE OF AUTHORIZING OFFICIAL
TITLE

CERTIFICATION: Signature is required if certification is being made to the registered establishments that data on products with these labeler codes are being furnished to Food and Drug Administration by private label distribution.

FORM FDA 2656 (3/92) PREVIOUS EDITION IS OBSOLETE.

NOTICE: This report is required by law (21 C.F.R. 207.20). Failure to report can result in imprisonment for not more than one year and/or a fine of not more than $1,000, or both. (FD&C Act, Section 303.)

PAGE OF PAGES.

Public reporting burden for this collection of information is estimated to average 30 minutes per response, including the time for reviewing instructions, searching existing data sources, gathering and maintaining the data needed, and completing and reviewing the collection of information. Send comments regarding this burden estimate or any other aspect of this collection of information, including suggestions for reducing this burden to:

Reports Clearance Officer, PHS
Hubert H. Humphrey Building, Room 721-B
200 Independence Avenue, S.W.
Washington, DC 20201
Attn. PRA

and to:

Office of Management and Budget
Paperwork Reduction Project (0910-0045)
Washington, DC 20503

Please DO NOT RETURN your questionnaire to either of these addresses.

Form Approved: OMB No. 0910-0045. Expiration Date: December 31, 1990. See OMB Statement on Reverse.

DEPARTMENT OF HEALTH AND HUMAN SERVICES
PUBLIC HEALTH SERVICE
FOOD AND DRUG ADMINISTRATION
DRUG PRODUCT LISTING
(In accordance with Public Law 92-387)

NAME AND ADDRESS OF FIRM

LABELING REVISION
CHANGE OF:
☐ RTE OF ADMIN ☐ INDICATION
☐ NAME/DOSE/STR/ INGR
☐ OTHER (Specify)

FOR FDA USE | CONTROL NO. | RECORD ID

SEC	S	U	PRODUCT TRADE NAME OR CATALOG NAME	NATIONAL DRUG CODE: LABELER	PRODUCT
0 1					

FDA APPLICATION NO.	REPORT DATE: MO	DA	YR	TYPE RPRT	TYPES OF BUSINESS: OTHER (Specify)	PRODUCT TYPE: OTHER (Specify)	BNDD	LEGAL STATUS	SCHED	PROF USE	PRODUCT DISCONTINUED: OTHER (Specify)	BASIS OF CONCENTRATION: WHOLE NUMBERS	DECIMAL	UNIT

DOSAGE FORM	ROUTES OF ADMINISTRATION: 1	2	3	OTH	PT	SEC	S	U	SMPL	PKG CODE	PACKAGE SIZE	PACKAGE TYPE
						0 3						
						0 3						
						0 3						
						0 3						
						0 3						

INITIAL MARKETING DATE: MO	YEAR	MOST RECENT MARKETING DATE: MO	YEAR	DISCONTINUED DATE: MO	YEAR

NOTICE. This report is required by law (21 C.F.R. 207.20). Failure to report can result in imprisonment for not more than one year or a fine of not more than $1,000, or both. (FD&C Act, Section 303).

SEC	S	U	TYPE	PT	ESTABLISHED NAME OF PRODUCT AND/OR INGREDIENT(S) OR BIOLOGIC PROPER NAME, TEST OBJECTIVE/EQUIPMENT/REAGENT NAME, ETC.	FDA USE ONLY: INGREDIENT NO.	AMOUNT: WHOLE NUMBER	DECIMAL	UNIT
0 5									
0 5									
0 5									
0 5									
0 5									
0 5									
0 5									
0 5									
0 5									
0 5									

SEC	S	U	SITE OR FIRM ESTABLISHMENT REG NO.	MANUFACTURING SITE NAME OR REGISTERED FIRM NAME	STATE	FOREIGN COUNTRY	NDC LABELER CODE	SHORT NAME
0 7								
0 7								
0 7								

FORM FDA 2657 (7/90) **Previous edition is obsolete.**

PAGE OF PAGES.

Public reporting burden for this collection of information is estimated to average 30 minutes per response, including the time for reviewing instructions, searching existing data sources, gathering and maintaining the data needed, and completing and reviewing the collection of information. Send comments regarding this burden estimate or any other aspect of this collection of information, including suggestions for reducing this burden to:

Reports Clearance Officer, PHS
Hubert H. Humphrey Building, Room 721-B
200 Independence Avenue, S.W.
Washington, DC 20201
Attn: PRA

and to:

Office of Management and Budget
Paperwork Reduction Project (0910-0045)
Washington, DC 20503

Please DO NOT RETURN your questionnaire to either of these addresses

*U.S. Government Printing Office: 1990-261-200/11961

FIGURE 19.

Form Approved: OMB No. 0910–0045. Expiration Date: May 31, 1986.

DEPARTMENT OF HEALTH AND HUMAN SERVICES
PUBLIC HEALTH SERVICE
FOOD AND DRUG ADMINISTRATION
REGISTERED ESTABLISHMENTS' REPORT OF PRIVATE LABEL DISTRIBUTORS

FOR FDA USE — CONTROL NO. (4–9)

REPORTING FIRM — NAME (As shown on Form FD 2656, Line 2, Columns 61-100) 272/27 … 311 | ESTABLISHMENT REGISTRATION NO. 312/20 … 318 | REPORTING FIRM NDC CODE: LABELER 251/79 … 256, PRODUCT

LINE						
2	SITE ADDRESS — NUMBER AND STREET 101 … 138	CITY 139 … 158	STATE 159	ZIP CODE 161 … 165	FOREIGN COUNTRY 166 … 175	RPRT DATE MO YR 14/100
3	MAILING ADDRESS (If different than Line 2) — NUMBER AND STREET 176 … 213	CITY 214 … 233	STATE 234	ZIP CODE 236 … 240	FOREIGN COUNTRY 241 … 250	

LINE						
4	RECORD ID (4, 11 12, 15)	SEC 16 17: 0 1	S 18	U 19	TRADE NAME OR ESTABLISHED NAME UNDER WHICH PRODUCT IS MARKETED BY ANOTHER FIRM 20 … 83	
5	NDC CODE — LABELER 40/84, PRODUCT 90 … 93	SHORT NAME 46 … 60	FIRM NAME ON LABEL 61 … 100	SEC 16 17: 0 3	PACKAGE CODE 1 2 3 4 5 (21 22 21 21 21 21)	ZIP CODE
6	RECORD ID (4, 11 12, 15)	SEC 16 17: 0 1	S 18	U 19	TRADE NAME OR ESTABLISHED NAME UNDER WHICH PRODUCT IS MARKETED BY ANOTHER FIRM 20 … 83	
7	NDC CODE — LABELER 40/84, PRODUCT 90 … 93	SHORT NAME 46 … 60	FIRM NAME ON LABEL 61 … 100	SEC 16 17: 0 3	PACKAGE CODE 1 2 3 4 5 (21 21 21 21 21)	ZIP CODE
8	RECORD ID (4, 11 12, 15)	SEC 16 17: 0 1	S 18	U 19	TRADE NAME OR ESTABLISHED NAME UNDER WHICH PRODUCT IS MARKETED BY ANOTHER FIRM 20 … 83	
9	NDC CODE — LABELER 40/84, PRODUCT 90 … 93	SHORT NAME 46 … 60	FIRM NAME ON LABEL 61 … 100	SEC 16 17: 0 3	PACKAGE CODE 1 2 3 4 5 (21 21 21 21 21)	ZIP CODE
10	RECORD ID (4, 11 12, 15)	SEC 16 17: 0 1	S 18	U 19	TRADE NAME OR ESTABLISHED NAME UNDER WHICH PRODUCT IS MARKETED BY ANOTHER FIRM 20 … 83	
11	NDC CODE — LABELER 40/84, PRODUCT 90 … 93	SHORT NAME 46 … 60	FIRM NAME ON LABEL 61 … 100	SEC 16 17: 0 3	PACKAGE CODE 1 2 3 4 5 (21 21 21 21 21)	ZIP CODE

FORM FDA 2658 (6/83) PREVIOUS EDITION IS OBSOLETE. PAGE OF PAGES.

NOTICE. This report is required by law (21 C.F.R. 207.20). Failure to report can result in imprisonment for not more than one year or a fine of not more than $1,000 or both. (FD&C Act, Section 303).

FIGURE 20.

DEPARTMENT OF HEALTH & HUMAN SERVICES

Memorandum

Date _____ FDA No._____

From   Medical Products Quality Assurance Staff (HFO - 26)

Subject   Drug Product Complaint

To   Bureau of_____ , HF_____

The attached complaint has been forwarded to us by

☐   This complaint does not appear to warrant immediate bureau investigation under existing GWQAP policy. We will respond to the complaining agency unless you advise us by COB_____that immediate bureau evaluation is appropriate.

Please inform us if any future bureau investigation of this complaint discloses adverse findings regarding the product and/or firm.

☐   This complaint warrants immediate evaluation by the bureau under existing GWQAP policy.

Please provide your preliminary or final evaluation by COB_____. The evaluation should comment on the suitability of the product for continued use. A preliminary response should also indicate any inspectional/analytical follow-up required, and whether the offending lot (s) should be suspended pending final evaluation.

REMARKS: _____

_____

_____

_____

_____

_____

_____

_____

                                       Drug Section
                                       Medical Products Quality Assurance Staff

cc: Complaint File
      Monitor

FORM FDA 2887a (5/82)

FIGURE 21.

395

1. RECALL INFORMATION

a RECALL NUMBER

b RECALLING ESTABLISHMENT

c RECALLED CODE(S)

d PRODUCT

2. PROGRAM DATA (CHECK BOX IF PREVIOUSLY SUBMITTED)
(DO NOT COMPLETE IF REPORTED UNDER FDA 2123.)

a. ACCOMP DISTRICT CODE	b HOME DISTRICT CODE	c. OPERATION CODE	d. OPERATION DATE		
			MO	DA	YR
			17		

e. CENTRAL FILE NUMBER OF RECALLING ESTABLISHMENT

f PAC CODE

g. EMPLOYEE			h. TYPE	# OF CHECKS	HOURS
HOME DIST.	POS. CLASS	NUMBER	VISITS		
			PHONE		

3. AUDIT ACCOUNTS

a DIRECT

PHONE NO _____

b. SUB-ACCOUNT (SECONDARY)

PHONE NO _____

c. SUB-ACCOUNT (TERTIARY)

PHONE NO _____

4. CONSIGNEE DATA   Contacted by:
☐ Phone   ☐ Visit   ☐ Other

a. NAME OF PERSON CONTACTED, TITLE, & DATE

b. TYPE CONSIGNEE
☐ Wholesaler   ☐ Physcian
☐ Retailer   ☐ Hospital   ☐ Other _____
☐ Processor   ☐ Pharmacy
☐ Consumer   ☐ Restaurant

c. DOES (DID) THE CONSIGNEE HANDLE RECALLED PRODUCT?
☐ YES   ☐ NO

5. NOTIFICATION DATA

a. FORMAL RECALL NOTICE RECEIVED?
(IF "NO" SKIP TO ITEM 6c)
☐ YES   ☐ NO   ☐ CANNOT BE DETERMINED

b. RECALL NOTIFICATION RECEIVED FROM:
☐ Recalling Firm
☐ Direct Account
☐ Sub-Account
☐ Other (Specify) _____

c. DATE NOTIFIED

d. TYPE OF NOTICE RECEIVED (e.g. letter, phone)

6. ACTION AND STATUS DATA

a DID CONSIGNEE FOLLOW THE RECALL INSTRUCTIONS? (IF "NO" DISCUSS IN ITEM 10 ACTION TAKEN UPON FDA CONTACT)
☐ YES   ☐ NO

b. AMOUNT OF RECALLED PRODUCT ON HAND AT TIME OF NOTIFICATION

c. CURRENT STATUS OF RECALLED ITEMS
☐ Returned   ☐ Destroyed
☐ Corrected   ☐ None on Hand
☐ Was Still Held For Sale/Use *
☐ Held For Return/Correction*
   * = Ensure Proper Quarantine/Action

d. DATE AND METHOD OF DISPOSITION

7. SUB-RECALL NEEDED?
Did Consignee Distribute to any other Accounts? (If "Yes" give Details in "Remarks" or Memo)
☐ YES   ☐ NO

8. AMOUNT OF RECALLED PRODUCT NOW ON HAND.

9. INJURIES/COMPLAINTS

IS CONSIGNEE AWARE OF ANY INJURIES, ILLNESS, OR COMPLAINTS?

☐ INJURY   ☐ COMPLAINT
☐ ILLNESS   ☐ NONE

IF ANSWER IS OTHER THAN "NONE" REPORT DETAILS IN A SEPARATE MEMO TO MONITORING DISTRICT AND COPY TO E.O.8 (HFC-162)

10. REMARKS (INCLUDE ACTION TAKEN IF PRODUCT WAS STILL AVAILABLE FOR SALE OR USE)

SIGNATURE OF CSO/CSI

DISTRICT

DATE OF CHECK

TO

DATE

SIGNATURE OF SCSO OR R&E COORDINATOR

ENDORSEMENT

FORM FDA 3177 (11/91)

RECALL AUDIT CHECK REPORT

*U.S.GPO:1991-0-312-208/41641

FIGURE 22.

396

Drug Quality Reporting System

DQRS

OMB# 0910-0024 2/29/92

DATE RECEIVED

1. PRODUCT NAME, DOSAGE FORM, STRENGTH, SIZE	**NDC** *(PLEASE PROVIDE, IF AVAILABLE)*

LABELER NO.	PRODUCT NO.	PKG. NO.

2. LOT NUMBER(S) AND EXPIRATION DATE(S)

3. NAME AND ADDRESS OF MANUFACTURER	4. NAME AND ADDRESS OF DISTRIBUTOR/LABELER

5. REPORTER'S NAME (Please print or type)	PROFESSION

6. PRACTICE LOCATION: NAME, ADDRESS, AND ZIP CODE   TELEPHONE NUMBER, AND AREA CODE

7. PROBLEM(S) NOTED OR SUSPECTED

NOTE: This is a voluntary reporting program authorized under Chapter V of the Food, Drug, and Cosmetic Act and your identity is provided to the Food and Drug Administration. A copy of your report will be forwarded to the respective manufacturer or distributor so that they can meet their obligation, (21CFR 211.198). You have the option of further restricting the disclosure of your identity.

By choosing "Anonymity Desired," your identification will be deleted from the copy provided to the respective manufacturer or distributor. In all cases, your identification will not be released to other parties under provisions of the Freedom of Information Act. If you wish to remain anonymous place an "X" in the box below.

SIGNATURE OF REPORTER		
	ANONYMITY DESIRED ☐	DATE

CALL OR **FAX** TOLL FREE — 24 HOURS A DAY — 7 DAYS A WEEK

1-800-FDA-1088

FDA 3318 (10/88)

PLEASE USE ADDRESS PROVIDED BELOW — JUST FOLD IN THIRDS, TAPE AND MAIL

NO POSTAGE
NECESSARY
IF MAILED
IN THE
UNITED STATES

BUSINESS REPLY MAIL
FIRST CLASS MAIL   PERMIT NO. 122   ROCKVILLE, MD

POSTAGE WILL BE PAID BY ADDRESSEE

The Food and Drug Administration
Drug Quality Reporting System
Suite 130
1055 First Street
Rockville MD 20850-9862

FIGURE 23.

397

Department of Health and Human Services
Public Health Service
Food and Drug Administration

$$\boxed{\text{NOTICE OF SEIZURE}}$$

TO: Date:

Notice is hereby given that, pursuant to Section 702(e)(5) of the Federal Food, Drug and Cosmetic Act (the Act), the following articles are being administratively seized:

There are reasonable grounds to believe that these articles are counterfeit and as such are subject to judicial seizure and condemnation under Section 304(a)(2) of the Act.

Proceedings will be instituted promptly in the Federal District Court under Section 304(a)(2) to place these articles under the jurisdiction of the Court.

Should you wish to defend any or all of these articles you may file a claim, stating your interest in the articles and your intent to defend them, and an answer, with the District Court following the filing of libel proceedings there.

_____
Investigator,   District
Food and Drug Administration

FORM FDA 3351 (7/89)

FIGURE 24.

398

COSMETICS

FDA 2511   Registration of Cosmetic Product Establishment

FDA 2512   Cosmetic Product Ingredient Statement

FDA 2512a   Cosmetic Product Ingredient Statement

FDA 2513   Cosmetic Raw Material Composition Statement

FDA 2513a   Cosmetic Raw Material Composition Statement

FDA 2514   Notice of Discontinuance of Commercial Distribution of Cosmetic Product or Cosmetic Raw Material

FDA 2704   Cosmetic Product Experience Report

FDA 2706   Summary Report of Cosmetic Product Experience by Product Categories

COSMETIC PRODUCT INGREDIENT STATEMENT

OFFICIAL RECEIPT

DEPARTMENT OF HEALTH AND HUMAN SERVICES
PUBLIC HEALTH SERVICE
FOOD AND DRUG ADMINISTRATION
WASHINGTON D C 20204

BRAND NAME AND NAME OF COSMETIC PRODUCT

TO:

FDA CPIS NO. F

REGISTRATION DATE / /

THIS STATEMENT IS ☐ COMPLETE ☐ INCOMPLETE
(If incomplete, Form FDA 2515 is attached)

FOR FDA USE ONLY

[1] Assignment of an FDA Cosmetic Product Ingredient Statement Number (FDA CPIS No.) does not denote in any way approval of the firm or the cosmetic product by the Food and Drug Administration. Any representation in labeling or advertising that creates an impression of official approval because of such filing or such number will be considered misleading. 21 CFR 720.9

DEPARTMENT OF HEALTH AND HUMAN SERVICES
PUBLIC HEALTH SERVICE
FOOD AND DRUG ADMINISTRATION
WASHINGTON, D.C. 20204

COSMETIC PRODUCT INGREDIENT STATEMENT

(In accordance with 21 CFR 720)

Read Instructions Booklet Before Completing. Type entries in CAPITAL LETTERS.

Form Approved: OMB No. 0910-0030. Expiration Date: March 31, 1992. See Reverse.

TYPE OF SUBMISSION: ☐ ORIGINAL SUBMISSION ☐ AMENDED SUBMISSION

NOTE: This report is authorized by Public Law 21 U.S.C. 371(a), 21 CFR 720. While you are not required to respond, your cooperation is needed to make the results of this voluntary program comprehensive, accurate and timely.

FOR FDA USE ONLY ON ORIGINAL SUBMISSIONS

FDA CPIS NO. (1 - 8)   REGISTRATION DATE (9 - 16)

ID NO. (17 - 19) 110

1. NAME OF MANUFACTURER/PACKER/DISTRIBUTOR (On label) (20 - 54)

2. DATE OF CHANGE (55 - 62) / /

3. NAME OF PARENT COMPANY (If any) (63 - 97)

4. KIND OF BUSINESS (98 - 100) ☐ MFR ☐ PKR ☐ DISTR

5. STREET ADDRESS (101 - 125)

6. CITY (126 - 140)

7. STATE (141 - 152)

8. ZIP CODE (153 - 157)

9. COUNTRY (If other than USA) (158 - 177)

10. DATE OF CHANGE (178 - 185) / /

11. NAME OF MANUFACTURER/PACKER (Private Labeler) (186 - 220)

12. DATE OF CHANGE (221 - 228) / /

13. NAME OF PARENT COMPANY (If any) (229 - 263)

14. STREET ADDRESS (264 - 288)

15. CITY (289 - 303)

16. STATE (304 - 315)

17. ZIP CODE (316 - 320)

18. COUNTRY (If other than USA) (321 - 340)

19. DATE OF CHANGE (341 - 348) / /

BRAND NAME (55 - 62)

20. BRAND NAME AND NAME OF COSMETIC PRODUCT (22 - 91)

220

	21. PRODUCT CODE (92 - 94)	22. TYPE OF ACTION (95 - 104)	23. DATE OF ACTION (105 - 112)
01			/ /
02			/ /
03			/ /
04			/ /
05			/ /
06			/ /
07			/ /
08			/ /

115

24. TYPED NAME AND TITLE OF AUTHORIZED INDIVIDUAL (20 - 74)

25. COMPANY (75 - 76)

26. SIGNATURE AND DATE

FORM FDA 2512 (4-89)   (CONTINUE COSMETIC PRODUCT INGREDIENT STATEMENT ON FORM FDA 2512a)   PART 1 — MASTER FILE COPY   Page ___ of ___ Pages

---

Public reporting burden for this collection of information is estimated to average 10 minutes per response, including the time for reviewing instructions, searching existing data sources, gathering and maintaining the data needed, and completing and reviewing the collection of information. Send comments regarding this burden estimate or any other aspect of this collection of information, including suggestions for reducing this burden to:

Reports Clearance Officer, PHS
Hubert H. Humphrey Building, Room 721-H
200 Independence Avenue, S.W.
Washington, DC 2020   Attn: PRA

and to:

Office of Management and Budget
Paperwork Reduction Project (0910-0030)
Washington, DC 20503

FIGURE 25.

Form Approved; OMB No. 0910-0030 Expiration Date: March 31, 1992 See Reverse

DEPARTMENT OF HEALTH AND HUMAN SERVICES
PUBLIC HEALTH SERVICE
FOOD AND DRUG ADMINISTRATION
Washington, D.C. 20204

COSMETIC PRODUCT INGREDIENT STATEMENT
(In accordance with 21 CFR 720)

TYPE OF SUBMISSION (Check one)
☐ Original Submission
☐ Amended Submission

REGISTRATION DATE (9-16)

FDA CPIS NO (1 - 8)

I.D. NO. (17-18)
230

INGRED NO	1 COMMON, UUSUAL, OR CHEMICAL NAME (22 - 85)	5 FDA CRMCS NO (112-119) R	6 TRADE NAME (120-154)	7 COMPANY NAME (155-189)	2 CAS REGISTRY NO (86-94)	3 TYPE OF ACTION (95-103)	8 CNFDL (190)	9 KIND INGRED (191)	4 DATE OF ACTION (104-111)	12 USE LEVEL MIN (194) MAX (195)
01										
02										
03										
04										
05										
06										
07										
08										
09										
10										

FORM FDA 2512a (6-89) Previous Edition Is Obsolete This Form Must Be Securely Attached to FDA2512.   **PART 1 - MASTER FILE COPY**

NOTE: This report is authorized by Public Law 21 U.S.C. 371(a); 21 CFR 720. While you are not required to respond, your cooperation is needed to make the results of this voluntary program comprehensive, accurate, and timely.

Public reporting burden for this collection of information is estimated to average 20 minutes per response, including the time for reviewing instructions, searching existing data sources, gathering and maintaining the data needed, and completing reviewing the collection of information. Send comments regarding this burden estimate or any other aspect of this collection of information, including suggestions for reducing this burden to:

Reports Clearance Officer, PHS
Hubert H. Humphrey Building, Room 721-H
200 Independence Avenue, S.W.
Washington, DC 2020   Attn: PRA

and to:

Office of Information and Regulatory Affairs
Office of Management and Budget
Washington, DC 20503

Page _____ of _____ Pages

FIGURE 26.

DEPARTMENT OF HEALTH AND HUMAN SERVICES
PUBLIC HEALTH SERVICE
FOOD AND DRUG ADMINISTRATION
Washington, D C 20204

NOTICE OF DISCONTINUANCE OF COMMERCIAL DISTRIBUTION
OF COSMETIC PRODUCT OR COSMETIC RAW MATERIAL

(In accordance with 21 CFR 720)

NOTE: This report is authorized by Public Law 21 U.S.C. 371(A); 21 CFR 720. While you are not required to respond, your cooperation is needed to make the results of this voluntary program comprehensive, accurate, and timely

Form Approved: OMB No. 0910-0029.
Expiration Date: January 31, 1989

1 FDA REGISTRATION NUMBER (1 - 8)

  a. CPIS NO.   F_____

     or

  b. CRMCS NO.   R_____

2 REGISTRATION DATE (9 - 16)

     __ __ / __ __ / __ __

ID NUMBER (17 - 19)   220

3 NAME OF MANUFACTURER/PACKER/DISTRIBUTOR

PROD NO. (20-21)	4 BRAND NAME AND NAME OF PRODUCT/TRADE NAME OF COSMETIC RAW MATERIAL (22 - 91)	5. DATE DISCONTINUED (92 - 99)
01		/ /
02		/ /
03		/ /
04		/ /
05		/ /
06		/ /
07		/ /
08		/ /
09		/ /
10		/ /

6. COMMENTS *(If any)*

7. TYPED NAME AND TITLE OF AUTHORIZED INDIVIDUAL

8. SIGNATURE AND DATE

FORM FDA 2514 (7/86) PREVIOUS EDITION IS OBSOLETE   **PART 1 - MASTER FILE COPY**   Page___of___Pages

FIGURE 27.

DEPARTMENT OF HEALTH AND HUMAN SERVICES
PUBLIC HEALTH SERVICE
FOOD AND DRUG ADMINISTRATION
WASHINGTON, D.C. 20204

COSMETIC PRODUCT EXPERIENCE REPORT
(In accordance with 21 CFR 730)

Read
Instructions
before
completing
form
Please type
entries

Form Approved: OMB Number 0910-0047
Expiration Date: April 30, 1989

FOR FDA USE ONLY

FDA NA NUMBER (1-5)

NOTE: This report is authorized by law 21 U.S.C. 371(a), 21 CFR 730. While you are not required to respond, your cooperation is needed to make the results of this voluntary program comprehensive, accurate and timely.

1. NAME OF MANUFACTURER/PACKER/DISTRIBUTER (On label)	2. SIGNATURE AND DATE

C.
(6)

10. BRAND NAME AND NAME OF COSMETIC PRODUCT (7-76)

11. PRODUCT CATEGORY CODE (77-79)

12. FDA CPIS NUMBER (80-87)

F_____

☐ PENDING   ☐ NOT FILED

FOR FDA USE ONLY (88-89)

13. YEAR COVERED (91-92)

19 ☐

14. SCREENING PROCEDURE (93)

☐ 1 PREVIOUSLY SENT
☐ 2. ATTACHED
☐ 3 NONE

J.
(6)

FOR FDA USE ONLY (7-14)

(15-19)

15. TOTAL NUMBER OF EXPERIENCES (20-24)

16. ESTIMATED UNITS DISTRIBUTED (25-32)

17. NUMBER OF EXPERIENCES REQUIRING PROFESSIONAL MEDICAL ATTENTION (49-52)

18. REMARKS

19. CONFIDENTIALITY REQUESTED   ☐   (Check this box if you wish to request confidentiality for the information given in items 10, 12, 15, 16, 17, and 18, and refuse to submit the information except on a confidential basis

FORM FDA 2704 (8/86)   PREVIOUS EDITION IS OBSOLETE   White - Master File Copy,   Canary - Data Processing Copy,   Pink - Registrant's Copy

FIGURE 28.

403

DEPARTMENT OF HEALTH AND HUMAN SERVICES
PUBLIC HEALTH SERVICE
FOOD AND DRUG ADMINISTRATION
WASHINGTON, D.C. 20204

Read
instructions
before
completing
form.
Please type
entries.

Form Approved: OMB Number 0910-0047
Expiration Date: April 30, 1989

FOR FDA USE ONLY

FDA NA NUMBER (1-5)

SUMMARY REPORT OF COSMETIC PRODUCT EXPERIENCE
BY PRODUCT CATEGORIES

(In accordance with 21 CFR 730)

A.
(6)

1. NAME OF MANUFACTURER/PACKER/DISTRIBUTER (On label) (7-41)

2. STREET ADDRESS (Or Box No.) (42-66)

B.
(6)

3. CITY (7-31)

4. STATE (32-33)

5. ZIPCODE (34-38)

6. COUNTRY (If other than USA) (39-58)

7. NAME AND ADDRESS OF REPORTING COMPANY (If other than above)

8. TYPED NAME AND TITLE OF AUTHORIZED INDIVIDUAL

9. SIGNATURE AND DATE

FOR FDA USE ONLY

FDA NA NO. (1-5)

NOTE: This report is authorized by law USC 371 (a); 21 CFR 730. While you are not required to respond, your cooperation is needed to make the results of this voluntary program comprehensive, accurate, and timely.

The information below should reflect Product Experiences reported on Forms FDA 2704 as well as Estimated Units Distributed of those products for which no experiences were reported.

E.
(6)

10. YEAR COVERED (8-9)
19 ☐

11. SCREENING PROCEDURE (10)
☐ 1. PREVIOUSLY SENT   ☐ 2. ATTACHED   ☐ 3. NONE

F.
(6)

12. PRODUCT CATEGORY CODE (7-9)	13. TOTAL EXPERIENCES (If any) (10-14)	14. ESTIMATED UNITS DISTRIBUTED (15-23)	12. PRODUCT CATEGORY CODE (7-9)	13. TOTAL EXPERIENCES (If any) (10-14)	14. ESTIMATED UNITS DISTRIBUTED (15-23)	12. PRODUCT CATEGORY CODE (7-9)	13. TOTAL EXPERIENCES (If any) (10-14)	14. ESTIMATED UNITS DISTRIBUTED (15-23)

15 CONFIDENTIALLY REQUESTED   ☐   (Check this box if you wish to request confidentiality for the information given in Items 12, 13, and 14 and refuse to submit the information except on a confidential basis.

FORM FDA 2706 (8/86) PREVIOUS EDITION IS OBSOLETE   White - Master File Copy, Canary - Data Processing Copy, Pink - Registrant's Copy

FIGURE 29.

DEVICES

FDA 2519f   Medical Device & Laboratory Product
Problem Reporting Program

FDA 2891   Initial Registration of Device Establishment

FDA 2891a   Annual Registration of Medical Device
Establishment

FDA 2892   Medical Device Listing

FDA 3322   Medical Device Report

Form Approved: OMB No. 0910-0143

Medical Device & Laboratory Product Problem Reporting Program

DATE RECEIVED

ACCESS NO

1. PRODUCT IDENTIFICATION:

Name of Product and Type of Device
(Include sizes or other identifying characteristics and attach labeling, if available)

Manufacturer's Name _____

Manufacturer's City, State, Zip Code _____

Is this a disposable item?   YES ☐   NO ☐

Lot Number(s) and Expiration Date(s) (if applicable)

Serial Number(s)

Manufacturer's Product Number and/or Model Number

2. REPORTER INFORMATION:

Your Name _____   Today's Date _____

Title and Department _____

Facility's Name _____

Street Address _____

City _____ State _____ Zip _____ Phone ( ) _____ Ext: _____

3. PROBLEM INFORMATION:

Date event occurred _____

Please indicate how you want your identity publicly disclosed:

No public disclosure ☐

To the manufacturer/distributor ☐

To the manufacturer/distributor and to anyone who
requests a copy of the report from the FDA ☐

This event has been reported to: Manufacturer ☐   FDA ☐

Other _____

If requested, will the actual product
involved in the event be available for
evaluation by the manufacturer or FDA?   YES ☐   NO ☐

Problem noted or suspected (Describe the event in as much detail as necessary. Attach additional pages if required. Include how and where the product was used. Include other equipment or products that were involved. Sketches may be helpful in describing problem areas.)

RETURN TO
United States Pharmacopeia
12601 Twinbrook Parkway
Rockville, Maryland 20852
Attention: Dr. Joseph G. Valentino

OR

CALL TOLL FREE ANYTIME
1-800-638-6725
IN THE CONTINENTAL UNITED STATES

FORM FDA 2519f (3/85)

FIGURE 30.

Medical Device & Laboratory
Product Problem
Reporting Program

What Is It?

An easy-to-use and nationally established program to report problems with medical devices, radiological devices and laboratory equipment used in health care. The program is funded by the Food and Drug Administration (FDA) and coordinated by the United States Pharmacopeia (USP).

Is It Effective?

Since its inception in 1973, the program has been successful in identifying and initiating many product design improvements and other corrective actions that have resulted from reports submitted by health care professionals.

What Kinds of Problems?

Anything is reportable that you consider to be a problem with the quality, performance, or safety of any device or piece of equipment used in medical care.

How Does It Work?

Reports may be submitted by completing the self-mailing form on the reverse side, or by calling the toll-free number indicated below.* USP forwards copies of these reports to FDA and the manufacturer for review and possible action. You may receive feedback from FDA and the manufacturer on your observations.

By request, USP can delete your name on the manufacturer's and/or FDA's copy.

Call Toll Free Anytime
1-800-638-6725

REMEMBER TO USE ANY IN-HOUSE
REPORTING PROCEDURES

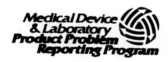

NO POSTAGE
NECESSARY
IF MAILED
IN THE
UNITED STATES

BUSINESS REPLY MAIL
FIRST CLASS PERMIT NO. 40, ROCKVILLE, MD.

Postage will be paid by addressee:

DR. JOSEPH G. VALENTINO
The U.S. Pharmacopeial Convention, Inc.
12601 Twinbrook Parkway
Rockville, Maryland 20852

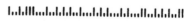

FIGURE 30 (continued).

DEPARTMENT OF HEALTH AND HUMAN SERVICES
PUBLIC HEALTH SERVICE
FOOD AND DRUG ADMINISTRATION
INITIAL REGISTRATION OF DEVICE ESTABLISHMENT
(Shaded Areas Are For FDA Use Only)

Form Approved, OMB No. 0910-0059
Expiration Date   March 31, 1993

VALIDATION

1 REGISTRATION NO.

RETURN THIS FORM TO: Food and Drug Administration, Center for Devices and Radiological Health, Device Registration and Listing Branch (HFZ-342), 1390 Piccard Drive, Rockville, Maryland 20850

Public reporting burden for this collection of information is estimated to average 1 hour per response, including the time for reviewing instructions, searching existing data sources, gathering and maintaining the data needed, and completing and reviewing the collection of information. Send comments regarding this burden estimate or any other aspect of this collection of information, including suggestions for reducing this burden to.

Reports Clearance Officer, PHS
Hubert H. Humphrey Building, Room 721-B
200 Independence Avenue, S W
Washington, DC 20201
Attn. PRA

and to

Office of Management and Budget
Paperwork Reduction Project (0910-0059)
Washington, DC 20503

Please DO NOT RETURN your questionnaire to either of these addresses

NOTE: This form is authorized by Section 510 of the Food, Drug and Cosmetic Act (21 U S C 360). Failure to report this information is a violation of Section 301(p) of the Act (21 U S C 331 (p)). Persons who violate this provision may, if convicted, be subject to a fine or imprisonment or both. The submission of any report that is false or misleading in any material respect is a violation of Section 301 (q) (2) (21 U S C 331 (q) (2)) and may be a violation of 18 U S C 1001

SECTION A

2. ESTABLISHMENT NAME		3 RECORD DATE
		(Mo.) (Day) (Yr)

4. NUMBER AND STREET	5 CITY	6 STATE	7 ZIP CODE

8. FOREIGN COUNTRY	9. ESTABLISHMENT TYPE (See Instruction Booklet) C D E M R S T U X	10 PREPRODUCTION REGISTRATION ☐ YES ☐ NO

SECTION B

11. OWNER/OPERATOR	12 OWNER/OPERATOR ID

13 NUMBER AND STREET	14 CITY	15 STATE	16 ZIP CODE

17. FOREIGN COUNTRY	18 TELEPHONE NUMBER · IF DIFFERENT FROM THAT OF OFFICIAL CORRESPONDENT (Area Code) (Number)

SECTION C

19. OFFICIAL CORRESPONDENT	20. TELEPHONE NUMBER (Area Code) (Number)

21. BUSINESS NAME	

22. NUMBER AND STREET	23 CITY	24 STATE	25 ZIP CODE

26. FOREIGN COUNTRY	27 FAX NUMBER (Area Code) (Number)

SECTION D

28. OTHER BUSINESS TRADING NAMES
(Enter any other name which the establishment in field #2 uses. Do not list Registered trademarks or names of private label distributors. This is usually any name such as a brand name which is not the firm name).

SEQ	ESTABLISHMENT NAME	SEQ	ESTABLISHMENT NAME
S01		S03	
S02		S04	

29. CERTIFYING AGENT (Typed Name)	30 TITLE AND PHONE NUMBER (Area Code) (Number)

SECTION E

31. SIGNATURE OF OFFICIAL CORRESPONDENT	32 TITLE

FORM FDA 2891 (3/92)   PREVIOUS EDITIONS ARE OBSOLETE

FIGURE 31.

DEPARTMENT OF HEALTH AND HUMAN SERVICES
PUBLIC HEALTH SERVICE
FOOD AND DRUG ADMINISTRATION
ANNUAL REGISTRATION OF MEDICAL DEVICE ESTABLISHMENT

A | Type of Submission (mark one (X) only) | ☐ No Change | ☐ No Longer Device Establishment
| | ☐ Correction | ☐ Out of Business

REGISTERED ESTABLISHMENT INFORMATION

B | CORRECTIONS TO REGISTERED ESTABLISHMENT INFORMATION

Business Name

Address

Address

City | State

Zip | Country

ESTABLISHMENT TYPES (If information below is inaccurate, correct in column to right)

☒ ... Distributor   ☐ Contract Sterilizer   ☐ Rebuilder/Refurbisher   ☐ Repkgr/Relabeler
... Manufacturer   ☐ Specification Dev   ☐ Contract Mfr

C | CORRECTIONS TO ESTABLISHMENT TYPE (To correct, mark (X) all which currently apply)

☐ Initial Distributor   ☐ Contract Sterilizer   ☐ Rebuilder/Refurbisher   ☐ Repkgr/Relabeler
☐ Manufacturer   ☐ Specification Dev   ☐ Contract Mfr

OWNER/OPERATOR INFORMATION

D | CORRECTIONS TO OWNER/OPERATOR INFORMATION

Business Name

Address

Address

City | State

Zip | Country

Phone No (   ) | Ext

OTHER BUSINESS TRADING NAMES

E | CORRECTIONS TO TRADING NAMES - If name on left has errors, write corrected name on line to its right; If no longer used, write "DELETE". Write new names last, preceded by an asterisk.

OFFICIAL CORRESPONDENT INFORMATION

F | CORRECTIONS TO OFFICIAL CORRESPONDENT INFORMATION

Name of Individual

Business Name

Address

Address

City | State

Zip | Country

Phone No (   ) | Ext

G | SIGNATURE OF OFFICIAL CORRESPONDENT | TITLE OF OFFICIAL CORRESPONDENT | DATE SIGNED

Form FDA 2891a (2-91) | Part 2 - Complete and Return | Form Approved OMB No. 0910-0060, Expiration Date

164618 | 12-31-92

FIGURE 32.

408

Form Approved: OMB No. 0910 0201 Expiration Date: June 30, 1992

DEPARTMENT OF HEALTH AND HUMAN SERVICES
PUBLIC HEALTH SERVICE
FOOD AND DRUG ADMINISTRATION
MEDICAL DEVICE REPORT

To: Center for Devices and Radiological Health
Office of Compliance and Surveillance, HFZ-351
1390 Piccard Drive
Rockville, MD 20850

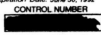

CONTROL NUMBER

Notes: Data elements identified by an asterisk (*) are not required to be reported under 21 CFR 803.24(c).
Shaded areas are for FDA use only.

ACCESS NO. FDA   DATE RECEIVED BY FDA   DATE SUBMITTED   ENCLOSURES

YES ☐   NO ☐

DEVICE IDENTIFICATION

1. BRAND NAME

2. COMMON NAME

3. MODEL NO.

4. CATALOG NO.

5. FIRM'S REFERENCE NO.*

6. LOT NO.

7. SERIAL NO.

8. METHOD OF MARKETING APPROVAL: (Check One)

510(k)* ☐   No. K-

PMA ☐   No. P-

☐ PREAMENDMENT EXEMPTED

9. TYPE OF SUBMITTAL (Enter Choice)

☐

A. 5-day Initial Facsimile (Death or Injury)
B. 15-day Initial Report (Malfunction)
C. 15-day Follow-up (Death or Injury)
D. Additional Information
    (As promised in Item 46 below, or response to FDA letter)
E. Supplemental Information (Unrequested)

If B, C, D or E is entered above, enter FDA Assigned Access:

M-

DOMESTIC FIRM SITE

10. FIRM NAME (Manufacturing Location or Responsible Importer)

11. REGISTRATION NO.*

12. TYPE
M-DOMESTIC MFR.
I-U.S. IMPORTER

13. ADDRESS   14. CITY   15. STATE   16. ZIP

CONTACT PERSON

17. CONTACT NAME   18. PHONE

19. FIRM NAME   20. REGISTRATION NO.*

21. ADDRESS   22. CITY   23. STATE   24. ZIP

FOREIGN MFR.

25. FIRM NAME (If Not Manufactured in the U.S.)   26. REGISTRATION NO. (IF AVAILABLE)*

27. CONTACT NAME

28. ADDRESS

29. CITY   30. COUNTRY   31. POSTAL CODE

INCIDENT INFORMATION

32. DATE OF EVENT

33. TYPE OF REPORT
D - DEATH
I - SERIOUS INJURY
M - MALFUNCTION

34. TYPE OF INJURY (Enter letter)*
A, B, C, D, E,
F, G, H, Z

35. NUMBER OF PERSONS AFFECTED

SOURCE OF REPORT

36. NAME   37. TITLE

38. FACILITY NAME   39. PHONE*

40. FACILITY ADDRESS

41. CITY   42. STATE   43. COUNTRY   44. ZIP (OR POSTAL CODE)   45. DATE MFR/IMPORTER ALERTED*

ADD. INFO.

46. TO BE SUBMITTED
☐ Y-YES
  N-NO

47. DATE TO BE SUBMITTED

48. NATURE OF INFORMATION (Analysis, labeling, etc.)

Page ☐1☐ Of ☐

FDA 3322 (4/91)

See OMB Disclosure Statement on Reverse

Public reporting burden for this collection of information is estimated to average 4 hours per response, including the time for reviewing instructions, searching existing data sources, gathering and maintaining the data needed, and completing and reviewing the collection of information. Send comments regarding this burden estimate or any other aspect of this collection of information, including suggestions for reducing this burden to:

Reports Clearance Officer, PHS   and to: Office of Management and Budget
Hubert H. Humphrey Building, Room 721-B   Paperwork Reduction Project (0910-0201)
200 Independence Avenue, S.W.   Washington, DC 20503
Washington, DC 20201
Attn: PRA

Please DO NOT RETURN this form to either of these addresses.

FIGURE 33.

METHADONE

FDA 2632   Application for Approval of Use of Methadone in a Treatment Program

FDA 2633   Medical Responsibility Statement for Use of Methadone in a Treatment Program

FDA 2634   Annual Report for Treatment Program Using Methadone

FDA 2635   Consent to Methadone Treatment

FDA 2636   Hospital Request for Methadone Detoxification Treatment

FDA 2654   Methadone Program Application Control Record

DEPARTMENT OF HEALTH AND HUMAN SERVICES
PUBLIC HEALTH SERVICE
FOOD AND DRUG ADMINISTRATION

**APPLICATION FOR APPROVAL OF USE OF
METHADONE IN A TREATMENT PROGRAM**

Form Approved; OMB No 0910 0140
Expiration Date: December 31 1990.
See Reverse for OMB Statement.

DATE OF SUBMISSION

NOTE: *This form is required by 21 CFR 291.505 pursuant to Sec. 303, Controlled Substances Act (21 USC 823) and Section 4, Comprehensive Drug Abuse Prevention and Control Act of 1970 (42 USC 275(a)). Failure to report can result in a recommendation for the suspension or revocation of the Narcotic Treatment Program registration.*

NAME OF PROGRAM *(Name of primary dispensing Location)*

ADDRESS OF PRIMARY DISPENSING LOCATION *(Include Zip Code)*

TELEPHONE NO. *(Include Area Code)*

NAME AND ADDRESS OF PROGRAM SPONSOR *(Include Zip Code)*

TELEPHONE NO *(Include Area Code)*

APPROXIMATE NUMBER OF PATIENTS TO BE TREATED AT ANY GIVEN TIME

PROGRAM FUNDING SOURCES *(Check each appropriate agency and attach the address of each)*

☐ NIDA
☐ LEAA
☐ CETA
☐ NIMH
☐ CLIENT FEE
☐ BUREAU PRISONS
☐ U S. COURTS
☐ OTHER *(Specify)*

☐ VETERANS ADMINISTRATION
☐ STATE GOVERNMENT
☐ CITY AND COUNTY GOVERNMENT
☐ INDIAN HEALTH SERVICE
☐ PUBLIC HEALTH INSURANCE
☐ PRIVATE HEALTH INSURANCE
☐ PRIVATE CHARITIES

Commissioner
Food and Drug Administration
5600 Fishers Lane
Division of Scientific Investigations (HFD-342)
Rockville, Maryland 20857

Dear Sir:

As the person responsible for this program, I submit this application in duplicate for approval to use methadone in a program for detoxification and/or maintenance treatment for narcotic addicts in accordance with 21 CFR 291.505, standards for Drugs Used for Treatment of Narcotic Addicts. A copy of this application has been sent to the State authority within which State the program is located. I understand that FDA and State approvals are necessary to obtain a registration from the Drug Enforcement Administration (DEA).

I. I have a copy of, or access to 21 CFR 291 505, Drugs Used for Treatment of Narcotic Addicts. I have read, understand and will comply with the standards established under that regulation which governs the treatment of narcotic addiction with methadone.

II. I have a copy of or access to 42 CFR Part 2, Confidentiality of Alcohol and Drug Abuse Patient Records, published June 9, 1987. I have read and understand the requirements to maintain the confidentiality of alcohol and drug abuse treatment patient records. I agree to protect the identity of all patients in accordance with the regulation.

III. I shall comply with the security standards for the distribution and storage of controlled substances, including methadone, as required by 21 CFR 1301, Registration of Manufacturers, Distributors, and Dispensers of Controlled Substances.

IV. A patient record system will be established to document and monitor patient care in this program. It shall be maintained so as to comply with the Federal and State reporting requirements relevant to methadone treatment. A drug dispensing record will be maintained to show dates, quantity, and batch or code marks of the drug administered or dispensed, traceable to specific patients. This drug dispensing record must be retained for a period of three years from the date of dispensing. A patient treatment record will be maintained for each patient. It will contain a signed "Consent for Methadone Treatment" (Form FDA 2635), the date of each visit, the results of each urinalysis, a description of any significant physical or psychological disability, the type of any rehabilitative and counseling efforts employed, an account of the patient's progress and other relevant aspects of the patient's treatment.

V. Attached is a description of the organizational structure of this program which includes the name and complete address of any central administration or larger organizational structure to which this program is responsible.

FORM FDA 2632 (2/90)   PREVIOUS EDITION IS OBSOLETE

FIGURE 34.

VI. The Form FDA 2633, "Medical Reponsibility Statement for Use of Methadone in a Treatment Program," is completed and submitted in duplicate to the Food and Drug Administration and the State authority by each licensed physician authorized to administer or dispense methadone. Attached is a list of other persons employed by the program who are licensed by law to administer or dispense narcotic drugs, even if they are not presently responsible for administering or dispensing the drug.

VII. A medical director will be designated to assume reponsibility for administering all medical services performed by the program. If a medical director is reponsible for more than one program, the feasibility of such an arrangement will be documented and submitted to the Food and Drug Administration. Within three weeks of any replacement of the medical director, notification will be sent to the Food and Drug Administration and the State authority.

VIII. This program shall provide a comprehensive range of medical and rehabilitative services to its patients. The addition, modification or deletion of any program services will be reported to the Food and Drug Administration

IX. Attached is a diagram and a description of the program's physical facilities which demonstrate that such facilities are sufficiently spacious and well maintained to provide all necessary program services.

X. Attached are the names, addresses, and description of each hospital, institution, clinical laboratory or other facility used by this program to provide necessary medical and rehabilitative services. The Food and Drug Admin-istration and State authority will be advised within three weeks of the addition or deletion of any facilities which provide service other than administering or dispensing of medication.

XI. Any new dispensing site for this program, including medication units shall be approved by the Food and Drug Administration and the State authority prior to its use. The Food and Drug Administration and State authority shall be notified within three weeks of the deletion of any facility used to dispense methadone.

XII. I agree to adhere to all the rules, directives, and procedures, set forth in 21 CFR 291.505, and any regulation regarding the use of methadone which may be promulgated in the future. I shall inform other individuals who work in this treatment program of the provisions of this regulation, and monitor their activities to assure compliance with the provisions. If I am replaced, the Food and Drug Administration and the State authority will be notified within three weeks.

XIII. I understand that failure to abide by the rules, directives, and procedures described above may cause a suspension or revocation of approval of my registration by the Drug Enforcement Administration.

Signature _____
(Program Sponsor)

_____
(Printed or typed name)

_____
(Date)

FIGURE 34 (continued).

DEPARTMENT OF HEALTH AND HUMAN SERVICES
PUBLIC HEALTH SERVICE
FOOD AND DRUG ADMINISTRATION
MEDICAL RESPONSIBILITY STATEMENT FOR USE
OF METHADONE IN A TREATMENT PROGRAM
(Completed by each physician licensed to dispense/administer
methadone under an approved program)

Form Approved; OMB No. 0910-0140
Expiration Date: December 31, 1990.

DATE

NOTE: *This form is required by 21 CFR 291.505 pursuant to Sec. 303, Controlled Substances Act (21 USC 823) and Section 4, Comprehensive Drug Abuse Prevention and Control Act of 1970 (42 USC 275(a)). Failure to report can result in a recommendation for the suspension or revocation of the Narcotic Treatment Program registration.*

NAME OF PROGRAM *(Name of primary dispensing location)*

ADDRESS OF PRIMARY DISPENSING LOCATION *(Include City, State, Zip Code)*

TELEPHONE NO. *(Include Area Code)*

I. The undersigned agrees to assume responsibility for the administration and dispensing of methadone under the above identified program and to abide by the required standards for methadone detoxification and maintenance treatment described in 21 CFR 291.505, standards for Drugs Used for Treatment of Narcotic Addicts; Conditions for Use of Methadone. I have read and understand the treatment standards established by the regulation.

II. I have read and understand 42 CFR Part 2, Confidentiality of Alcohol and Drug Abuse Patient Records, published June 9, 1987. I agree to protect the identity of all patients in accordance with this regulation.

III. If I am, or should become medical director, I will assume responsibility for administering all medical services performed by the program and ensure that the program is in compliance with all Federal, State and local laws and regulations regarding medical treatment of narcotic addiction.

PHYSICIAN FURNISHING MEDICAL SERVICES AT THIS LOCATION

IS THE PHYSICIAN ALSO A MEDICAL DIRECTOR   ☐ YES   ☐ NO

STATE MEDICAL LICENSE NO.

DEA CONTROLLED SUBSTANCES REGISTRATION NO.

TYPED OR PRINTED NAME

SIGNATURE

Public reporting burden for this collection of information is estimated to average 1 hour per response, including the time for reviewing instructions, searching existing data sources, gathering and maintaining the data needed, and completing and reviewing the collection of information. Send comments regarding this burden estimate or any other aspect of this collection of information, including suggestions for reducing this burden to:

Reports Clearance Officer, PHS
Hubert H. Humphrey Building, Room 721-H
200 Independence Avenue, S.W.
Washington, DC 20201
Attn: PRA

and to:

Office of Management and Budget
Paperwork Reduction Project (0910-0140)
Washington, DC 20503

FORM FDA 2633 (1/90)   PREVIOUS EDITION IS OBSOLETE.

FIGURE 35.

DEPARTMENT OF HEALTH AND HUMAN SERVICES	DATE
PUBLIC HEALTH SERVICE FOOD AND DRUG ADMINISTRATION **CONSENT TO METHADONE TREATMENT** *(Provisions of this form may be modified to conform to any applicable State law)*	

NAME OF PATIENT

NAME OF PRACTITIONER EXPLAINING PROCEDURES

NAME OF PROGRAM MEDICAL DIRECTOR

I hereby authorize and give my voluntary consent to the above named Program Medical Director and/or any appropriately authorized assistants he may select, to administer or prescribe the drug methadone as an element in the treatment for my dependence on heroin or other narcotic drugs.

The procedures necessary to treat my condition have been explained to me and I understand that it will involve my taking daily dosages of methadone, or other drugs, which will help control my dependence on heroin or other narcotic drugs.

It has been explained to me that methadone is a narcotic drug which can be harmful if taken without medical supervision. I further understand that methadone is an addictive medication and may, like other drugs used in medical practice, produce adverse results. The alternative methods of treatment, the possible risks involved, and the possibilities of complications have been explained to me, but I still desire to receive methadone due to the risk of my return to the use of heroin or other drugs.

The goal of methadone treatment is total rehabilitation of the patient. Eventual withdrawal from the use of all drugs, including methadone, is an appropriate treatment goal. I realize that for some patients methadone treatment may continue for relatively long periods of time but that periodic consideration shall be given concerning my complete withdrawal from methadone use.

I understand that I may withdraw from this treatment program and discontinue the use of the drug at any time and I shall be afforded detoxification under medical supervision.

I agree that I shall inform any doctor who may treat me for any medical problem that I am enrolled in a narcotic treatment program, since the use of other drugs in conjunction with methadone may cause me harm.

I also understand that during the course of treatment, certain conditions may make it necessary to use additional or different procedures than those explained to me. I understand that these alternate procedures shall be used when in the Program or Medical Director's professional judgment it is considered advisable.

(See reverse of this sheet for additional consent elements)

FORM FDA 2635 (10/89)

FIGURE 36.

FEMALE PATIENTS OF CHILD-BEARING AGE	PATIENTS UNDER 18 YEARS OF AGE
To the best of my knowledge, I ☐ am ☐ am not pregnant at this time. Besides the possible risks involved with the long-term use of methadone, I further understand that, like heroin and other narcotic drugs, information on its effects on pregnant women and on their unborn children is at present inadequate to guarantee that it may not produce significant or serious side effects. It has been explained to me and I understand that methadone is transmitted to the unborn child and will cause physical dependence. Thus, if I am pregnant and suddenly stop taking methadone, I or the unborn child may show signs of withdrawal which may adversely affect my pregnancy or the child. I shall use no other drugs without the Medical Director or his assistants' approval, since these drugs, particularly as they might interact with methadone, may harm me or my unborn child. I shall inform any other physician who sees me during my present or any future pregnancy or who sees the child after birth, of my current or past participation in a narcotic treatment program in order that he/she may properly care for my child and me. It has been explained to me that after the birth of my child I should not nurse the baby because methadone is transmitted through the milk to the baby and this may cause physical dependence on methadone in the child. I understand that for a brief period following the birth, the child may show temporary irritability or other ill effects due to my use of methadone. It is essential for the child's physician to know of my participation in a narcotic treatment program so that he/she may provide appropriate medical treatment for the child. All the above possible effects of methadone have been fully explained to me and I understand that at present, there have not been enough studies conducted on the long term use of the drug to assure complete safety to my child. With full knowledge of this, I consent to its use and promise to inform the Medical Director or one of his/her assistants immediately if I become pregnant in the future.	The patient is a minor, _____ years of age, born, _____. The risks of the use of methadone have been explained to (me/us) and (I/we) understand that methadone is a drug on which long term studies are still being conducted and that information on its effects in adolescents is incomplete. It has been explained to (me/us) that methadone is being used in the minor's treatment only because the risk of (his/her) return to the use of heroin is sufficiently great to justify this treatment. (I/We) declare that participation in the narcotic treatment program is wholly voluntary on the part of both the parent(s)/ guardians(s)) and the patient and that methadone treatment may be stopped at any time on (my/our) request or that of the patient. With full knowledge of the potential benefits and possible risks involved with the use of methadone in the treatment of an adolescent, (I/we) consent to its use upon the minor, since (I/we) realize that otherwise (he/she) shall continue to be dependent upon heroin or other narcotic drugs.

I certify that no guarantee or assurance has been made as to the results that may be obtained from methadone treatment. With full knowledge of the potential benefits and possible risks involved, I consent to methadone treatment, since I realize that I would otherwise continue to be dependent on heroin.

SIGNATURE OF PATIENT	DATE OF BIRTH	DATE
SIGNATURE OF PARENT(S) OR GUARDIAN(S)	RELATIONSHIP	DATE
SIGNATURE OF WITNESS		DATE

FIGURE 36 (continued).

Form Approval; OMB No. 0910-0140
Expiration Date: December 31, 1990.
See Reverse for OMB Statement.

DEPARTMENT OF HEALTH AND HUMAN SERVICES PUBLIC HEALTH SERVICE FOOD AND DRUG ADMINISTRATION **HOSPITAL REQUEST FOR METHADONE DETOXIFICATION TREATMENT**	FOR FDA USE ONLY
	HOSPITAL NO.
	DATE

NOTE: This form is required by 21 CFR 291.505 pursuant to Sec. 303, Controlled Substances Act (21 USC 823) and Section 4, Comprehensive Drug Abuse Prevention and Control Act of 1970 (42 USC 275(a)). Failure to report can result in a recommendation for the suspension or revocation of the Narcotic Treatment Program registration.

NAME OF HOSPITAL

ADDRESS (include City, State, Zip Code)	TELEPHONE NO. (include Area Code)

NAME OF PHARMACIST RESPONSIBLE FOR RECEIVING AND SECURING SUPPLIES OF METHADONE

NUMBER OF BEDS IN HOSPITAL	NUMBER OF BEDS COMMITTED TO METHADONE TREATMENT (May be expressed in parts, such as tenths)	ANTICIPATED NUMBER OF GRAMS OF METHADONE FOR NARCOTIC ADDICT TREATMENT NEEDED ANNUALLY

Commissioner
Food and Drug Administration
Division of Scientific Investigations (HFD-342)
5600 Fishers Lane
Rockville, Maryland 20857

Dear Sir:

As hospital administrator, I submit this request for approval to receive supplies of methadone to be used for detoxification treatment in accordance with 21 CFR 291.505. I understand that the failure to abide by the requirements described below may result in suspension or revocation of registration to receive shipments of methadone pursuant to the Controlled Substances Act of 1970, as amended by the Narcotic Addict Treatment Act of 1974.

I. A general description of the hospital including specialized treatment facilities and nature of patient care to be undertaken is attached.

II. Methadone or narcotic addict treatment will be administered or dispensed only for detoxification treatment of hospitalized patients. I understand that the approval of this application is not necessary to permit the hospital to maintain or detoxify a person as an adjunct to medical or surgical treatment of conditions other than addiction.

III. Accurate records shall be maintained showing dates, quantity, and batch or code marks of the drugs used for inpatient detoxification treatment. The records shall be retained for a period of three years.

IV. The Food and Drug Administration, the National Institute on Drug Abuse, and the State authority may inspect supplies of the drug and evaluate compliance with applicable parts of 21 CFR 291.505. The identity of the patient will be kept confidential (except when it is necessary to make follow-up investigations on adverse effect information related to the drug, when the medical welfare of the patient would be threatened by a failure to reveal such information, or when it is necessary to verify records relating to approval of the hospital or any portion thereof). The confidentiality requirements or 42 CFR Part 2 shall be followed.

TYPED OR PRINTED NAME OF HOSPITAL ADMINISTRATOR	SIGNATURE OF HOSPITAL ADMINISTRATOR	DATE

FORM FDA 2636 (2/90)   PREVIOUS EDITION IS OBSOLETE.

Public reporting burden for this collection of information is estimated to average 10 minutes per response, including the time for reviewing instructions, searching existing data sources, gathering and maintaining the data needed, and completing and reviewing the collection of information. Send comments regarding this burden estimate or any other aspect of this collection of information, including suggestions for reducing this burden to:

Reports Clearance Officer PHS   and to.   Office of Management and Budget
Hubert H. Humphrey Building, Room 721-H   Paperwork Reduction Project (0910-0140)
200 Independence Avenue, S W   Washington, DC 20503
Washington, DC 20201
Attn: PRA

FIGURE 37.

Drug Enforcement Administration Forms and Applications

DEA-41	Registrants Inventory of Drugs Surrendered
DEA-82	Notice of Inspection of Controlled Premises
DEA-104	Voluntary Surrender of Controlled Substances Privileges
DEA-106	Report of Theft or Loss of Controlled Substances
DEA-222	Controlled Substances Order Form—Schedules I and II (see page 61)
DEA-222A	Requisition for Form DEA-222
DEA-224	New Application for Registration under Controlled Substances Act of 1970 (for retail pharmacy, hospitals/clinics, practitioner, teaching institution).
DEA-225	New Application for Registration under Controlled Substances Act of 1970 (for manufacturers, wholesalers, distributors, importers, exporters, and most research activities).
DEA-226	Application for Reregistration for retail pharmacy, hospitals/clinics, practitioners, teaching institutions.
DEA-363	Registration for Narcotic Treatment Programs

The following schedule is an inventory of controlled substances which is hereby surrendered to you for proper disposition.

FROM: *(Include Name, Street, City, State and ZIP Code in space provided below).*

Signature of applicant or authorized agent

Registrant's DEA Number

Registrant's Telephone Number

NOTE: Registrants will fill in Columns 1, 2, 3, and 4 Only.

NAME OF DRUG OR PREPARATION	Number of Containers	CONTENTS (Number of grams, tablets, ounces or other units per container)	Controlled Substance Content, (Each Unit)	FOR DEA USE ONLY DISPOSITION	QUANTITY	
					GMS.	MGS.
1	*2*	*3*	*4*	*5*	*6*	*7*
1						
2						
3						
4						
5						
6						
7						
8						
9						
10						
11						
12						
13						
14						
15						
16						

DEA Form — 41
(Mar. 1980)

Previous edition may be used.

* See instructions on reverse side.

FIGURE 1.

NAME OF DRUG OR PREPARATION	Number of Con-tainers	CONTENTS (Number of grams, tablets, ounces or other units per con-tainer)	Con-trolled Sub-stance Con-tent (Each Unit)	FOR DEA USE ONLY		
				DISPOSITION	QUANTITY	
					GMS.	MGS.
	2	3	4	5	6	7
17						
18						
19						
20						
21						
22						
23						
24						

The controlled substances surrendered in accordance with Title 21 of the Code of Federal Regulations, Section 1307.21, have been received

in _____ packages purporting to contain the drugs listed on this inventory and have been: **(1) Forwarded tape-sealed without opening;

(2) Destroyed as indicated and the remainder forwarded tape-sealed after verifying contents; (3) Forwarded tape-sealed after verifying contents.

DATE _____ 19 ____   DESTROYED BY: _____

** Strike out lines not applicable.   WITNESSED BY: _____

INSTRUCTIONS

1. List the name of the drug in column 1, the number of containers in column 2, the size of each container in column 3, and in column 4 the controlled substance content of each unit described in column 3; e.g., morphine sulfate tabs., 3 pkgs., 100 tabs., 1/4 gr. (16 mg.) or morphine sulfate tabs., 1 pkg., 83 tabs., 1/2 gr. (32 mg.), etc.

2. All packages included on a single line should be identical in name, content and controlled substance strength.

3. Prepare this form in quadruplicate. Mail two (2) copies of this form to the Special Agent in Charge, under separate cover. Enclose one additional copy in the shipment with the drugs. Retain one copy for your records. One copy will be returned to you as a receipt. No further receipt will be furnished to you unless specifically requested. Any furhter inquiries concerning these drugs should be addressed to the DEA District Office which serves your area.

4. There is no provision for payment for drugs surrendered. This is merely a service rendered to registrants enabling them to clear their stocks and records of unwanted items.

5. Drugs should be shipped tape-sealed via prepaid express or registered mail to Special Agent In Charge, Drug Enforcement Administration, of the DEA District Office which serves your area.

PRIVACY ACT INFORMATION

AUTHORITY: Section 307 of the Controlled Substances Act of 1970 (P.L. 91-513).

PURPOSE: To document the surrender of controlled substances which have been forwarded by registrants to DEA for disposal.

ROUTINE USES: This form is required by Federal Regulations for the surrender of unwanted Controlled Substances. Disclosures of information from this system are made to the following categories of users for the purposes stated.

    A. Other Federal law enforcement and regulatory agencies for law enforcement and regulatory purposes.

    B. State and local law enforcement and regulatory agencies for law enforcement and regulatory purposes.

EFFECT: Failure to document the surrender of unwanted Controlled Substances may result in prosecution for violation of the Controlled Substances Act.

FIGURE 1 (continued).

U.S. DEPARTMENT OF JUSTICE
DRUG ENFORCEMENT ADMINISTRATION

NOTICE OF INSPECTION OF CONTROLLED PREMISES	DEA USE ONLY
	FILE NUMBER

NAME OF INDIVIDUAL		TITLE
NAME OF CONTROLLED PREMISES		DEA REGISTRATION NO.
NUMBER AND STREET		DATE
CITY AND STATE	ZIP CODE	TIME *(Initial inspection)*

STATEMENT OF RIGHTS

1. You have a constitutional right not to have an administrative inspection made without an administrative inspection warrant.
2. You have the right to refuse to consent to this inspection.
3. Anything of an incriminating nature which may be found may be seized and used against you in a criminal prosecution.
4. You shall be presented with a copy of this Notice of Inspection.
5. You may withdraw your consent at any time during the course of the inspection.

ACKNOWLEDGEMENT AND CONSENT

I, _____ have been advised of the above Statement of Rights
(Name)

by DEA _____ , who
(Title and Name)

has identified himself/herself to me with his/her credentials and presented me with this Notice of Inspection containing a copy of sections 302(f) and 510(a), (b) and (c) of the Controlled Substances Act (21 U.S.C. 822(f) and 21 U.S.C. 880(a), (b) and (c), printed hereon, * authorizing an inspection of the above-described controlled premises. I hereby acknowledge receipt of this Notice of Inspection. In addition, I hereby certify that I am the _____
(President) (Manager) (Owner)

for the premises described in this Notice of Inspection; that I have read the foregoing and understand its contents; that I have authority to act in this matter and have signed this Notice of Inspection pursuant to my authority.

I understand what my rights are concerning inspection. No threats or promises have been made to me and no pressure of any kind has been used against me. I voluntarily give consent for inspection of these controlled premises.

_____
(Signature)

WITNESSES:

_____
(Date)

_____   _____
(signed)   (date)

_____   _____
(signed)   (date)

* See reverse

DEA Form — **82**
(June 1982)   Previous edition, dated 2/74 is Obsolete.

FIGURE 2.

420

SEC. 302. (f) The Attorney General is authorized to inspect the establishment of a registrant or applicant for registration in accordance with the rules and regulations promulgated by him.

SEC. 510. (a) As used in this section, the term "controlled premises" means—

(1) places where original or other records or documents required under this title are kept or required to be kept, and

(2) places, including factories, warehouses, or other establishments, and conveyances, where persons registered under section 303 (or exempted from registration under section 302(d)) may lawfully hold, manufacture, or distribute, dispense, administer, or otherwise dispose of controlled substances.

(b)(1) For the purpose of inspecting, copying, and verifying the correctness of records, reports, or other documents required to be kept or made under this title and otherwise facilitating the carrying out of his functions under this title, the Attorney General is authorized, in accordance with this section, to enter controlled premises and to conduct administrative inspections thereof, and of the things specified in this section, relevant to those functions.

(2) Such entries and inspections shall be carried out through officers or employees (hereinafter referred to as "inspectors") designated by the Attorney General. Any such inspector, upon stating his purpose and presenting to the owner, operator, or agent in charge of such premises (A) appropriate credentials and (B) a written notice of his inspection authority (which notice in the case of an inspection requiring, or in fact supported by, an administrative inspection warrant shall consist of such warrant), shall have the right to enter such premises and conduct such inspection at reasonable times.

(3) Except as may otherwise be indicated in an applicable inspection warrant, the inspector shall have the right—

(A) to inspect and copy records, reports, and other documents required to be kept or made under this title;

(B) to inspect, within reasonable limits and in a reasonable manner, controlled premises and all pertinent equipment, finished and unfinished drugs and other substances or materials, containers, and labeling found therein, and, except as provided in paragraph (5) of this subsection, all other things therein (including records, files, papers, processes, controls, and facilities) appropriate for verification of the records, reports, and documents referred to in clause (A) or otherwise bearing on the provisions of this title; and

(C) to inventory any stock of any controlled substance therein and obtain samples of any such substance.

(4) Except when the owner, operator, or agent in charge of the controlled premises so consents in writing, no inspection authorized by this section shall extend to—

(A) financial data;

(B) sales data other than shipment data; or

(C) pricing data.

(c) A warrant under this section shall not be required for the inspection of books and records pursuant to an administrative subpena issued in accordance with section 506, nor for entries and administrative inspections (including seizures of property)—

(1) with the consent of the owner, operator, or agent in charge of the controlled premises;

(2) in situations presenting imminent danger to health or safety;

(3) in situations involving inspection of conveyances where there is reasonable cause to believe that the mobility of the conveyance makes it impracticable to obtain a warrant;

(4) in any other exceptional or emergency circumstance where time or opportunity to apply for a warrant is lacking; or

(5) in any other situations where a warrant is not constitutionally required

FIGURE 2 (continued).

421

After being full advised of my rights, and understanding that I am not required to surrender my controlled substances privileges, I freely execute this document and choose to take the actions described herein.

☐ In view of my alleged failure to comply with the Federal requirements pertaining to controlled substances, and as an indication of my good faith in desiring to remedy any incorrect or unlawful practices on my part;

☐ In view of my desire to terminate handling of controlled substances listed in schedule(s) _____ ;

I hereby voluntarily surrender my Drug Enforcement Administration Certificate of Registration, unused order forms, and all my controlled substances listed in schedule(s) _____ as evidence of my agreement to relinquish my privilege to handle controlled substances listed in schedule(s)_____ . Further. I agree and consent that this document shall be authority for the Administrator of the Drug Enforcement Administration to terminate and revoke my registration without an order to show cause, a hearing, or any other proceedings, (and if not all controlled substances privileges are surrendered, be issued a new registration certificate limited to schedule(s)_____).

I waive refund of any payments made by me in connection with my registration.

I understand that I will not be permitted to order, manufacture, distribute, possess, dispense, administer, prescribe, or engage in any other controlled substance activities whatever, until such time an I am again properly registered.

NAME OF REGISTRANT *(Print)*	ADDRESS OF REGISTRANT	
SIGNATURE OF REGISTRANT OR AUTHORIZED INDIVIDUAL	DATE	DEA REGISTRATION NO.

WITNESSES:

NAME AND DATE	TITLE
NAME AND DATE	TITLE

DEA Form — 104
(Sept. 1976)   Previous edition dated 1/74 is OBSOLETE.   DOJ

PRIVACY ACT INFORMATION   DEA-104

AUTHORITY: Section 301 of the Controlled Substances Act of 1970 (PL 91-513)

PURPOSE: Permit voluntary surrender of controlled substances.

ROUTINE USES: The Controlled Substances Act Registration Records produces special reports as required for statistical analytical purposes. Disclosures of information from this system are made to the following categories of users for the purposes stated:
A. Other Federal law enforcement and regulatory agencies for law enforcement and regulatory purposes.
B. State and local law enforcement and regulatory agencies for law enforcement and regulatory purposes.
C. Persons registered under the Controlled Substances Act (Public Law 91-513) for the purpose of verifying the registration of customers and practitioners.

EFFECT: Failure to provide the information will have no effect on the individual.

FIGURE 3.

U.S. DEPARTMENT OF JUSTICE / DRUG ENFORCEMENT ADMINISTRATION

REPORT OF THEFT OR LOSS OF CONTROLLED SUBSTANCES

OMB APPROVAL
No. 1117-0001

Federal Regulations require registrants to submit a detailed report of any theft or loss of Controlled Substances to the Drug Enforcement Administration.
Complete the front and back of this form in triplicate. Forward the original and duplicate copies to the nearest DEA Office. Retain the triplicate copy for your records. Some states may also require a copy of this report.

DEA MANUAL AUTHORITY:
Diversion Investigators 5124
FFS: 630-02

1. NAME AND ADDRESS OF REGISTRANT (Include ZIP Code)

ZIP CODE

2. PHONE NO. (Include Area Code)

3. DEA REGISTRATION NUMBER

2 ltr. prefix   7 digit suffix

4. DATE OF THEFT OR LOSS

5. PRINCIPAL BUSINESS OF REGISTRANT (Check one)

1 ☐ Pharmacy   5 ☐ Distributor
2 ☐ Practitioner   6 ☐ Methadone Program
3 ☐ Manufacturer   7 ☐ Other (specify)
4 ☐ Hospital/Clinic

6. COUNTY IN WHICH REGISTRANT IS LOCATED

7. WAS THEFT REPORTED TO POLICE?
☐ YES   ☐ NO

8. NAME AND TELEPHONE NUMBER OF POLICE DEPARTMENT (Include Area Code)

9. NUMBER OF THEFTS OR LOSSES REGISTRANT HAS EXPERIENCED IN THE PAST 24 MONTHS ?

10. TYPE OF THEFT OR LOSS (Check one and complete items below as appropriate)

1 ☐ Night break-in   3 ☐ Employee pilferage   5 ☐ Other (Explain)
2 ☐ Armed robbery   4 ☐ Customer theft   6 ☐ Lost in transit (Complete Item 14)

11. IF ARMED ROBBERY, WAS ANYONE:

KILLED ? ☐ No ☐ Yes (How many) _____
INJURED ? ☐ No ☐ Yes (How many) _____

12. PURCHASE VALUE TO REGISTRANT OF CONTROLLED SUBSTANCES TAKEN ?
$

13. WERE ANY PHARMACEUTICALS OR MERCHANDISE TAKEN ?
☐ No ☐ Yes (Est. Value)
$

14. IF LOST IN TRANSIT, COMPLETE THE FOLLOWING:

A. Name of Common Carrier

B. Name of Consignee

C. Consignee's DEA Registration Number

D. Was the carton received by the customer ?
☐ Yes ☐ No

E. If received, did it appear to be tampered with ?
☐ Yes ☐ No

F. Have you experienced losses in transit from this same carrier in the past ?
☐ No ☐ Yes (How Many) _____

15. WHAT IDENTIFYING MARKS, SYMBOLS, OR PRICE CODES WERE ON THE LABELS OF THESE CONTAINERS THAT WOULD ASSIST IN IDENTIFYING THE PRODUCTS ?

16. IF OFFICIAL CONTROLLED SUBSTANCE ORDER FORMS (DEA-222) WERE STOLEN, GIVE NUMBERS

17. WHAT SECURITY MEASURES HAVE BEEN TAKEN TO PREVENT FUTURE THEFTS OR LOSSES ?

DEA Form — **106**
(Dec. 1985)

Previous edition dated 3/83 is OBSOLETE.

CONTINUE ON REVERSE

FIGURE 4.

LIST OF CONTROLLED SUBSTANCES LOST

Trade Name of Substance or Preparation	Name of Controlled Substance in Preparation	Dosage Strength and Form	Quantity
Examples: Desoxyn	Methamphetamine Hydrochloride	5 Mg Tablets	3 x 100
Demerol	Meperidine Hydrochloride	50 Mg/ml Vial	5 x 30 ml
Robitussin A-C	Codeine Phosphate	2 Mg/cc Liquid	12 Pints
1.			
2.			
3.			
4.			
5.			
6.			
7.			
8.			
9.			
10.			
11.			
12.			
13.			
14.			
15.			
16.			
17.			
18.			
19.			
20.			
21.			
22.			
23.			
24.			
25.			
26.			
27.			
28.			
29.			
30.			
31.			
32.			
33.			
34.			
35.			
36.			
37.			
38.			
39.			
40.			
41.			
42.			
43.			
44.			
45.			
46.			
47.			
48.			
49.			
50.			

I certify that the foregoing information is correct to the best of my knowledge and belief.

Signature _____   Title _____   Date _____

☆ U.S. Government Printing Office: 1985—491-809/45006

FIGURE 4 (continued).

UNITED STATES DEPARTMENT OF JUSTICE
DRUG ENFORCEMENT ADMINISTRATION
P.O. Box 28083
CENTRAL STATION
WASHINGTON, D.C. 20005
For INFORMATION, Call: 202 254 - 8255

See "Privacy Act" Information on reverse

(Jul, 1982) – 224   OMB No. 1117 0014

NEW
APPLICATION FOR REGISTRATION
UNDER
CONTROLLED SUBSTANCES ACT OF 1970

Please PRINT or TYPE all entries.

No registration may be issued unless a completed
application form has been received (21 CFR 1301.21).

| CITY | STATE | ZIP CODE |

● FEE MUST
ACCOMPANY
APPLICATION

THIS BLOCK
FOR DEA
USE ONLY

REGISTRATION CLASSIFICATION: Submit Check or Money Order Payable to the DRUG ENFORCEMENT ADMINISTRATION in the Amount of $ 60.00.

1 BUSINESS ACTIVITY: (Check ☑ ONE only)

A ☐ RETAIL PHARMACY   B ☐ HOSPITAL/CLINIC   C ☐ PRACTITIONER
(Specify Medical Degree, e.g.,
DDS, DO, DVM, MD, etc.)

D ☐ TEACHING INSTITUTION
(Instructional purposes only)

2 SCHEDULES (Check ☑ all applicable schedules in which you intend to handle controlled substances. See Schedules on Reverse of Instruction Sheet.)

SCHEDULE II   SCHEDULE III   SCHEDULE III   SCHEDULE IV   SCHEDULE V
☐ NARCOTIC   ☐ NONNARCOTIC   ☐ NARCOTIC   ☐ NONNARCOTIC   ☐

3 ☐ CHECK HERE IF YOU REQUIRE ORDER FORMS.

4 ALL APPLICANTS MUST ANSWER THE FOLLOWING:

(a) Are you currently authorized to prescribe, distribute, dispense, conduct research, or
otherwise handle the controlled substances for which you are
applying, under the laws of the State or jurisdiction in which you are operating
or propose to operate?

☐ YES State License Number(s)

☐ NOT APPLICABLE   ☐ PENDING

(b) Has the applicant ever been convicted of a crime in connection with controlled substances
under State or Federal law, or ever surrendered or had a DEA registration revoked,
suspended or denied, or ever had a State professional license or controlled substance
registration revoked, suspended, denied, restricted or placed on probation ?
☐ YES   ☐ NO

(c) If the applicant is a corporation, association, partnership, or pharmacy, has any officer,
partner, stockholder or proprietor been convicted of a crime in connection with
controlled substances under State or Federal law, or ever surrendered or had a DEA
registration revoked, suspended or denied, or ever had a State professional license or
controlled substance registration revoked, suspended, denied, restricted or placed on
probation ?   ☐ YES   ☐ NO   ☐ NOT APPLICABLE

IF THE ANSWER TO QUESTIONS 4(b) or (c) is YES, include a statement using the space
provided on the REVERSE of this part.

● ATTACH CHECK HERE ●

5 CERTIFICATION FOR FEE EXEMPTION

☐ CHECK THIS BLOCK IF INDIVIDUAL NAMED HEREON IS A FEDERAL,
STATE, OR LOCAL OFFICIAL.

The Undersigned hereby certifies that the applicant herein is an officer or employee of a Federal,
State or local agency who, in the course of such employment, is authorized to obtain, dispense,
or prescribe controlled substances or is authorized to conduct research, instructional activity or
chemical analysis with controlled substances, and is exempt from the payment of this application
fee.

Signature of Certifying Official _____   Date _____

Print or Type Name _____

Print or Type Title _____

Name of Institution or Agency _____

WARNING: SECTION 843(a)(4) OF TITLE 21, UNITED STATES CODE, STATES THAT
ANY PERSON WHO KNOWINGLY OR INTENTIONALLY FURNISHES FALSE
OR FRAUDULENT INFORMATION IN THIS APPLICATION IS SUBJECT TO
IMPRISONMENT FOR NOT MORE THAN FOUR YEARS, A FINE OF NOT
MORE THAN $30,000.00 OR BOTH.

Mail the Original and 1 copy with FEE to the above address.   Retain 3rd copy for your records.

SIGN ▶
HERE

Signature of applicant or authorized Individual _____   Date _____

Print or Type Name Here - Sign Below   Applicant's Business Phone No.

Title (If the applicant is a corporation, institution, or other entity, enter the TITLE
of the person signing on behalf of the applicant (i.e., President, Dean, Procurement
Officer, etc...))

FIGURE 5.

425

● **Explanation for answering "Yes", to question(s) 4(b) through (c).**

Applicants who have answered "yes" to questions 4(b) or (c) are required to submit a statement explaining such response(s). The space provided below should be used for this purpose and must be separately signed.

▲ _____ Date

PRINT or TYPE Name Here · Sign Below

▲ _____

Signature

PRIVACY ACT INFORMATION

AUTHORITY: Section 302 and 303 of the Controlled Substances Act of 1970 (PL 91-513)

PURPOSE: To obtain information required to register applicants pursuant to the Controlled Substances Act of 1970

ROUTINE USES: The Controlled Substances Act Registration Records produces special reports as required for statistical analytical purposes. Disclosures of information from this system are made to the following categories of users for the purposes stated:

    A. Other Federal law enforcement and regulatory agencies for law enforcement and regulatory purposes

    B. State and local law enforcement and regulatory agencies for law enforcement and regulatory purposes

    C. Persons registered under the Controlled Substances Act (Public Law 91-513) for the purpose of verifying the registration of customers and practitioners

EFFECT: Failure to complete form will preclude processing of the application

FIGURE 5 (continued).

426

Legal Citations of Major Laws Affecting Drugs/Cosmetics/Devices in the United States

The list that follows contains in chronological sequence some of the more familiar and frequently cited federal legislative enactments pertaining to drugs, medical devices, and cosmetics.

Each act lists either its formal or unofficial name (e.g., Food, Drug, and Cosmetic Act, Durham-Humphrey Amendments), legal citation expressed in different ways (e.g., P.L., U.S.C.), the date of enactment, and the name of the president of the United States who held office at the time. In addition, a brief description of each law is provided.

Pure Food and Drugs Act

P.L. 59-384   21 U.S.C. 1-15
34 STAT. 768 (1906)   June 30, 1906
Theodore Roosevelt

Prohibited interstate commerce of misbranded and adulterated food and drugs.

Food, Drug, and Cosmetic Act

P.L. 75-717   21 U.S.C. 301
52 STAT. 1040 (1938)   June 25, 1938
Franklin Delano Roosevelt

• Extended coverage to cosmetics and medical devices
• Required predistribution clearance for safety of new drugs that an approved New Drug Application (NDA) mandated before a manufacturer could commercially distribute a new drug
• Eliminated Sherley Amendment requirement to prove intent to defraud in drug misbranding cases
• Provided for tolerances for unavoidable poisonous substances
• Authorized standards of identity, quality, and fill of container for foods
• Authorized factory inspections
• Added the remedy of court injunction to previous remedies of seizure and prosecution

Durham-Humphrey Amendments

P.L. 82-215   21 U.S.C. 353
65 STAT. 648 (1951)   October 26, 1951
Harry S. Truman

Requires that drugs that cannot be safely used without medical supervision must be dispensed only by prescription of a licensed practitioner, and prohibits refills of prescriptions without express consent of the prescriber. The Amendments also provide guidance to the pharmacist as to what minimal information must be included on the prescription label.

Hazardous Substances Act

P.L. 86-613   15 U.S.C. 1261
74 STAT. 372 (1960)   July 12, 1960
Dwight D. Eisenhower

Regulates the distribution and sale of packages of hazardous substances intended or suitable for household use.

Color Additive Amendments

P.L. 86-618   21 U.S.C. 376 (1982)
74 STAT. 397 (1960)   July 12, 1960
Dwight D. Eisenhower

Allows FDA to establish, by regulation, the conditions of safe use for color additives in foods, drugs, and cosmetics, and to require manufacturers to perform the necessary scientific investigations to establish safety for their intended uses.

Kefauver-Harris Drug Amendments

P.L. 87-781   21 U.S.C. 301 et seq.
76 STAT. 780 (1962)   October 10, 1962
John F. Kennedy

• Assures greater degree of safety and strengthens new drug clearance procedures. For the first time, drug manufacturers were required to prove to FDA the effectiveness of their products before marketing them

- Transfers jurisdiction over medical advertising of prescription products from the FTC to FDA
- Extends FDA's inspection authority over establishments in which prescription drugs are manufactured, processed, packed or held to include records, files, papers, controls, and facilities
- Requires that facilities, methods, and control procedures used by manufacturers conform to "current good manufacturing practices"
- Establishes "full disclosure" under which the most vital, up-to-date and reliable information about a prescription drug was required in its labeling, in the form of a package insert
- Adds more extensive control for clinical investigations by strengthening FDA's authority governing human testing of new drugs

Freedom of Information Act

P.L. 89-487
80 STAT.   July 4, 1966
Lyndon B. Johnson
Amends Section 3 of the Administrative Procedure Act; also known as the Public Information Act of 1966. Provides public access to information and documents, with some exceptions, possessed by federal agencies in the conduct of their business.

Fair Packaging and Labeling Act

P.L. 89-755   15 U.S.C. 1451
80 STAT. 1296 (1966)   July 1, 1967
Lyndon B. Johnson
Regulates various aspects of the packaging and labeling of consumer products. Basically, the law applies to those who distribute consumer products in interstate commerce. Requires that products be honestly and informatively labeled and packaged. Empowers FDA to enforce provisions of the law which affect food, drugs, cosmetics, and medical devices.

Comprehensive Drug Abuse Prevention and Control Act (Controlled Substances Act)

P.L. 91-513   21 U.S.C. 801 et seq.
84 STAT. 1242 (1970)   October 27, 1970
16 CFR 1700
Richard M. Nixon
Title I pertains to treatment and rehabilitation of drug abusers; Title III relates to the import and export of controlled substances. Title II regulates the manufacture, production, distribution, marketing, prescribing, dispensing, storage and inventory, and record-keeping of controlled substances.

Poison Prevention Packaging Act

P.L. 91-601   15 U.S.C. 1471
84 STAT. 1670   December 30, 1970
Richard M. Nixon
Its basic purpose was to provide special packaging to protect children from serious personal injury or illness that could result from handling, using, or ingesting certain toxic or harmful household substances and certain OTC Rx drug products.

Drug Listing Act

P.L. 92-387   21 U.S.C. 31 et seq.
86 STAT. 559 (1972)   August 16, 1972
Richard M. Nixon
The amendment was enacted because the FDA did not know or have available the means to construct a list of commercially available drug products (Rx and OTC) marketed in the United States, and therefore could not maintain surveillance over their manufacture and/or distribution, except by periodic inspection of registered establishments.

The purpose of the Act and the regulations is to provide the FDA with a current list by pharmacological category, of manufactured, prepared, compounded, processed and "repackaged" human and veterinary drugs and drug products, blood, and blood products, biological and in-vitro diagnostic products (drugs) in commercial distribution in the United States, whether or not they are involved in interstate commerce.

The list of products must contain the brand name (if any), generic name (if any), a quantitative list of the active ingredients, and the National Drug Code (NDC). Labeling and representative samples of advertisements must be submitted also. All inactive ingredients may be required, as well as all advertisements if such is necessary to carry out the purposes of the FDC Act.

The NDC provides for uniform drug classification and permits retrieval of computer based information.

All manufacturers must register annually with the FDA.

Each registrant (manufacturer, processor), including foreign manufacturers of drugs imported into the United States, must report to FDA twice each year (June and December) any new products introduced to the market and any product previously listed which have been discontinued (withdrawn from market).

Failure to file the semi-annual report, when it is required, may result in withdrawal of a new drug application (Section 505e), and is a prohibited act under the FDC Act (Section 301 (p)).

Medical Device Amendments of 1976

P.L. 94-295   21 U.S.C. 360
90 STAT. 539 (1976)   May 28, 1976
Gerald R. Ford
Assures the safely and effectiveness of medical devices, including certain diagnostic and laboratory products, and (2) upgrade the regulatory authority over such devices intended for human use. In addition, the amendments require:
- Classification of all devices with graded regulatory requirements
- Establishment registration
- Device listing
- Premarket approval
- Investigational device exemptions (IDE)
- Good manufacturing practice (GMP) regulations
- Records and reporting requirements
- Preemption of state and local regulation of devices
- Performance standards
- Statutory criteria for the determination of safety and effectiveness

Orphan Drug Act

P.L. 97-414   21 U.S.C. 360 et seq.
96 STAT. 2049 (1983)   January 4, 1983
Ronald W. Reagan

The Orphan Drug Act, some provisions of which are incorporated into the Federal Food, Drug, and Cosmetic Act, encourages the development of needed products whose marketing would not otherwise be profitable. It provides various incentives to stimulate the development of drugs, biologicals and products for rare diseases or medical conditions. A rare disease or condition is defined as one affecting fewer than 200,000 people in the United States, or one affecting more than this number if there is no reasonable expectation that the cost of developing the drug will be recovered from its sales in the United States. Further, the Orphan Drug Act commits the FDA to provide written recommendation for the nonclinical and clinical investigations of a drug or a biologic product to treat a rare disease or condition. Also, the Orphan Drug Act directs FDA to encourage the sponsor to conduct studies that permit the inclusion of all patients with the disease or condition that the drug is intended to treat.

Drug Price Competition and Patent Term Restoration Act

P.L. 98-417   21 U.S.C. 355
98 STAT. 1585 (1984)   September 24, 1984
Ronald W. Reagan

There are two titles which concern new drugs. Title 1, which amended Section 505 of the Federal Food, Drug, and Cosmetic Act, codifies FDA's authority to accept abbreviated new drug applications (ANDAs) for generic versions of drug products first approved after 1962. Prior to Title 1, ANDAs were only permitted under FDA regulations for generic versions of drug products first approved between 1938 and 1962. (The FDA can approve ANDAs for drugs without the submission of safety and effectiveness data if they are generically equivalent to brand name drugs already proved to be safe and effective.) Title II requires FDA's involvement in the process to allow holders of patents for drugs, biologics, medical devices, food, and color additives to obtain up to five years of patent life long during FDA's regulatory review of a product. (Patent protection ordinarily lasts 17 years, but some of this time is often lost while products are evaluated prior to approval. Title II permits up to five years of this time to be restored but limits the total time to no more than 14 years.)

Federal Anti-Tampering Act

P.L. 98-127   18 U.S.C. 1365
97 STAT. 831   October 13, 1983
Ronald Reagan

Amended the U.S. Code to establish penalties for threatening to tamper with an article subject to the FD&C Act in a manner to create risk of death or bodily injury.

Drug Export Amendments

P.L. 99-660   21 U.S.C. 382
100 STAT. 3743 (1986)   November 14, 1986
Ronald W. Reagan

Provides for the export of new ("pipeline") drugs and biologics not yet approved by the Food and Drug Administration for sale or distribution in the United States. Products may be shipped only to twenty-one specific countries where the products have been approved already and are legal, and are manufactured, processed, and packaged in conformance with good manufacturing practices.

Prescription Drug Marketing Act of 1987

P.L. 100-293   21 U.S.C. 301 et seq.
102 STAT. 95 (1987)   April 22, 1988
Ronald W. Reagan

Is intended to reduce public health risks from adulterated, misbranded, subpotent, expired, or counterfeit drug products that enter the marketplace through drug diversion. The law provides that prescription drug products manufactured in the United States and exported can no longer be reimported, except by the product's manufacturer. It also establishes restrictions on sales of prescription drug products and samples. Samples of prescription drug products may be distributed only if a licensed prescriber requests them. Other distribution channels for samples specified in the law are permissible, provided records are maintained. Under the law, wholesale distributors must be licensed by the state and meet uniform standards. Penalties for violations of the law are also identified. According to FDA's advisory guidelines on the statute, the law will permit hospitals to return drug products, provided the return is made to manufacturer or wholesaler and provided written notice is secured that the goods were received (for manufacturers) or the good were destroyed or returned to the manufacturer (for wholesalers).

Generic Animal Drug and Patent Term Restoration Act

P.L. 100-670   21 U.S.C. 301 et seq.
102 STAT. 3971 (1988)   November 16, 1988
Ronald W. Reagan

Omnibus Budget Reconciliation Act of 1990 (OBRA '90)

P.L. 101-508
104 STAT. 138 (1990)   November 5, 1990
George H. W. Bush

The Act became effective January 1, 1993 and affects *Medicaid* patients. Requires that pharmacists maintain a written record about patients and their drug therapy. The law provides for prospective (ProDUR) and retrospective (RDUR) drug utilization review, and education and intervention programs. In addition, the law mandates that an *offer* be made to counsel the patient or caregiver. An *offer* may be conveyed by an unlicensed person on behalf of the pharmacist, however, only a pharmacist (or pharmacy intern) may counsel.

Transplants Amendments Act

P.L. 101-616   42 U.S.C. 201
104 STAT. 3279 (1990)   November 16, 1990
George H. W. Bush

Safe Medical Devices Act

P.L. 101-629   21 U.S.C. 301 et seq.
104 STAT. 451 (1990)   November 8, 1990
George H. W. Bush

Expands and strengthens the regulation of medical devices. Requires postmarketing surveillance via "user reports," new 510k requirements, and FDA recall authority with civil penalties. Permits the use of Premarket Approval (PMA) to approve subsequent (generic) devices and orphan device exemption. Requires manufacturer of Class III devices introduced into commerce before 1976 to submit safety and efficacy date by 1995.

Anabolic Steroids Control Act

P.L. 101-647	21 U.S.C. 801
104 STAT. 4851 (1990)	November 29, 1990
George H. W. Bush	

Mandates that anabolic steroids be classified as Schedule III controlled substances to minimize their non-medical use, and to restrict their abuse and illegal trafficking.

Generic Drug Enforcement Act

P.L. 102-282	21 U.S.C. 301 et seq.
106 STAT. 149 (1992)	June 1, 1992
George H. W. Bush	

Commonly referred to as the Debarment Act. Provides the Food and Drug Administration (FDA) with new authority to ensure the integrity of generic drug applications, and to deal with corrupt conduct in the U.S. pharmaceutical industry. The Act authorizes the FDA to debar individuals and firms, impose fines, suspend distribution and temporarily deny approval of drugs subject to an abbreviated new drug application (ANDA) and withdraw approval of an ANDA due to corrupt conduct associated with the approval process.

Prescription Drug User Fee Act

P.L. 102-571	21 U.S.C. 321
106 STAT. 4491 (1992)	October 29, 1992
George H. W. Bush	

Provides for fees to be paid FDA by manufacturers to enhance the (shorten time) review for new drug or biologic applications, drug products, and manufacturing establishments, covered by the Food, Drug, and Cosmetic Act approval process.

Dietary Supplement Health and Education Act

P.L. 103-147	21 U.S.C. 321
108 STAT. 4325	October 25, 1994
William J. Clinton	

Dietary supplements, defined broadly, are now a special class of foods and will not be subject to FDA's "food additive" jurisdiction. This dramatic legal change assures that dietary supplements will not require FDA "food additive" pre-marketing clearance. Consequently, FDA has the burden of proof to establish that a dietary supplement is either adulterated or misbranded.

In addition, the law with regard to "labeling" is modified. Scientific publications and other types of information marketed with dietary supplements will not be defined as "labeling" as long as certain conditions are met. Ingredient labeling requirements for dietary supplements are also modified. The law also establishes a category of "new dietary ingredients" that are subject to greater regulatory scrutiny than "old dietary ingredients" (dietary ingredients marketed in the U.S. prior to October 15, 1994).

Perhaps the most dramatic change results from the explicit Congressional authorization for marketers of dietary supplements to make certain "structure/function" labeling claims. While it is not entirely clear which claims come within the "structure/function," the law assuredly expands the range of legally permissible claims.

Also, the law creates two regulatory agencies that will focus on dietary supplement regulations. *First,* a Presidential Commission within the executive branch, the Commission on Dietary Supplement Labels, is authorized to study and provide recommendations for the regulation of dietary supplement label claims. *Second,* the law authorizes the creation of the Office of Dietary Supplements (within the National Institutes of Health), designed to promote scientific studies regarding the health benefits of dietary supplements.

Although the law accords the dietary supplement industry with many new protections from FDA regulation, many aspects of dietary supplement regulation are nevertheless unchanged. The only overt revocation of existing law is the requirement that FDA withdraw its advance notice of proposed rulemaking regarding suggested procedures for regulating dietary supplements. The Nutrition Labeling and Education Act of 1990 ("NLEA") and implementing regulations are still applicable to the dietary supplement industry to the extent they are not specifically contradicted by the law. Furthermore, FDA may still regulate a dietary supplement product *as a drug* if the product labeling contains "drug" claims. Dietary supplement claims are also still subject to FDA action if they are false or misleading. The Federal Trade Commission retains jurisdiction over dietary supplement **advertising** and the laws that the FTC enforces have not been altered by this law.

The Food and Drug Administration (FDA) Modernization Act of 1997

P.L. 105-115	21 U.S.C. 301 et seq.
111 STAT. 2296	November 21, 1997
William J. Clinton	

Prescription Drug User Fees

The act reauthorizes, for five more years, the Prescription Drug User Fee Act of 1992 (PDUFA). In the past five years, the program has enabled the agency to reduce to 15 months the 30-month average time that used to be required for a drug review before PDUFA. This accomplishment was made possible by FDA managerial reforms and the addition of 696 employees to the agency's drugs and biologics program, which was financed by $329 million in user fees from the pharmaceutical industry.

FDA Initiatives and Programs

The codified initiatives include measures to modernize the regulation of biological products by bringing them in harmony with the regulations for drugs and eliminating the need for establishment license application; eliminate the batch certification and monograph requirements for insulin and antibiotics; streamline the approval processes for drug and biological manufacturing changes; and reduce the need for environmental assessment as part of a product application.

The act also codifies FDA's regulations and practice to increase patient access to experimental drugs and medical devices and to accelerate review of important new medications. In addition, the law provides for an expanded database on clinical trials which will be accessible by patients. With the sponsor's consent, the results of such clinical trials will be included in the database. Under a seprate provision, patients will receive advance notice when a manufacturer plans to discontinue a drug on which they depend for life support or sustenance, or for a treatment of a serious or debilitating disease or condition.

Information on Off-Label Use and Drug Economics

The law abolishes the long-standing prohibition on dissemination by manufacturers of information about unapproved uses of drugs and medical devices. The act allows a firm to disseminate peer-reviewed journal articles about an off-label indication of its product, provided the company commits itself to file, within a specified time frame, a supplemental application based on appropriate research to establish the safety and effectiveness of the unapproved use.

The act also allows drug companies to provide economic information about their products to formulary committees, managed care organizations, and similar large-scale buyers of health-care products. The provision is intended to provide such entities with dependable facts about the economic consequences of their procurement decisions. The law, however, does not permit the dissemination of economic information that could affect prescribing choices to individual medical practitioners.

Pharmacy Compounding

The act creates a special exemption to ensure continued availability of compounded drug products prepared by pharmacists to provide patients with individualized therapies not available commercially. The law, however, seeks to prevent manufacturing under the guise of compounding by establishing parameters within which the practice is appropriate and lawful.

Risk-Based Regulation of Medical Devices

The act complements and builds on FDA's recent measures to focus its resources on medical devices that present the greatest risks to patients. For example, the law exempts from premarket notification Class I devices that are not intended for a use that is of substantial importance in preventing impairment of human health, or that do not present a potential unreasonable risk of illness or injury. The law also directs FDA to focus its postmarket surveillance on higher risk devices, and allows the agency to implement a reporting system that concentrates on a representative sample of user facilities—such as hospitals and nursing homes—that experience deaths and serious illnesses or injuries linked with the use of devices.

Finally, the law expands an ongoing pilot program under which FDA accredits outside—so-called "third party"—experts to conduct the initial review of all Class I and low-to-intermediate risk Class II devices. The act, however, specifies that an accredited person may not review devices that are permanently implantable, life-supporting, life-sustaining, or for which clinical data are required.

Food Safety and Labeling

The act eliminates the requirement of FDA's premarket approval for most packaging and other substances that come in contact with food and may migrate into it. Instead, the law establishes a process whereby the manufacturer can notify the agency about its intent to use certain food contact substances and, unless FDA objects within 120 days, may proceed with the marketing of the new product. Implementation of the notification process is contingent on additional appropriations to cover its cost to the agency. The act also expands procedures under which FDA can authorize health claims and nutrient content claims without reducing the statutory standard.

Standards for Medical Products

While the act reduces or simplifies many regulatory obligations of manufacturers, it does not lower the standards by which medical products are introduced into the market place. In the area of drugs, the law codifies the agency's current practice of allowing in certain circumstances one clinical investigation as the basis for product approval. The act, however, does preserve the presumption that, as a general rule, *two* adequate and well-controlled studies are needed to prove the product's safety and effectiveness.

In the area of medical devices, the act specifies that FDA may keep out of the market products whose manufacturing processes are so deficient that they could present a serious health hazard. The law also gives the agency authority to take appropriate action if the technology of a device suggests that it is likely to be used for a potentially harmful unlabeled use.

How to Make a Freedom of Information Act Request to FDA

The Freedom of Information Act (FOI) allows anyone to request information from FDA records not normally prepared for public distribution. Certain materials that are prepared for public distribution—such as press releases, consumer publications, speeches, and congressional testimony—are available from FDA without having to file an FOI request. Simply contact the appropriate FDA office. Also, consumers can ask questions about FDA related matters by writing to:

Consumer Inquiries Office (HFE-88)
Food and Drug Administration
5600 Fishers Lane
Rockville, MD 20857

How to Make an FOI Request

The Freedom of Information Act pertains only to existing records and is not a research service that compiles information not already available and identifiable. Make your request specific enough to locate the record in a reasonable period of time. Separate requests should be submitted for each firm or product involved.

All FOI requests should be in writing and must be addressed to:

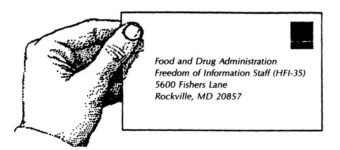

Food and Drug Administration
Freedom of Information Staff (HFI-35)
5600 Fishers Lane
Rockville, MD 20857

Your letter should include the following:
• Your name, address and telephone number;
• A statement of the records being sought, identified as specifically as possible. A request for specific information that is releasable to the public can be processed much more quickly than a request for "all information" on a particular subject. Also, a more specific and limited request will cost less for search, review, and duplication fees.

Fees

Since FOI requesters may have to pay fees covering some or all of the cost of processing a request, you may want to mention the maximum dollar amount you are willing to pay. If the fees will exceed this amount, FDA will contact you before filling the request. The current fee schedule for commercial requests is:
• *Search and review time:* Varies ($11, $23 or $41 per hour), depending on the level of FDA employee filling the request;
• *Photocopying:* 10 cents/page for standard-size paper or the actual cost per page for odd-size paper;
• *Microfiche:* 50 cents per fiche;
• *Certifications:* $10 each;
• *Computer charge:* actual cost for time involved.

For noncommercial requests, such as representatives of educational institutions, public interest groups and the news media, fees are charged only for duplication (with no charge for the first 100 pages). Consumers are charged for search time and duplication (with no charge for the first two hours of search time and the first 100 pages of duplication).

Do not send payment with your request. You will be billed if the total charges are $10 or more. FDA does not accept credit cards. Payment must be made by check or money order.

433

MEDWATCH—The FDA Medical Products Reporting Program

FDA, in June 1993, launched MEDWATCH, the new, streamlined Medical Products Reporting Program. MEDWATCH is designed to facilitate and improve reports from health professionals about serious adverse reactions and product defects associated with medications, devices, and nutritional products. These reports are essential to FDA's postmarketing surveillance efforts.

"MEDWATCH is not just a new FDA system," Commissioner David A. Kessler, M.D., said. "It is a way of making reporting second nature for health professionals. Physicians, pharmacists, nurses, and others who care for patients are the first to know when a drug or medical device does not perform as it should. The sooner they report it to FDA, the faster the agency can analyze the problem and take corrective action."

Report to MEDWATCH only if one or more of the following occurs:

• *Death*—If an adverse reaction to a medical product is a suspected cause of a patient's death.

• *Life-threatening hazard*—If the patient was at risk of dying at the time of the adverse reaction or if it is suspected that continued use of a product would cause death (examples: pacemaker breakdown or failure of an intravenous (IV) pump that could cause excessive drug dosing).

• *Hospitalization*—If a patient is admitted or has a prolonged hospital stay because of a serious adverse reaction (example: a serious allergic reaction to a product such as latex).

• *Disability*—If the adverse reaction caused a significant or permanent change in a patient's body function, physical activities, or quality of life (examples: strokes or nervous system disorders brought on by drug therapy).

• *Birth defects, miscarriage, stillbirth, or birth with disease*—If exposure to a medical product before conception or during pregnancy is suspected of causing an adverse outcome in the child (example: malformation in the child caused by the acne drug Accutane, or isotretinoin).

• *Needs intervention to avoid permanent damage*—If use of a medical product required medical or surgical treatment to prevent impairment (examples: burns from radiation equipment or breakage of a screw supporting a bone fracture).

FDA emphasizes that it is not necessary to *prove* that a medical product caused an adverse reaction—a suspected association is sufficient reason to make a report.

MEDWATCH also needs to know about suspected contamination, questionable stability, defective components, and poor packaging or labeling of FDA-regulated medical products.

Although drug and device manufacturers must report adverse events associated with their products, the voluntary reports the agency receives from health professionals are often the first indication that a newly marketed product does not perform as it should. FDA depends on these reports to safeguard public health, since clinical trials that precede product approval typically include safety data for a limited patient population. Once on the market, the much wider use of the drug or medical device occasionally reveals serious safety concerns that did not emerge in the clinical trials.

FDA has published a guide for health professionals entitled *The FDA Desk Guide for Adverse Event and Product Problem Reporting*. The guide contains examples of types of events to report and completed sample forms, as well as blank forms with instructions. A copy of the guide, as well as additional reporting forms, can be obtained by calling 1-800-FDA-1088.

The agency also plans to make a sustained effort to keep health professionals informed about how MEDWATCH reports have led to changes in products or their use. It will encourage medical, pharmacy, dental, and nursing schools to include in their curricula lectures on adverse event and product problem recognition and reporting.

MED**W**ATCH

THE FDA MEDICAL PRODUCTS REPORTING PROGRAM

For **VOLUNTARY** reporting
by health professionals of adverse
events and product problems

Page ____ of ____

PLEASE TYPE OR USE BLACK INK

A. Patient information

1. Patient Identifier	2. Age at time of event: or _____ Date of birth:	3. Sex ☐ female ☐ male	4. Weight ____ lbs or ____ kgs
In confidence			

B. Adverse event or product problem

1. ☐ **Adverse event** and/or ☐ **Product problem** (e.g., defects/malfunctions)

2. **Outcomes attributed to adverse event** (check all that apply)

☐ death ____ (mo/day/yr)
☐ life-threatening
☐ hospitalization – initial or prolonged

☐ disability
☐ congenital anomaly
☐ required intervention to prevent permanent impairment/damage
☐ other: ____

3. Date of event (mo/day/yr)	4. Date of this report (mo/day/yr)

5. **Describe event or problem**

6. **Relevant tests/laboratory data, including dates**

7. **Other relevant history, including preexisting medical conditions** (e.g., allergies, race, pregnancy, smoking and alcohol use, hepatic/renal dysfunction, etc.)

C. Suspect medication(s)

1. **Name** (give labeled strength & mfr/labeler, if known)

#1 ____

#2 ____

2. Dose, frequency & route used #1 #2	3. Therapy dates (if unknown, give duration) from/to (or best estimate) #1 #2

4. **Diagnosis for use (indication)**

#1 ____

#2 ____

5. **Event abated after use stopped or dose reduced**

#1 ☐ yes ☐ no ☐ doesn't apply

#2 ☐ yes ☐ no ☐ doesn't apply

6. Lot # (if known) #1 #2	7. Exp. date (if known) #1 #2

8. **Event reappeared after reintroduction**

#1 ☐ yes ☐ no ☐ doesn't apply

#2 ☐ yes ☐ no ☐ doesn't apply

9. **NDC #** (for product problems only)

__ – __ – __

10. **Concomitant medical products and therapy dates** (exclude treatment of event)

D. Suspect medical device

1. **Brand name**

2. **Type of device**

3. **Manufacturer name & address**

4. **Operator of device**
☐ health professional
☐ lay user/patient
☐ other: ____

6.
model # ____
catalog # ____
serial # ____
lot # ____
other # ____

5. **Expiration date** (mo/day/yr)

7. **If implanted, give date** (mo/day/yr)

8. **If explanted, give date** (mo/day/yr)

9. **Device available for evaluation?** (Do not send to FDA)
☐ yes ☐ no ☐ returned to manufacturer on ____ (mo/day/yr)

10. **Concomitant medical products and therapy dates** (exclude treatment of event)

E. Reporter

1. **Name & address**   phone # ____

2. Health professional? ☐ yes ☐ no	3. Occupation	4. Also reported to ☐ manufacturer ☐ user facility ☐ distributor

5. **If you do NOT want your identity disclosed to the manufacturer, place an " X " in this box.** ☐

Mail to: MED**W**ATCH
5600 Fishers Lane
Rockville, MD 20852-9787

or FAX to:
1-800-FDA-0178

FDA

FDA Form 3500

Submission of a report does not constitute an admission that medical personnel or the product caused or contributed to the event.

FIGURE 1.

Medical Products Regulated by FDA

The MEDWATCH reporting program depends on the alertness and responsiveness of health professionals to learn of product problems and adverse events associated with medical products regulated by FDA. Because MEDWATCH uses the same form for all reports, it is no longer necessary to know which part of FDA is responsible for a particular product. Nevertheless, knowing which products are included makes reporting easier:

• Drugs are primarily articles intended for use in the diagnosis, cure, mitigation, treatment, or prevention of disease in humans, or articles (other than food) intended to affect the structure or function of the body.

• Biological products include any virus, therapeutic serum, toxin, antitoxin, vaccine, blood, blood component or derivative, allergenic product, or analogous product applicable to the prevention, treatment, or cure of the diseases or injury to humans. Vaccines are the only biological products not included in the MEDWATCH program. Vaccine problems should be reported to the Vaccine Adverse Experience Reporting System (VAERS).

• Medical devices include products with an intended use similar to a drug, but that do not achieve any of their primary intended purposes by chemical action in or on the body or by being metabolized.

• Special nutritional products include dietary supplements, infant formulas, and medical foods.

Products on which to report include, but are not limited to, drugs such as antibiotics, steroids, and antiarrhythmics; biological and therapeutic sera toxins, antitoxins, blood, and blood components or derivatives; medical devices such as heart valves, latex gloves, kidney dialysis machines; and medical foods such as the low nitrogen products used by patients with severely reduced renal function.

Serious adverse experiences with major food additives such as artificial sweeteners and preservatives should also be reported to FDA.

What Is a Product Problem?

Product problems (defective or malfunctioning) should be reported when there is a concern about the quality, performance, or safety of any medication or device.

Problems with product quality may occur during manufacturing, shipping, or storage. They include product contamination; defective components; poor packaging or product mix-up; questionable stability; device malfunctions; and labeling concerns.

With drugs, the pharmacist is often the first to recognize a product quality problem. Nurses are often the first to recognize a problem with a medical device. Report these suspicions to FDA through MEDWATCH.

Examples:

• A customer returned to the pharmacy after purchasing a bottle of a liquid antacid and complained about the foul odor coming from the product when it was opened. The pharmacist took note of the terrible odor and also observed that the plastic bottle container was distended. The customer was given a similar product to replace this antacid. Next, the pharmacist checked the storeroom stock and checked the lot numbers of the affected product. Then the FDA was contacted to relay this drug product quality concern and to provide the necessary facts to investigate this production lot.

• While stocking a box of 15 mL bottles of Syrup of Ipecac, a pharmacy technician noticed that one translucent bottle labeled as Syrup of Ipecac had a much brighter color than the rest. FDA was immediately contacted through its voluntary reporting program. Within one day an investigation was under way. It was discovered that the translucent product was not Syrup of Ipecac but another agent, that while not toxic would not produce the desired effect of Syrup of Ipecac if used to treat a case of poisoning. The investigation of this labeling mix-up resulted in the product being recalled.

• A pharmacist observed that a 5 mL unit bottle of diphenhydramine syrup made a rattling noise when shaken. After removing the seal, it became obvious that the noise was caused by loose glass fragments floating in the syrup. Recognizing the life-threatening nature of this product if swallowed, FDA was contacted. An FDA investigator picked up the samples and initiated an investigation at the manufacturer. The results revealed a problem with the production of glass bottles. This report resulted in a nationwide recall of the product.

• A nurse noted a frayed cable leading to the pendant (hand control) of a hospital bed. An investigation showed that the wiring was faulty and had a tendency to fray at this point of entry into the pendant housing. This presented a potential electric shock and/or fire hazard. A recommendation of recall affected 33,155 pendants in distribution.

Table 1
Advice about Voluntary Reporting

Report experiences with:
- medications (drugs or biologics)
- medical devices (including in-vitro diagnostics)
- special nutritional products (dietary supplements, medical foods, infant formulas)
- other products regulated by FDA

Report SERIOUS adverse events. An event is serious when the patient outcome is:
- death
- life-threatening (real risk of dying)
- hospitalization (initial or prolonged)
- disability (significant, persistent or permanent)
- congenital anomaly
- required intervention to prevent permanent impairment or damage

Report even if:
- you're not certain the product caused the event
- you don't have all the details

Report product problems—quality, performance or safety concerns such as:
- suspected contamination
- questionable stability
- defective components
- poor packaging or labeling
- therapeutic failures

How to report:
- just fill in the sections that apply to your report
- use section C for all products except medical devices
- attach additional blank pages if needed
- use a separate form for each patient
- report either to FDA or the manufacturer (or both)

Important numbers:
- 1-800-FDA-0178 to FAX report
- 1-800-FDA-7737 to report by modem
- 1-800-FDA-1088 for more information or to report quality problems
- 1-800-822-7967 for a VAERS form for vaccines

If your report involves a serious adverse event with a device and it occurred in a facility outside a doctor's office, that facility may be legally required to report to FDA and/or the manufacturer. Please notify the person in that facility who would handle such reporting.

Confidentiality: The patient's identity is held in strict confidence by FDA and protected to the fullest extent of the law. The reporter's identity may be shared with the manufacturer unless requested otherwise. However, FDA will not disclose the reporter's identity in response to a request from the public, pursuant to the Freedom of Information Act.

How to Make a MedWatch Report

FDA offers several ways for health professionals or consumers to submit MedWatch reports:
- **Online**—Go to the MedWatch Website at *www.fda.gov/medwatch/* and follow the instructions for submitting a report electronically.
- **By mail**—Use the postage-paid MedWatch form, which includes the address. Many health professionals keep the form in stock. To get a copy, call MedWatch at 1-800-332-1088, and one will be sent by mail or fax. You also can download the software for printing out the form through MedWatch's Website, *www.fda.gov/medwatch/*. Or the agency will send a copy of the software on disk. Call 301-443-0117.
- **By fax**—You can submit a completed form to MedWatch's fax number, 1-800-332-0178.

Reports of serious adverse reactions or problem products also may be made to product manufacturers, where, by law, they must be reported to FDA.

If you have any questions about the reporting process, call 1-800-332-1088; press "0" or wait on the line. Or send questions by e-mail to *medwatch@bangate.fda.gov.*

Answers to Questions

CHAPTER 1—The Legislative Process

1–c	2–d	3–d	4–d	5–a	6–a	7–b	8–b
9–e	10–b	11–b	12–b	13–b	14–d	15–d	16–a
17–a	18–c	19–a	20–d	21–b	22–b	23–b	

CHAPTER 2—The Judicial System

1–d	2–e	3–c	4–e	5–d	6–c	7–d	8–c
9–c	10–b	11–a	12–b	13–e	14–e	15–d	16–e
17–a	18–d	19–b	20–a	21–d	22–b	23–d	24–d
25–d	26–a	27–a	28–d	29–c	30–b	31–d	32–c
33–d	34–b						

CHAPTER 3—The Compendia and the *USP DI*

1–d	2–c	3–b	4–b	5–e	6–b	7–c	8–b
9–e	10–e	11–a	12–c	13–e	14–c	15–c	16–c
17–e	18–b	19–b	20–a	21–c	22–d	23–e	24–c
25–b							

CHAPTER 4—The Controlled Substances Act

MISCELLANEOUS

1–d	2–e	3–e	4–a	5–a	6–c	7–d	8–c
9–e	10–a	11–b					

SCHEDULES OF CONTROLLED SUBSTANCES

1–a	2–b	3–d	4–a	5–b	6–e	7–c	8–c
9–a	10–d	11–c	12–a	13–c	14–c	15–e	16–a
17–a							

SCHEDULE II

1–a	2–d	3–d	4–e	5–e	6–b	7–d	8–e
9–d	10–e	11–d	12–d	13–c	14–c	15–c	

SCHEDULES III AND IV

1–b	2–e	3–d	4–e	5–e

SCHEDULE V

1–b	2–b	3–d	4–a	5–b	6–b	7–e	8–a
9–b	10–e	11–a	12–c	13–b	14–c		

REGISTRATION

1–e	2–b	3–e	4–d	5–c	6–e	7–d	8–c
9–d	10–c	11–e	12–c	13–a	14–a	15–c	

ORDER FORMS

1–d	2–c	3–a	4–a	5–d	6–c	7–c	8–e
9–c	10–e	11–e	12–c	13–d	14–b	15–d	16–e
17–d	18–a	19–d	20–d	21–d	22–d	23–c	24–b
25–e	26–c	27–a	28–c	29–d	30–c	31–d	32–b
33–e							

INVENTORY

1–a	2–d	3–d	4–e	5–a	6–d	7–e	8–e
9–e	10–a						

CHAPTER 5—Poison Prevention Packaging Act

1–b	2–c	3–d	4–d	5–d	6–d	7–d	8–a
9–e	10–d	11–d	12–a	13–e	14–c	15–b	16–e
17–b	18–e	19–e	20–c	21–e	22–c	23–e	

CHAPTER 6—Medical Device Law

1–d	2–b	3–c	4–d	5–c	6–c	7–c	8–c
9–d	10–a	11–e	12–b	13–a	14–a	15–c	16–e
17–d	18–a	19–e	20–c	21–c	22–b	23–a	

CHAPTER 7—Drug Recalls

1–b	2–c	3–a	4–e	5–b	6–e	7–c	8–c
9–a	10–d	11–c	12–a	13–c	14–e	15–c	

CHAPTER 8—**Expiration Dating**

1–d	2–d	3–b	4–d	5–c	6–e	7–e	8–d
9–b	10–d	11–a	12–d				

CHAPTER 9—**Drug Law**

1–e	2–b	3–e	4–d	5–e	6–d	7–d	8–c
9–d	10–e	11–a	12–a	13–d	14–b	15–b	16–c
17–c	18–d	19–d	20–d	21–c	22–d	23–c	24–d
25–c	26–d	27–c	28–c	29–d	30–e	31–d	32–e
33–d	34–c	35–b	36–b	37–d	38–d	39–d	40–c
41–b	42–d	43–b	44–d	45–e	46–c	47–e	48–d
49–b	50–c	51–a	52–a	53–e	54–c	55–b	56–d
57–c	58–b	59–e	60–e				

CHAPTER 10—**National Drug Code**

1–c	2–b	3–d	4–c	5–a	6–b	7–e	8–b
9–d	10–c	11–a	12–c	13–d			

CHAPTER 11—**U.S. Postal Regulations**

1–b	2–a	3–e	4–c	5–c

CHAPTER 12—**Cosmetics**

1–d	2–b	3–d	4–d	5–c

CHAPTER 13—**Anabolic Steroids**

1–a	2–c	3–b	4–e	5–d	6–e	7–c	8–e
9–d	10–d	11–c	12–b	13–c	14–b		

CHAPTER 14—**Prescription Drug Marketing Act of 1987**

1–b	2–d	3–d	4–e	5–b,d,e,g,j

CHAPTER 15—**Narcotic Treatment Programs (Methadone)**

1–d	2–b	3–b	4–d	5–c	6–e	7–e	8–d
9–a	10–b	11–c	12–d	13–c	14–e	15–d	16–a
17–c							

CHAPTER 16—**The Orange Book**

1–c	2–b	3–b	4–a	5–d	6–a	7–c	8–a
9–d	10–b	11–a	12–a	13–c	14–d	15–c	16–b
17–a	18–d	19–d	20–d				

CHAPTER 19—**Federal Anti-Tampering Act**

1–b	2–a	3–c	4–b	5–b	6–c

CHAPTER 21—**Color Additives**

1–b	2–d	3–e	4–a	5–b	6–c	7–c	8–e
9–d	10–d						

CHAPTER 22—**Food and Drug Administration**

1. Answer a: Spam is a meat product. The U.S. Department of Agriculture is responsible for regulating meat (and poultry) products.

2. Answer c: Insect repellents are regulated as pesticides by the Environmental Protection Agency.

Both aspirin and shampoos that get rid of lice are drugs; eye shadow and lipstick are cosmetics; all are regulated by FDA.

3. Answer c: Oven cleaners are regulated by the Consumer Product Safety Commission.

Canned tomatoes and spaghetti are regulated as foods by FDA. Tolerances for pesticide residues in foods are established by EPA, but FDA is responsible for ensuring that these tolerances are not exceeded on foods (except for meat, poultry and certain egg products, which are under USDA's jurisdiction). FDA enforces a ban on the sale and distribution of turtles less than 4 inches long, the size most often sold as pets. Pet turtles frequently carry *Salmonella* bacteria, which may cause severe diarrhea in children and adults. Baby turtles were sold as pets in the United States until 1975, when the National Centers for Disease Control and Prevention determined that the bacterial contamination could not be prevented by any known treatment.

4. Answer d: Smoke detectors—both photoelectric and ionization chamber types—are regulated by the Consumer Product Safety Commission. The radioactive source used in the ionization chamber detector is naturally occurring, not electronic and, therefore, is not a substance that would be regulated by FDA.

Under the FD&C Act, FDA is responsible for protecting consumers from unnecessary exposure to radiation emitted from electronic products. (These provisions were originally separate from the FD&C Act and were referred to as the Radiation Control for Health and Safety Act. They were later incorporated into the FD&C Act when the Safe Medical Devices Act of 1990 was enacted.) MRI diagnostic equipment is regulated as a medical device under the FD&C Act. Laser products used in lumber mills must conform to an FDA standard that ensures their safety. This standard applies to all laser products, whether medical, industrial or consumer.

5. Answer c: The only advertisements over which FDA has direct jurisdiction are those for prescription drugs. FTC oversees advertising for other FDA-regulated products.

TV sets are regulated under the radiological health provisions of the FD&C Act. Over-the-counter and prescription drugs, as well as human biological products (such as vaccines and blood products), are regulated by FDA.

6. **Answer a:** Baby pacifiers are regulated by CPSC unless they are marketed with health claims, in which case they are under FDA's jurisdiction.

Food-contact articles, including baby bottle nipples, ceramic ware intended for food use, and coffee mugs, are regulated by FDA. So are eye charts, which, as diagnostic products, are considered to be medical devices.

7. **Answer a:** Illegal use of heroin is the responsibility of the Drug Enforcement Administration, the key federal agency that polices illicit, or "street," drugs. (If heroin were being studied for medical uses, FDA would regulate it as an investigational drug.)

Barbiturates are subject to abuse and thus may, potentially, wind up on the "street," bringing them under DEA's purview. However, barbiturates have legitimate medical uses, and FDA is responsible for ensuring they are properly manufactured and labeled. FDA regulates methadone as a drug, and methadone maintenance treatment programs are monitored under regulations promulgated by both FDA and the National Institute on Drug Abuse (NIDA). Medicinal oxygen is regulated by FDA as a drug. Animal drugs, including veterinary tetracycline, are regulated by FDA.

8. **Answer e:** Hair dryers are regulated by CPSC.

Kidney dialysis machines and tongue depressors, as different as they are in complexity, are both considered to be medical devices. FDA regulates nonfluoridated toothpastes as cosmetics, and fluoridated toothpastes as drugs.

9. **Answer a:** Labels on beer and other malt beverages, distilled spirits (liquors), and wines are regulated by the Bureau of Alcohol, Tobacco and Firearms under the Federal Alcohol Administration Act.

Ground coffee, coffee beans, rabbit meat, and canned tuna are all regulated by FDA as food.

10. **Answer a:** Home canning equipment, under a memorandum of understanding between FDA and CPSC, is regulated by CPSC.

FDA's jurisdiction includes the facilities where the products it regulates are stored, such as food and drug warehouses. Hearing and dispensing establishments are bound by specific FDA regulations that impose conditions for the sale of hearing aids. The regulations attempt to prevent misrepresentation

and ensure adherence to proper medical standards. Regarding exporting drugs, FDA continues to have authority over its regulated products even when they are exported.

11. **Answer c:** The FD&C Act specifically excludes soap from its definition of cosmetics. CPSC regulates this product.

All of the other choices are defined as cosmetics and, therefore, are regulated by FDA.

12. **Answer a:** A vaccine for horses is a veterinary biological product. FDA does not have jurisdiction over veterinary biologics. The Virus, Serum, and Toxin Act gives this responsibility to USDA.

The FD&C Act gives FDA authority over pet foods and drugs, which would include veterinary penicillin, medicated feeds, and bird feed. The Public Health Service Act confers on FDA the authority to regulate the interstate movement of psittacine birds (parrots, cockatoos, macaws, parakeets, and other birds in the psittacine family).

13. **Answer a:** The safety of public drinking water (tap water) is protected by EPA, as decided in an agreement between that agency and FDA.

FDA has jurisdiction over bottled water, which is considered a food under the FD&C Act. The remaining choices are also defined as foods.

14. **Answer b:** Child-proof packaging authority, addressed under the Poison Prevention Packaging Act, was delegated to CPSC.

Tamper-resistant packaging, which is required for certain OTC drugs, cosmetics, and medical devices, is FDA's responsibility. Food packaging materials, such as plastic containers and candy boxes, are subject to regulation as food additives under the FD&C Act because of the possibility that they may leach their chemical constituents into the food product. These potential additives are referred to as indirect food additives. A container bearing a drug product is considered to be a component of that drug, and FDA, therefore, requires that it be appropriate for that drug.

15. **Answer a:** The animal counterpart of a cosmetic is commonly referred to as a "grooming aid." Cosmetics, as defined in the FD&C Act, apply only to human use. Therefore, products intended for cleansing or promoting attractiveness of animals are not subject to FDA control.

An artificial limb for dogs is regulated as a veterinary medical device. While such products do not require FDA approval, they do come under the purview of the FD&C Act.

They may not bear labeling that is false or misleading, nor may they be otherwise misbranded or adulterated. The laser scanner must comply with the standard. Mercury vapor lamps, most often used to light streets, gymnasiums, sports arenas, banks, and stores, must be maintained properly to be safe. With some types of mercury vapor lamps, if the outer envelope is broken and the lamp continues to operate, intense, harmful ultraviolet radiation is emitted. An FDA standard ensures that this lighting is safe. Finally, FDA regulates vitamin C tablets as food supplements.

CHAPTER 23—**Ipecac Syrup**

1–*a*   2–*d*   3–*a*

CHAPTER 27—**Patient Package Inserts**

1–*e*   2–*b*   3–*b*   4–*e*   5–*e*